ROCK STRESS

PROCEEDINGS OF THE INTERNATIONAL SYMPOSIUM ON ROCK STRESS
KUMAMOTO/JAPAN/7-10 OCTOBER 1997

ROCK STRESS

Edited by
KATSUHIKO SUGAWARA & YUZO OBARA
Department of Civil Engineering and Architecture, Kumamoto University, Japan

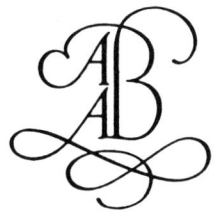

A.A.BALKEMA/ROTTERDAM/BROOKFIELD/1997

Acknowledgements

The Organizing Committee of the International Symposium on Rock Stress gratefully acknowledges the financial contributions of: The Ministry of Education, Science, Sports and Culture, Japan; The Centennial Anniversary Association, Faculty of Engineering, Kumamoto University, Japan.

The Proceedings of the International Symposium on Rock Stress are published using a Grant-in-Aid for Publication of Scientific Research Results presented by the Ministry of Education, Science, Sports and Culture, Japan.

The texts of the various papers in this volume were set individually by typists under the supervision of each of the authors concerned.

Authorization to photocopy items for internal or personal use, or the internal or personal use of specific clients, is granted by A.A.Balkema, Rotterdam, provided that the base fee of US$1.50 per copy, plus US$0.10 per page is paid directly to Copyright Clearance Center, 222 Rosewood Drive, Danvers, MA 01923, USA. For those organizations that have been granted a photocopy license by CCC, a separate system of payment has been arranged. The fee code for users of the Transactional Reporting Service is: 90 5410 901 7/97 US$1.50 + US$0.10.

Published by
A.A.Balkema, P.O.Box 1675, 3000 BR Rotterdam, Netherlands (Fax: +31.10.413.5947)
A.A.Balkema Publishers, Old Post Road, Brookfield, VT 05036-9704, USA (Fax: 802.276.3837)

ISBN 90 5410 901 7
© 1997 A.A.Balkema, Rotterdam
Printed in the Netherlands

Table of contents

Preface — XIII

Organization — XV

Special lectures

The importance of rock stress measurement and its interpretation for rock disposal of hazardous waste — 3
O. Stephansson

Measuring rock stress and rock engineering in Japan — 15
K. Sugawara

Keynote presentations

Fault dynamics – Dynamic triggering of fault slip — 27
H. P. Rossmanith & K. Uenishi

Borehole breakouts and core disking as tools for estimating in situ stress in deep holes — 35
B. C. Haimson

The regional stress field and its heterogeneity — 43
F. H. Cornet

Stress measurements by borehole pressurization and its potential for future rock engineering projects in Japan — 51
Y. Mizuta

Methods for stress measurement

Rock stress determinations at great depth using the modified doorstopper gauge — 59
P. M. Thompson, R. Corthésy & M. H. Leite

Some aspects of a stress calculation model for deep measurements using the modified doorstopper cell — 65
M. H. Leite, R. Corthésy, D. E. Gill & R. S. Read

Use of the modified doorstopper-IAM combination as a stress-meter 71
R. Corthésy, M.H. Leite, D.E. Gill & D. Nguyen

Improvement in accuracy of the conical-ended borehole technique 77
Y. Obara & K. Sugawara

Applicability of the compact overcoring method for initial stress measurement in highly cracked bedrock 83
N. Demboya, A. Fukuhara, Y. Obara & K. Sugawara

Improvement on hollow inclusion technique and its application to in situ stress measurement in four Chinese metal mines 89
M. Cai, L. Qiao, C. Li, B. Yu & S. Wang

Comparison of the results of stress measurements determined by various methods at the Kamaishi mine 95
H. Matsui, T. Sato, K. Sugihara & N. Nakamura

Numerical simulations of overcoring stress measurements in elastoplastic rocks 101
A. Giraud, F. Homand, J.F. Shao & A. Nechnech

Conventional hydrofrac method in arbitrarily oriented stress fields 107
A. Sato, T. Ito & K. Hayashi

Material non-linearity and alteration of breakdown pressures in hydraulic fracturing 111
P.A. Nawrocki & M.B. Dusseault

Estimation of in-situ stress state by the measurement of the wall displacement during hydraulic fracturing and injection tests at Kamioka mine 117
T. Takehara, T. Yamaguchi, M. Kuriyagawa, H. Ishihara & M. Yamashita

Hydrofracturing stress measurement in granitic rock with scarce joints 121
K. Shin, B. Zhang, F. Li & S. Okubo

Influence of fracture aperture and normal stiffness on the reopening pressure in classical hydraulic fracturing stress measurements 127
J. Rutqvist & O. Stephansson

Studies on rockmass stress measurement by parallel-borehole-controlled fracturing 133
W. Chou, H. Cheng & J. Sun

Modelling experiments on rockmass stress measurement by controlled fracturing 137
W. Chou, H. Cheng & J. Sun

A proposal of geo-stress measurement technique by plate fracturing 143
T. Yokoyama & A. Nakanishi

In situ stress measurement using the ANZI stress cell 149
K.W. Mills

A case study of pressuremeter tests for measurement of stresses in sedimentary soft rock ground 155
K. Tani & Y. Yoshida

Initial stress estimation in rock using ultrasonic *S.Kobayashi, T.Yamaguchi & T.Yoshikawa*	161
Residual stress in rock core samples and stress state at great depths *T.Ito, K.Watanabe & K.Hayashi*	167
Estimation of stress state in the deep portion of the Osaka plane *Y.Fujiwara, M.Horie, Y.Ito, Y.Hirakawa, Z.Xue & K.Sugawara*	171
Differential strain curve analysis to estimate stress state around Soultz EPS-1 well *Y.Oikawa, I.Matsunaga & S.Miyazaki*	177
Laboratory investigation of controls of stress history on ASR response *D.F.Wang, N.Yassir, J.Enever & P.J.Davies*	181
Determination of in situ stress using DRA and AE techniques *M.Utagawa, M.Seto & K.Katsuyama*	187
Numerical 2D-simulation of memory effects in rocks around a borehole *V.L.Chkouratnik & A.V.Lavrov*	193
Three-dimensional simulation of memory effects in rock samples *A.V.Lavrov*	197

Interpretation of rock stresses

Interpretation of stress measurements in a Provence mine using a block modelling *F.Homand & M.Souley*	205
Recent advances in the interpretation of the overcoring test *K.Fouial, M.Alheib & P.Bigarre*	211
Data processing in rock stress measurement *S.Zhang, M.Yang, J.Zhang & J.Jia*	217
A geostatistical approach to evaluate differences in results between hydraulic fracturing and overcoring *J.Andersson & C.Ljunggren*	223
Validation of far field overcore stress measurement data using an integrated geomechanical analysis *W.F.Bawden & J.D.Tod*	229
On determination of large scale stresses and moduli *A.N.Galybin, A.V.Dyskin & R.J.Jewell*	235
Sound velocity as a measure of small stress change *O.Sano, T.Murakami, Y.Tanaka & Y.Mizuta*	241
Estimation of regional in-situ stress field controlling subsurface fracture system by using microseismic multiplets *H.Moriya, H.Niitsuma, J.T.Rutledge & M.Fehler*	247

Development of high sensitivity borehore strainmeters and application for rock mechanics and earthquake prediction study 253
H.Ishii, T.Yamauchi & F.Kusumoto

Estimation of far-field stresses from borehole strainmeter observations 259
H.Ishii, G.Chen & Y.Ohnishi

Determination of the in-situ stresses at Sellafield, UK: A case study 265
A.S.Batchelor, K.A.Kwakwa, A.J.Proughten & N.Davies

Interpretation of rock fracture phenomena

On rock stress in rockburst risk assessment of deep gold mines 279
X.-T.Feng, M.Seto, K.Katsuyama, M.Özbay & S.Webber

Crack kinematics and stress intensity factors by acoustic emission 283
M.C.Muzo, M.Ohtsu & H.P.Rossmanith

Simulation of borehole breakout using fracture mechanics models 289
B.Shen, X.Tan, C.Li & O.Stephansson

In-situ stresses in the North Sea from careful analysis of breakouts and fracturing data 299
A.S.Batchelor & K.A.Kwakwa

Concrete structures cracking survey by video image processing 305
M.J.Rouis, M.Zairi & M.S.Bouhlel

Crack angle dependence of initial yield stress and stress concentration in rocks 309
G.-C.Jeong, T.Seiki & Y.Ichikawa

Effect of normal stiffness and strain rate on the shear strength of soft joints 315
B.Indraratna & A.Haque

Effect of surface roughness on peak and residual shear stress of irregular rock joints 321
S.Du, T.Esaki, Y.Jiang & J.Sun

Relaxation of shear stress along rock discontinuity 327
N.H.Tubagus, K.Fukui & S.Okubo

Penetration experiment of rocks by use of TBM roller bit with aiming the fast execution: Effect of bit shape 333
H.Takahashi, S.Suzuoki, N.Hatakeyama, S.Nunomura & Y.Shimizu

Borehole instability – New drilling tool technology for stability control 339
J.C.Rowley

A tensile principal stress analysis for estimating three-dimensional in-situ stresses from core discing 343
K.Matsuki, K.Hongo & K.Sakaguchi

State of stress in the earth's crust

Stress measurements by the hydraulic fracturing in the 1995 Hyogoken-nanbu earthquake source region
H.Ito, Y.Kuwahara & O.Nishizawa — 351

Estimation of in-situ stresses from ASR and DSCA measurements on drilled cores in the 1995 Hyogoken-nanbu earthquake source region
H.Ito, O.Nishizawa, Z.Xue & O.Sano — 355

Stress measurements with core samples by AE-DRA methods in the 1995 Hyogoken-nanbu earthquake source region
R.Kudo, T.Yokoyama, H.Ito, Y.Kuwahara, O.Nishizawa & K.Yamamoto — 359

A geomechanical model of crustal waveguides dynamics
Yu.I.Kuznetsov & A.V.Karakin — 363

The general characteristics of the stress state in the various parts of the earth's crust
Ö.Aydan & T.Kawamoto — 369

Relation of in-situ stress field to seismic activity as inferred from the stresses measured on core samples
K.Yamamoto, H.Yamamoto & Y.Yabe — 375

Statistical models of geomechanical processes in multiscale cracked geological media
A.V.Karakin & Yu.I.Kuznetsov — 381

The relation between geological features and the stress state of the earth's crust in Central Japan
T.Seiki, Ö.Aydan & T.Kawamoto — 385

Rock stress measurements in the Hong Kong region
H.H.Choy, C.F.Chan, W.K.Pun & L.S.Cheung — 391

Influence of a fault and a dyke on stress distribution at two project sites in India
S.Sengupta, D.Joseph, C.Nagaraj & A.Kar — 397

Stress state in the Urals earth crust and its relationship with geological and tectonic evolution
A.V.Zoubkov & Y.I.Liepin — 403

Intergranular cracking and relaxation of stress in deep crystalline rock as a result of physico-chemical influence of water
M.Z.Abdrakhimov & V.Yu.Traskin — 409

Application of rock stress measurements in mining

Determination of stress and strain fields around a horizontal fold and some applications in mining geomechanics: Correct and incorrect problems
V.Iv.Dimova — 417

Evaluation of the effect of mine's rock bolts using a finite elements computer modeling
J.A.Ardito & G.De-La-Sota — 423

Influence of initial stress on rock slope stability   429
K. Kaneko, M. Kato, Y. Noguchi & N. Nakamura

Physical changes due to reservoir compaction – A finite element solution   435
Y. B. Sukirman

Insitu stress measurement and its application in mining – Case studies of Indian mines   441
P. Sharma

Characteristics of in-situ stress state and control methods of ground pressure in Jinchuan nickel mine   447
T. Liu & C. Zhou

Some experiences on rock stress measurements and its application in mining   451
F. Fujimura, A. C. Campos Fernandes & C. M. Nieble

Evaluation of rock stress in the mines of Kolar Gold Fields – A seismological approach   457
C. Srinivasan, P. C. Jha & N. M. Raju

Possibility of estimating in-situ stress of virgin coal field using acoustic emission technique   463
M. Seto, V. S. Vutukuri & D. K. Nag

A review of recent in-situ stress measurements in United Kingdom Coal Measures strata   469
P. B. Cartwright

Stability of interpanel-pillar due to longwall mining   475
K. Matsui, H. Shimada & M. Ichinose

Experimental study on the relation between in-situ stress and permeability of coal   479
T. Yamaguchi, X. M. Zhang, Y. Oikawa, T. Narita & H. Kobayashi

Application of rock stress measurements in civil engineering

Significance of in-situ stress measurement in the practice regarding engineering projects   485
F. Li

Rock stress measurement for design of underground powerhouse and considerations   491
Y. Ishiguro, H. Nishimura, K. Nishino & K. Sugawara

Two-dimensional elastic analysis for a circular tunnel lining in the pre-deformed ground due to initial stresses – An approach to quantitative evaluation of the load bearing capacity of the surrounding rock mass   499
H. Kiyama, H. Fujimura, T. Nishimura & Y. Ikezoe

Induced stress measurements in damaged region around a tunnel   505
A. Hirata, M. Yamamoto, T. Inaba & Y. Obara

In site measurement of geostresses in a tunnel of Nanning-Kunming railway   511
Z. Fang & S. Bai

Rock stress changes during excavation of a large underground cavern   515
K. Kudoh, T. Koyama & Y. Komatsuzaki

Affect of thermal hysteresis on rock mass around openings for storage of heated water   521
Y. Inada, N. Kinoshita, T. Ueda & K. Yamada

Rock stress behavior of large cavern in underground excavation 527
K. Ohno & A. Yada

Optimum locations for displacement measurements in underground openings to determine 533
in situ stress by means of back analysis
N. Shimizu, H. Kakihara, K. Nakagawa & S. Sakurai

Application of in situ stresses measured by hydraulic fracturing to a tunnel design in Korea 539
S.-O. Choi & H.-S. Shin

Rock behavior estimated by field measurements during large underground cavern excavation 545
Y. Uchita, Y. Hirakawa & T. Ishida

Author index 551

Preface

The International Symposium on Rock Stress – RS Kumamoto'97 – was held at the Kumamoto City Auditorium and the Kumamoto City International Center, Kumamoto, Japan, from October 7 to 10, 1997. The Symposium was organized by Kumamoto University, the West Japan Rock Engineering Society and the Mining and Materials Processing Institute of Japan, in collaboration with the Ministry of Education, Science, Sports and Culture, Japan.

This 1997 Symposium followed the International Symposium on Rock Stress and Rock Stress Measurements held in Stockholm, Sweden, in September 1-3, 1986. Thus, RS Kumamoto'97 was the principal forum for a critical review of research in progress and of engineering achievements since the last symposium in all areas of rock stress and rock stress measurement, as practiced in civil, mining, petroleum, earthquake and environmental engineering, and energy development, as well as in geology and geophysics.

The proceedings entitled Rock Stress contain two special lectures, four keynote addresses given by renowned researchers, and 84 research papers presented by 251 authors from 21 countries. The wide variety of topics covered by the papers range from fundamental research to actual industrial applications, and are grouped in the proceedings according to the subject matter under the following headings:
– Methods for stress measurement;
– Interpretation of rock stresses;
– Interpretation of rock fracture phenomena;
– State of stress in the earth's crust;
– Application of rock stress measurements in mining;
– Application of rock stress measurements in civil engineering.

Knowledge of rock stress is of fundamental importance in a wide range of engineering activities. The methods and techniques for in situ rock stress measurement were focused on as the fundamental principals which are common in all areas. Numerous case examples of rock stress measurements were presented, as well as theoretical studies of rock stress for the interpretation of rock stress and rock fracture phenomena, and to clarify the state of stress in the earth's crust. The applications of rock stress measurements in various engineering areas were also presented and discussed, including the safe and economic excavation design in civil and mining engineering, stress-related instability problems of underground openings, dams, slopes, stopes, tunnels and deep wellbores, the interpretation for hot dry rock geothermal energy projects and radioactive waste disposal, and the prediction research of earthquakes. Special emphasis was given to a rapidly growing international activity in the development of potential techniques available at a great depth and/or in complicated geology, and data acquisition and processing techniques which are applicable to engineering practices.

The Organizing Committee wishes to sincerely thank the authors for their valuable contributions and hopes that the information relayed with this volume will be of use to scientists and engineers who are concerned with rock stress and measurements of rock stress.

It is our honor, to acknowledge the great contributions Prof. Dr K.Kaneko, Prof. Dr Y.Mizuta, Prof. Dr T.Esaki, Prof. Dr J.Otani and Prof. Dr A.Hirata have made to the organization of the symposium.

Kumamoto, October 1997
Katsuhiko Sugawara & Yuzo Obara

Organization

ORGANIZING COMMITTEE

Katsuhiko Sugawara, Kumamoto University, Japan, Chairman
Yuzo Obara, Kumamoto University, Japan, Co-chairman
Katsuhiko Kaneko, Hokkaido University, Japan, Co-chairman
Yoshiaki Mizuta, Yamaguchi University, Japan, Vice-chairman
Tetsuro Esaki, Kyushu University, Japan, Vice-chairman
Jun Otani, Kumamoto University, Japan, Secretary General
Ömer Aydan, Tokai University, Japan
Kouhei Furukawa, Yamaguchi University, Japan
Kazuo Hayashi, Tohoku University, Japan
Satoshi Hibino, Central Research Institute of Electric Power Industry, Japan
Atsuo Hirata, Kumamoto Institute of Technology, Japan
Yoshinori Inada, Ehime University, Japan
Yoji Ishijima, Hokkaido University, Japan
Hideo Kiyama, Tottori University, Japan
Shouichi Kobayashi, Kyoto University, Japan
Katsuaki Koike, Kumamoto University, Japan
Michio Kuriyagawa, National Institute for Resources and Environment, Japan
Kikuo Matsui, Kyushu University, Japan
Kouji Matsuki, Tohoku University, Japan
Kouji Nakagawa, Yamaguchi University, Japan
Seisuke Okubo, The University of Tokyo, Japan
Michito Ohmi, Kumamoto University, Japan
Yuzo Ohnishi, Kyoto University, Japan
Masayasu Ohtsu, Kumamoto University, Japan
Toshiaki Saito, Kyoto University, Japan
Jiro Yamatomi, The University of Tokyo, Japan

ADVISORY COMMITTEE

John A. Hudson, Imperial College, UK
Peter K. Kaiser, Laurentian University, Canada
Toshikazu Kawamoto, Aichi Institute of Technology, Japan
Chung-In Lee, Seoul National University, Korea
Hi-Keun Lee, Seoul National University, Korea
Yuichi Nishimatsu, The University of Tokyo, Japan
Shunsuke Sakurai, Kobe University, Japan
Ove Stephansson, Royal Institute of Technology, Sweden

SPECIAL LECTURERS

Ove Stephansson, Royal Institute of Technology, Sweden
Katsuhiko Sugawara, Kumamoto University, Japan

KEYNOTE LECTURERS

Hans P. Rossmanith, Technical University of Vienna, Austria
Bezalel C. Haimson, University of Wisconsin, USA
François H. Cornet, Institut de Physique du Globe de Paris, France
Yoshiaki Mizuta, Yamaguchi University, Japan

Special lectures

The importance of rock stress measurement and its interpretation for rock disposal of hazardous waste

Ove Stephansson
Department of Civil and Environmental Engineering, Royal Institute of Technology, Stockholm, Sweden

ABSTRACT: This paper presents a list of activities where the knowledge of *in situ* stress is required in order to engineer, construct and control an underground, hazardous waste repository. The importance of rock stress measurements and their accurate interpretation for waste disposal in rocks are exemplified with a series of case studies of existing and potential repositories disposals of industrial and hazardous wastes. The strategy and programme for stress measurement for waste repositories are highlighted with respect to timing; methods available for use; number of measurements; and the accuracy and uncertainty in measurements.

1 INTRODUCTION

Increasing public concern for the environment during the past decades has led to the reassessment of surface disposal of hazardous waste because of its potential for contaminating otherwise groundwater and soil. With increased governmental regulation and related safety assessment, disposal of hazardous waste is now stringently controlled in order to avoid accidents and thus protect human health and the environment. The scientific and engineering professions have endeavoured to meet the steadily increasing requirements for safe associated with disposal of hazardous waste. As a consequence, an active community of professionals, dedicated to solving problems and improving technologies associated with deep disposal of hazardous waste, has been established.

The application of appropriate solutions to the disposal of hazardous waste depends on momentous political decision-making, in the knowledge that any decision in this domain is likely to be definite and irreversible. This heavy burden must be borned not only by the political decision-makers but also by those who are responsible for providing the scientific basis for the decisions.

The political decisions need to be based, above all, on scientific judgements. It follows, therefore, that the decisions taken by the politicians will be dependent upon the quality of the work that has been conducted by the researchers and engineers to whom the preparatory work is entrusted. This is the situation where scientists and engineers in rock mechanics and rock engineering enter the scene.

Rock engineering is concerned with the investigation, design, construction and performance of engineered structures built on, in or of rock. It involves engineering applications of the science of rock mechanics (Brown, 1993). Storage facilities for hazardous materials are suggested to be located in rocks at great depth. That calls for an understanding of stresses in rocks and rock masses. The understanding of stresses is essential in order to provide boundary conditions to the storage facility; it provides the means to make a proper design and to analyse the mechanical response and possible failure of the rock mass; and it sheds some light on how fluids flow underground. The disposal facility, independent of the exact type, must be located and oriented so its long-term stability is guaranteed, the operation is safe and the reaction between the waste and the geological medium is kept at a minimum.

This contribution will first present rock engineering activities which require in depth knowledge of virgin stress state. Thereafter, the importance of rock stress measurement and their interpretation for underground storage of hazardous waste will be demonstrated for several examples: a) a silo for operational radioactive waste, b) a deep repository for spent nuclear fuel, c) a repository for toxic waste in an abandon mine, and d) injection disposal of hazardous and industrial waste in deep boreholes. Applying stresses in rock engineering for disposal of hazardous waste and the role of *in situ* stresses in the planning, construction and control of underground repository will also be discussed. Further, recommendations for stress measurement programs related to waste disposal in competent rocks are presented.

2 IMPORTANCE OF ROCK STRESS FOR DISPOSAL OF HAZARDOUS WASTE

In the recent book by Amadei and Stephansson (1997) on rock stress and its measurement they pointed out and exemplified the importance of knowing the *in situ* state of stress in the Earth's crust when dealing with rocks and rock masses in civil, mining and petroleum engineering and energy development.

A list of activities where knowledge of *in situ* stress is required in the engineering and control of an underground hazardous waste repository is presented in Table 1.

The magnitude and orientation of the stresses determine the orientation, geometry, dimension, sequence of excavation, heat loading rate in case of HLW waste of a repository, and independent of siting depth. When selecting a shallow underground excavation for low and intermediate radioactive waste, as the SFR facility at Forsmark, Sweden, where the virgin stresses are relatively low in comparison with the rock strength, the ultimate goal is to make a design where stress concentrations are kept at a minimum. Here the compressive stresses in the wall of the openings should be as low as possible and regions of tensile stress should be avoided. This approach is sometimes called the 'harmonic hole' concept (Amadei & Stephansson, 1997). On the contrary, when designing underground excavations at large depth where virgin stresses are high and close to the strength of the rock mass the depth wise location, orientation and shape of cross section become crucial for a safe construction with long term performance. As pointed out by Fairhurst (1968) and Hoek & Brown (1980) the 'harmonic hole concept' is not recommended when the virgin stresses are high. Instead the shape should be selected so that zones of high stress are concentrated in sharp corners and the zones have the smallest possible extension.

There are in many cases great advantages in locating an underground waste repository in an abandon mine since rock conditions, including the state of stress and the overall stability, ought to be satisfactory known.

Drilling and boring tunnels in highly stressed rock masses is known to give problems. Negative correlation between the rate of penetration in rotary drilling with increasing stress has been reported by Myrvang et al. (1993). Boring tunnels in highly stressed rock masses is known to create major problems with trapped full-face tunnel-boring machines and squeezing rock masses. The rock failure and the trapped boring machine at the Yacambú Quibor tunnel in Venezuela can serve as an example.

Rock burst and mine seismicity are essentially examples of rock failure due to the alteration of the virgin stress state by mining an opening in a rock mass. Several mining factors including the depth of mining, mine geometry, and the rate and volume extracted can influence the redistribution of *in situ* stresses and hence the occurrence of rockbursts and mine seismicity. Equally important are surface topography, rock type, geological structures and the magnitude and orientation of the virgin stresses. Mines or sites known for seismicity and rock bursts have to be rulled out as candidates for underground waste repositories.

Rock stress measurements are often performed to give input data to numerical modelling carried out for the design of underground structures with respect to deformation, strength of the openings and design of proper reinforcements. According to the US Nuclear Regulatory Commission (10CFR60),

Table 1. Activities in underground waste disposal requiring knowledge of the *in situ* stress.

Location and orientation of underground excavations (tunnel, cavern, deposition hole, shaft) and mines (stoop, haulage, shaft)
Prediction and performance of drilling and blasting
Prediction and performance of tunnel boring
Prediction of rock bursts
Design of support systems
Fluid flow and contaminant transport in the near field and far field
Coupled thermo-hydro-mechanical-chemical processes; T-H-M-C couplings

Section 60.10 and 60.21, *in situ* stresses should be measured at a potential site, before and during the construction of a repository. The strategy for stress measurement at a potential site will be presented in Chapter 4.

Rock permeability is without doubt the key parameter in any model of fluid flow and transport through rocks. The permeability is determined by the pore structure of the rock mass and the pores can be located within the rock matrix and/or in the joints and fractures of the rock mass. Several models exist that relate rock permeability to porosity and pore structure. In principle they can be grouped into: (1) tube, channel and fracture network models; and (2) models utilising the concept of hydraulic radius (Jamtveit and Yardley, 1997). Any process that changes the pore structure effects the permeability. Rock stress is certainly the most important factor for changing permeability of structures belonging to the first group of pores (tubes, channels and fracture networks). Flow through single fracture under normal and shear stress is presented by Tsang and Stephansson (1996) and characterisation of possible fluid flow paths for fracture system, based on combinatorial topology and percolation theory, are presented by Jing and Stephansson (1997).

An important consequence of the storage and transport of fluids in rocks is that it gives rise to significant coupling between mechanical, hydrological, thermal and chemical processes. Such coupled processes can effect significantly the performance of structures and processes engineered in an underground repository. Coupling between fluid pressure and mechanical stresses is the classical concept of effective stress in soil and rock mechanics. Thermo-mechanical stresses will be generated heat generating waste is placed into the bedrock. Both convective transports of heat by fluids and heat conduction are important mechanisms in the coupled processes.

The need to isolate hazardous waste from the biosphere in the geological disposal emphasises the importance of coupled processes in rocks. To demonstrate effective isolation it is necessary to have the capability to model and predict the effects of coupled processes on waste isolation over very long periods of time. The coupling of thermo-hydro-mechanical (THM) process has been studied in the project titled 'Development of Coupled THM Models and Their Validation Against Experiments' (DECOVALEX). The first phase of the international co-operative project has yielded three major benefits: (1) encouraged the development of coupled THM codes by the different national research teams and provided peer review resulting advice to each other; (2) defined both simple and realistic benchmark test (BMT) problems, so that research teams could verify their codes and compare computational results with those from other teams; and (3) collected and documented major laboratory and field test cases (TC), so that research teams could use them to perform validation studies of their models and codes. Result of the first phase of the DECOVALEX project has been presented in a special issue of the International Journal for Rock Mechanics & Mining Science (Stephansson, 1995) and in a book in the series Development in Geotechnical Engineering, 79 (Stephansson, Jing & Tsang, 1996). Studies of the fully T-H-M-C coupling, where chemical processes are included (see Table 1) will become the next step in the development of models for predicting the effects of waste isolation over very long periods of time.

3 EXISTING AND POTENTIAL REPOSITORIES FOR HAZARDOUS WASTE

The importance of rock stress measurements and their interpretation for underground storage of hazardous waste will be exemplified with a description of an existing repository for low and intermediate radioactive waste under the sea and potential repositories and disposal of industrial and hazardous waste. The following examples have been selected:

1. Cavern for radioactive operational waste; SFR, Forsmark, Sweden;
2. Deep repository for spent nuclear fuel; KBS 3 (Sweden) and POSIVA (Finland);
3. Toxic waste (Hg and Cd) in an abandon mine;
4. Deep injection disposal of hazardous and industrial waste in deep boreholes.

3.1 *Cavern for radioactive operational waste*

The final repository for radioactive operational waste, called SFR, is situated near the Forsmark Nuclear Power Station. SFR is a facility for the final disposal of the short-lived low- and intermediate-level waste that arises in Sweden. It has a current capacity of 60,000 cubic metres of waste. The repository is situated in granitic rocks at a depth of about 50 m beneath the sea bed. The depth of the sea at the site is about 5 m. SFR consists of five rock caverns (one silo and four vaults) of differing design according to the type of waste to be emplaced. Intermediate-level waste is deposited in the 50 m high concrete silo. The space between the silo wall and the rock mass is filled with a mixture of bentonite clay and sand to seal against water flow, Fig.1.

The waste is placed by remote control in vertical shafts in the silo, which are subsequently backfilled with concrete. Excavation of the silo was performed by drilling and blasting against a central shaft and muck loading from a transport tunnel entering the bottom of the silo. Rock reinforcement, grouting and installation of rock monitoring instruments were performed in the roof of the silo.

Rock stress measurements were conducted from three boreholes prior to the excavation. One hole Kb 7, was drilled from a platform at the sea level, 300 m Southeast of the silo. The other two holes Kb20 and Kb 21, were drilled from tunnels into the site of the silo prior to excavation, Table 2.

Table 2. Stress data at SFR silo for intermediate-level radioactive waste. After Stille & Fredriksson, 1988.

Bh No	Level	σ_1 MPa	σ_3 MPa	Direct degree	σ_V MPa
Kb 7	+460	11.9	3.2	131	6.2
	+430	16.7	8.3	117	6.3
	+400	17.0	7.6	134	2.9
	+360	17.1	11.5	54	3.7
Kb21	+430	5.2	2.3	162	1.4
	+435	5.7	1.9	129	0.6
	+440	21.1	5.0	156	0.9
	+445	7.9	3.0	144	-1.4
Kb22	+425	8.3	3.2	157	-2.3
	+430	7.3	4.2	159	0.7

Stress measurement results with overcoring at the shallow depth in Forsmark show a typical scatter in magnitude and orientation (Table 1). This is favourable with respect to the design of the roof of the silo, namely that the magnitudes are moderate and the orientation is scattered. For the purpose of calculations Stille and Fredriksson (1988) used the following stress field

- Maximum horizontal stress: 10 MPa
- Minimum horizontal stress: 5 MPa
- Vertical stress: 2-3 MPa.

3.2 Deep repository for spent nuclear fuel

The deep geological disposal of radioactive wastes is a common concept for all nations that have extensive programmes for production of energy by nuclear power. SKB in Sweden and POSIVA in Finland plan to site and build a deep repository for spent nuclear fuel from the Swedish and Finnish nuclear power stations, respectively. The ongoing deep repository work consists of studies of the design of the disposal system and the deep repository. Such studies are being carried out in stages, with an increasing degree of detail, to provide background data for studies of environmental consequences, siting requirements and effects on the local economy and infrastructure. The repository system must achieve three safety functions:

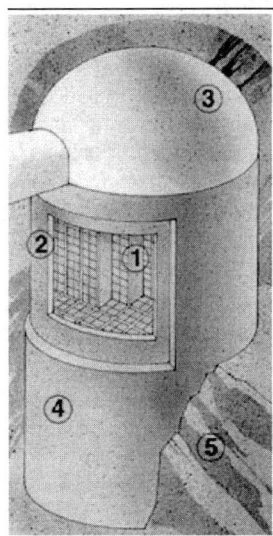

Figure 1. Intermediate-level radioactive waste is deposited in the 50 m high concrete silo at SFR. 1. Waste, 2. Silo of concrete, 3. Backfill of sand and bentonite, 4. Buffer of bentonite, 5. Rock mass.

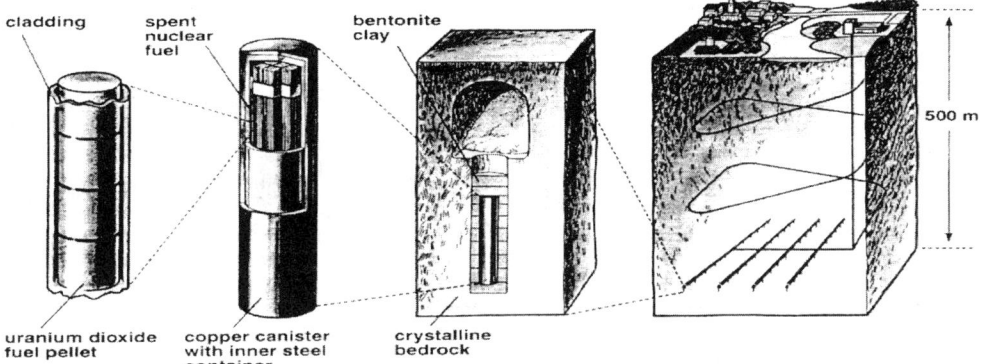

Figure 2. Multiple safety barriers in the KBS-3 concept of SKB, Sweden.

- isolation
- retention and retardation
- dilution and dispersion

in that order. Figure 2 illustrates how the safety functions are applied in the KBS-3 concept of SKB, Sweden.

The canister (copper/steel), the buffer material and the bedrock are three barriers tending to isolate the spent fuel. If the barriers happen to fail and the fuel comes in contact with the groundwater than the barrier work in order to retard and retain the hazardous radionuclides. The fuel itself has a low solubility in groundwater as well as the actinides. The buffer material prevents water movements and sorbs radionuclides. Granitic rocks in the Precambrian shield areas have reducing chemistry, slow groundwater flow and are able to sorb dissolved nuclear species.

The long-term stability of a repository is determined by the virgin state of stress, the orientation of stress, the stress gradient with depth and the rocks mechanical properties. Tolppanen et al. (1995) have performed an interesting study on how to prevent possible failure around the excavations of a deep repository at three potential sites in Finland. They made use of hydraulic stress measurements conducted in semi-vertical boreholes at each site and determined the state of stress at three different depths for each site (300, 500 and 800 metres), see Table 3.

Numerical analyses were performed for two different concepts with vertical and horizontal

Table 3. Principle stress magnitude (mean value) and standard deviation at three sites in Finland. After Tolppanen et al., 1995.

Depth (m)	σ_H (MPa)	s (MPa)	σ_h (MPa)	s (MPa)	σ_v (MPa)
Olkiluoto					
300	12	-	9	-	8
500	24	2.5	14	1.4	14
800	43	2.4	23	0.8	22
Kivetty					
300	29	-	15	-	8
500	32	6.9	17	3.3	14
800	35	3.2	19	1.6	22
Romuvaara					
300	19	-	9	-	8
500	29	-	15	-	14
800	46	8.0	24	2.7	22

deposition hole by using the three-dimensional distinct element code 3DEC. For interpretation of the critical stages of the rock mass at the depth of the repository the brittle rock strength criterion developed by Martin (1997) was applied. The sectors of elastic deformation, stable crack growth, unstable crack growth and immediate shear failure and related limits of crack initiation (σ_{ci}), unstable cracking (σ_{cd}) and peak strength (σ_c) were defined from uni-axial compressive testing of core samples. The envelopes defined in the σ_1-σ_2 space were applied in the interpretation of the 3DEC analyses (Fig. 3).

In the interpretation of the results from stress measurements and rock mechanical testing,

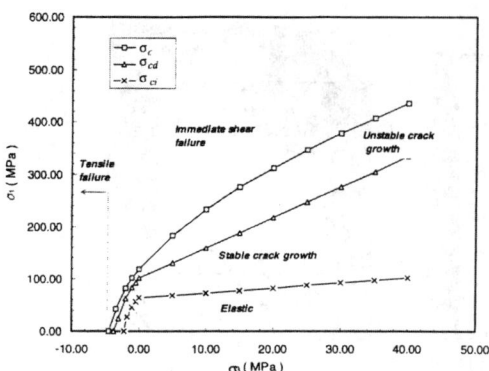

Figure 3. Strength envelopes used in the interpretation of results from the 3DEC analyses, Olkiluoto mica gneiss. After Tolppanen et al., 1995.

Table 4. Repository depth where no immediate shear failure appears at the wall of the deposition hole for the candidate sites in Finland. After Tolppanen et al., 1995.

CONCEPT	HORIZONTAL DEPOSITION HOLE		VERTICAL DEPOSITION HOLE	
Direction of principal stress	$\sigma_H \perp$ Hole	$\sigma_H \perp$ Hole	$\sigma_H \perp$ Hole & $\sigma_H \perp$ Tunnel	$\sigma_H \perp$ Hole & $\sigma_H \perp$ Tunnel
Olkiluoto, MGn	800 m	>800 m	550 m	700 m
Kivetty, PGrDr	>800 m	>800 m	300 m	500 m
Romuvaara, MGn	750 m	>800 m	400 m	500 m
Romuvaara, TonGn	>800 m	>800 m	700 m	>800 m

maximum stress at the wall of the deposition hole and the roof of the deposition tunnel is plotted as a function of one of the measured stress components, (Fig. 4).

The range of measured stresses at three different depth and the given boundaries of elastic deformation, stable and unstable crack growth and shear failure are presented for two different ratios of Fig. 4. Repository depth where no immediate shear failure appears at the wall of the deposition hole for σ_H/σ_V and the case where the maximum horizontal stress is directed perpendicular to the tunnel axis.

For the given stress ratios immediate shear failure will occur in the roof of the tunnel and the wall of the deposition hole for a repository located at the depth of 800 metres. Stable crack growth will develop around the openings at a repository depth of 500 metres, cf. Fig. 4. The crack initiation is calculated to reach 20-75 cm from the surface of the openings and the shear failure will reach a depth of about 2 cm.

From this study Tolppanen et al. (1995) were able to define the depth limits of the three potential repository sites in Finland, (Table 4). In addition they found that the concept of horizontal deposition hole gives more stable mechanical conditions and that for both concepts the best stability is achieved when tunnel axes are oriented parallel to the direction of the major horizontal stress.

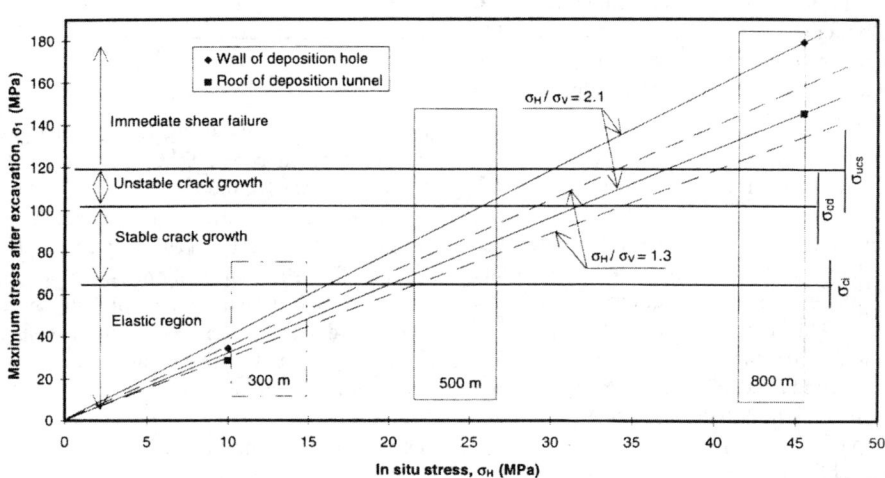

Figure 4. Interpretation of 3DEC results from Olkiluoto site, Finland. Maximum stress after excavation in the roof of the tunnel and wall of the deposition hole versus measured maximum horizontal stress is shown for three depths and two stress ratios. After Tolppanen et al., 1995.

The method of conducting three-dimensional numerical analyses using measured rock stress data for boundary conditions and laboratory data about strength and deformability for the interpretation of stability are a promising methodology to determine the stability field of repository openings. However, the study by Tolppanen et al. (op.cit.) does not include the additional stress components from the heat generation of the waste and the swelling pressure of the high-compacted bentonite in the deposition hole.

A rock mechanics study was performed for the SITE-94 project initiated by the Swedish Nuclear Power Inspectorate (SKI), (Hansson et al., 1995, 1996). The objectives were to investigate the mechanical influence of repository excavation, swelling pressure of the bentonite, thermal loading by the spent fuel and a complete glaciation cycle on the stability and safety of a hypothetical nuclear waste repository, in both far- and near-field scales. The Äspö Hard Rock Laboratory test site was used as the target site for regional and local geology, *in situ* stress data and material properties to the modelling. The far-field study treated the rock mass as an assembly of discrete blocks defined by 23 major faults and fracture zones. From the numerical results using 3DEC, it was found that the maximum temperature of 48 degrees would be reached 200 years after the emplacement of the waste canisters. The average increase of maximum principle stress due to thermal loading is 9.5 MPa horizontally and 20.2 MPa in vertical direction due to glaciation. These stresses are superimposed on the virgin stress in the bedrock and therefore are likely to shift the stability fields as presented in Fig. 4.

3. 3 Toxic waste in an abandon mine - a potential site at Stripa Mine, Sweden.

In 1994 the Swedish Government decided to stop the use of mercury (Hg) and that by year 2000 the dilution must stop and the metal be phased out to protect the environment. The task to collect free mercury and clean up products containing mercury was given to the Swedish Environmental Protection Agency. The collection of Hg from industry, government and private organisations has been very successful. In September 1997 the Agency will present a plan for the final disposal of the collected mercury. The most likely solution for Sweden is a deep repository in hard rocks whereby the toxic waste is placed back into its natural geochemical cycle. In addition the surrounding rock mass will prevent the waste from reaching the biosphere.

In designing a repository for mercury the mobility of the substance has to be kept low by minimising the groundwater flow to reduce the leaching of the mercury compounds. A deep repository is characterised by a low flow and a stable geochemical environment. The low rate of flow allows the existing minerals in the surrounding rocks to buffer the groundwater at this depth and the reducing condition gives a low solubility of the waste. In addition a deep repository will offer a stable mechanical environment and will protect the waste from human intrusion, external loading from glaciations, earthquakes, erosion, sea level changes and post-glacial uplift.

The abandon Stripa Mine in Central Sweden is suggested as a site for disposal of mercury and other toxic waste metals like cadmium and scrap from iron casting etc. Iron ore mining at Stripa was active for more than 200 years. In 1976 the mining ceased and one year later the mine was opened for research in association with the Swedish-American Co-operative Program on Radioactive Waste Storage in Mined Caverns in Crystalline Rock (1977-1980) and later the OECD/NEA International Stripa Project (1980-1992). At present the mine is shut down, the pumps are stopped and the groundwater level is rising.

The tunnels in Stripa granite where the former research took place are at levels 336 and 385m and have a total volume of 11.000 cubic metres. Adding the drifts ramps and transport tunnels with cross sections of 12 to 20 square meters, than the total volume of the repository is about 46.000 cubic metres. The state of stress is of utmost importance for the long-term stability and integrity of the potential repository.

The state of stress at the Stripa mine has been studied through a program of hydraulic fracturing and overcoring stress measurements performed both in one 381 m deep vertical borehole, SBH-4, drilled from the surface and from several short boreholes drilled around the heater experiment drift at 336 m level in the Swedish-American Research Program (Doe et al., 1983). Results by the two methods applied in SBH-4 agreed well on orientation of the maximum horizontal stress and on the interpolated stresses for the depth of the test site at 336 m level. Near-field stress measurements were conducted with

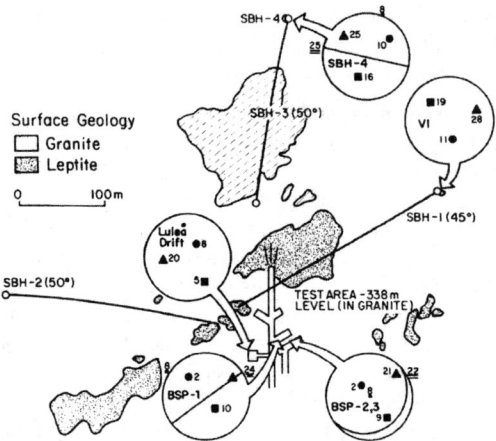

Figure 5. Stereographic projection showing average magnitude and orientations of principle stress (overcoring) and maximum horizontal stress (hydrofracturing). σ1=triangle; σ2=square; σ3=circle. Hydraulic fracture orientation is shown as planes and the magnitude is doubled underlined. After Doe et al., 1983.

hydraulic fracturing and four different overcoring methods. All results agreed on the magnitude and direction of the stresses. The average directions and magnitudes of the stresses determined in the near- and far-field are presented in a stereographic projection, see Fig. 5.

The maximum stress direction at Stripa rotates from Northwest in the far field to Northeast in the near-field, cf. Fig. 5. This rotation is likely to be due to the influence of the mine as a whole rather than to the experimental drifts.

During the Stripa Project, rock characterisation tools and methods were applied to obtain data to describe the geohydrology of the Stripa mine and its surroundings. The Site Characterisation and Validation (SCV) programme was one of the principle components of Phase 3 of the Stripa Project with the aim to characterise a previously undisturbed block of saturated, fractured granite. *In situ* stress measurements were made in nine boreholes in three locations with hydrofracturing and overcoring. The results of these measurements showed that the maximum stress is almost horizontal and oriented WSW-ENE (Fig. 6).

The measurements that were made in the late stage of the Stripa Project (DBH-1, DBH-2 and DBH-3) were generally consistent with the orientation and magnitude observed from previous measurements, cf. Figs. 5 & 6. Considering the total

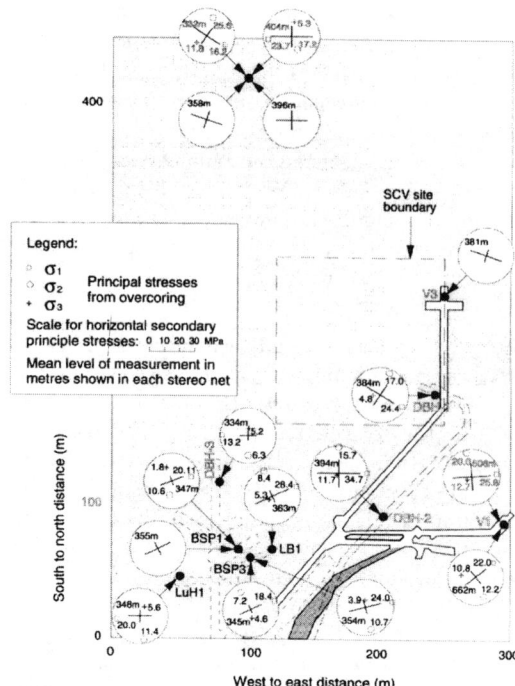

Figure 6. Plan view of *in situ* stress measurements conducted in Stripa mine during 1977-1990. After Gnirk, 1993.

set of measurements, the maximum principle at the 385m level of the SCV site was estimated to have a magnitude of 24.4 MPa and to be oriented N75W. The minimum principle stress was estimated to be vertical and of magnitude 10 MPa and the intermediate principle stress to be 16 MPa. The result is in fair agreement with the average state of stress at this depth in the Fennoscandian Shield as recorded in the Fennoscandian Rock Stress Data Base (Stephansson et al., 1986).

From this analysis we can conclude that at Stripa mine there exist a far-field stress different in orientation from the near-field stress. The magnitudes of stresses are moderate and fairly consistent over a relatively large area at the depth interval 330 to 400 metres and the stress state and stresses versus depth are in accordance with the average state of stress in the Fennoscandian Shield. Stability problems never occurred during the operation of the research projects in the hard and competent Stripa granite. From these findings we can conclude that the requirement for mechanical stability and integrity of a repository for toxic waste in the Stripa mine are fulfilled. Additional studies of the geohydrology, ground-water chemistry and fluid transport will show wheather or not the site is suitable as a repository for mercury and other toxic metals.

3.4 Deep injection disposal of hazardous and industrial waste in deep boreholes.

During the past 50 years, many industries have elected to dispose parts of their hazardous and industrial liquid wastes in sedimentary formations deep below the Earth's surface. By the 1980s, nearly 42 million cubic meters of hazardous wastehad been injected in deep formations in the United States alone. In the former Soviet Union, large volumes of exceedingly radioactive liquid waste from plutonium recovery facilities were being injected into structurally isolated sedimentary formations on an interim basis while alternative means of disposal remained under development. These sentences are quoted from the preface of a recent publication on deep injection disposal of hazardous and industrial waste (Apps & Tsang, 1996).

Cooper and Lyle (1996) reported that since the U. S. Environmental Protection Agency (EPA) began to implement stringent underground-injection-control (UIC) regulations in early 1980s, no instances of Class I well failures have affected underground water resources of drinking water. In addition the authors presented a long list of geological and geophysical studies and siting criteria that are needed to eliminate the potential risk for disposal into formations that may outcrop or recharge near-surface or usable waters in the vicinity of a disposal facility. They emphasise that the most effective method for investigating the geologic suitability of arrestment and confining layers with respect to *in situ* fracture properties is a specialized form of well testing which they call *in situ* stress testing or microfracture test. This method is in principal conventional hydraulic fracturing stress measurement (see Amadei & Stephansson, 1997, Chapter 4) with relatively short test duration (1-10 min per injection cycle) and low fluid rates (1-50 l/min). A straddle-packer assembly and a downhole shut-in tool are used with high-resolution, and downhole pressure gages collect data. The data are then analysed to determine formations breakdown pressure, re-opening pressure, fracture propagation and aperture, and shut-in pressure equal to fracture-closure pressure.

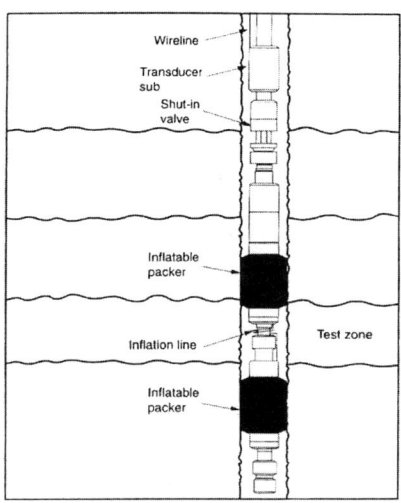

Figure 7. Wireline straddle-packer assembly for *in situ* stress testing at hazardous disposal well sites. After Cooper & Lyle, 1996.

The conventional tool configuration for microfracture testing includes two inflatable packers separated by a perforated short-tubing joint (sub), see Fig. 7. The perforated pipe (sub) maintain communication between the test interval, the pressure gage, and the workstring. The assembly can be controlled by wireline or a multi-hose system from the surface. These tools currently available offer several advantages over conventional tubing-conveyed equipment.

Slurry fracturing is reported to be success-fully used in the Western Canadian Sedimentary basin for large volume disposal of an inert, low toxicity, fine-grained oily quartzose sand (Dusseault et al., 1996). Slurry injection is intended for inert granular terminal wastes without gas generation or decomposition and offers an alternative to landfills and other methods of surface storage.

4 STRATEGY AND PROGRAM FOR STRESS MEASUREMENT IN WASTE REPOSITORIES

Recommendations for stress measurement programs related to site location of nuclear waste repository in hard rocks are presented by Doe et al. (1983). The need for estimating *in situ* stresses from knowledge of structure geology, rock anisotropy, topography etc. prior to measurement campaigns in the field is strongly advocated by Amadei and Stephansson (1997, Chapter 2). In addition they present data on accuracy and uncertainty in stress measurements for the majority of measuring techniques. In the following sections the strategy and program for stress measurement in waste repositories are presented with respect to:

- Timing and strategy of stress measurements;
- Methods available for use;
- Number of measurements;
- Accuracy and uncertainty in measurements.

4.1 *Timing and strategy of stress measurements*

1. Before measuring virgin stresses with any of the existing methods available, an attempt should be made to obtain an estimate of the *in situ* stress field using existing techniques presented by Amadei & Stephansson (1997, Chapter 2).

2. Stress measurements should be performed prior to the construction and be a part of the early borehole exploration programme for a potential repository site.

3. The goal of the stress measuring programme should be to determine the stress magnitude and orientation at the depth of a repository or the injection level for a hazardous disposal well site. Results can be obtained either by a) performing a large number of tests at the depth of the potential repository, or b) performed a number of tests at a range of depths and than use linear regression to determine the stress magnitude and direction at the level of the repository or disposal level. Notice that this calls for borehole which extend well below the repository or disposal level.

4. The first stress measurements from boreholes drilled from the surface can be used to qualify a candidate site. If stress magnitudes, stress ratios and stresses versus depth are too high then the site will be disqualified.

5. Results from first stress measurements can be used to design the initial shafts and rock characterisation facilities.

4.2 *Methods to use*

1. The hydraulic fracturing method in combination with Hydraulic Pressurisation of Pre-existing Fractures - HTPF method is recommended for the first stress measurements in surface boreholes.

2. If data on focal mechanisms or other stress or strain data exists in the site area an integrated stress determination is recommended.

3. During shaft sinking surface hole measurements should be confirmed using reliable overcoring methods such as CSIRO HI cell or cells where there exist long experience and reliable calibrations.

4. During site characterisation, design and construction of a repository reliable overcoring methods should be used.

4.3 *Number of measurements*

1. Given the scatter in the stress measurements and the scale effect, it is important to have performed enough measurements so a mean value and confidence interval can be defined. At best, and in good quality to very good quality rock conditions, rock stresses can be determined with an error of ± 10-20% for their magnitude and an error of ± 10-20 degrees for their orientation. For poor quality rocks no confidence intervals can be established.

2. For determining stress magnitudes in good quality rock, 20 measurements are recommended to define the mean values within 10% of the maximum stress value and 15 measurements are sufficient to define the stress orientation within 20 degrees.

4.4 *Accuracy and uncertainty in measurements*

1. The accuracy of an instrument to measure stress has to be assessed by controlled laboratory tests where the measured stress is compared with the applied stresses.

2. Natural uncertainties in rock stresses are due to variations in stresses from point to point in the rock mass. Analytic solutions for the analysis of strain measurements with overcoring methods should be applied in anisotropic rocks.

3. Measurement-related uncertainties are best avoided by using well-established methods and techniques and using measurement teams with long experience.

4. Data analysis-related uncertainties may be created due to non-linear or inelastic response, time-dependent response, yielding of the rock after

drilling and inhomogeneities at the scale of the overcore sample or at the level of hydraulic fracturing.

Presentation of stress measurement data should include error bars or confidence intervals, with mean value and standard deviation, for both stress magnitude and stress orientation. For examples see Amadei & Stephansson (1997, Chapter 3).

5 REFERENCES

Amadei, B. & O. Stephansson 1997. *Rock stress and its measurement*. London: Chapman & Hall.

Apps, J.A. & C.-F. Tsang 1996. Preface. In J.A. Apps & C.-F. Tsang (eds), *Deep injection disposal of hazardous and industrial waste*. San Diego: Academic Press.

Brown, E.T. 1993. The nature and fundamentals of rock engineering. In J.A. Hudson (ed), *Comprehensive Rock Engineering, Vol. 1*, 1-23. Oxford: Pergamon Press.

Cooper, K.J. & R.R.Lyle 1996. *In situ* stress measurement at hazardous disposal well sites: Field application. In J.A. Apps & C.-F. Tsang (eds), *Deep injection disposal of hazardous and industrial waste*. San Diego: Academic Press.

Doe, T.W. et al. 1983. *In situ* stress measurements at the Stripa mine, Sweden. Technical Information Report No. SAC-44. Berkeley: Lawrence Berkeley Laboratory.

Dusseault, et al. 1996. Disposal of granular solid wastes in the Western Canadian Sedimentary basin by slurry fracture injection. In J.A. Apps & C.-F. Tsang (eds), *Deep injection disposal of hazardous and industrial waste*: 725-742. San Diego: Academic Press.

Fairhurst, C. 1968. Methods of determining in-situ rock stresses at great depth. *Tech. Rep. No.1-68*. Omaha, Nebraska: Corps of Engineers.

Gnirk, P. 1993. OECD/NEA International Stripa Project; Overview Volume II, Natural Barriers. Stockholm: SKB.

Hansson, H., B. Shen, O. Stephansson & L. Jing, 1995. SITE-94. Rock mechanics modelling for the stability and safety of a nuclear waste repository. Executive summary. SKI Report 95:41. Stockholm: Swedish Nuclear Power Inspectorate.

Hoek, E. & E.T. Brown 1980. *Underground excavations in rock*. London: Inst. Mining and Metallurgy.

Jamtveit, B. & W.D. Yardley 1997. Fluid flow and transport in rocks: an overview. In B. Jamtveit & B. Yardley (eds), *Fluid Flow and Transport in Rocks*: 1-14. London: Chapman & Hall.

Jing, L. & O. Stephansson 1997. Network topology and homogenisation of fractured rocks. In B. Jamtveit & B. Yardley (eds), *Fluid Flow and Transport in Rocks* London: Chapman & Hall.

Martin,C.D. 1997. Brittle rock strength failure: Laboratory and *in situ*. In *Proc. Int. Soc. Rock Mech. 8th Congress,Sept 1995, Vol 3*: 1033-1040.. Rotterdam: Balkema.

Myrvang, A., S.E. Hansen & T. Sörensen 1993. Rock stress redistribution around an open pit mine in hardrock. *Int. J. Rock Mech. Min. Sci. & Geomech. Abstr.* 30:1001-1004.

Stephansson, O. 1995. Introduction to special issue on thermo-hydro-mechanical coupling in rock mechanics. *Int. J. Rock Mech. Min. Sci. & Geomech. Abstr.* 32: 387-535.

Stephansson, O., P. Särkkä & A. Myrvang 1986. State of stress in Fennoscandia. In O. Stephansson (ed), *Rock Stress and Rock Stress Measurements*:21-32. Luleå: Centek Publishers.

Stephansson, O., L. Jing & C.-F. Tsang 1996. *Coupled Thermo-Hydro-Mechanical Processes of Fractured Media; Mathematical and Experimental Studies*. Amsterdam: Elsevier.

Stille, H. & A. Fredriksson 1988. Measurements,calculations and stability prognoses at the SFR undersea repository for low- and medium level nuclear waste. *Tunneling and Underground Space Technology,* 3: 277-282.

Tolppanen, P., E. Johansson & M. Hakala, 1995. Rock mechanical analyses of *in situ* stress/strength ratio at the TVO investigation sites Kivetty, Olkiluoto and Romuvaara. *Report YJT-95-11,* Helsinki: Nuclear Waste Commission of Finnish Power Co.

Tsang, C.-F. & O. Stephansson 1996. A conceptual introduction to coupled thermo-hydro-mechanical processes in rocks. In O. Stephansson et al. (eds), *Coupled Thermo-Hydro-Mechanical Processes of Fractured Media*: 1-24. Amsterdam: Elsevier.

Measuring rock stress and rock engineering in Japan

K. Sugawara
Department of Civil Engineering and Architecture, Kumamoto University, Japan

ABSTRACT: Importance of in situ stress measurements is discussed, as well as the engineering requirements, presenting the topics of rock engineering in Japan, the stress-related stability problems and the future rock engineering projects. Excellent developments of the stress relief method and the hydraulic method are briefly reviewed, and subsequently the in situ stresses measured by means of the stress relief method are presented and analyzed to clarify the non-homogeneity due to geological heterogeneity and inevitable sliding on faults, and the characteristics of the near-surface in situ stress field in the Japanese island arcs situated on an active border at which the Pacific plate and the Philippine sea plate are driving beneath the Eurasian plate.

1 INTRODUCTION

Knowledge of rock stress is of importance in civil, mining, petroleum and earthquake engineering and energy development, as well as in geophysics and geology. However, an exact prediction of the in situ stresses and their spatial variation is very difficult, since the current stress state is the end product of a series of past geological events. Further, rock mass is rarely homogeneous and continuous, then stresses vary from place to place. For instance, the horizontal stress can vary from one layer to the next in stratified rock formations, which is common in sedimentary as well as the volcanic rock masses in Japan, due to changes in rock stiffness. In situ stresses not only vary in space but also with time due to the tectonic events and geological process. Thus, the rock stress measurement in situ is an only means presently available to evaluate the in situ stress field which is required for analysis and design of rock structures, such as caverns, stopes, tunnels, slopes and etc.(Sugawara, 1993; Amadei & Stephansson, 1997).

In the present paper, to make clear the importance of rock stress and rock stress measurements in situ, rock engineering activities in Japan will be firstly described, including future projects. Subsequently, in situ stress field of the Japanese Isles is presented, as well as the current researches on the methods for rock stress measurement. Analyzing the trends of in situ stress field, it is discussed how the near-surface in situ stresses depend on geological discontinuities such as faults, and on the tectonic activities.

2 ROCK ENGINEERING IN JAPAN

2.1 *Large Rock Caverns Construction*

Many large rock caverns have been constructed also in Japan, for pumped-storage power generation and crude oil storage. The pumped-storage power plants of high-head and large capacity have been developed since the 1970s in the pursuit of enhanced economic efficiency, and the scale of cavern becomes greater. For instance, the Kazunogawa powerhouse cavern under construction in the Yamanashi prefecture at a depth of about 500m is 54m high, 34m wide and 210m long, having an egg-shaped cross section. The crude oil storage plants were constructed at Kuji, Kikuma and Kushikino in 1994, and each plant has a capacity from 1.5 to 1.75 million kilo liters.

In the large rock caverns construction, the stability of the cavern is the most important problem. Since the behavior of rock mass surrounding the cavern in response to the excavation is deeply depending upon the state of in situ stresses and geological conditions, it is essential to select a favorable location. While avoid large fault or fracture zones, the large size of the cavern makes it inevitable that some weak rock formations and unfavorable joints will intersect with the cavern or be present in the vicinity of it. Thus, the scrupulous rock engineering survey is required to design the cavern layout and the reinforcement system. Usually, the stability analysis using FEM and/or various numerical methods are performed, basing on initial rock stress measurements and in situ experiments of the rock mass properties, and the observational design and construction procedure is applied in the excavation stage to decide the suitable amount of the reinforcement (Hibino et al., 1977).

One criterion used for determining the orientation of large rock cavern is the minimization of stress concentrations and deformation. Mimaki (1976) and Mimaki & Matsuo (1986) have presented two case examples of the design of the pumped-storage power house cavern, where it has been decided to orient the caverns with their axes parallel to the maximum horizontal in situ stress, as illustrated in Figure 1.

The mushroom shape is the predominant form of the power house caverns in Japan. This has recently been replaced by the egg-shaped one. The modified egg-shaped cross section has been adopted for the crude oil storage, with the reinforcement system of shotcrete and rock bolts. In the crude oil storage plants, the water barrier method was successfully applied to prevent gas and oil leakage. At present, underground LPG storage plants are being planned, and a feasibility study on deep underground seawater pumped-storage power generation system has been initiated, as well as the research on compressed air storage (Sugawara, 1996).

2.2 Mining and Limestone Quarrying

In mining engineering, in situ stresses need to be taken into account when selecting mining methods and designing stopes, pillars and support systems. Stress-related stability problems in Japan clearly increased with depth. For instance, the Japanese coal mines met with various problems in the past, such as gas outburst and coal burst, at the depth greater than about 500m. The occurrence of coal burst has been correlated with the depth of mining, mine geometry and the rate of the extraction (Kimura et al., 1982), and governed by predominant fault systems (Kaneko et al., 1988).

The stability problem of stopes can also be found in volcanic regions, that is to a large extent governed by the thermal stress. For instance, the geothermal gradient at the Toyoha mine in Hokkaido island is 200~300°C/km, and the rock temperature at working site reaches up to 160°C at the deepest level. In the Hishikari mine in Kyushu island, a new gold mine, is now operated under the rock temperature of 80°C in maximum.

Stability problems may also be found in limestone quarrying in steep mountainous regions. Since the lime stone deposits usually form steep mountains and lie on schalstein of susceptible to weathering, final slopes are built up with leaving limestone as a cover rock to prevent the weathering of schalstein or weak rock formations. A huge rock slope, 3km to 4km in length and over 500m in height, is expected to be appeared in the final stage. In such a region, the influence of topography on the in situ stress field is very significant (Sugawara, 1996).

2.3 Tunneling

Stress-related stability problems have also be found when conducting tunnels in mountainous regions. At the Kan-Etsu tunnel, which has been constructed by means of the full-face NATM with large machines, a systematic rock bolting has been applied normal to the cutting face as the preventives to remove the risk of rock bursts predicted by the AE monitoring and

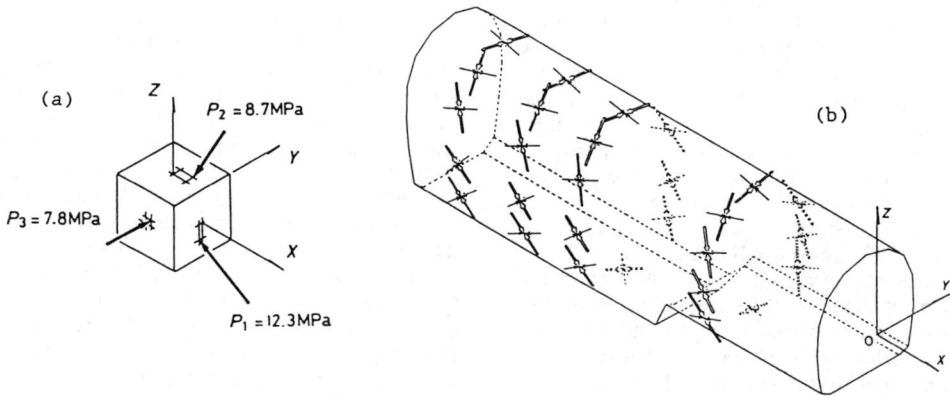

Figure 1 Three-dimensional elastic stress analysis of the Imaichi power house cavern using the boundary element method. (a) Measured in situ stress field, (b) distribution of tangential principal stresses on the cavern wall.

the focus analysis. On the other hand, at the Enasan tunnel of 8.6km long, through the 182 prominent faults in the steep mountain zone, many efforts have been made to overcome the high stress and large deformation of rock, and a large quantity of water.

At present, for the further expansion of transportation network, such as the Shinkansen network, the superconducting magnetic levitation railtrack system, the cross-Japan expressway system, the 2nd Tomei expressway and the 2nd Meishin expressway, it is discussed how to build large tunnels of significant length and cross-section, overcoming high in situ stresses and geological difficulties in mountainous regions near steep valley walls (Sugawara, 1996).

2.4 Geothermal Energy Extraction

Geothermal energy extraction is an engineering field of energy development where borehole stability and rock stresses are intimately related. It is an attractive idea to extract heat energy from hot dry rock(HDR). Although the concept is simple, its implementation presents an interesting challenge to rock engineering (Sugawara, 1996).

The research to develop HDR geothermal system has been promoted and conducted in Japan by the field experiments at Hijiori, Higashi-Hachimantai and Ogachi. Although the field experiments have demonstrated the potential for energy production, no HDR power plant is realized yet, because hot water circulation system is still not fully understood and consequently could not be designed in the rock engineering base. The interaction of in situ stresses with other rock mass properties and the effects of in situ stresses on flow and pressure in fractures is particularly important in understanding fluid flow mechanism, and in predicting the effectiveness of hydraulic injections which are common in the HDR geothermal energy systems.

2.5 Others

A clear understanding of in situ stresses is also vital for the storage of nuclear waste in rock, which is of great concern all over the world. The objective is to isolate the radionuclides while they remain radiologically significant. The most likely mechanism for migration of radionuclides away from a geological repository is by solution in groundwater, and the minimal groundwater movement is required to result in a long transit time back to the environment. In particular, it should be required that there is no likelihood of natural disruptive events such as earthquakes, because Japan is subject to severe seismic and geothermal activities (Sugawara, 1996). It can be pointed out that the tightness of a rock mass due to large enough in situ stresses have to be taken into account in repository site suitability, selection and characterization.

In situ stresses are important to geologists and geophysicists in order to understand the mechanism of plate tectonics and various geological processes, including earthquakes. Since the Japanese Isles are situated on an active border at which the Pacific plate and the Philippine sea plate are driving beneath the Eurasian plate, Japan is subject to severe seismic and geothermal activities as previously described. Thus, the crustal stresses is an important subject in geology and geophysics and also in earthquake engineering.

3. RESEARCH ON STRESS RELIEF METHOD

Research on the stress relief method in Japan has a long history (Hiramatsu & Oka, 1968; Suzuki & Ishijima, 1968; Sugawara & Obara 1993). Many excellent methods have been developed, but some of them are not usually used. The current developments are reviewed in the following, with historical topics.

The Shin-Takasegawa project, for the construction of a pumped-storage power plant, is considered to present a breakthrough. This is because a systematic investigation of initial rock stress was introduced for the first time, using a borehole deformation method. The continuous measurement system was developed for monitoring the changes in deformation due to overcoring, then the reliability of measurements was evidently improved. At present, this system is used in all of the stress relief methods in Japan.

A systematic measurement of the induced rock stress by the excavations was firstly performed in the Imaichi project, to clarify the stress concentration within the ground arch (Mimaki & Kudoh, 1984), and to verify the strength of rock mass (Sugawara et al., 1986), using the doorstopper system and the hemispherical-ended borehole technique (Sugawara & Obara, 1986).

The borehole deformation method developed by the Central Research Institute of the Electric Power Industry is one of the widely used methods in Japan. Using an eight-element borehole deformation gauge, the diametral and diagonal components of borehole deformation are measured within a single borehole, which are sufficient for determining the complete state of in situ stresses (Kanagawa et al., 1986a).

Doorstopper system (Leeman, 1969) was studied by Oka et al.(1976) and Kameoka (1978), and they developed the eight-element strain cell, to reduce the number of boreholes required for determining the complete state of in situ stresses from three to two. This has been used in the mining field and deep tunnels (Saito et al., 1983).

Hemispherical-ended borehole technique presented by Sugawara et al.(1985) is based on a principle much similar to the doorstopper system, apart from the shape of the borehole bottom. Measuring the

16-element of induced strain on the hemispherical bottom surface in a borehole, the complete state of stress is back-analyzed by the theory of elasticity. A modification has been proposed by Kobayashi et al. (1987), and consists of gluing strain gages at the end of a conical borehole. Sakaguchi et al. (1992) have refined the conical-ended borehole technique by increasing the number of strain measurement. The 24 element conical strain cell as shown in Figure 2 has been presented, as well as the 16 element conical strain cell. Moreover, to reduce the time, effort and cost for the in situ strain measurement, Sugawara et al. (1992) have developed the compact overcoring method, in which the overcoring is conducted using a thin-wall diamond bit of special make having a diameter of 76mm.

The combination of the conical-ended borehole technique and the compact overcoring method has been tested by Obara et al.(1994, 1995a), Jang et al. (1994), Tamai et al.(1994) and Sugawara & Obara (1995). A case example in Figure 3 clearly shows that the existence of faults affect the magnitude and orientation of in situ stresses. This suggests that the in situ measurement of stress jumps characteristics and non-homogeneous stress fields occurring while crossing or due to the vicinity of discontinuities such as faults provide the important and valuable data for the back-analysis of the geometry and characteristics of them (Obara et al. 1995b).

4 RESEARCH ON HYDRAULIC METHOD

Hydraulic method can be divided into the hydraulic fracturing method (Fairhurst,1964; Haimson, 1978), the hydraulic tests on preexisting fractures (HTPF) method (Cornet, 1986), and the sleeve fracturing method (Stephansson, 1983). Hydraulic fracturing method has successfully been combined with the HTPF method by Mizuta et al.(1987), to decide the complete state of in situ rock stresses.

Since 1978, the stress measurements by means of the hydraulic fracturing method have been conducted to investigate the stress state in relation to earthquake prediction in Japan (Tsukahara, 1983). For instance, stress magnitude and orientations were measured in 19 boreholes of depth from 100m to 900m, to derive an outline of the stress state related to the crustal structure as well as the crustal movement around the Kanto-Tokai area (Tsukahara & Ikeda, 1987).

In situ stress evaluation by means of the hydraulic fracturing method have also been promoted by the

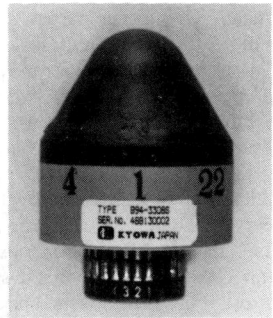

Figure 2 The 24 element conical strain cell.

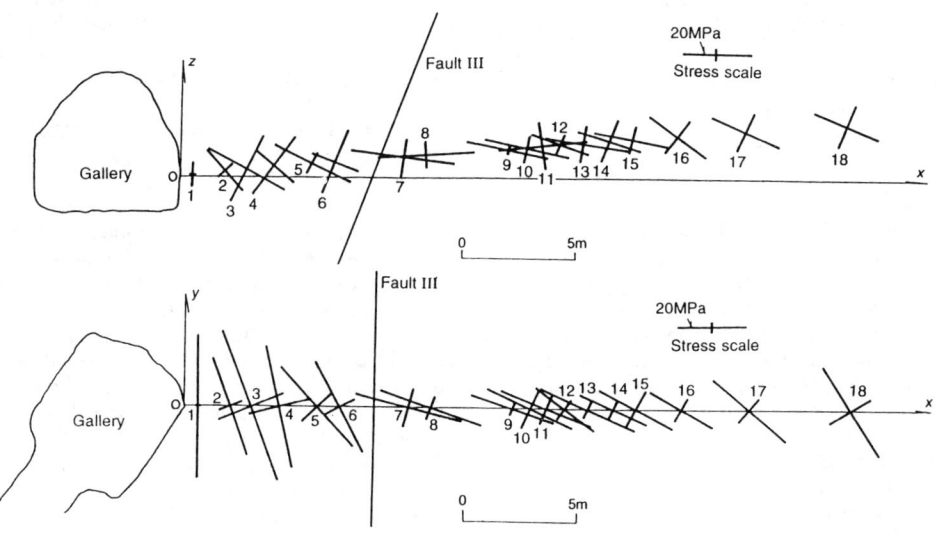

Figure 3 Principal stresses measured by means of the compact overcoring method.
(a) Vertical cross-section, (b) plan view.

HDR projects. Excellent developments associated with the HDR projects in Japan can be found in Hayashi & Abe (1984), Mizuta et al. (1985), Kuriyagawa et al.(1989), Matsunaga et al. (1989), Hayashi et al. (1989), Hayashi & Sakurai (1989), Ito & Hayashi (1991, 1992), among many others.

The sleeve fracturing method has been improved by Serata & Kikuchi (1986) and Sakuma et al. (1989) for stress measurements at shallow depth, and the fracture process has been investigated by Sugawara et al. (1987) basing on the linear fracture mechanics.

5 STRESSES IN THE JAPANESE ISLANDS

5.1 *Maximum Horizontal Stress Directions*

Japanese Isles are situated as shown in Figure 4 on an active border at which the Pacific and Philippine sea plates are driving beneath the Eurasian plate. The biggest island, called Honshu, is divided into two segments, the southwestern and the northeastern, by the Fossa Magna (Sugimura, 1972). The former is further subdivided into two units, the outer and the inner, by the Median tectonic line (Huzita, 1980).

The outer unit has a zonal structure. It consists of the Sanbagawa metamorphic zone (crystalline schists immediately neighboring the Median tectonic line), the Chichibu zone (Carboniferous sedimentary rock formations) and the Shimanto zone (Cretaceous to Tertiary sedimentary rocks). The northern border of the Shimanto zone in the outer unit is, in Figure 5, represented by a broken curve running parallel to the Median tectonic line. The inner unit has a similar zonal structure. Directly beside the Median tectonic line, there is a belt of Cretaceous sedimentary rocks and then the Ryouke metamorphic zone to the north. These consist of granite and gneiss. Northern fringe of the inner unit is a volcano-sedimentary complex zone of the Neogene period, called the Green tuff zone, of which the border is indicated by a broken curve of parallel to the Median tectonic line.

The northern part of the northeastern segment is divided into the eastern side and the western side by a north-south broken line e-f. The eastern side is an accretionary prism which comprises granites and Paleozoic to Mesozoic formations. The western side is called the Green tuff zone, since it mainly consists of green tuff of submarine eruption origin from the Neogene period. The Green tuff zone is clearly compressed in the E-W direction. Many difficulties in rock engineering are associated with the clastic rock formations in the green tuff area and also in the younger volcanic and volcano-sedimentary rocks having cooling joints still open. Large heaves and heavy squeezing after stress relief often cause the severe engineering problems.

Maximum horizontal stress directions measured using the stress relief methods are as illustrated in Figure 6. From the tectonic activity of the Pacific plate, the northwestern segment may be expected to be compressed in the E-W direction. However, the stress directions measured in the east zone of the Fossa Magna are mostly in the N-S direction. This clearly proves that the in situ stress field of the northeastern segment is affected by both the Pacific plate and the Philippine sea plate. Moreover, It is noteworthy that the stress directions in the eastern side of the broken curve e-f are generally in the N-S direction, while the stress orientations in the western side are generally in the E-W direction. In relation to

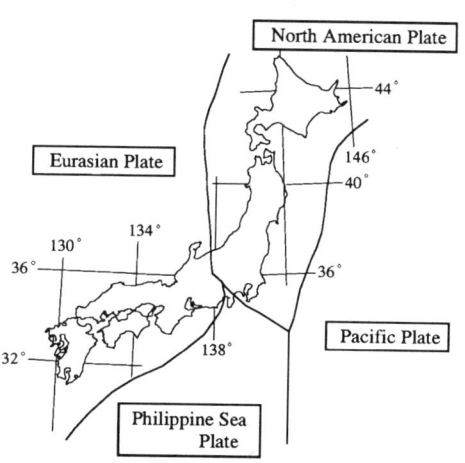

Figure 4 Four main islands of Japan and global plate tectonics.

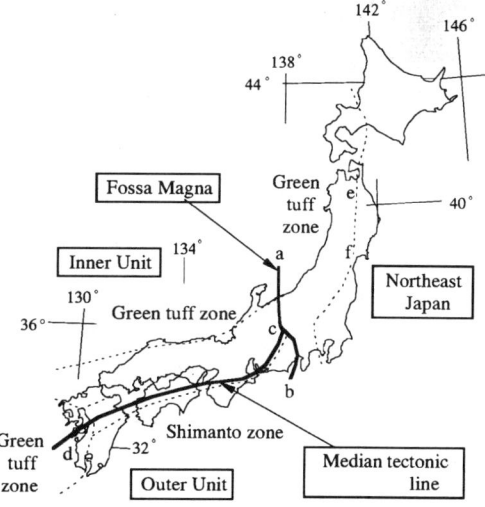

Figure 5 Outline of geological structure of Japan.

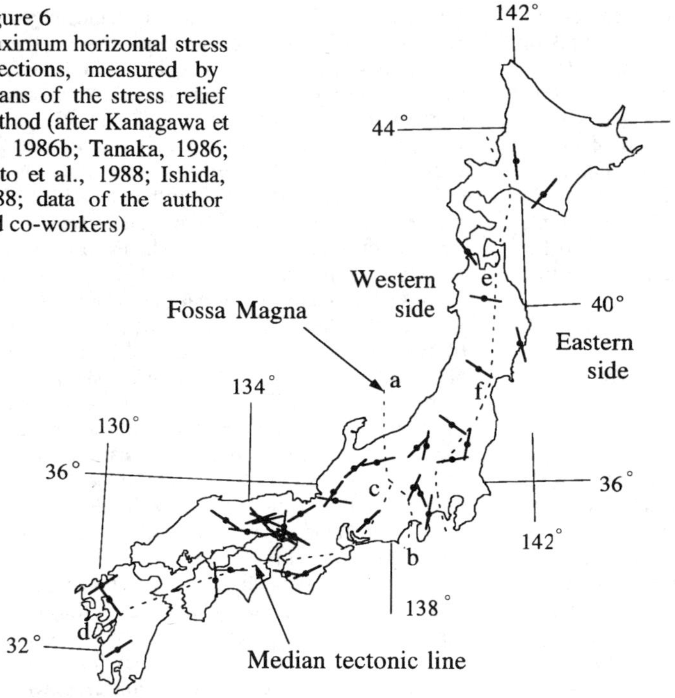

Figure 6
Maximum horizontal stress directions, measured by means of the stress relief method (after Kanagawa et al., 1986b; Tanaka, 1986; Saito et al., 1988; Ishida, 1988; data of the author and co-workers)

the southwestern segment, it can be noted that the stress directions measured in the outer and inner units are nearly parallel to the Median tectonic line.

The global trends of the in situ stress orientation is considered to be of importance in understanding the mechanism of the plate tectonic and its effect on the near-surface in situ stress field in Japan.

5.2 Increase of Stresses with Depth

The vertical stress σ_V observed is given in Figure 7, as a function of the depth z below surface. The mean vertical stress $\sigma_{V\,mean}$ has been computed as shown in the figure by Sugawara et al. (1995a) This means that $\sigma_{V\,mean}$ coincides with the overburden pressure. In relation to the deviation: $\sigma_V - \sigma_{V\,mean}$, Haung & Sugawara (1996) have shown from a more detail examination that the absolute value of it has a peak at a depth of about 1km.

The ratio, called k, of the average horizontal stress $\sigma_{Haverage}$ to the vertical stress σ_V is shown in Figure 8, as a function of the depth. Although the ratio k is greater than unity at shallow depths, this becomes less than unity and approaches a constant value at great depths. Brown & Hoek (1978) have firstly set out the limiting envelope curves of the observed ratio k. The curve of $k = 0.1/z + 0.3$ in the figure is the one stated by Brown & Hoek as the lower limit for the observed data, and the curve of $k = 1.5/z + 0.5$ represents the upper limit. In Figure 8, the Japanese data (solid circle) are distributed along the lower limit curve of k, and some of them are below it.

McCutchen(1982) has analyzed theoretically the empirical trends presented by Brown & Hoek, using a simple model of a self-gravitating spherical shell which is situated on a massive and un-yielding interior body. From the equilibrium of the elastic shell on the boundary condition of zero displacement at the base of the shell, it has been shown that the value of k can increase with increasing the basement depth, and that the lower limit curve presented by Brown & Hoek corresponds to a basement depth of 33.73km. This model suggests that Japan is situated on a shallow basement.

Sugawara et al. (1995a) have set out new limits by proposing the modified isotropic spherical shell model. In Figure 8, these are given by the two thin curves. These well fit in with the limits of the ratio observed. Sugawara & Jang (1996) have proposed the average horizontal compressive strain $\varepsilon_{Haverage}$ as a parameter to indicate the locality of the horizontal restriction. The thin curves in Figure 8 are defined by $\varepsilon_{Haverage}$=0.0002 and 0.002, respectively.

The maximum horizontal stress σ_{Hmax} and the minimum horizontal stress σ_{Hmin} are shown in Figure 9. The amount of scatter in the observed values is considered to be significant. Curves I and II are the non-linear limiting envelopes of σ_{Hmax} and σ_{Hmin}, respectively. In reference to the curve I, it may be significant that it has a peak at z =1km. With regard to the curve II, it is noteworthy that there is a stress

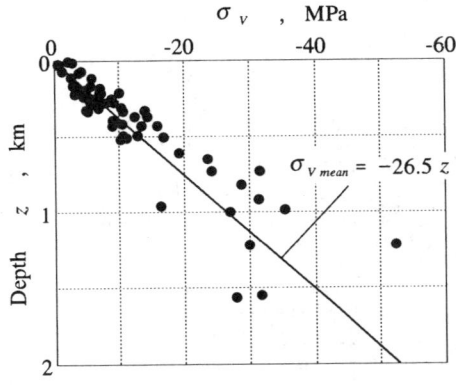

Figure 7 Variation of the vertical stress observed by means of the stress relief method.

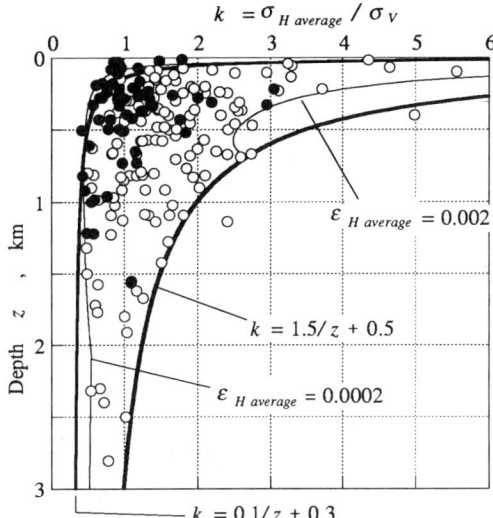

Figure 8 The ratio k as a function of the depth z.

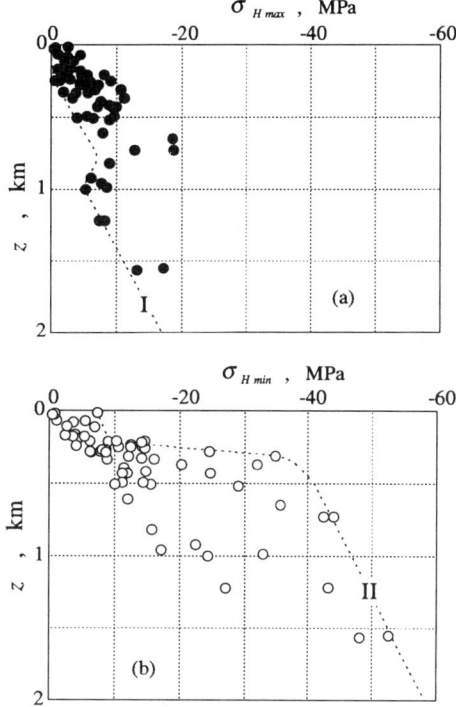

Figure 9 Variation of the horizontal stresses.
(a) The maximum horizontal stress;
(b) the minimum horizontal stress.

jump at $z=0.2\sim0.3$km. Such a nonlinearity of the limiting envelope curves I and II is considered to be a remarkable characteristic of the near-surface in situ stress field of Japan.

5.3 *Influence of Faults*

The nonlinearity and the stress jump characteristics mentioned above is considered to be closely related to the disturbance due to near-surface fault systems. In order to assess the stress disturbance caused by inevitable sliding on faults, the numerical analysis is presented in the following, which has been carried out using the displacement discontinuity method (Crouch & Starfield, 1983). Effects of the gravity and tectonic thrust have been considered, assuming that the fault plane is frictionless and no-tension.

A two-dimensional model is indicated in Figure 10, as well as the initial stress condition for the computation. The 60 degrees dipping fault system intersects with the flat ground surface of stress free, and consists of the shallow faults of 0.433km in depth and the deep faults of 1.039km in depth, having a constant horizontal interval of 0.45km. As shown in the figure, the initial stresses are defined by $\sigma_H = \sigma_o + 0.44\sigma_V$ and $\sigma_V = -26.5z$, where σ_o is the horizontal stress on the ground surface, that is a parameter to represent the amount of the horizontal restriction. In this model analysis, the stresses on fault planes are improved through the iteration until they satisfy the assumption of frictionless and no-tension.

The analyzed results in the case of $\sigma_o = 0$, are as in Figures 11(a) and 12(a). The displacement arrow diagram shows clearly that the normal sliding mode is prominent on the deep faults. The principal stress diagram indicates that the gravity faulting results in the vertical stress concentration at the upper side of the tips of the deep faults. The disturbance of the in situ stress field is as shown in Figure 13(a), where the horizontal normal stresses at the selection points arranged in a regular manner between the central two deep faults are compiled as a function of the depth. Comparison of Figure 13(a) and Figure 9(a) shows that the results of computation have a scatter pattern much similar to the measurement. The similarity may give a proof of the fact that the gravity faulting plays an important role in determining the distribution of σ_{Hmax}. The gravity fault results in a slight increase of the horizontal stress in the shallow region, and the accompanied decrease of it in the deeper region.

Effects of the tectonic thrust on the 60 degrees dipping fault system have been analyzed by reducing the magnitude of σ_o, step by step. An example is shown in Figures 11(b) and 12(b). The displacement arrow diagram shows clearly that the reverse sliding mode is prominent on the deep faults. The principal stress diagram shows that the tectonic thrust results

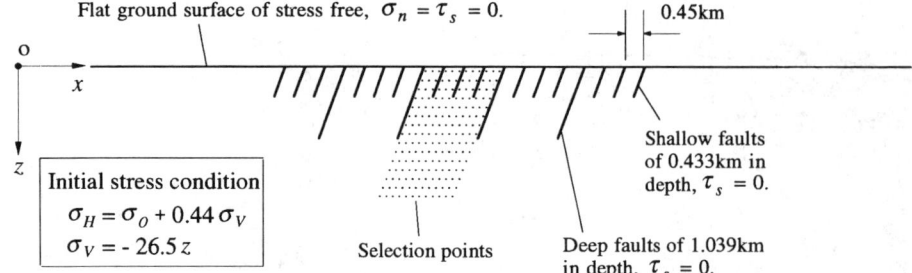

Figure 10 A faulted ground model for the displacement discontinuity method analysis.

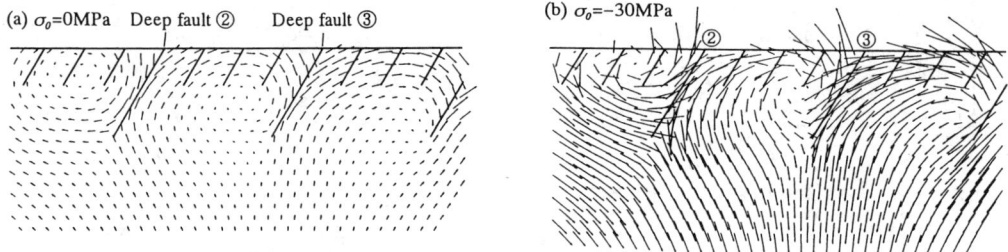

Figure 11 The displacement arrow diagram. (a) $\sigma_o = 0$, (b) $\sigma_o = -30$MPa.

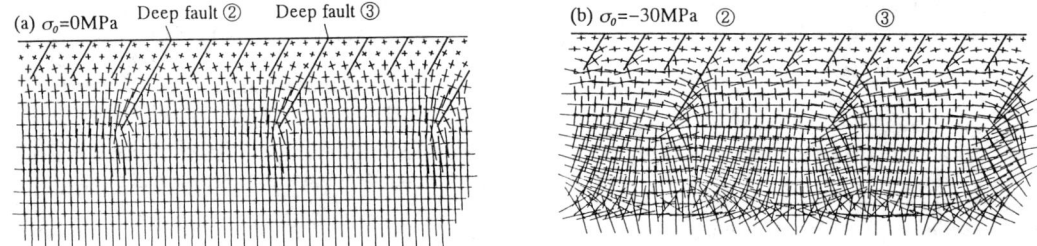

Figure 12 The principal stress diagram. (a) $\sigma_o = 0$, (b) $\sigma_o = -30$MPa.

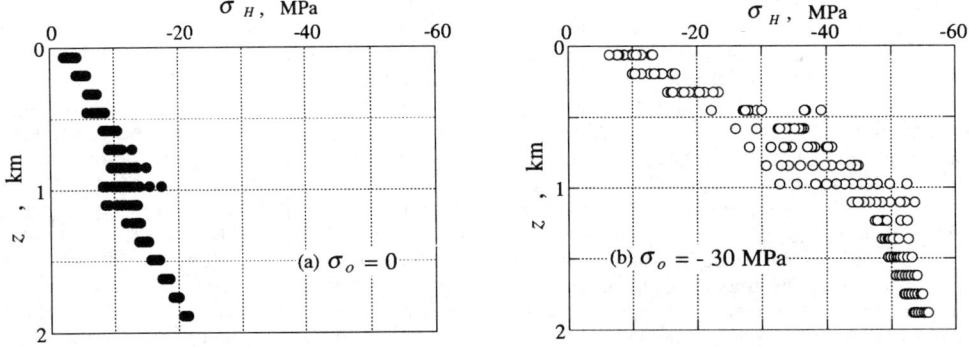

Figure 13 The horizontal stresses at the selection points as a function of the depth.
(a) $\sigma_o = 0$, (b) $\sigma_o = -30$MPa.

in the horizontal stress concentration at the tips of the deep faults. The distribution of the horizontal normal stresses at the selection points compiled in Figure 13(b) clearly indicates that the stress relaxation can appear in the vicinity of the ground surface. Such a near-surface stress relaxation may be a reason of the non-homogeneity and stress jump characteristics of the limit envelope curve II.

6 CONCLUDING REMARKS

Current rock engineering activity in Japan has been reviewed to make clear the importance of the knowledge of the in situ stress and the in situ stress measurements, as well as the engineering requirements for them. Rock engineering for large rock caverns construction in Japan has been described, as well as the stress-related stability problems in mining and limestone quarrying, and the problems in tunneling in the steep mountainous regions and in the clastic rock masses in the Green tuff area, and also in the younger volcanic and volcano-sedimentary rocks. Moreover, it has been described that the interesting challenge to rock engineering is required for the geothermal energy extraction from hot dry rock and the storage of nuclear waste, as well as for understanding the mechanism of the plate tectonics and various geological processes, including earthquakes. Subsequently, the excellent developments of the stress relief method and the hydraulic method in Japan have been reviewed with the historical topics on in situ stress measurements.

The trends of the in situ stresses in the Japanese islands have been presented by compiling the data of in situ stress measurement by means of the stress relief method. The horizontal stress directions have been discussed to be generally harmonic with the tectonic movements of the Pacific plate and the Philippine sea plate. The limiting envelope curves of the ratio k of the average horizontal stress to the vertical stress have been analyzed, as well as the non-linear limiting envelope curves of the maximum and minimum horizontal stresses.

In particular, it has been clarified that the presence of the stress jump in the lower limiting envelope curves of the minimum horizontal stress is the remarkable characteristics of the near-surface in situ stress field of Japan. The disturbance of stress caused by the inevitable sliding on the faults has been analyzed by the displacement discontinuity method, and it has been clarified that the effects of adjacent faults are significant in understanding the non-linearity of the near-surface in situ stress field in Japanese islands and its stress jump characteristics. These indicate that the in situ stresses are closely depending upon the stiffness of the rock masses, and upon the loads due to the gravity and the tectonic movements.

REFERENCES

Amadei, B. & Stephansson, O. 1997. *Rock Stress and its Measurement*: 96-104, London: Chapman & Hall.
Brown, E. T. & E. Hoek 1978. Trends in relationships between measured in-situ stresses and depth. *Int. J. Rock Mech. Min. & Geomech. Abstr.* 15: 211-215.
Cornet, F. H. 1986. Stress determination from hydraulic tests on preexisting fractures - the HTPF method, *Proc. Int. Symp. Rock Stress and Rock Stress Measurements*, Stockholm, pp.301-312.
Crouch, S. L. & A. M. Starfield 1983. *Boundary element methods in solid mechanics*. London: George Allen & Unwin Ltd.
Fairhurst, C. 1964. Measurement of in-situ rock stresses with particular reference to hydraulic fracturing, *J. Rock Mech. Eng. Geol.* 2: 129-147.
Haimson, B. C. 1978. The hydrofracturing stress measuring method and recent field results, *Int. J. Rock Mech. Min. Sci. & Geomech. Abstr.* 15: 167-178.
Haung, X. & K. Sugawara 1996. Analysis and considerations of the effect of faults on initial rock stress. *J. Min. Mater. Inst. Jpn.* 112: 289-294.
Hayashi, K. & H. Abe 1984. A new method for the measurement of in situ stress in geothermal fields, *J. Geothermal Res. Soc., Jpn.* 6(3): 203-212.
Hayashi, K., T. Ito and H. Abe 1989. In situ stress determination by hydraulic fracturing - a method employing an artificial notch, *Int. J. Rock Mech. Min. Sci. & Geomech. Abstr.* 26: 197-202.
Hayashi, K. & I. Sakurai 1989. Interpretation of hydraulic fracturing shut-in curves for tectonic stress measurements, *Int. J. Rock Mech. Min. Sci. & Geomech. Abstr.* 26: 477-482.
Hibino S., M. Hayashi, T. Kanagawa and M. Motojima 1977. Forcast and measurement of the behaviour of rock masses during underground excavation works, *Field Measurements in Rock Mech.*: 2, 935-948. Rotterdam: Balkema.
Hiramatsu, Y. & Y. Oka 1968. Determination of the stress in rock unaffected by boreholes or drifts, from measured strains or deformations. *Int. J. Rock Mech. Min. Sci.* 5: 337-353.
Huzita, K. 1980. Role of the median tectonic line in the quaternary tectonic of the Japanese islands, *Mem. Geol. Soc. Jpn.* 18: 129-153.
Ishida, T. 1988. Study on the initial stress state in rock mass, *Ph.D. Thesis*, Kyoto University.
Ito, T. & K. Hayashi 1991. Physical background to the breakdown pressure in hydraulic fracturing tectonic stress measurements, *Int. J. Rock Mech. Min. Sci. & Geomech. Abstr.* 28: 285-293.
Ito, T. & K. Hayashi 1992. Characteristics of shut-in curves in hydraulic fracturIng stress measurements, *Geother. Res. Coun. Trans.* 16: 651-556.
Jang, H., Y. Obara and K. Sugawara 1994. Rock stress measurement in a granitic massif by means of the conical-ended borehole technique, *Proc. of Int. Forum of Resouses Engineering*, Seoul, pp.256-261.
Kameoka, Y. 1978. Study on rock stress measurement by relieving the stress on a borehole bottom surface, *Ph.D. Thesis*, Kyoto University.
Kanagawa, T., S. Hibino and T. Ishida 1986a. In-situ stress measurements by over-coring method, Development of 8-element gauge for 3-dimensional estimation. *CRIEPI Rep.* E385033.
Kanagawa, T., S. Hibino, T. Ishida, M. Hayashi and Y. Kitahara 1986b. In situ stress measurements in the Japanese island: Overcoring results from a multi-element gauge used at 23 sites, *Int. J. Rock Mech. Min. & Geomech. Abstr.* 23: 29-39.
Kaneko, K., K. Sugawara and Y. Obara 1988. Rock Stress and Microseismicity in a Coal Burst District, *Proc. 2nd Int. Symp. Rockbursts and Seismisity in Mine*, Minneapolis, pp.247-256.

Kimura, O., K. Sugawara and K. Kaneko, 1982. Study on the Controlling of Coal Burst in Miike Mine, *Proc. of 7th Int. Strata Control Conf.*, Liege, Vol.1, pp.431-451.

Kobayashi, S., N. Nishimura and K. Matsumoto 1987. Displacements and strains around a non-flat-end borehole, *Proc. 2nd Int. Symp. on Field Measurements in Geomech.*, Kobe, Vol.2, pp.1079-1084.

Kuriyagawa, M., H. Kobayashi, I. Matsunaga, T. Yamaguchi and K. Hibiya 1989. An Application of hydraulic fracturing to three-dimensional in situ stress measurement, Tochigi, Japan, *Int. J. Rock Mech. Min. Sci. & Geomech. Abstr.* 26: 587-593.

Leeman, E. R. 1969. The doorstopper and triaxial rock stress measuring instruments developed by the CSIR, *J. S. Afr. Inst. Min. Metall.*, 69: 305-339.

Matsunaga, I., M. Kuriyagawa and S. Sasaki 1989. In situ stress measurements by the hydraulic fracturing method at Imaichi pumped storage power plant, Tochigi, Japan, *Int. J. Rock Mech. Min. Sci. & Geomech. Abstr.*, 26: 203-209.

McCutchen, W. R. 1982. Some elements of a theory for in-situ stress. *Int. J. Rock Mech. Min. Sci. & Geomech. Abstr.* 19: 201-203.

Mimaki, Y. 1976. Design and construction of a large underground power station. *Design and Construction of Underground Structures*: 115-125. Tokyo: The Japan Society of Civil Engineers.

Mimaki, Y. & K. Kudoh 1984. Measurements of rock stress and the design criteria of additional supporting system at the opening, *Proc. of the 16th Symp. Rock Mech.*, Tokyo, pp.275-279.

Mimaki, Y. & K. Matsuo 1986. Investigation of asymmetrical deformation behaviour at the horseshoe-shaped large cavern opening. *Proc. of Int. Symp. Large Rock Caverns*, Helsinki, Vol.2, pp.1337-1348.

Mizuta, Y., M. Kuriyagawa, H. Kobayashi and I. Matsumura 1985. Hydraulic fracturing experiments at the sites in hot ground in relation to geothermal heat extraction and improvement of underground environment, *Proc. 4th Int. Bureau of Mine Thermophysics*, Burton-on-Trent, U.K., part II. 2.21.

Mizuta, Y., O. Sano, S. Ogino and H. Katoh 1987. Three dimensional stress determination by hydraulic fracturing for underground excavation design, *Int. J. Rock Mech. Min. Sci. & Geomech. Abstr.* 24: 15-29.

Obara, Y., K. Sugawara and T. Takehara 1994. Rock stress measurement by stress relieving in Japan, *Proc. of MMIJ/ AusIMM Joint Symp.*, Ube, pp.425-432.

Oka Y., Y. Hiramatsu, T. Saito and K. Sugawara 1976. The observation equations obtained from three-dimensional stress analysis and some examples of stress determination by this method. *J. Min. Metall. Inst. Jpn.* 92: 1-6.

Obara, Y., K. Sugawara and K. Sakaguchi 1995a. Rock stress measurements by the conical-ended borehole technique using the compact overcoring, *Proc. of Int. Congress of ISRM*, Tokyo, pp.145-148.

Obara, Y., H. Jang, K. Sugawara and K. Sakaguchi 1995b. Measurement of stress distribution around fault and considerations, *Proc. of 2nd Int. Symp. on Mechanics of Jointed and Faulted Rock*, Vienna, pp.483-488.

Saito, T., K. Tsukada, E. Inami, H. Inoma and Y. Ito 1983. Study on rockbursts at the face of a deep tunnel, the Kanetsu tunnel in Japan being an example, *Proc. 5th Int. Congr. Rock Mech.*, Melbourne, D: pp.203-206, Rotterdam: Balkema.

Saito, T., T. Ishida, M. Terada and T. Tanaka 1988. The general tendency of initial stress state in Japan with the data of in-situ measurements: *Proc. Jpn. Soc. Civil Engineers* III-9, 394: 71-78.

Sakaguchi, K., Y. Obara, T. Yamanaka and K. Sugawara 1992. Accuracy of rock stress measurement by means of conical-ended borehole technique. *J. Min. Mater. Inst. Jpn.* 108: 455-460.

Sakaguchi, K., T. Takehara, Y. Obara, T. Nakayama and K. Sugawara 1994. Rock stress measurement by means of the compact overcoring method. *J. Min. Mater. Inst. Jpn.* 110: 331-336.

Sakaguchi, K., X. Huang, Y. Noguchi and K. Sugawara 1995. Application of Conical-ended Borehole Technique to Discontinuous Rock and Considerations: *J. Min. Mater. Inst. Jpn.* 111, 5: 283-288.

Sakuma, S., S. Kikuchi, Y. Mizuta and S. Serata 1989. In-situ stress measurement by double fracturing. *Proc. Jpn. Soc. Civil Eng.* 406:87-96.

Serata, S. & S. Kikuchi 1986. A diametral deformation method for in stitu stress and rock property measurement, *Int. J. Min. Geol. Eng.* 4: 15-38.

Stephansson, O. 1983. Rock stress measurement by sleeve fracturing, *Proc. 5th Int. Congr. Rock Mech.*, Melbourne, F: pp.129-137. Rotterdam: Balkema.

Sugawara, K., Y. Obara, H. Okamura and Y. Wang 1985. The determination of the complete state of stress in rock by the measurement of strains on a hemispherical borehole-bottom. *J. Min. Metall. Inst. Jpn.* 101: 277-282.

Sugawara, K., Y. Obara, M. Akimoto and T. Aoki 1986. Stability Estimation of Large Rock Cavern by In-situ Stress Measurements, *Proc. Int. Symp. on Engineering in Complex Rock Formations*, Beijing, Vol.1, pp.135-141.

Sugawara K. and Y. Obara 1986. Measurement of In-situ Rock Stress by Hemispherical-ended Borehole Technique, *Int. J. Mining Science and Technology*: 3, 287-300.

Sugawara, K., Y. Obara and H. Araki 1987. Sleeve Fracturing for Determining Rock Stresses, *Proc. 7th Japan Symp. on Rock Mech.*, Tokyo, pp.181-186.

Sugawara, K., K. Sakaguchi, Y. Obara, T. Nakayama and H. Jang 1992. Rock stress measurement and Numerical approach for cavern designing. *J. Korean Rock Mechanics Society.* 2, 1, 164-176.

Sugawara, K. 1993. Initial Stress. *Rock Mechanics*: 357-383, Tokyo: Maruzen.

Sugawara, K. & Y. Obara 1993. Measuring Rock Stress: Case Examples of Rock Engineering in Japan: *Comprehensive Rock Engineering*: 3, 533-552. Oxford: Pergamon Press.

Sugawara, K. & Y. Obara 1995. Rock stress and rock stress measurements in Japan, *Proc. of Int. Workshop on Rock Stress Measrement at Great Depth*, Tokyo, pp.1-6.

Sugawara, K., H. Jang and X. Huang 1995. Analysis of observed initial stress by the isotropic spherical shell theory and considerations. *J. Min. Mater. Inst. Jpn.* 111: 913-918.

Sugawara, K & H. K. Jang 1996. Evaluation of initial rock stress by the orthotropic spherical shell model, *Proc. 2nd NARMS*, Montreal, 1: pp.905-912. Notterdam: Balkema.

Sugawara, K. 1996. Rock engineering activity on mining and construction in Japan, *Proc. of Korea-Japan Joint Symp. on Rock Engineering*, Soeul, pp.15-24.

Sugimura, A. 1972. Plates boundaries around Japan, *Kagaku* (Tokyo), 42: 192-202.

Suzuki, K. & Y. Ishijima 1968. Theory and practice of rock stress measurement by borehole deformation method. *J. Soc. Mater. Sci. Jpn.* 17, 856-862.

Tamai, A., T. Kaneda and T. Mimaki 1994. Measurement of in-situ initial stress and excavation-induced stress changes in the vicinity of underground opening, *Proc. 1st NARMS*, Austin, pp.377-384. Rotterdam: Balkema.

Tanaka, Y. 1986. State of crustal stress inferred from in situ stress measurements. *J. Phys. Earth* 34: 57-70.

Tsukahara, H. 1983. Stress measurements utilizing the hydraulic fracturing technique in the Kanto-Tokai area, Japan, *Proc. Hydraulic Fracturing Stress Measurements*, Monterey, pp.18-27. Washington, DC: National Academy Press.

Tsukahara, H. & R. Ikeda 1987. Hydraulic fracturing stress measurements and in situ stress field in the Kanto-Tokai area, Japan. *Tectonophys.* 135: 329-345.

Keynote presentations

Fault dynamics – Dynamic triggering of fault slip

H.P.Rossmanith & K.Uenishi
Institute of Mechanics, Vienna University of Technology, Austria

ABSTRACT: The results of experimental and numerical investigations on the interaction of a Rayleigh pulse with a partially contacting interface under static normal and shearing pre-stress are presented. Utilizing dynamic photoelasticity in conjunction with high speed cinematography, the evolution of time-dependent isochromatic fringe patterns associated with Rayleigh pulse-interface interaction has been recorded. Numerical simulations by means of a finite difference wave propagation simulation program have been performed for quantitative analysis of the problem. Energy transmission and reflection coefficients for Rayleigh pulse interaction have been calculated. The experimental and numerical results have been compared and discussed.

KEYWORDS: Contact Mechanics, Dynamic Faulting, Dynamic Photoelasticity, Finite Difference Method, Interface Slip, Mohr-Coulomb Condition, Rayleigh Wave Interaction

1 INTRODUCTION

Ever since the publication in 1885 of his work on surface waves in elastic solids, Lord Rayleigh's (John William Strutt) surface waves have played a major role in many fields of engineering. At the end of his short mathematical paper (Rayleigh 1885) he observed: „It is not improbable that the surface waves here investigated play an important part in earthquakes, and in the collision of elastic solids. Diverging in two dimensions only, they must acquire at a great distance from the source a continually increasing preponderance."

Giants in physics such as H. Lamb (1904), J. Jeans, H. Jeffreys, and A.E.H. Love (1911) worked out the path of the Rayleigh waves induced by earthquakes along the interface of elastic media in the earth's crust and generalized the theory of surface waves in solids. The presence of these Rayleigh waves in earthquake shocks was verified with seismographs (Ash & Paige 1985).

While studying the effect on the propagation of Rayleigh waves of a thick layer on a semi-space, Love discovered that some solutions of the wave equation depended on the properties of both media, and Stoneley (1924) clarified the nature of these peculiar solid-solid surface waves which are guided by the interface. Wide ranging earthquake research stimulated by the 1885 paper by Lord Rayleigh resulted in extensive studies by Japanese researchers in surface layer wave propagation (Sezawa 1927a,b, Nakano 1925).

Solid-liquid interface surface waves come in two varieties. One, called Stoneley wave, is a true interface wave, which decays exponentially away from the interface in both media and carries most of its energy in the liquid phase. The other wave is a leaky Rayleigh wave which has most of its energy in the solid, propagates along the interface with attenuation radiating energy into the liquid phase. Curved interfaces have a very pronounced effect on the behavior of solid-liquid interface surface waves.

The effect of surface defects of any sort (cracks, scratches, irregularities, humps, deposits, etc.) on the propagation of Rayleigh waves is to scatter some of the energy. The Rayleigh wave is then attenuated due to these scattering effects (Viktorov 1967). For various industrial reasons theoretical and experimental investigations have been performed to characterize the effect of surface finishing processes of a metal (planing, milling, grinding, polishing, etc.) on the attenuation of Rayleigh surface waves (Bykov & Shneider 1960).

Isolated surface defects and their effect on Rayleigh wave propagation and attenuation has been the subject of a large number of theoretical and experimental studies. Dynamic photoelasticity in conjunction with high speed photography has proven particularly useful in these studies. Transmission and reflection coefficients for R-wave interaction with corners (acute and re-entrant) and surface breaking features (cracks and slots) have been calculated on the basis of isochromatic fringe patterns recorded (Lewis & Dally 1970, Henzi & Dally 1971, Dally 1977, Rossmanith & Dally 1983a,b, Rossmanith 1984, Rossmanith 1985, Rossmanith & Knasmillner 1989).

Interfaces come in a large number of different forms and shapes. They can be classified in various ways but the interface conditions always play a decisive role. From a mathematical point of view the straight interface is the easiest to handle. Curved and undulating interfaces pose series problems with respect to taking into account the geometrical shape. Perfectly bonded and perfectly lubricated interfaces have been dealt with in most papers. However, geological interfaces such as faults and man-made shear zones due to mining operations in rock mass deviate from these idealized representatives. In addition, real interfaces most often have an intermediate layer of varying thickness embedded and the material qualities of this sandwiched zone have a strong influence on the propagation and attenuation behavior of the interface waves.

A particularly complex situation occurs when the interface quality becomes inhomogeneous or even anisotropic. In fact, partial delamination of a joint surface between two rock blocks introduces a highly complex connectivity structure and the study of the effect of this bond pattern on wave propagation requires extensive numerical simulation effort (Sutton & Balluffi 1995).

The conditions along a geological fault can vary widely with respect to their mechanical properties. Usually, within the fault zone a layer of material (ranging from air, water, weak mud to quartzite) is present which controls the reflection, transmission and refraction of surface waves.

Although, at present, a large body of information is available, there is still a large discrepancy between the theoretical investigations of highly idealized geometrical configurations and actual observations. In addition, only very limited special cases do allow closed form analytical solutions.

The interaction of Rayleigh surface waves with partially contacting surfaces preloaded due to normal and shearing stresses seems to have escaped the scrutiny of researchers. This kind of phenomenon occurs in mining induced seismicity and on smaller scales in non-destructive testing as well as in testing of micro-electronic devices.

In this contribution an experimental and numerical simulation study is presented of the interaction of a Rayleigh surface wave with contacts. The results of this contribution will assist in an improved understanding of the mechanism of dynamic interface instability caused by the passage of a Rayleigh (R-) pulse.

2 CHARACTERISTICS OF RAYLEIGH PULSES

The wave system generated by the rapid application of a concentrated line load or by the detonation of an exploding line charge includes two bulk waves (a longitudinal or P-wave and a transverse or shear or S-wave) and two Rayleigh-pulses (R-waves) propagating in opposite directions along the surface of the elastic half-space. These R-waves propagate in a non-dispersive fashion and carry much more energy than the related bulk waves (Rayleigh 1885, Lamb 1904).

The stress and strain field associated with a plane R-pulse of arbitrary shape can be analytically represented in terms of one complex potential (Cardenas 1983). Deriving the stress field from the complex potential, one can draw the characteristic isochromatic fringe pattern (contours of maximum in-plane shear stress) which pertains to a R-pulse. A typical theoretically predicted isochromatic fringe pattern is shown in Figure 1(1) with the R-pulse propagating from the left to the right.

The fact that the disturbance is largely confined to a thin layer adjacent to the free surface implies that a thin layer deposited on the surface will have a strong effect on the propagation and attenuation behavior of the surface wave. If the wave disturbance propagates along a filled fault there will be strong interaction between the wave disturbance and the interfacially embedded layer, commonly called gauge layer.

The particle displacement associated with the same R-pulse, shown in Figure 1(2), is entirely retrograde. Whereas, in a harmonic Rayleigh wave, the particles undergo closed loop movements, this is not the case for a R-pulse where the trace of the material particles motion may not form a closed loop during the passage of the pulse.

The displacement vector of a material particle displaced due to the leading (trailing) part of the R-pulse points toward to the exterior (interior) of the half-space. At the surface, the displacement field

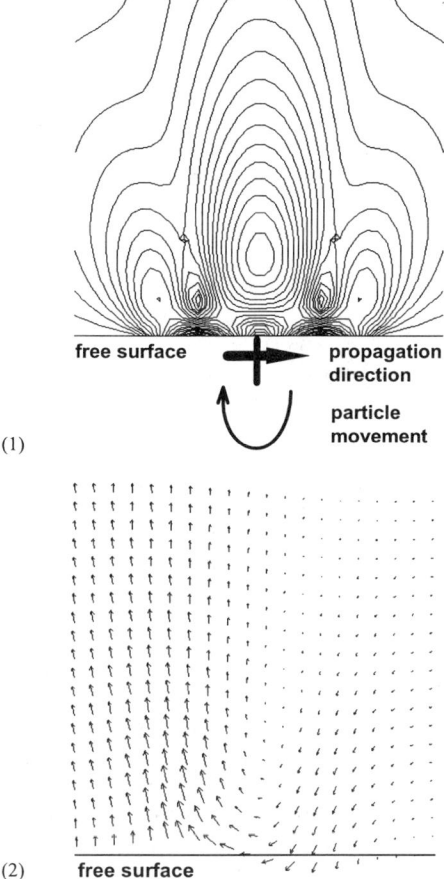

(1)

(2) free surface

Figure 1. A R-pulse propagating from the left to the right along a free surface.
(1) isochromatic fringe patterns (contours of maximum shear stress); and
(2) vector representation of particle movements.

generates a moving hump followed by a trough. In the present problem of a compressive line force, the resulting displacement vector, upon passage of the R-pulse, is oriented into the body.

3 LABORATORY EXPERIMENTS

3.1 *Experimental set-up*

Dynamic photoelasticity in conjunction with high speed photography is employed to analyze the interaction between a R-pulse and a statically pre-loaded, non-welded, partially contacting interface. Photo-

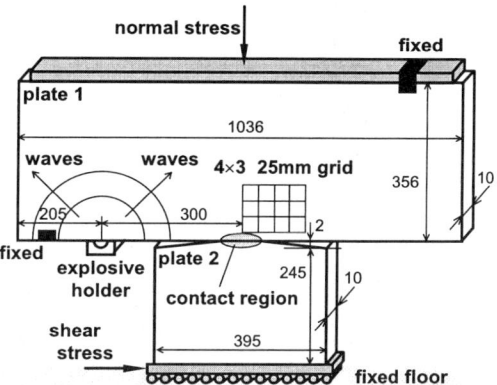

Figure 2. The experimental model set-up for R-pulse interaction investigation [all lengths in mm].

elasticity is well documented in the literature and detailed descriptions can be found in the text-books by Dally and Riley (1978), Kuske and Robertson (1974), or in a recent handbook edited by Kobayashi (1993).

The experimental model is schematically shown in Figure 2. The model consists of two plates of Araldite B (a transparent, birefringent, homogeneous and isotropic polymeric material) which initially are in contact over a region of fixed length. The dimensions of the plates are $1036 \times 356 \times 10 mm^3$ and $395 \times 247 \times 10 mm^3$. Care is taken in selecting the size of the plates so as to prevent reflected waves from impinging upon the region of contact and altering the results.

The upper surface of the plate 2 (lower plate) is given a very blunt double wedge cut such that only the central section of the surface will initially be in contact with the upper plate (plate 1). Three contact configurations will be investigated in detail:

(1) single contact: one contact of 55mm length;
(2) two small contacts of 12.5mm length each; and
(3) three small contacts of 12.5mm length with two gaps (symmetrically arranged) each.

The three geometrically different contact configurations are schematically shown in Figure 3.

Non-welded, i.e. imperfect interface conditions apply across the contact region. During the interaction process the contact will be diminished or enforced depending on the relative position of the R-pulse with respect to the contact region.

The two plates are statically pre-loaded in compression and shear. The static pre-load combination between compressive and shear traction is chosen

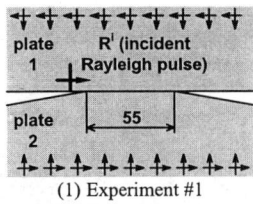

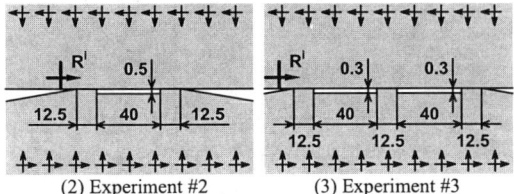

Figure 3. Three different geometries of the contact region [all lengths in mm]:
(1) Experiment #1: One long (55mm) contact;
(2) Experiment #2: Two small (12.5mm) contacts; and
(3) Experiment #3: Three small (12.5mm) contacts.

such that the contact conditions in the contact region induce a limiting state of equilibrium (stick) where any increase of the shear traction in the same direction will cause slip in the contact region.

A small amount of explosive (240mg of PbN_6) is detonated on a free section of the lower surface of plate 1 at a distance 300mm from the center of the contact region. A classical Rayleigh pulse isochromatic fringe pattern is generated in plate 1. For scale reasons a grid with 25mm spacing is attached to the side of plate 1 facing the camera.

Using circularly polarized monochromatic light, optical interference produces isochromatic fringe patterns due to the birefringence in the material. The order of interference is related to the state of stress in the model by the stress-optic law (Dally & Riley 1978), which depends on the difference of the principal stresses, the material fringe value and the model thickness. A Cranz-Schardin type multiple spark gap camera is used to record the dynamic fringe patterns. The camera is triggered by the detonation of a micro-explosive. The exposure of the first negative occurs after a selected delay period. Twentyfour frames are recorded at discrete times during the dynamic event at a framing rate of 120,000 frames per second. A short exposure time of 200ns is necessary to obtain sharp photographic images of the rapidly moving fringe patterns.

3.2 *Experiment #1: single contact*

First, the interaction of a R-pulse with a single contact zone at a (non-welded) interface is investigated. The two half-planes are statically pre-loaded by compression and shear. The magnitude of static compressive stress at the center of the contact region is selected at 0.1MPa. The incident R-pulse generated by the impulsive detonation has a length of 75mm (as compared to the contact length of 55mm) and exhibits a maximum horizontal normal stress of 3.5MPa on the free surface.

Figure 4 shows a sequence of three isochromatic fringe patterns illustrating the dynamic wave interaction process. The R-pulse propagates from the lhs to the rhs and thereby interacts with the contact region. A relative time scale t has been introduced; the clock measures the time elapsed from the instance of maximum stress amplification at the lhs edge of the contact region.

3.2.1 *Stress amplification at the lhs edge*

Figure 4(1) pertains to the event where the incident R-pulse impinges upon the lhs edge of the contact region and thereby amplifies the stress field. The strength (expressed by the fringe order) of the stress singularity associated with diffraction about the lhs edge is larger than that about the rhs edge where, in this phase of the interaction process, the dynamic effect is still negligible. The stress amplification at the lhs is due to retrograde motion of particles on the free surface [Fig.1(2)] where the leading part of the incident R-pulse induces a back- and downward movement of the particles [Fig.4(1)]. The surface particles which are already in contact move together towards the lower plate 2, and thus increase the stresses about the lhs edge.

3.2.2 *Stress cancellation at the lhs edge*

The trailing part of the R-pulse induces a retrograde motion of the surface particles. This back- and upwardly oriented movement [Fig.4(2)] of the receding particles may lead to a stress reduction, possibly followed by complete cancellation of the stress singularity if the surfaces separate during a later stage of the interaction process. In fact, at a later stage shown in Figure 4(2), the structure of the wave interaction pattern has changed considerably. The fringe patterns about the lhs diffraction edge now show a very small amplitude of the stress singularity.

3.2.3 *Interface slip*

When the incident R-pulse approaches the rhs diffraction edge of the contact region, as shown in Figure 4(3), partial wave energy transmission occurs across the interface into the lower plate 2. Receding

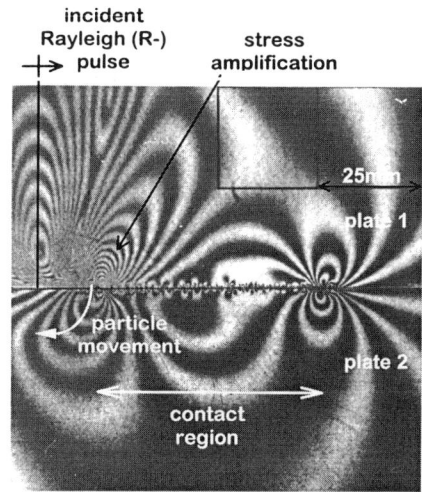

(1) $t = 0\mu s$

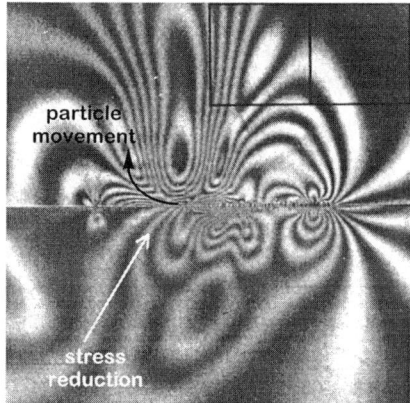

(2) $t = 39\mu s$

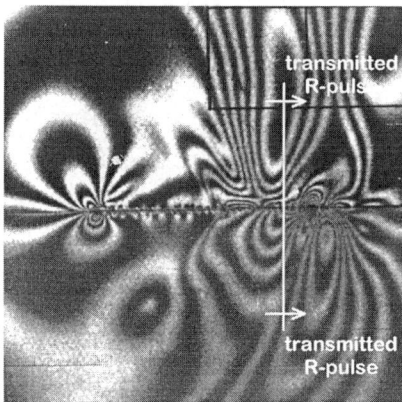

(3) $t = 64\mu s$

Figure 4. Sequence of isochromatic fringe patterns showing Rayleigh pulse interaction with a single contact (Exp. #1)

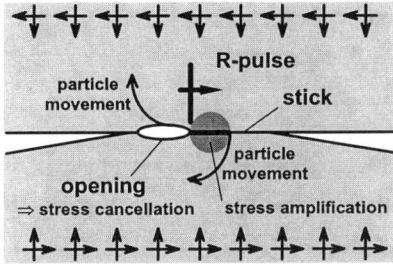

Figure 5. Interface slip and opening caused by a Rayleigh (R-) pulse.

contact of the surface particles in the trailing part of the R-pulse leads to the fact, that there are no corresponding fringes in the lower plate 2.

During the phase covering the time between the diffraction of the incoming R-pulse about the lhs edge of the contact region and the diffraction of low amplitude waves about the rhs edge of the contact region the details of the physical wave diffraction and wave emergence process are still fairly unclear. The isochromatic fringe patterns as well as numerical simulation studies allow the identification of a radiated shear wave and the diffracted, transmitted and reflected R-pulses in both the upper and lower plates. Theoretically, the R-pulse ceases to exist in the contact region and there must be other kinds of generalized interface waves which carry the energy across and along the contact region to enable the re-formation of R-pulses on the rhs edge of the contact region.

In summary, the retrograde motion, especially the down- and upward movement of the particles in the incident R-pulse, plays an important role in the wave interaction and contact separation process as shown in Figure 5.

3.3 Experiments #2 and #3: multiple contacts

In order to investigate the effect of multiple contacts on Rayleigh wave scattering a double [Exp. #2 in Fig 3(2)] and triple [Exp. #3 in Fig 3(3)] contact system will be investigated. Smaller contact lengths are chosen.

In Figure 6 isochromatic fringe patterns pertaining to two particular phases of the interaction process allow a comparison between similar dynamic situations occurring in the double (lhs column) and triple (rhs column) contact experiment. The phases shown pertain to the stages where

(1) the maximum stress amplification at the lhs edge of the first contact is observed; and

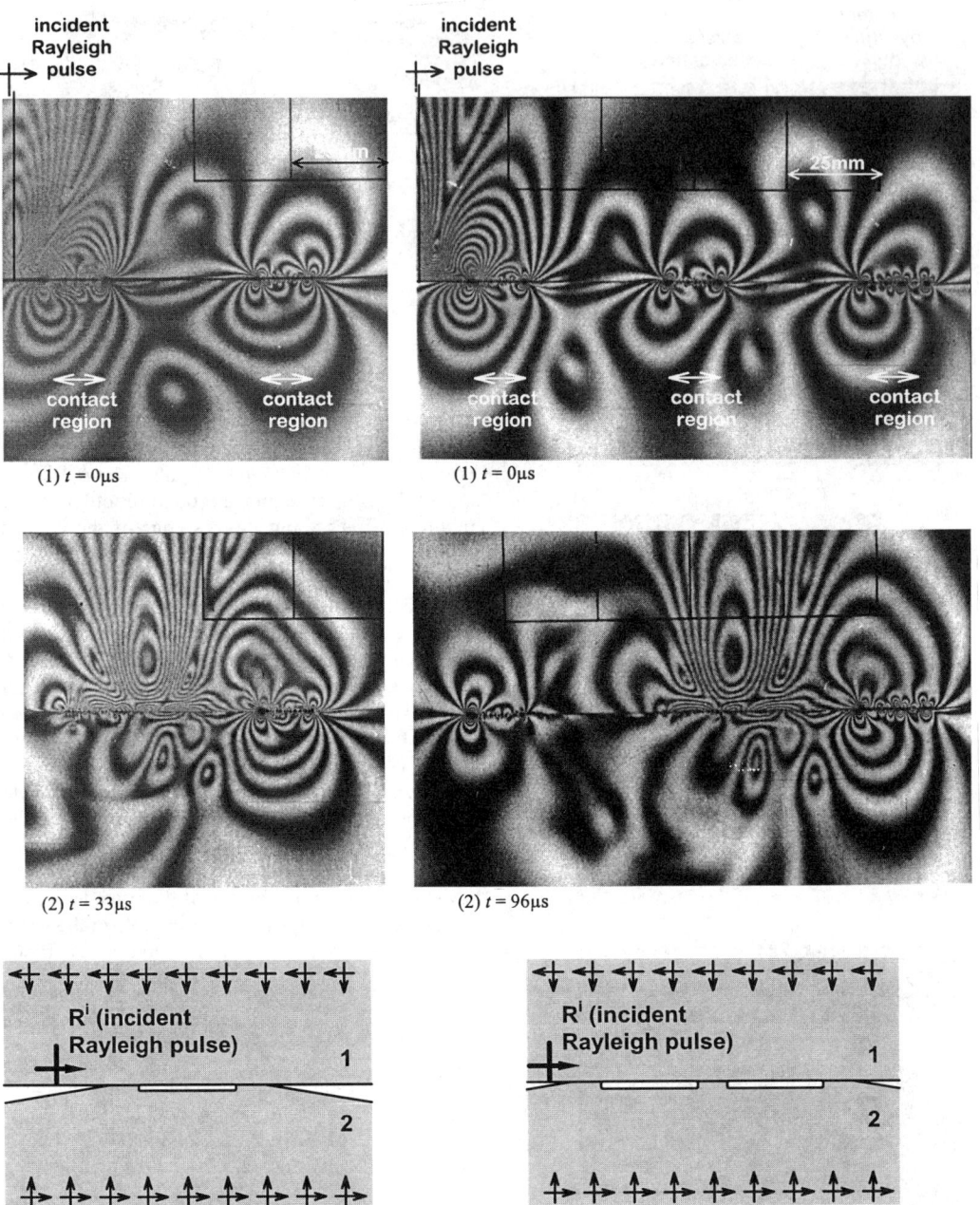

Figure 6. Snapshots of isochromatic fringe patterns obtained by experiments.
Left column: Experiment #2 (two contacts); and
Right column: Experiment #3 (three contacts).

(2) the transmitted Rayleigh pulse approaches the last contact section.

The overall characteristic features of the dynamic wave interaction patterns, i.e. stress amplification and reduction due to the Rayleigh pulse, basically appear to be similar in both experiments. However, the amplitude of the transmitted R-pulse shown in Experiment #3 (2) (i.e. after passing through two

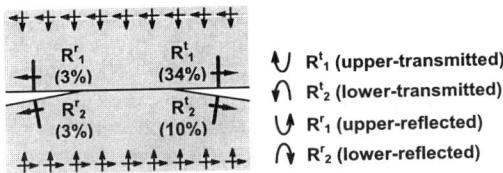

	R^t_1 (upper-transmitted)
	R^t_2 (lower-transmitted)
	R^r_1 (upper-reflected)
	R^r_2 (lower-reflected)

Figure 7. Partition of the energy contained in the incident R-pulse.

Table 1. Relative energy in the upper-transmitted R-pulse.

Number of contacts	One		Two	Three
Length of contacts	55mm	12.5mm	12.5mm×2	12.5mm×3
Relative energy contained in R^t_1	34%	61%	43%	31%

contacts) is smaller than that in Experiment #2 (2) (i.e. after the interaction with one contact). This indicates that each individual interaction reduces the energy of the incident/transmitted Rayleigh pulse by generating diffracted R-pulses and bulk waves in the upper and lower half-planes.

4 NUMERICAL SIMULATIONS

The dynamic R-pulse interaction problems discussed above have been simulated using a finite difference wave propagation simulator SWIFD (Rossmanith & Uenishi 1995, 1996). In these numerical simulations, dynamic contact is considered to occur under plane stress conditions, and the R-pulse is assumed to interact with an interface which is characterized by a Mohr-Coulomb friction criterion with the coefficient of friction being 0.3. The interface is pre-compressed and the tensile strength (tensile cut-off) of the interface segment is set to 650Pa.

Waves are generated in the upper plate by a blast load $p(t)$ which is prescribed in the form $p(t) = A \exp(1-t/t_o) \, t/t_o \, (t > 0)$, where the parameters A and t_o characterize the amplitude and duration of the loading pulse. In the following some quantitative aspects of these interaction problem will be discussed.

4.1 Wave energy partition

It is informative to evaluate the energy related transmission and reflection coefficients for the interaction of a Rayleigh pulse with a contact region. As this information cannot be obtained solely from isochromatic fringe patterns the entire interaction process is numerically simulated to obtain the displacement data necessary for the calculation of these coefficients. Some of the numerical results are schematically shown in Figure 7 for the case of a single contact.

The results indicate that about one half of the energy initially contained in the incident R-pulse has been radiated in the form of bulk waves into the far-field, and only 34% of the total energy is transmitted in the form of a new R-pulse, marked R^t_1 in Figure 7, along the free surface. Note, that the energy carried by the reflected R-pulses is relatively small as compared with the energy carried along in the transmitted R-pulses.

Table 1 shows the relative energies contained in the upper-transmitted R-pulse, R^t_1, for the three different contact configurations. The results show that any increase in the length and the number of the contact sections reduces the energy transmitted along the contact region in plate 1.

5 CONCLUSIONS

The purpose of this study was to obtain an improved understanding of the interaction between a Rayleigh pulse and a partially contacting interface. A series of experiments using dynamic photoelasticity in conjunction with high speed cinematography have provided better understanding of the R-pulse-induced instability of a statically pre-stressed interface. The analytically predicted retrograde particle motion in a R-pulse is shown to play an important role in the wave-interface interaction process. The SWIFD finite difference simulator has provided quantitative information on the interaction process.

ACKNOWLEDGMENTS

The authors kindly acknowledge the support of the Austrian National Science Foundation under Project P 10326-GEO. The experiments were performed at the Fracture and Photomechanics Laboratory at Vienna University of Technology under the guidance of R.E. Knasmillner.

REFERENCES

Ash, E.A. & Paige, E.G.S.(eds) 1985. *Rayleigh-Wave Theory and Application*. Springer Series on

Wave Phenomena, Berlin: Springer-Verlag.
Bykov, N.S. & Shneider, Yu.G. 1960. An experimental investigation of the effect of surface quality on the attenuation of surface waves. *Akustik Zh.* 6(4): 501-503.
Cardenas-Garcia, J.F. 1983. *On Rayleigh Waves and Rayleigh Wave Extension of Surface Micro-Cracks*. Ph.D. Thesis: Mechanical Engineering Department, University of Maryland.
Dally, J.W. 1977. Dynamic photoelastic studies of stress wave propagation. Proc. IUAM-Conf. on Elastic Wave Propagation, Toronto.
Dally, J W. & Riley, W.F. 1978. *Experimental Stress Analysis*. New York: McGraw-Hill.
Henzi, A.N. & Dally, J.W. 1971. A photoelastic study of stress wave propagation in a quarter-plane. *Geophysics* 26,2:296-310.
Kobayashi, A.S. 1993. *Handbook on Experimental Mechanics*. SEM, Bethel CT, USA.
Kuske, A. & Robertson, G. 1974. *Photoelastic Stress Analysis*. New York: John Wiley & Sons.
Lamb, H. 1904. On the propagation of tremors over the surface of an elastic solid. *Phil. Trans. Roy. Soc. London* A 203: 1-42.
Lewis, D. & Dally, J.W. 1970. Photoelastic analysis of Rayleigh wave propagation in wedges. *J.of Geophysical Research* 75, 17: 3387-3398.
Love, A.E.H. 1911. *Some Problems in Geodynamics*. Cambridge London: University Press.
Nakano, H. 1925. On Rayleigh waves. *Japan. J. Astron. Geophys.* 2, 233.
Rayleigh, Lord 1885. On waves propagating along the plane surface of an elastic solid. *Proc. London Math. Soc.* 17: 4-11.
Rossmanith, H.P. & Dally, J.W. 1983a. Rayleigh wave interaction with inhomogeneities - Part I: Near surface cavity and inclusion. *Strain* 19, 7-13.
Rossmanith, H.P. & Dally, J.W. 1983b. Rayleigh wave interaction with inhomogeneities - Part II: The buried cavity and inclusion. *Strain* 19, 159-171.
Rossmanith, H.P. 1984. Fracture initiation by Rayleigh-wave diffraction. *Theor. & Appl. Fract. Mech.* 1, 257-269.
Rossmanith, H.P. 1985. Elastic wave interaction with a cracked quarter-plane. *Meccanica* 20: 127-135.
Rossmanith, H.P. & Knasmillner, R.E. 1989. Diffraction of Rayleigh waves at surface irregularities. *Appl.Mech.Rev.* 24,11, Part 2, S223-232.
Rossmanith, H.P. & Uenishi, K. 1995. *SWIFD User's Manual Version 1995*. Vienna: SWIFD Development Center, Fracture- and Photo-Mechanics Laboratory, Institute of Mechanics, Vienna University of Technology.
Rossmanith, H.P. & Uenishi, K. 1996. PC software assisted teaching and learning of dynamic fracture and wave propagation phenomena. In H.P. Rossmanith (ed.), *Teaching and Education in Fracture and Fatigue*: 253-262. London: E & FN SPON/Chapman & Hall.
Sezawa K.1927a. On the propagation of Rayleigh waves on plane and spherical surfaces. *Bull. Earthquake Res. Inst. (Tokyo)* 2, 21-28.
Sezawa K.1927b. Dispersion of elastic waves propagated on the surface of stratified bodies and on curved surfaces. *Bull. Earthquake Res. Inst. (Tokyo)* 3, 1-18.
Stoneley, R 1924. Elastic waves at the surface of two solids. *Proc. Roy. Soc. A,* 106, 416-428.
Sutton, A.P. and Balluffi, R.W. 1995. *Interfaces in Crystalline Materials*. Oxford: Clarendon Press.
Uenishi, K., Rossmanith, H.P. & Knasmillner, R.E. 1997. Interaction of a Rayleigh pulse with non-uniformly contacting interfaces. To appear in: *The Proceedings of the International Conference on Materials and Mechanics '97* (July 20-22 1997, Tokyo).
Viktorov, I.A. 1967. *Rayleigh and Lamb Waves*. New York: Plenum Press.

Rock Stress, Sugawara & Obara (eds)© 1997 Balkema, Rotterdam, ISBN 90 5410 901 7

Borehole breakouts and core disking as tools for estimating in situ stress in deep holes

Bezalel C. Haimson
Geological Engineering Program, University of Wisconsin, Madison, Wis., USA

ABSTRACT: Borehole breakouts and core disking result from rock failure during drilling and coring. Both phenomena are closely related to the state of far-field stress. Our experimental results show that breakout and core disk dimensions could indeed be used to obtain an estimate of a far-field principal stress if the other two principal stresses are independently known.

1 INTRODUCTION

A number of methods of direct measurement of in situ stresses at great depths have been advanced over the years, the most commonly accepted and frequently used being hydraulic fracturing (Haimson 1978). However, the use of hydraulic fracturing is often prohibitive both financially and technically at great depths (beyond 1-2 km), high temperatures (beyond 100°C), or in hostile environments such as when unstable rock conditions prevail. Bell and Gough's (1979) finding that 4-arm dipmeter logging showed consistent bearing of oil-well breakouts (borehole cross-section elongations resulting from rock failure) over a large part of Alberta, which they attributed to breakout propensity to be aligned with the direction of the least in situ horizontal stress σ_h, was pivotal in the development of a new technique for assessing crustal stress orientation. The borehole-breakout technique has revolutionized our ability to map crustal stress directions over extended areas of the globe, including regions that had not been subjected to any direct stress measurements (M.L. Zoback, 1992). Moreover, the phenomenon of borehole breakouts, being an expression of mechanical failure of the rock, is potentially a valuable indicator of in situ stress magnitudes as well. Use of borehole breakouts is considerably more economical for collecting stress data than direct in situ measurements, and it may be the only technique available for collecting stress information under some conditions of depth, rock physical state, and temperature.

Core disking is a phenomenon by which core recovered from drilling into hard rock subjected to high in situ stresses is split up into many nearly-identical slices similar to a loaf of bread. Field evidence suggests that core disking in vertical holes can be related to high horizontal stresses (Natau et. al, 1989). No laboratory experiments have been conducted to our knowledge to examine the core disking phenomenon and its characteristic 'saddle shape' under a truly triaxial state of stress. Several numerical modelings have been carried out, most of them in 2-D. Sugawara et. at. (1978) introduced a linear elastic axisymmetric 2-D finite element model to simulate core disking at the bottom of a drilled hole. They obtained stress contours around the kerf area as a function of the applied load, and concluded that core disking occurs in the region of high tension. Lehnhoff et. al. (1982) employed a similar 2-D finite element program, but introduced the effect of anisotropic horizontal stresses through the application of Fourier series to the axisymmetric model. An extensive numerical investigation of core disking was undertaken by Dyke (1989). He conducted a 3-D boundary element analysis, assuming linear elastic behavior, to calculate stresses and vertical extension strains around the borehole and drill kerf geometry. Failure of the core was

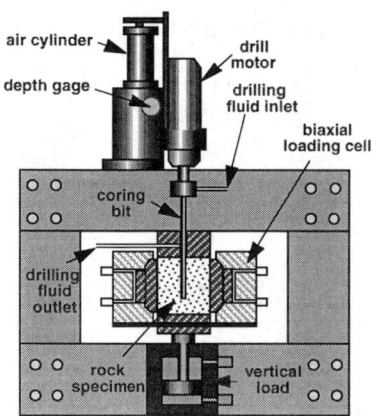

Figure 1. Profile of drilling-loading machine enabling the drilling of vertical boreholes through block specimens subjected to polyaxial far-field stresses.

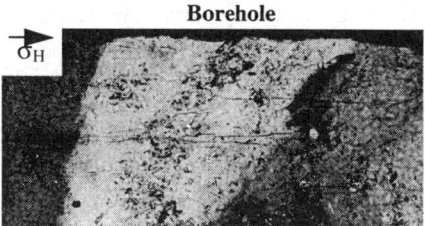

Figure 2. Thin section showing trans-crystalline multiple extensile cracks subparallel to borehole wall and σ_H prior to breakout failure (granite).

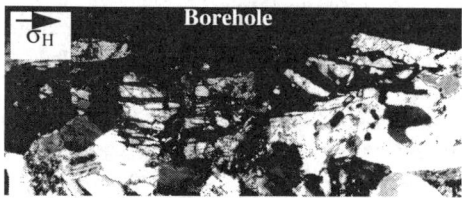

Figure 3. Intensified cracking. buckling and spalling of the crack-bounded flakes at the borehole wall as σ_H increases (granite).

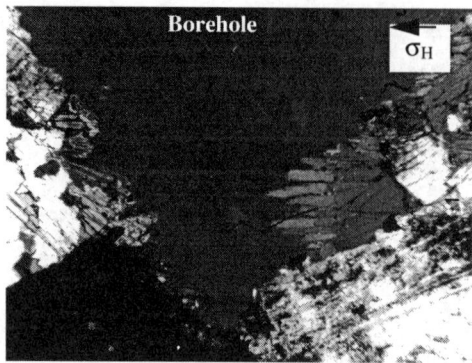

Figure 4. Typical 'V' shaped breakout showing remnants of buckled and sheared-off flakes. (granite).

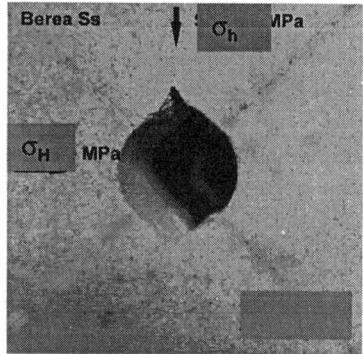

Figure 5. Typical "V" shaped breakout in well-consolidated Berea sandstone,

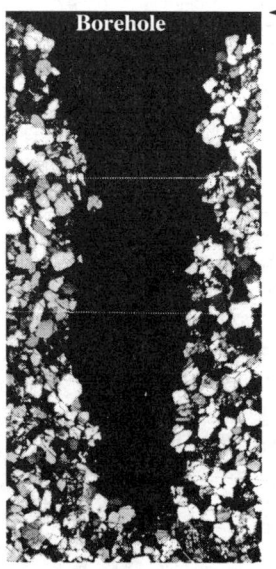

Figure 6. Elongated breakout in high porosity Berea sandstone, suggesting non-dilatational failure resulting from grain debonding.

found to initiate at the kerf surface in the direction of σ_h and propagate downward to form the characteristic "saddle shape" (or 'potato chip') geometry.

This paper reviews the experimental work carried out at the University of Wisconsin over the last decade in the area of borehole breakouts and core disking. The method employed was to simulate field conditions as realistically as possible, by core-drilling vertical holes in rock blocks already subjected to a general anisotropic state of far-field stress.

2 BOREHOLE BREAKOUT AND DISKING EXPERIMENTS

We have conducted laboratory vertical core-drilling experiments exploring the mechanism of breakout and disk formation, and the relationship between far-field principal stresses and breakout location and dimensions, as well as between far-field stresses and core-disk thickness and shape. Rectangular rock blocks (11x11x11 cm^3) were subjected to a general state of far-field stress such that $\sigma_H > \sigma_h \neq \sigma_v$. The vertical stress σ_v was applied by a hydraulic ram; the horizontal stresses were produced through a biaxial cell (Haimson and Lee, 1995). While applying the preset far-field stresses, a central borehole of radius R = 11 mm was drilled along the vertical axis of the specimen using a diamond coring bit. Water was typically used as the bit coolant. The experimental test setup is shown in Figure 1.

To date we have carried out such experiments in three clastic rocks (Alabama limestone, Cordova Cream limestone, and Berea sandstone) and two crystalline rocks (Lac du Bonnet and Westerly granites). This paper summarizes some of the important results of this investigation with respect to both breakouts and core disking, emphasizing their relationship to in situ stress.

3 BREAKOUT FAILURE MECHANISM

The failure mechanism leading to breakouts was studied by examining thin sections of selected specimens under a petrographic microscope with a polarized light source.

The clearest mechanism of failure leading to breakouts is exhibited by the granite specimens. By varying the preset far-field stresses between drilling tests, we obtained boreholes showing different stages of breakout formation. In boreholes drilled under far-field stresses less than critical, no damage could be observed on the borehole surface. However, thin sections of cross sections of such boreholes exhibit considerable microstructural damage. In the two zones surrounding the intersection of the borehole with the springline of σ_h families of extensile microcracks are noticed subparallel to σ_H (Figure 2). Moreover, these microcracks are obviously intra- and trans-crystalline. The density of the subparallel microcracks is higher just behind the borehole wall, where the tangential stress attains a higher compressive value, and the radial stress approaches zero. The microcracks separate thin layers of rock flakes subparallel to σ_H direction.

At somewhat higher far-field stresses boreholes begin to develop breakouts. Thin sections here depict the mechanism of spalling that help create breakouts (Figure 3). Previously developed microcracks continue to dilate and grow, coalescing with other fractures, or branching into multiple cracks forming a complex network of discontinuities. Rock flakes bounded by adjacent microcracks form. Those near the borehole wall buckle, break off and fall into the borehole, leaving end cantilevers still attached to the borehole wall.

As flakes fall off the stress is redistributed around the new free surface of the hole. This contributes to the instability of the next layer, which also spalls off, continuing the breakout process. The cantilevers of broken rock left on both ends limit the span of the next spall. This process continues such that each detached and spalled layer away from the borehole wall has a successively smaller span. Eventually, the span becomes too small to permit buckling, and the breakout stabilizes revealing a deep and pointed V-shape (Figure 4). Lee and Haimson (1993) demonstrate that the laboratory induced breakouts in Lac du Bonnet granite are practically identical to those observed in the field on a much larger scale, strongly suggesting no size effect biasing our laboratory results.

The mechanism of breakout failure in softer rocks such as sandstones and limestones is less obvious, and appears to depend largely on the difference in fracture toughness between the grains and the matrix material. In limestones and well consolidated sandstone the final breakout appearance is similar to that in granite (Figure 5), although microcracks observed in thin sections are of two types: transgranular as in granite, and intergranular (preferring propagation within the weaker matrix and bypassing the tougher grains).

In the case of less consolidated, more permeable, Berea sandstone a surprisingly and fundamentally different breakout shape was obtained (Figure 6). The rough breakout surface indicates that whole grains were left intact and failure was confined to that of the matrix only. The apparent mechanism of failure is one of grain debonding and spalling without the dilatant behavior accompanying extensile microcracking (Bessinger et al, 1995). Dilatant failure, such as in granite, creates a radial pressure on the grains, thus inducing tangential extension of microcracks; grain debonding, on the other hand, contributes additional tangential stress to the layer behind and no radial stress and thus brings about new grain debonding due to failure of the surrounding matrix material. The process continues in this manner, propagating the breakout in a direction perpendicular to that of σ_H.

4 BREAKOUTS AND IN SITU STRESS

The most obvious behavior, common to all rocks, is the consistent breakout alignment along the far-field σ_H direction (Figure 4). This result validates the assumption made by Bell and Gough (1979) and others based on field logging results of borehole breakouts, and verifies that breakouts are reliable principal stress direction indicators.

Another observation that is common to all rock types tested is that for each σ_h magnitude tested, proportional increases were recorded in both breakout depth and width with rising maximum horizontal stress σ_H. Plotting breakout span θ_b and normalized depth r_b/R as functions of σ_H for each level of σ_h suggests approximate linear relationships (examples are shown in Figures 7 and 8). Moreover, within each of the plots the slopes of the fitted lines do not differ significantly.. The implication of these results is that, provided an estimate of one of the two horizontal principal stresses is available, the logging of breakout dimensions could be used to assess the magnitude of the other principal stress from plots such as Figures 7 or 8.

Quantitative methods for calculating the maximum horizontal far-field stress σ_H from the logged span of the breakout have been suggested based on the assumptions that rock is linear-elastic and isotropic, and that at the boundary of the breakout the state of stress is in limit equilibrium with the strength of the rock. Using the well known Kirsch solution, the principal stresses σ_{rr}, $\sigma_{\theta\theta}$, σ_{zz} at point of breakout and borehole intersection are given by:

$$\sigma_{rr} = P_w$$
$$\sigma_{\theta\theta} = \sigma_H + \sigma_h - 2(\sigma_H - \sigma_h)\cos 2\Theta_b - P_w \quad (1)$$
$$\sigma_{zz} = \sigma_v - 2\nu(\sigma_H - \sigma_h)\cos 2\Theta_b$$

where P_w is the wellbore fluid pressure, ν is the Poisson's ratio, $\Theta_b = \frac{1}{2}(\pi - \theta_b)$, and θ_b is the angular span of the breakout.

The far-field vertical stress σ_v can be calculated from the density of the overlying rock. The least horizontal stress σ_h can be estimated from simplified hydraulic fracturing tests or leak-off tests. If breakout span is assessed from borehole logging, and rock strength criterion is established, it is then possible to determine σ_H from equations (1).

Commonly, rock strength of hard rock is assumed to be represented by the Mohr-Coulomb criterion ($\sigma_1 = A + B\sigma_3$), which is based on the premise that the intermediate principal stress has no effect on compressive strength (Jaeger and Cook, 1979). However, triaxial tests which are used to determine this criterion render it strictly valid only for the case in which $\sigma_1 > \sigma_2 = \sigma_3$. von Mises, Nadai and others have contended that the strength criterion of brittle materials are functions of all three principal stresses. Mogi (1971) provided the most convincing empirical evidence that the ultimate strength of brittle rock increases not only with the least compressive stress σ_3 but also with the intermediate stress σ_2. He found that the strength criterion can be expressed as:

$$\tau_{oct} = f_1(\sigma_2^m) \quad \text{or:}$$
$$\frac{1}{3}\sqrt{(\sigma_1 - \sigma_2)^2 + (\sigma_2 - \sigma_3)^2 + (\sigma_3 - \sigma_1)^2} = f_1[\tfrac{1}{2}(\sigma_1 + \sigma_3)] \quad (2)$$

where f_1 is a monotonically increasing nearly-linear function. We call equation (2) 'Mogi's polyaxial strength criterion'.

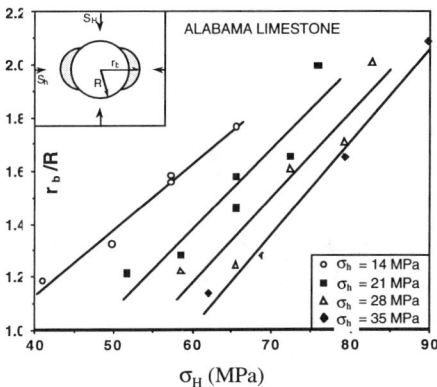

Figure 7. Example of relationship between logged breakout depth r_b (normalized by borehole radius R) and σ_H for different values of the other far-field stresses.

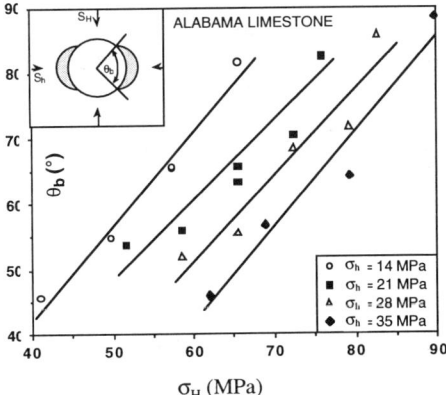

Figure 8. Example of relationship between logged breakout span θ_b and σ_H for different values of the other far-field stresses.

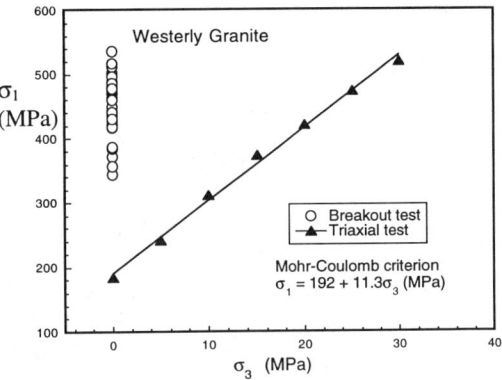

Figure 9. Example of Mohr-Coulomb criterion as obtained from triaxial tests, and the critical stress condition at failure at the intersection of borehole and breakout

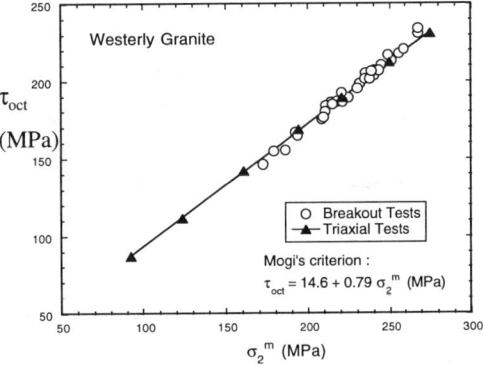

Figure 10. Example of Mogi criterion criterion as obtained from triaxial tests, and the critical stress condition at failure at the intersection of borehole and breakout

At the University of Wisconsin we have undertaken to verify which of the above strength criteria applies in the case of breakout failure in two granites (Lac du Bonnet and Westerly). Both criteria were obtained strictly from triaxial tests. From knowledge of the applied far-field stresses in our laboratory tests and from the measurement of the average angular breakout span θ_b for each tested specimen, we were able to calculate the critical principal stresses at the breakout ends on the borehole wall i.e. at $\Theta_b = \frac{1}{2}(\pi - \theta_b)$. We then compared the stresses at Θ_b with the strength of the respective granite for the particular state of stress.

As mentioned above, the Mohr-Coulomb criterion is the generally used expression of strength of hard rock under triaxial stresses. However, σ_1 versus σ_3 diagrams (Figure 9) show that the breakout results do not at all correlate with the Mohr-Coulomb criterion, suggesting that the Mohr-Coulomb criterion is not appropriate for the condition of stress leading to breakouts.

On the other hand, plotting the same experimental results in the form of octahedral shear stress τ_{oct} versus the mean stress σ_2^m on planes striking in σ_2 direction suggests rather strongly that for the two tested granites Mogi's criterion as established by our

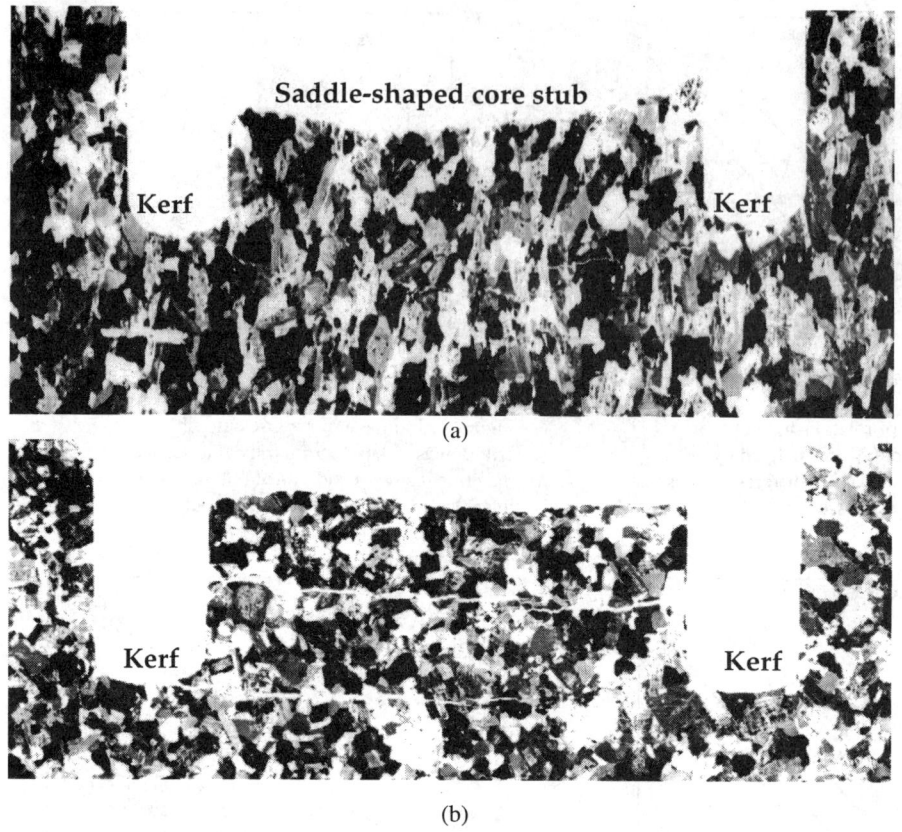

Figure 11. Two profiles of the bottom of a core-drilled hole in Westerly granite, (a) along σ_h and (b) along σ_H. Note that in (b) the tensile cracks parting future disks are practically horizontal; in (a) both the top surface and the crack at the root of the core stub are inclined downward towards the center, so as to form the eventual trough or saddle shape.

triaxial tests is the appropriate borehole failure criterion to be used in relating breakout dimensions to far-field stress(Figure 10.

Our experimental results are of fundamental importance. First, they show in a rather dramatic way that the indiscriminate use of the Mohr-Coulomb criterion for stress conditions beyond those used to establish experimentally the criterion is unwarranted. Secondly, they suggest that at least in the two tested granites one of the in-situ horizontal principal stresses can be assessed if the other two principal stresses, the breakout span θ_b, and the borehole failure criterion in terms of τ_{oct} versus σ_2^m are known (Haimson and Song, 1995).

5 CORE DISKING MECHANISM

Large far-field horizontal stresses brought about failure not only at the borehole wall (resulting in breakouts), but also in the base of the core, giving rise to disking. Disking was induced in all rocks tested, but so far we have studied only those obtained in the two granites. Core disks were nearly identical in shape and thickness within the same hole. The failure mechanism leading to disking was studied from thin sections of vertical cross-sections in the kerf area along the axis of the borehole. Vertical cross sections of a borehole cut along the directions of σ_h and σ_H are shown in Figure 11. Core tensile fractures initiated below the coring-bit-created kerf extend toward the axis of the core with a slight downward tilt in the direction of σ_h. In the σ_H

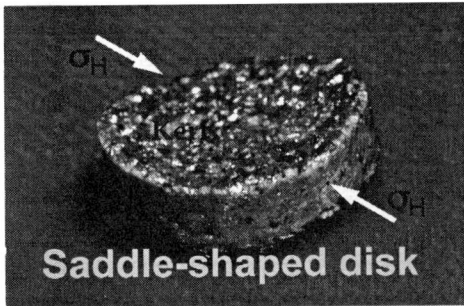

Figure 12. A typical core disk showing the familiar saddle shape with trough axis aligned with σ_H direction.

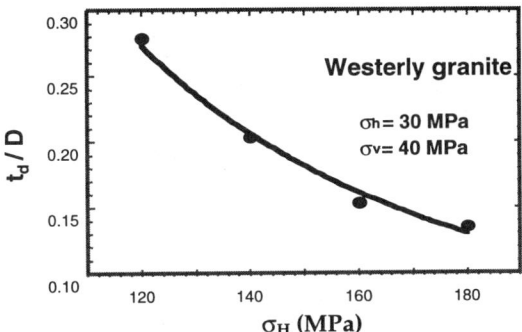

Figure 13. Example of the relationship between disk thickness t_d (normalized by core diameter) and σ_H for given σ_h and σ_v.

direction the same cracks are practically horizontal. As drilling advanced, these fractures open resulting in saddle-shaped disks having a trough axis oriented in the σ_H direction (Figure 12).

6 CORE DISKING AND IN SITU STRESS

The consistency of the trough-axis orientation reinforces the suggestion that disks recovered from oriented cores could be used as indicators of the in situ σ_H direction. In addition, our laboratory tests suggest that disk thickness is indicative of the level of the applied stress. Careful measurement of core-disk dimensions shows that for given magnitudes of σ_h and σ_v the thickness decreases monotonically with increasing σ_H. (Figure 13). As described above, σ_h and σ_v are often easier to estimate from the density of the overburden and the results of simple leak-off tests. Our tests indicate that in such cases σ_H magnitude and direction could be estimated from the average disk thickness and trough axis attitude, provided extracted oriented-core is disked and the relationship between thickness and σ_H is established.

7 CONCLUSIONS

Breakouts in granite result from extensile parallel microcracking behind the borehole wall in two opposite zones aligned with the direction of σ_h. Rock flakes bounded by two adjacent microcracks at the borehole wall tend to part due to crack-related expansion in the σ_h direction. Buckling of these flakes creates spalling and leaves cantilevers of rock on one or both sides of the breakout. These cantilevers help create the breakout 'V'-shape. Core disking and its saddle shape are the result of subhorizontal extensile cracks at the root of the drilled core. The trough of the saddle is aligned with the direction of σ_H, making the disk an excellent indicator of far-field principal horizontal stress azimuths.

Measured breakout dimensions can be potentially used as indicators of σ_H magnitude. In particular, knowledge of the breakout span and the correct rock strength criterion can be used to calculate one of the principal stresses if the other two are independently assessed. Disk thickness decreases in a linear fashion as the level of σ_H is raised (for given σ_h and σ_v) and may also provide a basis for estimating the maximum horizontal stress.

The usefulness of core disking is in being complementary to breakouts both for establishing principal stress directions and for indicating far-field stress magnitudes. Together with breakouts, core disking can provide limits on in situ stress levels and help assess the maximum horizontal stress from the measurement of characteristic dimensions.

ACKNOWLEDGMENTS: Much of the work reported here was funded by NSF grant EAR-9405836, and was carried out by graduate students C. Herrick, M. Lee, and I. Song.

REFERENCES

Bell, J.S. and D.I. Gough 1979. Northeast-southwest

compressive stress in Alberta: evidence from oil wells, *Earth and Planetary Sc. Letters*, 45:475-482.

Bessinger, B.A., Z. Liu, and N.G.W. Cook 1995. Laboratory borehole breakout patterns in non-dilatational geologic media: the formation of fractures orthogonal to the maximum compressive stress, *EOS Trans. Am. Geoph. U.* 76:F556.

Dyke, C. G. 1989. Core disking: its potential as an indicator of principal in situ stress directions. in V. Maury & D. Fourmaintraux (eds.), *Rock at Great Depth*: 1057-1064. Rotterdam: Balkema.

Haimson, B. C. 1978. The hydrofracturing stress measuring method and recent field results. *Int. J. Rock Mech. Min. Sci. and Geomech, Abstr.*, 15:167-178.

Haimson, B.C. and M.Y. Lee 1995. Estimating in situ stress conditions from borehole breakouts and core disking-experimental results in granite, *Proceedings of the International Workshop on Rock Stress Measurement at Great Depth*, K. Matsuki and K. Sugawara (Eds.), in the 8th International Congress on Rock Mechanics, Balkema Publ., Tokyo, 3 (in press).

Haimson, B.C. and I. Song 1995. A new borehole failure criterion for estimating in situ stress from breakout span, *The 8th International Congress of Rock Mechanics*, T. Fuji (Ed.), Tokyo, Japan, 341-3346,

Jaeger, J. C. and N. G. W. Cook 1979. *Fundamental of Rock Mechanics*. Chapman and Hall.

Lee M. Y. and B. C. Haimson 1993. Borehole breakouts in Lac du Bonnet granite: a case of extensile failure mechanism, *Int. J. Rock Mech. Min. Sci.* 30:1039-1045.

Lehnhoff, T. F., B. Stefansson, K. Thirumalai, and T. M. Wintezak 1982. The core disking phenomenon and its relation to in situ stress at Hanford, Technical Report SD-BWI-TI-085, Rockwell Hanford Operations, Washington.

Mogi, K. 1971. Fracture and flow of rocks under high triaxial compression. *J. Geophys. Res.* 76:1255-1269,

Natau, O., G. Borm, and Th. Rockel 1989. Influence of lithology and geological structure on the stability of the KTB pilot hole in V. Maury & D. Fourmaintraux (eds.), *Rock at Great Depth*: 1487-1490. Rotterdam: Balkema.

Sugawara, K., Saito, T., Hiramatsu, Y., Kameoka, Y., and Y. Oka 1978. A study on core disking of rock, *Japan Mining Industry Society Journal*. 94: 797-803.

Zoback, M.L. 1992. First- and second-order patterns of stress in the lithosphere: The world stress map project. *J. Geophys. Res.* 97:11703-11728,

The regional stress field and its heterogeneity

F.H.Cornet
Institut de Physique du Globe de Paris, France

ABSTRACT :Some evaluation of the stress field at sismogenic depth can be obtained from the analysis of focal plane solutions of natural earthquakes. Such an analysis assumes that the stress field at depth is homogeneous and varies proportionately with depth. Results from induced seismicity analysis have shown that in fact the stress field may be locally heterogeneous near active fault zones so that results from the sole inversion of focal plane solutions may not be accurate. This shortcoming may be overcome by integrating focal plane solutions with deep borehole measurements. Observations suggest that simple linear models for extrapolating borehole stress measurements to sismogenic depth are appropriate when the rock mass is homogeneous and topographic effects are negligible. These models imply a smoothing out of local stress heterogeneity and therefore cannot be used directly for analyzing hydromechanical coupling effects associated with forced fluid flow.

1. INTRODUCTION

A comprehensive review of the various methods proposed for determining the stress field at depth has been compiled recently (Cornet, 1993). Many of these methods imply measurements in boreholes while some others are based on indirect observations linked to seismic waves generation and/or propagation. Many of them involve some simplifying hypothesis concerning the relative orientation of the principal stress directions, the continuity and/or the uniformity of the stress field, the homogeneity and/or the isotropy of the material, etc... None of them yields directly the complete stress tensor at a given point and the stress determination always ends up being some kind of inversion process which often requires, implicitly or explicitly, some parameterisation of the regional stress field.

In this paper we define first the concept of local stress tensor and that of regional stress field. Then we discuss various parameterisation methods proposed for characterizing the regional stress field which have revealed efficient in regional stress determination. Finally we present practical cases where some heterogeneity in the regional stress field have been measured. These examples outline the merit and the limit of the validity of regional stress characterization by simple linear parameterisation.

2. DEFINITION OF THE REGIONAL STRESS FIELD

In continuum mechanics, the concept of stress is used for describing surface forces acting on and within a continuous body. If **t** is the force supported by a small surface **ds** of area da and normal **n**, and σ is the stress tensor defined at point **X** located at the center of **ds**, then :

$$\mathbf{t} = \sigma (\mathbf{X}) \mathbf{n} \, da \qquad (1)$$

t is called the stress vector, or surface traction, acting on **ds**. The components of the stress tensor σ may be assumed to be uniform over the area da when da is small. Clearly, for all materials, this concept looses its physical significance when da becomes too small. For homogeneous materials, the limiting scale is the molecular structure of the material. For rocks, the limiting scale is dictated by the structure of the rock matrix and possibly also by that of the rock mass. Thus, the first question that must be answered when dealing with stresses in rock mechanics, concerns the definition of the scale at which the concept of stress is to be applied.

The answer to this question is sought by referring to the concept of equivalent continuum material and to that of Elementary Representative Volume (ERV. When the rock can be assimilated to a continuum material, the ERV is the smallest volume for which there is equivalence between the idealized continuum material and the real rock. For crystalline and metamorphic rocks the definition of the ERV remains usually fairly simple. For example, for a granite, the ERV is about ten times the size of the largest crystal. But what is the ERV for a sedimentary rock formation made up of a suite of beds of shale and limestone the thickness of which varies in a random manner from a few millimeters to a few tens of centimeters ? It is assumed in this paper that an equivalent continuum material has been defined.

Although the concept of equivalent continuous material is necessary for the definition of stress, it is not sufficient. Let us consider the smallest cube surrounding the ERV and let x_1, x_2, x_3 be three axes of reference normal to its faces A_i, $i=1,..,6$ The two parallel faces normal to x_1 are indexed 1 and 4, the two faces normal to x_2, are indexed 2 and 5 and the two faces normal to x_3 are indexed 3 and 6. The resultant force supported by face A_i is called F_i, $i=1,...,6$. It has three components F_{ij}, $j=1,3$. This resultant force includes the forces supported by that part of A_i which passes through the solid and that part of A_i which passes through the fluids. The three components of the six resultant forces supported by the faces of the cube define a table of eighteen coefficients. These eighteen coefficients represent the components of a symmetrical stress tensor defined at point **X** located at the center of the cube only if:

$$F_{ij} = F_{(i+3)j} ; i,j = 1, 2, 3 \quad (2)$$
$$F_{ij} = F_{ji} ; i,j = 1, 2, 3 \quad (3)$$

Condition (2) implies that both the body forces acting on the cube and the gradient of the resultant surface forces are negligible. Condition (3) implies that the cube does not support any resultant moment. With these simplifying assumptions, the nine components

$$\sigma_{ij}(X) \equiv F_{ij}/A_i \; ; i, j = 1, 2, 3 \quad (4)$$

define the local stress tensor σ at **X**.

In short, the local stress tensor is defined at any point **X** in the rock mass by the components of the mean surface traction supported by the faces of the smallest cube which surrounds completely the ERV centered on point **X**. It involves all the forces acting on the equivalent continuum, those transmitted through the solid phases and those transmitted through the fluid phases. It cannot be used for the study of phenomena occurring at a scale smaller than that of the ERV. The ERV is the physical representation of the mathematical point; it may be considered as part solid and part fluid. It ranges usually from a few cubic centimeters to a few cubic meters

When the ERV gets too large, resultant moments and body forces cannot be neglected. When none of conditions (2) and (3) are satisfied, the concept of stress is not valid and stress measurements should not be attempted. When condition (2) is satisfied but condition (3) is not, the stress tensor as defined by Equation (4) is not symmetrical. In such cases, stress measurements should be interpreted with great care for classical interpretation methods lose their validity.

The complete determination of the local stress tensor requires the appraisal of six quantities, whether these correspond to the components of the tensor as expressed in a given frame of reference (generally North, East and vertical positive downward) or to the eigen values and the eigen vectors of the tensor (referred to as principal stress components σ_1, σ_2, σ_3, and principal stress directions).

When data are obtained within a small enough volume, stress variations are neglected. In many cases however, measurements are too distant from each other for neglecting stress variations. The variation of the stress tensor over large domains, which is referred to as the regional stress field, is characterized by six functions of the spatial coordinates. Hence, interpretation of stress measurements conducted over large volumes implies some approximation of the regional stress field.

3. CHARACTERIZATION OF THE REGIONAL STRESS FIELD

3.1 Principality and magnitude of the vertical stress component

A very common practice in rock mechanics is to assume that the vertical direction is a principal direction for the natural regional stress field and that the vertical stress component is equal to the weight of overburden. The validity of this hypo-

thesis rests on a few prerequisite conditions:
- The ground surface is perpendicular to a principal stress direction. Accordingly, in flat regions, the vertical direction is principal, at least at the ground surface. But in mountainous area the vertical direction is not a principal direction in the vicinity of ground surface and the domain in which the stress field is influenced by topography may be quite large, depending on the mountain range.
- Even if the ground surface is horizontal the vertical direction may not be a principal direction away from ground surface because of the influence of the structure of the formation. For example, Amadei et al. (1996) address the case of various laterally restrained anisotropic rock masses which are assumed to exhibit an elastic response to the effect of gravity forces. Their results suggest that for these conditions the principal directions may be strongly off the vertical direction. More generally, if the formation involves inclined, or folded, layered rocks, it should be anticipated that the vertical direction is not principal.
- Active faults may induce local perturbations of the regional stress regime. For example Shamir et al. (1992) explain some local variability in orientation of the wellbore breakouts observed in the Cajon Pass borehole by slips on faults. A similar conclusion is reached by Scotti and Cornet (1993) concerning some local stress heterogeneities observed in a granite massif.

Surprisingly, despite all these reasons for perturbation, most results published in the literature suggest that indeed the vertical direction is a principal direction, at least in deep formations. However, it should be kept in mind that most deep stress determinations involve methods in which the vertical stress is assumed a-priori to be vertical. Only very few direct measurements concerning the verticality of one of the principal stress directions are indeed available. Some are discussed later in the paper.

Clearly, when the vertical direction is not a principal direction it is erroneous to assume that the vertical component of the local stress tensor is equal to the weight of overburden. But even if the vertical direction is principal this assumption may not be valid. This is the case for deep formations which are laying below zones where none of the principal stress directions are vertical so that some of the weight of the overburden is supported by lateral domains. This reason has been proposed by Cornet and Burlet (1992) to explain the low values obtained for the vertical stress component measured by the HTPF method in various mountainous environments.

Accordingly, although it is widely assumed that the vertical stress is principal and equal to the weight of overburden, it is wise to verify always the validity of this hypothesis before it is used for a stress determination. In fact a sound stress determination method should provide means to validate this hypothesis by direct measurements.

3.2. Parameterisation of the regional stress field

The simplest parameterisation is the linear expansion around a central value estimated at some point X_c within the volume of interest :

$$\sigma(X) = \sigma(X_c) + (x_1-x_{1c}) \alpha^{(1)} + (x_2-x_{2c}) \alpha^{(2)} + (x_3-x_{3c}) \alpha^{(3)} \quad (5)$$

where $\sigma(X)$ is the stress tensor at point X (with coordinates x_1, x_2 and x_3), while $\sigma(X_c)$ is the stress tensor at point X_c (with components x_{1c}, x_{2c}, x_{3c}) and $\alpha^{(1)}$, $\alpha^{(2)}$ and $\alpha^{(3)}$ are second order symmetrical tensors characterizing the stress gradients in the x_1, x_2 and x_3 directions. Equation (5) must satisfy equilibrium conditions as defined in (6)

$$\text{div } (\sigma(X)) - \rho(X) \mathbf{b} = 0 \quad (6)$$

where $\sigma(X)$ is the stress tensor which exists at point X; $\rho(X)$ is the rock density at point X; $\mathbf{b}$ is the gravity force. Equation (6) implies that :

$$\alpha_{11}^{(1)} + \alpha_{21}^{(2)} + \alpha_{31}^{(3)} = 0 \quad (7a)$$
$$\alpha_{12}^{(1)} + \alpha_{22}^{(2)} + \alpha_{32}^{(3)} = 0 \quad (7b)$$
$$\alpha_{13}^{(1)} + \alpha_{23}^{(2)} + \alpha_{33}^{(3)} - \rho(X) g = 0 \quad (7c)$$

where g is gravity.

Accordingly, a simple linear description of the regional stress field implies 21 parameters and in addition requires a description of the spatial variations of the rock density. This simple 3D description of the regional stress field has never been applied. It would require a satisfactory 3D sampling of the regional stress field but generally only one deep borehole is available for stress measurements. Only simplified versions of it have been considered in the literature.

The four parameter model of focal plane solutions inversion :

The only method presently available for estimating the stress field at seismogenic depths (say larger than 5 km) is based on an interpretation of focal plane solutions of natural or induced earthquakes (e.g. Vasseur et al., 1983; Gephart and Forsyth 1984; Julien and Cornet, 1987; Riveira and Cisternas, 1990). With these methods, the slip vector associated with each seismic event is assumed to be parallel to the resolved shear stress supported by the corresponding fault plane. Seismic events are assumed to be small enough and distant enough from each other so that they are characteristic of the natural « undisturbed » regional stress field. It is assumed in these methods that the stress field is uniform throughout the volume in which earthquakes have occurred. The stress field is parameterised in such a way that the eigen values can be expressed as :

$$\sigma_i = \sigma_1 + (\sigma_3 - \sigma_1) T_i ; \quad i = 1,2,3 \quad (8)$$

where $T_1 = 0$, $T_2 = R = (\sigma_2 - \sigma_1) / (\sigma_3 - \sigma_1)$, $T_3 = 1$.

The solution of the inverse problem yields the components of tensor **T**, namely the three Euler angles which characterize the principal stress directions and the factor R which provides some characteristics of the ellipticity of the regional stress field. These methods have been applied to events with depth differences of a few kilometers and horizontal distances equal sometimes to a few tens of kilometers. Clearly, for such a volume, the stress cannot be assumed to be uniform. Yet, according to the numerical criteria used for evaluating the significance of the inversion solutions, results seem often to be well constrained. This implies that for the cases where these methods have been applied :

$$\sigma(\mathbf{X}_c) = \alpha^{(1)} = \alpha^{(2)} = 0 ; \quad \alpha^{(3)} \neq 0 \quad (9)$$

In other words, these results suggest that, at depth of the order of 10 km, the stress components are essentially proportional to depth. The interest of the method is that no assumption is made as far the principal stress direction are concerned. And indeed, in many of the cases where the method has been applied, none of the principal directions were found to be vertical.

However, Yin and Cornet (1994) have shown that, when such a method is applied to microseismic events induced by water injections, some discrepancy is observed between principal stress determinations derived from focal plane solutions inversions and those derived from hydraulic tests interpretations. As will be mentioned later in the paper, the discrepancy comes from local stress heterogeneities which influence the inversion solution. For the case of induced seismcity, this difficulty has been solved by integrating focal mechanisms with results from hydraulic tests so that heterogeneous events can be identified.

Linear models for hydraulic tests in vertical boreholes :

In many instances, the stress field at depth is derived from hydraulic tests conducted in one single vertical borehole. Results are interpreted either according to the classical hydraulic fracturing theory (e.g. Haimson, 1993) ; or to the HTPF (Hydraulic Tests on preexisting Fractures) method (e.g. Cornet, 1993). When lateral variations can be neglected ($\alpha^{(1)} = \alpha^{(2)} = 0$), equilibrium conditions implies that $\alpha^{(3)}$ is characterized by only four parameters, i.e. one of its principal directions is vertical. Accordingly the stress field is represented by :

$$\sigma(\mathbf{X}) = \sigma(\mathbf{X}_c) + (x_3 - x_{3c}) \alpha^{(3)} \quad (10)$$

The most general model requires 8 parameters including four parameters for $\sigma(\mathbf{X}_c)$, since one principal stress is assumed to be vertical throughout the volume of interest. If $\sigma(\mathbf{X}_c)$ is defined at ground surface then the eigen value associated with the vertical direction is null and equation (10) implies 7 parameters. If the rock density is known within the volume of the measurements, the eigen value associated with the vertical direction for $\alpha^{(3)}$ is derived from the equilibrium conditions and only 6 parameters are necessary for describing the stress field. If in addition, the horizontal principal directions are assumed to remain constant throughout the volume of interest then the principal directions of $\alpha^{(3)}$ are known and only 5 parameters are implied by equation (10).

In practice, it has been very often observed that principal stress directions rotate in the upper 200 to 300 m (e.g., Cornet and Burlet, 1992) so that a 5 parameters model cannot be applied for interpolating superficial data to greater depth. For depths larger than 1000 m however, the magnitude of the components of $\sigma(\mathbf{X}_c)$ becomes often negligible as compared to the depth dependent terms. For example, in Central France, Scotti and Cornet (1994) found that the interpolation of deep borehole observations to seismogenic depth is satisfactory with a simple four parameter model which corresponds to the components of the vertical stress gradient. It assumes that one principal stress direction is vertical. It is different from the 4 parameter model of focal plane inversions.

Brudy et al. (1997) have conducted a stress determination down to 8 Km in central Europe (KTB site) from direct borehole observations including drilling induced fractures, borehole breakout orientations and hydraulic tests in borehole. They conclude that one principal component is indeed vertical for the complete depth range of investigation and that stress magnitudes vary linearly with depth. Accordingly, for these measurements, a 4 parameter model similar to that of Scotti and Cornet is found appropriate. These authors further observe that the stress magnitudes at the KTB site imply that the crust is very close to incipient failure according to a Coulomb failure criterion with zero cohesion and a friction coefficient close to 0.8.

Ten parameters models :

Ten parameters models have been introduced so as to avoid the hypothesis that one principal stress is vertical. It has been applied first for integrating focal plane solutions of induced seismicity with hydraulic test results (Yin and Cornet, 1994) for a depths ranging from 250 m to 900 m. In this model, the tensor $\sigma(\mathbf{X}_c)$ is characterized by its 6 components while the $\alpha^{(3)}$ tensor is characterized by 4 parameters, i.e. lateral stress variations are negligible ($\alpha^{(1)} = \alpha^{(2)} = 0$). Interestingly, for the site where the method has been applied, it has been found that indeed the vertical direction is principal.

A 10 parameter model has also been introduced for determining with the HTPF method the stress field along an inclined deep borehole drilled in granite, in a mountainous area (Cornet et al., 1997). In this case, all principal directions are unknown and, further, lateral stress gradients cannot be ignored. However, the borehole from which measurements were conducted exhibit constant dip and azimuth within the depth range of interest (between 850 m and 1150 m). Accordingly equation (5) has been written with the x_3 axis parallel to the borehole axis so that all points where measurements have been conducted exhibit the same x_1 and x_2 components. Within this frame of reference, the tensor $\mathbf{S}(\mathbf{X}_c)$ defined by :

$$\mathbf{S}(\mathbf{X}_c) = \sigma(\mathbf{X}_c) + (x_1 - x_{1c})\alpha^{(1)} + (x_2 - x_{2c})\alpha^{(2)} \quad (11)$$

is uniform throughout the volume where measurements have been conducted so that equation (5) can be rewritten :

$$\sigma(\mathbf{X}) = \mathbf{S}(\mathbf{X}_c) + (x_3 - x_{3c})\alpha^{(3)} \quad (12)$$

It implies 12 parameters. In this case, no constraint on the components of $\alpha^{(3)}$ can be derived from the equilibrium conditions. For this site, only 19 measurements were available and, further, four tests yielded 2 different fractures and did not bring, in consequence, a very strong constraint on the stress field. Accordingly, the 12 parameters model has been reduced to 10 with the additional hypothesis that one of the principal stress direction of $\alpha^{(3)}$ is parallel to one principal direction of $\mathbf{S}(\mathbf{X}_c)$. Results derived from this stress determination show that the borehole is in fact less than 20° off one of the principal stress direction. The orientation of the smallest of the two principal stress components which are sub perpendicular to the borehole axis has been found to be within 25° off that of a breakout observed within this depth range. Interestingly the maximum principal stress has been found to be inclined about 60° to the vertical direction. It corresponds to a stress concentration induced by the valley near the site

4. HETEROGENEITY IN THE REGIONAL STRESS FIELD

The simple linear parameterisation of the regional stress field described above is valid only when the rock mass is homogeneous. In some sedimentary formations, changes in material property with depth are accompanied with stress variations of very significant magnitude (e.g. Evans et al, 1989; Cornet and Burlet, 1992) and this raises some difficulty for extrapolating to greater depth measurements obtained within a certain depth interval. Determining the complete regional stress field over large depth ranges in such sedimentary formation remains an open problem.

Another difficulty is that of stress heterogeneity associated with major fracture or fault zones in an otherwise homogeneous formation. Classically, when stress measurements are conducted in deep boreholes with the HTPF method, attention is given to avoid conducting measurements in heavily altered zones. Experience shows that in most stress measurements campaign, more than 75 to 80 % of the measurements are consistent with a simple linear model for the regional stress field. However, often, altered zones are also zones of high hydraulic conductivity. Accordingly, when hydromechanical coupling is of concern, attention must be given to evaluating these heterogeneities.

Such an attempt has been undertaken at the Le

Mayet de Montagne granite test site where in situ experiments on forced fluid flow have been conducted. Results from induced seismicity and from HTPF stress measurements have been integrated so as to constrain a 10 parameter characterization of the regional stress field (Yin and Cornet, 1994). Data involved 23 HTPF tests at depth ranging from 250 m to 760 m and 83 focal mechanisms of events which occurred at depths ranging from 300 to 950 m. The solution, which shows that the vertical direction is indeed principal, is consistent with 21 of the HTPF tests and 70 % of the focal plane solutions. This implies that some of the seismic events occurred in zones of stress heterogeneity.

An attempt has been made to verify that, indeed, the zones of high fluid flow where some of the induced seismicity was observed were locally heterogeneous (Cornet and Yin, 1995). Results show that the normal stress supported by fractures located 15 to 20 m away from the flow zone are some 10 Mpa larger than the maximum principal stress evaluated at this depth with the 10 parameters solution. Such high stress concentrations cannot be explained by simple change in material property (Scotti and Cornet, 1994) but imply some stress concentration mechanism linked with some local slippage along the fracture zone. Accordingly this confirms results from the integrated stress determination which showed that some events were heterogeneous with the regional stress field. Interestingly however, many focal mechanisms of events located along the same fracture zone are homogeneous with the regional stress determination. This implies that the heterogeneity in the stress field is not evenly distributed within the fracture zone. More work is needed for modeling these stress concentrations processes.

The conclusion of these results is that the stress field within major fault zones is not well approximated from regional stress field determinations and this raises a difficulty for modeling effects of hydromechanical coupling in fractured rock mass.

The fact that active fault zones correspond to local stress heterogeneities has also been identified at much larger scales through an analysis of focal plane solutions of natural earthquakes (Vasseur et al., 1983; Scotti and Cornet, 1994). This implies that inversion of focal plane solutions of natural earthquakes for regional stress determinations may be biased, as are inversions of induced seismicity data. In order to avoid this difficulty, focal plane solutions should always be integrated with data from different origins so as to help identify zones of stress heterogeneity for which focal plane solutions are to be disregarded.

5. CONCLUSION

The regional stress field observed at depth greater than a few kilometers in homogeneous basement rocks seems to be reasonably well modeled by a four parameter model (proportional dependency with depth). In the upper 1000 m, in region of negligible topography, some rotation of the principal stress direction is often observed close to ground surface so that the modeling implies 7 or 10 parameters (linear dependency of depth). When topography becomes significant linear models have been found appropriate but the complete description of the local variations of the regional stress field requires 21 parameters. Because generally only one deep borehole is available for conducting stress measurements, these 21 parameters cannot be resolved and only the stress variations along the direction of the borehole axis can be determined.

These simplified models have revealed useful for extrapolating to greater depth results from direct measurements in boreholes and for estimating regional principal stress directions. However locally the stress may significantly differ from these simple models. In particular, it has been observed that the normal stress supported by preexisting fractures near major fracture zones may be much larger than the maximum principal stress estimated from the simple linear models. The modeling of these local heterogeneities remains to be done. Such modeling is required for predicting efficiently hydromechanical coupling effects associated with forced fluid flow in fractured rock masses.

ACKNOWLEDGMENTS

I thank very sincerely Pr. Sugawara for inviting me to prepare this keynote paper. It provided me with the opportunity to synthesize some experience with regional stress field parameterisation.

REFERENCES

Amadei B and O. Stephanson; 1996; Rock Stress and its Measurement, 512 p.; Chapman & Hall, London.

Brudy M., M.D. Zoback, K. Fuchs, J. Baumgartner and F. Rummel; 1997; Determination of stress orientation and magnitude to 8 Km depth in the KTB site, Germany; Jour. Geophys. Res., in press.

Cornet F.H.; 1993; Stresses in Rock and Rock Masses; Comprehensive Rock Engineering (Hudson ed.), vol. 3, ch.12, pp 297-327, Pergammon Press, Oxford

Cornet F.H.;1993; The HTPF and the Integrated stress determination methods; Comprehensive Rock Engineering (Hudson ed.); Vol 3, ch. 15, Pergammon Press, Oxford

Cornet F.H. and D. Burlet; 1992; Stress Field Determinations in France by Hydraulic Tests in Boreholes; Jour. Geophys. Res., vol. 97, nb B8, pp 11829-11850

Cornet F.H. and Yin Jianmin ; 1995; Analysis of Induced Seismicity for Stress Field Determination and Pore Pressure Mapping; Pageoph, vol. 145, nb 3/4, pp 677-700.

Evans K., T. Engelder and R.A. Plumb; 1989; Appalachian stress study 1. : A detailed description of stress variations in Devonian Shales of the Appalachian Plateau; Jou. Geophys. Res., vol. 94, pp 1729-1754

Gephart J. W. and D.W. Forsyth; 1984; An improved method for determining the regional stress tensor using earthquake focal mechanism data : Application to San Fernando Earthquake sequence; Jou. Geophys. Res., vol. 89, nb. B11, pp 9305-9320

Haimson B.; 1993; The hydraulic Fracturing stress measurement method; Comprehensive Rock Engineering (Hudson ed.), vol. 3, ch.14, , Pergammon Press, Oxford

Julien Ph. and F.H. Cornet; 1987; Stress determination from aftershocks of the Campania-Lucania earthquake of November 23, 1980; Ann. Geophys.,vol 5B, nb 3,pp 289-300

Riveira L and A. Cisternas; 1990; Stress tensor and fault plane solutions for a population of earthquakes; Bull. Seis. Soc. Am., vol.80, nb 3, pp 600-614

Scotti O. and F.H. Cornet; 1994; In situ stress fields and focal mechanism solutions in Central France; Geophys. Res. Let., vol. 21, nb 22, pp 2345-2348.

Shamir G.; M.D. Zoback and F.H. Cornet; 1990; Fracture induced stress heterogeneity : Examples from the Cajon Pass scientific drillhole near the San Andreas Fault, California; Rock Joints (Barton and Stephansson Edit.), pp 719-724; Balkema Publ. Rotterdam

Vasseur G., A. Etchecopar and H. Philip; 1983; Stress state inferred from multiple focal mechanisms; Ann. Geophys., vol.1, nb. 4/5, pp 291-298

Yin J.M. and F.H. Cornet; 1994; Integrated stress determination by joint inversion of hydraulic tests and focal mechanisms; Geophys. Res. Let.; vol. 21, nb 24, pp 2645-2648.

Rock Stress, Sugawara & Obara (eds) © 1997 Balkema, Rotterdam, ISBN 90 5410 901 7

Stress measurements by borehole pressurization and its potential for future rock engineering projects in Japan

Y. Mizuta
Department of Civil Engineering, Yamaguchi University, Japan

ABSTRACT: Three kinds of in-situ stress measurements by borehole pressurization, i.e. hydraulic fracturing, sleeve fracturing to create double fracture planes and sleeve fracturing to create single fracture plane were carried out in the two mines of Kamioka Mining & Smelting Co., Ltd., who offers one of the major test fields for studies on radioactive waste depository. Determination procedure of far field stress from the point stress measurement which is to contribute to further investigation on the behavior of rock around the fault in the mine which is regarded as a active fault and improved procedure using acoustic emission technique for accurate detection of fracture closing pressure are described.

1. INTRODUCTION

Numerical modelling has potential to illustrate rock stress distribution around the fault and thus one can determine the mechanical characteristics of the fault by adjusting the computed to the measured stress distribution. One of the important parameter for this modelling is the far field stress state which induced the initial stress of the concerning domain. The state of far field stress is described by the magnitudes and orientations and determination of those are not so easy. There are several in-situ stress measurement techniques which have been developed such as the overcoring and the hydraulic fracturing method. However, these measurements have usually been carried out near the earth surface. It means that the measured results may be affected by geometry of the surface boundary and only represent the state of stress at a point involving a relatively small volume of rock.

2. TRADITIONAL BUT UNJUSTIFIED ASSUMPTION

For the purpose of numerical modelling, the state of far field stress, often be assumed as :

$$\sigma_{z0} = \rho g z, \quad \sigma_{x0} = \sigma_{y0} = \frac{\nu}{1-\nu} \rho g z \quad (1)$$

where ρ is density of rock (kg/m³), z(m) is depth from the height of origin of the coordinate which can be arbitrarily, g is acceleration by gravity and ν is Poisson's ratio.

2.1 Stress determination by hydrofracturing at Tochibora Mine

In situ stress measurement by hydraulic fracturing method [1] was carried out at Site No.1(the site in a drift of Tochibora Mine). Three boreholes of different orientations, which were not laid on one plane, were used to determine three dimensional stress state. The vertical distance from the site to the surface is about 160 meters although the surface plane is steeply include. The magnitudes of six stress components which were determined by hydraulic fracturing tests are shown in Table 1.

Table 1 The six stress component s measured by hydrofracturing at site No.1(Tochibora site)

Most probable values (MPa)		Probability errors (MPa)
σ_E =2.24	±	0.49
σ_N =3.06	±	0.61
σ_V =3.08	±	1.25
σ_{EN} =-0.55	±	0.46
σ_{NV} =1.33	±	0.31
σ_{VE} =-0.17	±	0.66

E,N and V indicate North, East and upward Vertical

2.2 Numerical determination of site stress assuming far field stress

In order to determine the initial stress state at the site of stress measurement, numerical calculation by the boundary element method was carried out, assuming the far field stress state as Expression (1). Modelling was carried out by the procedure of Fictitious Stress Method. Fig. 1 shows the surface boundary divided into the triangular leaf elements. According to the procedure of indirect boundary element method, three components of tractions (uniform distributions of fictitious stress) over each element are determined first by solving $3N$ linear simultaneous equations, where N is the number of leaf element on the boundary. The simultaneous equations can be constructed by making the sum of each initial stress component on the boundary and each corresponding stress component induced by $3N$ tractions be zero for every leaf element [2]. Then the stress distribution around the boundary is calculated.

2.3 Comparison f the calculated stress with the measured stress

Fig. 2 shows the stress state on E plane, which was obtained by three dimensional numerical computation, provided that rock material is isotropic, homogeneous, elastic and specific weight of rock, $\rho g = 27.8$ kN/m³, is uniformly distributed over the model.

Fig. 3 shows the stress state on E plane, which was measured in-situ. It can be seen from Fig. 2 and Fig. 3 that the calculated stress is different from the measured stress state. It means that real horizontal stress components are greater than those given by Expression (1).

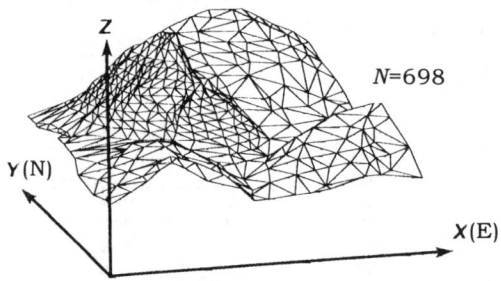

Fig.1 The model of the surface boundary divided into the triangular left elements.

3. DETERMINATION OF FAR FIELD STRESS FROM THE POINT STRESS MEASUREMENT

3.1 Determination procedure

Suppose that the real far field stress is described by $\sigma_{x0} = k_x \rho gz$, $\sigma_{y0} = k_y \rho gz, \cdots$, and $\sigma_{zx0} = k_{zx} \rho gz$.

If the concerning domain of rock mass is assumed to be isotropic, homogeneous and elastic, determination of the far field stress state can be carried out by the following procedure. First, for each of the six specified far field stress states,

$$\{\rho gz,0,0,0,0,0\},\{0,\rho gz,0,0,0,0\},\cdots,\{0,0,0,0,0,\rho gz\},$$

the corresponding stress state at the site can be calculated numerically by boundary element method. Then the factors related to the six components of far field stress, k_x etc., can be determined next, using the following formula:

$$\sigma = kA \qquad (2)$$

$$\sigma = \left\{(\sigma_{xa})_m,(\sigma_{ya})_m,(\sigma_{za})_m,(\tau_{xya})_m,(\tau_{yza})_m,(\tau_{zxa})_m\right\}^T$$

$$k = \left\{k_x,k_y,k_z,k_{xy},k_{yz},k_{zx}\right\}^T$$

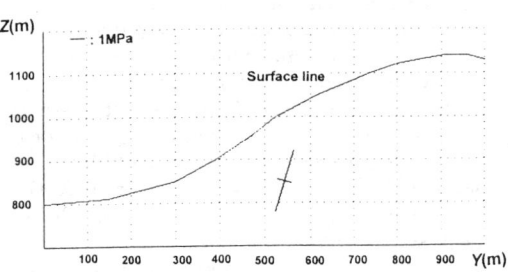

Fig.2 The calculated stress state in the planet perpendicular to E axis.

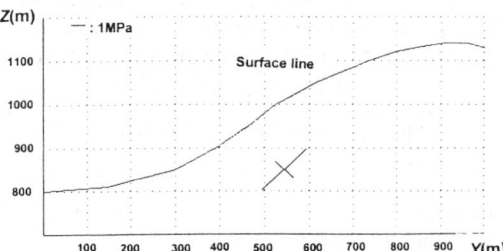

Fig.3 The measured stress state in the plane perpendicular to E axis.

$$A = \begin{bmatrix} (\sigma_{xa})_x & (\sigma_{xa})_y & (\sigma_{xa})_z & (\sigma_{xa})_{xy} & (\sigma_{xa})_{yz} & (\sigma_{xa})_{zx} \\ (\sigma_{ya})_x & (\sigma_{ya})_y & (\sigma_{ya})_z & (\sigma_{ya})_{xy} & (\sigma_{ya})_{yz} & (\sigma_{ya})_{zx} \\ (\sigma_{za})_x & (\sigma_{za})_y & (\sigma_{za})_z & (\sigma_{za})_{xy} & (\sigma_{za})_{yz} & (\sigma_{za})_{zx} \\ (\tau_{xya})_x & (\tau_{xya})_y & (\tau_{xya})_z & (\tau_{xya})_{xy} & (\tau_{xya})_{yz} & (\tau_{xya})_{zx} \\ (\tau_{yza})_x & (\tau_{yza})_y & (\tau_{yza})_z & (\tau_{yza})_{xy} & (\tau_{yza})_{yz} & (\tau_{yza})_{zx} \\ (\tau_{zxa})_x & (\tau_{zxa})_y & (\tau_{zxa})_z & (\tau_{zxa})_{xy} & (\tau_{zxa})_{yz} & (\tau_{zxa})_{zx} \end{bmatrix}$$

where $(\sigma_{xa})_m, (\sigma_{ya})_m, \cdots, (\tau_{zxa})_m$ are the stress components measured at the site (point a) and the column components, $(\sigma_{xa})_x$, etc., $(\sigma_{xa})_y$, etc., $(\sigma_{xa})_z$, etc., $(\sigma_{xa})_{xy}$, etc., $(\sigma_{xa})_{yz}$, etc. and $(\sigma_{xa})_{zx}$, etc. are the calculated stress components under the six specified far field stress state $\{\rho gz, 0, 0, 0, 0, 0\}$, $\{0, \rho gz, 0, 0, 0, 0\}$ $\cdots$, $\{0, 0, 0, 0, 0, \rho gz\}$, respectively.

3.2 Stress determination by double fracture method at site No.2

In-situ stress measurement by double fracture method [3] was carried out at site No.2 (the site in a drift of Mozumi Mine). The distance between Tochibora Mine and Mozumi Mine is about 8km. Mozumi Sukenobu Fault which is regarded as an active fault is 300m distant from the site. Three boreholes of different orientation, which were laid on one plane, were used to determine three dimensional stress state. The vertical distance from the surface is about 380 meters. The magnitudes of six stress components measured are shown in Table 2.

Table 2 The six stress components measured by double fracture method at site No.2(Mozumi site near Sukenobu Fault)

Most probable values (MPa)		Probability errors (MPa)
σ N =15.91	±	0.61
σ E =17.50	±	0.97
σ V =14.88	±	3.75
σ EN =-0.19	±	0.65
σ VE =-0.24	±	0.85
σ NV =-0.40	±	1.31

3.3 Numerical determination of real far filed stress

In order to determine the far field stress state of Kamioka district, the surface boundary above the site of stress measurement was divided into triangular leaf elements of Fictitious stress Method. Fig. 4 shows the numerical model.
At this time, the fault boundary was not included in the model. The coefficient matrix, A, was calculated next. Then, the factors of the far field stress, k, was determined by solving Equation (2). The values of k determined thus are shown in Table 3.

3.4 Numerical calculation of the stress state at site No.2

The point stress state at the site in Mozumi Mine, which is 300m distant from Mozumi Sukenobu Fault was calculated based on the far field stress

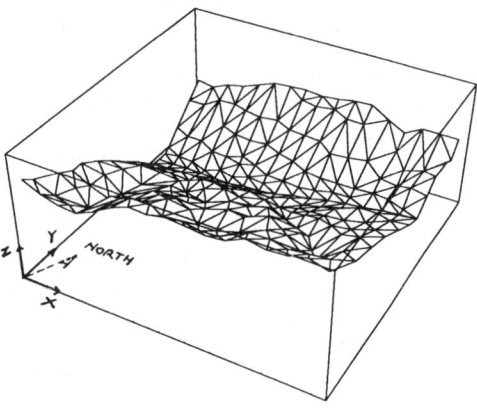

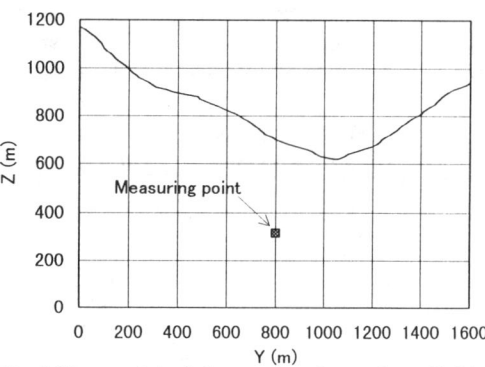

Fig.4 The model of the surface boundary divided into FSM elements.

factors, k. Fig. 4 shows the numerical modelling in which the surface boundary is divided into Fictitious stress elements (for further investigation in future, Mozumi Sukenobu Fault is divided into Displacement Discontinuity elements). The stress state calculated thus is shown in Table 3. It can be seen by comparison of the values in Table 2 with the values in Table 3 that the calculated point stress well agree with the measured point stress. It means that far field stress determination from point stress measurement in consideration of effect of the surface boundary geometry although rock material is assumed to be isotropic, homogeneous and elastic.

4. IMPROVED PROCEDURE FOR STRESS DETERMINATION BY SINGLE FRACTURE PROBE

In-situ stress measurement by using Single Fracture Probe developed by SGI (Serata Geomechanics Incorporation) was carried out at site No.3 (the site in Atotsugawa Drift of Mozumi Mine). One vertical borehole and one horizontal borehole were used to determine the stress components in rock around the drift. The depth of the site from the surface is about 1,000 meters.

4.1 Single fracture probe and AE sensor

As Fig. 5 shows, the established method for stress determination, which was prepared by SGI, is to detect fracture re-opening pressure from the relationship between fluid pressure in probe and diametral displacement in the direction perpendicular to the single fracture created by first pressurization.

Fig. 6 shows the configuration of the single fracture probe used. Three LVDTs are set along the probe axis. In the procedure for stress measurement using the horizontal borehole,

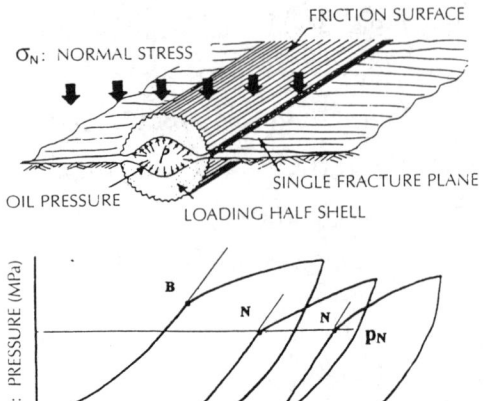

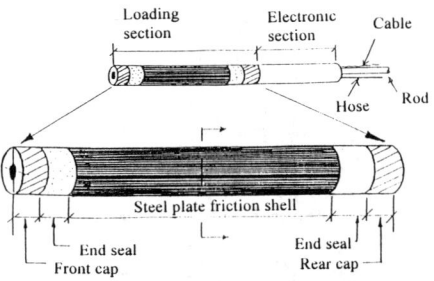

Fig.5 Illustration of creation of single fracture plane and determination of fracture re-opening pressure.

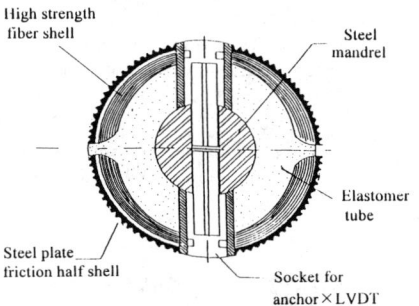

Fig.6 Configuration of the single fracture probe.

Table 3 The values of k determined and the calculated stress state at site No.2

far field stress factors (ρ g z)	stress state at the site (MPa)
k_x =0.6315	σ_x =16.31
k_y =0.5865	σ_y =17.09
k_z =0.9552	σ_z =14.89
k_{xy} =0.0117	σ_{xy} =0.72
k_{yz} =0.0556	σ_{yz} =-0.38
k_{zx} =-0.0357	σ_{zx} =0.27

The measured stress state is exactly equal to the calculated stress state.

however, acoustic emission detection was associated with recording of pressure, diametral deformation related to time. PZT sensors of special design for field use were attached around the borehole on the side wall of the drift by using fast hardening cement.

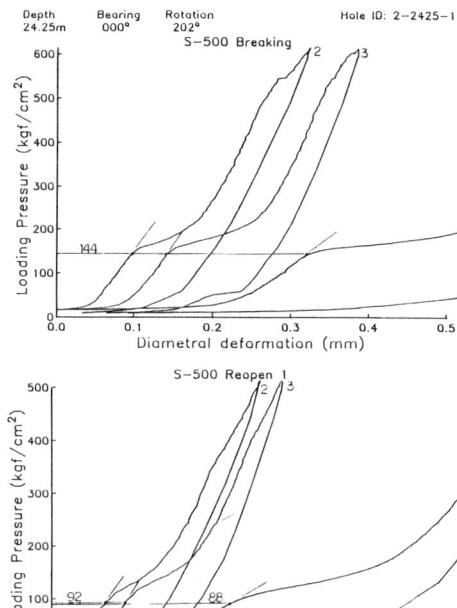

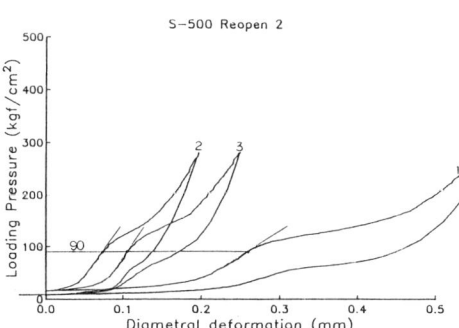

Fig.7 The example of the pressure-deformation curves obtained by fracturing test and two re-opening tests.

4.2 In-situ experiment at site No.3

Fig. 7 shows the examples of the pressure-deformation curves obtained by fracturing test and two re-opening tests, which were carried out at the section 24m deep from the mouth of the vertical borehole. In this case, the deviation points of the p-D curve, which is corresponding to the single fracture re-opening pressure, were clearly detected. This feature may depend on the stress state at the measuring point and the stress state

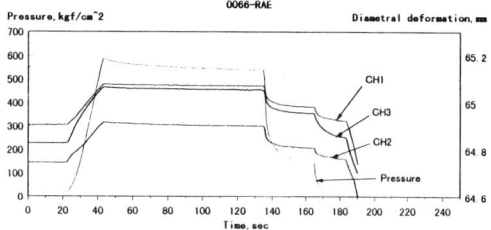

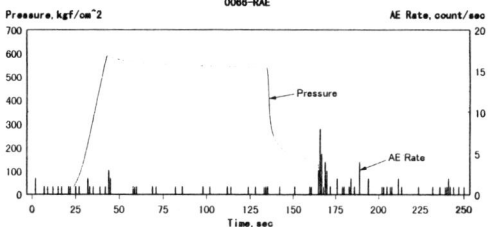

Fig.8 The deformation- time and AE rate-time records plotted over pressure-time record.

in the plane perpendicular to the borehole axis, i. e. horizontal plane was and static the magnitude of the stress were relatively small.

However, such a deviation point was not clearly shown on the p-D curves, which were obtained at the sections 0.66~2.54m deep from the mouth of the horizontal borehole. It may be because stress difference and the magnitude of the vertical stress component is quite large. In practice, horizontal fracture could not produced in the vertical borehole even the maximum pressure (70MPa) was applied since vertical stress component is too large due to association with stress concentration around the opening. In this case, therefore, detection of AE activity was associated to the experiment and the variation of AE event rate with time was represented over the pressure- time record.

Fig. 8 shows the diametral deformation-time and AE even rate-time records which are plotted over pressure-time record. Those were obtained from a re-opening test of the fracture created at the section 1.1m deep from the borehole mouth. In this test, fluid injection into the probe was done up to 43 seconds passage and fluid flow was stopped. After a while this condition was kept, the return valve was partly opened at 135 seconds passage and fully opened at 183 seconds passage. It is found from the curves that the single fracture closing pressure which is related to the stress component perpendicular to the fracture can be clearly shown by the point where AE rate significantly increase. Furthermore, It may be possible to detect the fracture closing pressure even from gradient changes of deformation-time curve and pressure-time itself.

CONCLUSION

Three kinds of in-situ stress measurements were carried out at three different sites, respectively. A stress state measured by Hydraulic Fracturing Method was compared with the calculated stress state based on the traditional assumption concerning to far field stress state. A procedure of numerical approach for determination of far field stress state from a point stress measurement was proposed. The far field stress state was determined through the procedure from the point stress state measured by the Double Fracture Method and applicability of the procedure was shown. The improved procedure for stress measurement by Single Fracture Probe was proposed and practical use of it was demonstrated. In conclusion, It was shown that the three kinds of borehole pressurization techniques have high potential as the stress measurement method.

ACKNOWLEDGEMENTS

Numerical works for determination of far field stress from point stress measurement were carried out by the graduate students (Mr. Sulistiant and Mr. Kido) of Department of Civil Engineering, Yamaguchi University. In-situ stress measurement by hydraulic fracturing method was supported by Research & Development Department (Director: Dr. Kato), NOF corporation and carried out by Dr. Kato, Dowa Engineering. In-situ stress measurements by double fracture method were supported by PNC and carried out by MINDECO (Mr. Shingu and Mr. Horinokuchi). In-situ AE experiments associated with fracturing tests by the single fracture probe were carried out by Nihon Public Co. Inc. (Mr. Nakayama, Mr. Tanaka and Mr. Kuwabara) in cooperation with MINDECO and Prof. Ishida, Department of Civil Engineering, Yamaguchi University. All of the experiments could be done with assistance by Kamioka Mining and Smelting Co. Ltd. (Mr. Fujii et al.). The author wish to thank those people.

REFERENCES

1. Mizuta,Y., Sano,O., Ogino,S. and Katoh,H., Three Dimensional Stress Determination by Hydraulic Fracturing for Underground Excavation Design, Int. J. Rock Mech. Min. Sci. & Geomech. abstr. Vol.24, No.1, 1987.
2. Kuriyama,K. et al, Three-dimensional Elastic Analysis by the Boundary Element Method with Analytical Integrations over Triangular Leaf Elements, Int. J. Rock Mech. Min. Sci. & Geomech. Abstr. Vol.32, No.1, 1995.
3. Serata,S., Sakuma,S., Kikuchi,S. and Mizuta,Y., Double Fracture Method of In Situ Stress Measurement in Brittle Rock, Rock Mechanics and Rock Engineering. 25,89-108, 1992.
4. Sulistianto,B., Kido,T. and Mizuta,Y., Determination of Far Field Stress from the Point Stress Measurement, a Numerical Approach, Shigen to Sozai (in contribution).

Methods for stress measurement

ated, constructed and tested during 1995 and
Rock stress determinations at great depth using the modified doorstopper gauge

P.M.Thompson
Whiteshell Laboratories, AECL, Pinawa, Man., Canada

R.Corthésy & M.H.Leite
Départements des Génies Civil, Géologique et des Mines, Ecole Polytechnique, Montréal, Qué., Canada

ABSTRACT:

AECL has developed a Deep Doorstopper Gauge System (DDGS) designed to allow doorstopper gauge overcoring tests at depths as great as 1,000 m in sub-vertical boreholes. The device utilizes an Intelligent Acquisition Module, a remote battery-powered datalogger that collects and stores strain data during a stress measurement test. This paper describes the DDGS and the results of the first series of tests conducted, including a successful test in a water-filled borehole at a depth of 518 m.

1 INTRODUCTION

An issue raised during environmental hearings into the concept of deep geological disposal of nuclear fuel waste in the Canadian Shield was the state of in situ stress in the rock at depth. Horizontal in situ stresses below a major thrust fault and fracture zone (Fracture Zone 2) at 270 m depth at the Underground Research Laboratory (URL) were anomalously high, and it was necessary to determine if these high stress magnitudes continued or returned to more normal levels with depth. Hydraulic fracturing had been unable to provide results because of an inability to generate vertical fractures, and previous attempts at deep overcoring had failed as a result of core discing.

In 1987, deep overcoring measurements using the Swedish State Power Board triaxial strain cell (Hiltscher et al. 1979) and the Deep Borehole Deformation Gauge (Thompson 1990) were attempted in the granite of the URL in Manitoba, Canada. No overcoring with these instruments was possible deeper than 358 m because of core discing resulting from high horizontal in situ stresses.

A promising instrument choice in high-stress environments is the so-called "doorstopper gauge" which is less susceptible to core discing problems than overcoring methods requiring a pilot hole. However, the standard doorstopper gauge is only suitable for short installations (approximately 20 m) in dry (i.e. self-draining or angled-up) boreholes.

AECL has applied a remote data logger/signal conditioner, developed by the Rock Mechanics Laboratory of École Polytechnique in Montréal, to the design of a Deep Doorstopper Gauge System (DDGS) for use to 1,000-m-depth. The DDGS was designed, constructed and tested during 1995 and 1996 and has achieved successful measurements at borehole depths as great as 518 m (943-m-depth from surface).

2 PRINCIPLE OF THE DEEP DOORSTOPPER GAUGE SYSTEM

The DDGS incorporates several features that enable it to be used for deep overcoring measurements:

1. It is used with a self-contained Intelligent Acquisition Module (IAM) developed by the Rock Mechanics Laboratory of École Polytechnique in Montreal. The IAM is a remote battery-powered data logger that remains attached to the doorstopper gauge during a stress measurement test. It is programmed by connecting it to a personal computer. Collected data is retrieved in the same way.

2. The concept of a "diving bell" is used to protect the base of the doorstopper gauge during installation (i.e. while it is being lowered down a water-filled borehole). An air pocket forms below the strain gauge rosette and it, together with adhesive smeared on the strain gauge face, remains dry until the moment of installation.

3. A specially formulated adhesive has been developed that has the properties (viscosity, pot-life, setting time, ability to bond to wet rock etc.) required for use in deep water-filled boreholes.

4. Components of the system have been designed to withstand pressures of 10 MPa, in order to allow use to depths of 1,000 m.

5. A gravity-based orientation system is incorporated in the design which allows remote measurement of installation orientation in sub-vertical installations.

6. Once the DDGS has bonded to the base of the test borehole, an automatic trigger release allows recovery of the installation weight, "diving bell", and orientation system using a wireline cable. Only the IAM inside a high-pressure housing, together with the doorstopper gauge, remain downhole during the overcore test drilling.

2.1 The Modified Doorstopper Gauge

The Modified Doorstopper Gauge (Corthésy and Gill, 1990) has been used for overcore testing at the URL for a number of years. A series of 14 tests were conducted in 1991 at the 420 Level of the URL. Unlike the standard doorstopper gauge, the Modified Doorstopper Gauge is hard-wired, allowing continuous monitoring of strains throughout the stress relief operation. During the testing at the 420 Level, it became apparent that the Modified Doorstopper Gauge could provide measurements in locations where instruments requiring pilot holes could not be used because of discing problems caused by high in situ stresses.

Prior to final design of the DDGS, a series of overcore tests using a Modified Doorstopper Gauge were tried in the upper part of a deep probe hole (PH1) to test the "diving bell" concept. Five tests were attempted between 33 and 34 m deep in the hole. Although none of the tests were successful, many lessons were learned (including correct flattening procedures during diamond drilling operations). It was determined that the "diving bell" concept was feasible, and final design of the DDGS prototype was undertaken.

2.2 The Intelligent Acquisition Module

The Intelligent Acquisition Module (IAM) is a self-contained sealed datalogger designed for structural and geological stress measurements using the Modified Doorstopper Gauge. The IAM utilizes open architecture supporting both real-time and data logging applications. It is fully supported by the GeoWind geotechnical data acquisition software (Microsoft Windows ™ compatible).

The cylindrical IAM has a diameter slightly larger than the doorstopper and an overall length of about 300 mm. It is attached directly to a Modified Doorstopper Gauge and is re-usable. Since it is battery operated, it allows continuous acquisition and logging of digitized measurements while the stress relief overcoring is in progress, without the need for a bulky signal cable running to the borehole collar. The IAM operates on a pair of standard 9 volt batteries. Minimum battery life is specified at 3 hours using alkaline batteries.

The standard housing for the IAM is a thin-walled aluminum cylinder only suitable for pressures of up to 0.5 MPa. The IAM housing was redesigned for the DDGS to allow use at greater depths. A thicker stainless steel housing was designed that was only open at one end, thus minimizing the number of seals required.

2.3 The Deep Doorstopper Gauge System

The main components of the DDGS are the IAM in a high-pressure housing; an outer "sliding sleeve with double O-ring seal" that, when extended below the doorstopper, acts as a "diving bell" protecting the doorstopper gauge rosette and adhesive from water; and an upper installation weight and gravity-based orientation device. The DDGS is installed inside HQ drill rods (77.8-mm-ID) into the HQ wireline core barrel by simply lowering it by wireline down the water-filled hole after applying adhesive to the face of the Modified Doorstopper Gauge. The annular space around the DDGS installation assembly controls the speed at which it travels down the borehole. A thin covering of open-cell foam rubber attached to the face of the gauge is used to allow a fairly thick coating of adhesive. The adhesive used with the DDGS is derived from silikal with added silanes and benzyl peroxide. Silica flour is added to increase viscosity.

When the DDGS reaches the bottom of the core barrel, a trigger mechanism is activated and the sliding sleeve is released from the IAM housing. The weight of the installation and orientation assembly then cause the IAM housing to descend inside the sliding sleeve, thus forcing the trapped air-pocket inside the sleeve to "burp" water away from the borehole bottom at the instant the Modified Doorstopper Gauge (with attached adhesive) is pressed onto the flattened borehole bottom. At the same time, the momentum of the upper portion of the installation assembly, which is spring-loaded, carries it down onto a free ball-bearing rolling on an aluminum disc inside the orientation device. The DDGS is designed for operation in non-vertical

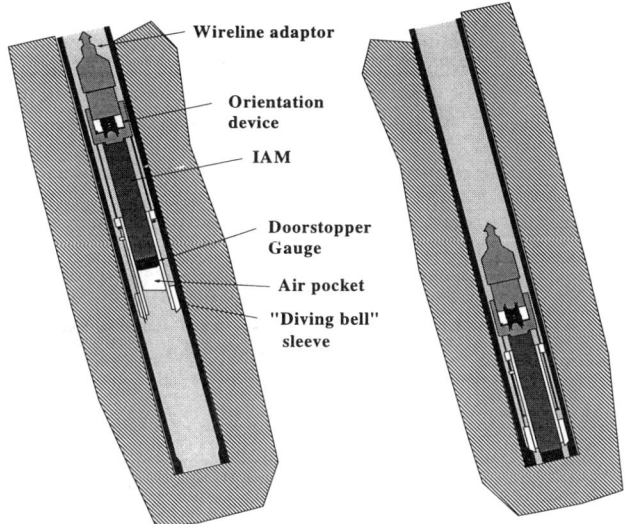
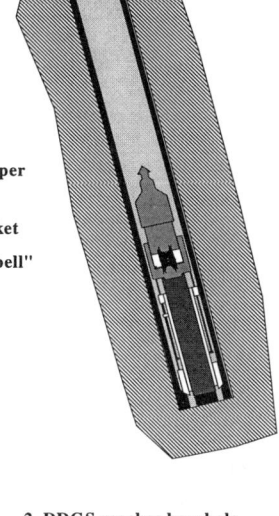
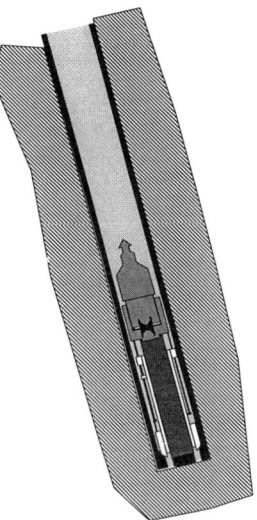

1. DDGS lowered down borehole by wireline just prior to installation

2. DDGS reaches borehole bottom; trigger is activated by base of core barrel and the sleeve is forced back over IAM housing allowing doorstopper gauge to be forced down through the air bubble to bond to borehole bottom.

3. Weight of wireline overshot and upper assembly compresseses the orientation spring and ball bearing leaving an imprint in the aluminum orientation disc corresponding to borehole invert.

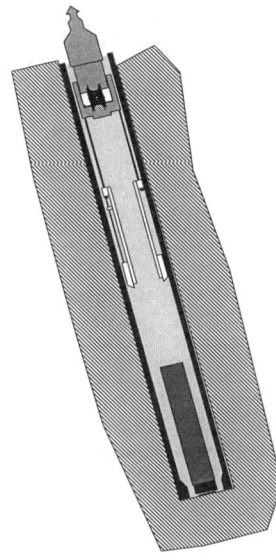
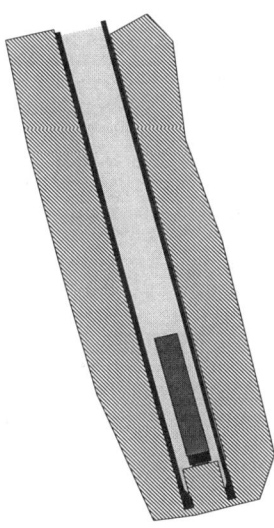

4. After glue has set, the installation assembly is retrieved by wireline cable, leaving the IAM and doorstopper gauge. The preprogrammed IAM starts datalogging at a set time.

5. The diamond drill is used to extend the borehole and the IAM records associated strains.

6. The overcore and IAM are retrieved in the core innertube. Biaxial pressure and Brazilian tensile testing are done to determine the elastic properties of the rock.

Figure 1. Operation of the Deep Doorstoppper Gauge

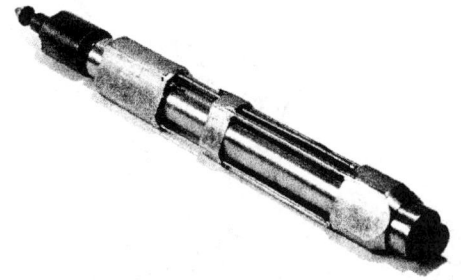

Figure 2. The Deep Doorstopper Gauge System

boreholes plunging at 80° or less, thus the ball bearing rests on the lowest side of the hole at the moment of impact. This results in an impression on the aluminum disc corresponding to the borehole invert. The operating principle of the DDGS is illustrated in Figure 1. The DDGS is shown in Figure 2.

Typically, the adhesive is allowed to set for 2 hours before the IAM timer activates the IAM to start collecting data. At that time, the wireline cable is pulled out of the hole retrieving the installation assembly, orientation device and sliding sleeve (which is attached by thin steel rods). If the adhesive has worked properly, only the doorstopper gauge and the IAM, in its high-pressure housing remain on the borehole bottom, and the overcoring can begin.

2.4 GeoWind Software

The manufacturer of the IAM has developed a software package, GeoWind, compatible with Microsoft's Windows 3.1™ environment. It allows the collection and display of real time data in a compatible format with other Windows' applications. GeoWind is used to program the IAM to start collecting data when overcoring is about to commence, typically 2.5 hours after the programming takes place. This allows time to install the DDGS, and for the glue to set. Scan rates are also programmable.

3 DEEP OVERCORING USING THE DDGS

The prototype DDGS was used to measure in situ stress conditions in URL borehole 413-002-PH1 collared at a depth of 440 m, and plunging at 76°. Testing took place between 1995 April and November. Initial testing consisted of commissioning and verifying that the various parts of the system (both mechanical and electronic) were functioning properly. Early dry runs measured the down-hole free fall velocity of the DDGS as 0.71 m/s. Travel to the base of the hole at a depth of 234 m took 5.5 minutes. This was deemed suitable in terms of adhesive pot life.

Early field tests indicated a number of areas that required further work. A silica gel pack was placed in the IAM during testing to absorb any moisture collecting due to condensation or minor leakage. Because of the high stresses expected to be imposed by water pressure in deep borehole installations, a stainless steel ring was potted around each doorstopper gauge to increase stiffness and prevent excessive deformation.

A major source of early problems was the battery choice and battery management electronics of the IAM design. The original IAM was designed in such a way that if either of the two batteries discharged below a certain level prior to downloading collected data, all collected data was lost. It was therefore extremely important that the batteries were not permitted to completely discharge prior to retrieval. After conferring with the manufacturer, the battery management system on the IAM was redesigned and a retrofit kit installed to allow more even battery usage. In the initial design, one of the two batteries was subjected to a greater current draw and would always discharge first. The retrofit kit wired both batteries in parallel so there was even usage of both batteries.

A thin annular space was machined between the aluminum battery case and the IAM housing to create a thermal barrier so that the heat generated by the electronics was not lost too quickly. A layer of thermally reflective foil was also used between the batteries and the IAM housing. These measures increased battery life.

The GeoWind software worked well. A 486 laptop computer was used to program and communicate with the IAM. Detailed procedures and checklists were developed during the testing program and are now used for all tests.

4 RESULTS

During the initial testing, five successful tests were obtained out of 43 attempts, for a success rate of 12%. While this is extremely low, it must be realized that there was no opportunity to properly commission the DDGS prior to field testing because of the overall schedule. Lessons learned during the testing, such as obtaining adequate

Table 1. In situ stresses measured in PH1-002-PH1 using the DDGS. E_1 and E_2 are the maximum and minimum moduli in the measurement plane. υ is the Poisson's ratio. θ is measured counterclockwise from top of hole (Azimuth 310°).

Borehole Depth (m)	Depth Below Surface (m)	E_1 (GPa)	E_2 (GPa)	(υ)	P (MPa)	Q (MPa)	θ
238.1	671.0	22.8	19.5	0.296	48.1	46.1	62°
238.7	671.6	32.0	28.0	0.224	60.5	59.8	7°
238.84	671.74	33.6	30.2	0.149	64.7	63.0	38°
409.9	837.7	49.5	35.8	0.153	70.6	65.0	56°
518.2	942.8	20.0	17.1	0.357	48.2	44.8	29°

battery life, should result in higher success rates in future applications. Failures were attributable to many reasons including inadequate battery life, premature tripping of the sliding sleeve release mechanism, debris on the hole bottom, seal failures, adhesive failures etc.

The strain recovery curves for the successful tests are quite remarkable considering the technical challenge of performing in situ stress measurements at these depths. The strain recovery curve for the test at 409.9 m is shown in Figure 3. The close agreement of the two strain invariants indicates accurate measurements.

Interpretation of the tests is described by Leite et al. 1996. The interpretation accounts for rock anisotropy and for the effect of hydrostatic pressure of water in the test borehole. The principal stresses in the plane perpendicular to the axis of the test borehole are contained in Table 1. This analysis assumes the stress component parallel to the borehole axis corresponds to the overburden stress calculated with a volumetric weight of 0.027 MN^3/m. Note that anisotropy is accounted for by determining the anisotropic elastic moduli in the plane perpendicular to the borehole axis.

These are the first successful in situ stress determinations below the 420 Level at the URL and add to the in situ stress database collected previously at the URL (Chandler et al. 1996). These results indicate that the maximum horizontal principal stress magnitude increases only slightly and that the ratio of the horizontal principal stresses approaches unity with depth.

This indicates that the high horizontal in situ stress magnitudes below thrust fault Fracture Zone 2 are a local anomaly resulting from tectonic forces associated with the fault. The stress magnitudes return to normal values with increasing depth below Fracture Zone 2.

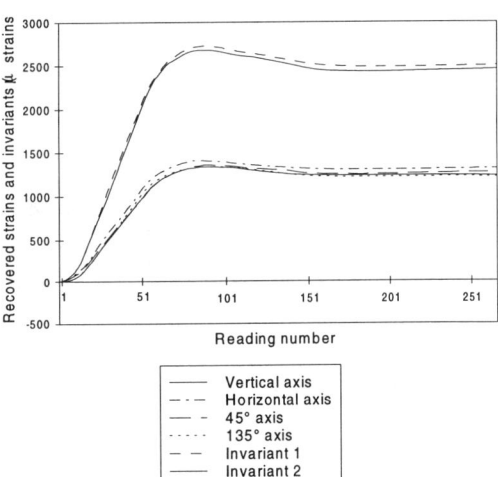

Figure 3. Strain recovery curves for 409.9 m

5 SUMMARY

The DDGS allows overcore in situ stress determinations in high-stress environments where core discing prevents the use of techniques requiring a pilot hole. Successful measurements have been obtained as deep as 518 m in a water-filled borehole plunging at 76°. The initial success rate of only 12% was attributed to commissioning and initial field testing of the concept. Higher success rates are expected in future as many lessons have been learned and improvements to the prototype have been made.

The deep overcoring measurements performed using the DDGS at the URL are the first successful in situ stress determinations below the 420 Level and indicate that the maximum horizontal principal stress magnitude trends slightly upward and that the ratio of the horizontal principal stresses approaches unity with depth.

Therefore the high horizontal in situ stress magnitudes below Fracture Zone 2 are considered to be a local anomaly resulting from tectonic forces associated with the fracture zone. The stress magnitudes return to normal values with increasing depth below the fracture zone.

As far as the authors are aware, these are the deepest successful overcoring stress determinations described in published literature.

ACKNOWLEDGEMENT

The research described in this paper has been jointly funded by AECL and Ontario Hydro under the auspices of the CANDU® Owners Group.

REFERENCES

Chandler, N.A., Read, R.S. & C.D. Martin 1996. In situ stress measurements for nuclear fuel waste repository design. *Proc. 2nd North American Rock Mechanics Symposium, Montréal, Vol. 1, p. 929-936.*

Corthésy, R. & D.E. Gill 1990. The modified doorstopper cell stress measuring technique. *Proc. of Conf. On Stresses in Underground Structures, Ottawa, Canada, p. 23-32.*

Corthésy, R., Gill, D.E. & M.H. Leite 1993. Doorstopper Stress Measurements at the 420 Level of the URL. *Final Report, C.D.T., École Polytechnique de Montréal; Project P1596.*

Hiltscher, R., Martna, J. & L. Strindell 1979. The measurement of triaxial rock stresses in deep boreholes and the use of rock stress measurements in the design and construction of rock openings. *Proc. 4th Int. Cong. Rock Mech., Montreux, Vol. 2., p. 227-234.*

Leite, M.H., Corthésy, R. & D.E. Gill 1996. Deep borehole stress measurements at the URL, Final Report, C.D.T., *École Polytechnique de Montréal; Project P1596.*

Thompson, P.M. (1990). A borehole deformation gauge for stress determinations in deep boreholes. *Proc. of 31st US Rock Mechanics Symposium, Golden, 1990 June, ISRM, p. 579-586.*

Some aspects of a stress calculation model for deep measurements using the modified doorstopper cell

Maria Helena Leite, Robert Corthésy & Denis E. Gill
Department of Civil, Geological and Mining Engineering, Ecole Polytechnique, Montréal, Qué., Canada

Rodney S. Read
Underground Research Laboratory, Atomic Energy of Canada Ltd, Canada

Abstract: A deep borehole stress measurement system has been developed jointly by the Rock Mechanics Laboratory at École Polytechnique in Montréal and Atomic Energy of Canada Ltd in Pinawa, Manitoba, based on the modified doorstopper technique. Since deep stress measurements are carried out in a single water-filled subvertical hole in order to minimize the drilling costs, the stress component parallel to the borehole axis has to be estimated or calculated by the RPR method. This stress calculation method is based on the shape of the strain recovery curve which can be affected by the pressure caused by the water column in the borehole and by the non linear elastic stress-strain relationships shown by the rock at the URL at the depths where the measurements were performed. This paper presents the results of a series of numerical analyses performed to assess the influence of these two factors on the shape of the strain recovery curves, on the magnitude of the recovered strains and on the stress concentration factors at the borehole bottom.

1 INTRODUCTION

Different stress measurement techniques have been used at the URL over the last fifteen years in order to evaluate their potential for the site characterization required in the design of spent fuel repository sites (Chandler et al., 1996). The stress measurements performed have clearly indicated that several distinct stress domains exist at the URL site, the deepest being characterized by high horizontal in situ stresses. As a consequence, overcoring techniques (CSIR triaxial cells, CSIRO cells and borehole deformation gauges) face the problem of core discing during stress relief.

The success obtained with the modified doorstopper strain cell measurement technique (which relies on coring and not overcoring to relieve the stresses) in previous measurements and the fact that this technique requires a very short drilling distance for total stress relief, led AECL to choose it for stress measurements in high stress zones. Moreover, the interpretation model developed by Corthésy et al. (1993) for the determination of stresses from modified doorstopper measurements can take into account the non-linear and anisotropic behavior of rocks resulting from stress induced micro-cracks.

Because of the lack of techniques allowing the accurate measurement of stresses in deep boreholes, AECL started a stress measurement program using the modified doorstopper technique in deep holes (more than 500 meters deep). These measurements are now possible due to a series of improvements to the modified doorstopper stress measurement technique (Leite et al., 1996; Thompson et al., 1997). One of the most significant improvements is the development of a down-the-hole conditioner/data logger or IAM for Intelligent Acquisition Module, developed at the Rock Mechanics Laboratory of École Polytechnique (Leite et al., 1996). Thanks to this data logger, continuous strain readings are obtained during stress relief drilling without a cable running through the drill rods. Technical data of the equipment and procedures used in this measurement program are given by Thompson et al. (1997).

The interpretation of the modified doorstopper stress measurements consists in calculating the partial 2D stresses using the recovered strains and the deformability parameters obtained from the biaxial and diametrical compression tests on the recovered cores. This requires assumptions on the stress-strain relationships of the material. Aspects such as non-linearity, heterogeneity and anisotropy of the stress-strain relationships can be considered in the stress calculation model used (Corthésy et al., 1993). The stresses at the borehole bottom are then converted to far field stresses using the stress concentration factors which depend on the Poisson's ratio. Finally, when measurements in three differently oriented boreholes are available, the partial 2D stresses from these three boreholes can be combined to give the complete 3D stress tensor without making any hypothesis concerning the stress component parallel to the borehole axis. If measurements in a single borehole are available, the stress component parallel to the borehole axis can be obtained with the RPR stress calculation method (Corthésy et al., 1994). This method is based on the fact that, for a given Poisson's ratio, there exists a relationship between two parameters called RPR (Recovered to Peak Ratio) and SR (Stress Ratio). The first is defined as the ratio between the mean strain invariants corresponding to the recovered and peak strains measured on the strain recovery curves. The second is the ratio between the far-field stress component parallel to the borehole axis and the far-field stress invariant in the plane perpendicular to the borehole axis.

Due to the high cost of drilling deep holes as those involved in the AECL stress measurement program, the execution of modified doorstopper stress measurements were limited to a single near vertical water-filled borehole. This practical limitation has three consequences as far as the interpretation method is concerned. First, a stress concentration factor relating the water pressure to the stresses at the borehole bottom has to be obtained. Secondly, the recovered strains monitored at the borehole bottom have to be corrected, since the presence of water under pressure during stress relief drilling will decrease their magnitude (expansion is considered positive). This decrease will also influence the magnitude of the peak strains and, possibly, the value of the RPR parameter used in the evaluation of the stress component parallel to the borehole axis by the RPR method. Finally, the water can eventually penetrate existing microcracks during stress relief drilling. As a consequence, the stress-strain relationships obtained by reloading the overcores can be different from those prevailing during the stress relief process.

The first two aspects are studied in the present paper as well as the influence of the non linearity of the stress strain relationships on the strain recovery curves.

2 INFLUENCE OF WATER PRESSURE

In order to evaluate the influence of water pressure on the stresses at the borehole bottom, finite element analyses have been performed with the program COSMOS/M from Structural Research Inc.
The geometry of the model is such that the borehole can be considered to be drilled in an infinite medium and the material is taken as linear elastic, homogeneous and isotropic. A constant water pressure of 5 MPa is applied to the borehole walls and bottom. This water pressure corresponds to the water column prevailing during a measurement in a 500 meter deep borehole.

If no water pressure is applied to the borehole walls and bottom, the stresses at the borehole bottom calculated from the recovered strains are related to the far-field stress components through the stress concentration factors in the following way (Rahn, 1984):

$$\bar{\sigma}_x = H_1 \sigma_x + H_2 \sigma_y + H_3 \sigma_z \qquad (1)$$

$$\bar{\sigma}_y = H_2 \sigma_x + H_1 \sigma_y + H_3 \sigma_z \qquad (2)$$

$$\bar{\tau}_{xy} = H_4 \tau_{xy} \qquad (3)$$

In this equation, the XY plane is the borehole bottom plane and the Z direction is parallel to the borehole axis; $\bar{\sigma}_x, \bar{\sigma}_y$ and $\bar{\sigma}_z$ are, respectively, the normal stresses in the X, Y and Z directions at the borehole bottom; $\bar{\tau}_{xy}$ is the shear stress in the XY borehole bottom plane; σ_x, σ_y, σ_z and τ_{xy} are corresponding far-field stresses; H_1, H_2 and H_3 are the stress concentration factors which depend on the Poisson's ratio at the measurement point.

When the borehole walls and the measurement plane are submitted to a hydrostatic pressure p_o, the normal stresses at the borehole bottom are given by:

$$\bar{\sigma}_x = H_1 \sigma_x + H_2 \sigma_y + H_3 \sigma_z - H_5 p_o \qquad (4)$$

$$\bar{\sigma}_y = H_2 \sigma_x + H_1 \sigma_y + H_3 \sigma_z - H_5 p_o \qquad (5)$$

where H_5 is the stress concentration factor for the hydrostatic water pressure. It has been obtained from finite element analyses which show that:

$$H_5 = 0.61 \nu + 0.1862 \qquad (6)$$

As long as the stress relief drilling simulation proceeds, the 5 MPa pressure is also applied to the overcore and the newly created borehole wall. For a given Poisson's ratio, a series of analyses are performed to simulate the stress relief drilling advance. During this phase, the recovered core is submitted to a hydrostatic pressure which will induce compressive strains in the plane of the borehole bottom while the stress relief drilling operation proceeds. As a consequence, the recovered strains reflect, on one hand, the relief of a far-field stress state and on the other hand, the applied water pressure.

The results of these analyses were used to produce normalized strain recovery curves corresponding to different Poisson's ratios. The strains are normalized by the Young's modulus used in the numerical analyses and the stress relief drilling distance is normalized by the borehole radius. Figure 1 shows these normalized strain recovery curves. Hence, for each measurement, corrected strain recovery curves can be obtained by adding to the measured in situ strains corresponding to a certain *drilling distance/borehole radius* ratio, the strain obtained from the normalized curve corresponding to the Poisson's ratio of the rock.

This value is obtained by multiplying the normalized strain by the average Young's modulus in the plane of the borehole bottom obtained from the biaxial reloading. Finally, since these values correspond to a water pressure of 5 MPa (numerical analyses), a linear regression is used to obtain the strains corresponding to the water pressure prevailing at the borehole bottom during drilling.

3 THE INFLUENCE OF NON LINEARITY OF THE STRESS-STRAIN RELATIONSHIPS ON THE RECOVERY CURVES

A series of numerical analyses were performed with FLAC, an explicit finite differences code from Itasca Consulting Group. FLAC was chosen for two main reasons: user-built stress-strain relationships can be implemented in a relatively simple way and the excavation process can be simulated by transforming elements of the grid into "null" elements. An axysimmetric model with 6000 elements was used for the analyses. The first step consisted in simulating the excavation of the borehole up to the measuring point. The stress relief operation was then simulated by progressively increasing the number of "null" elements located near the borehole wall until the final geometry shown in Figure 2 was reached.

The far-field stress state used for the analyses was arbitrarily chosen as $\sigma_x = \sigma_y = 80$ MPa and $\sigma_z = 50$ MPa. These stress components are principal stresses, the XY plane being perpendicular to the borehole axis and the Z axis being parallel to it.

Other than the far-field stresses, in a certain number of analyses, an internal pressure of 5 MPa was also applied to the borehole wall at all stages of the stress relief drilling process. In this way, the influence of the drilling water pressure could also be evaluated for the non linear elastic behavior of the material.

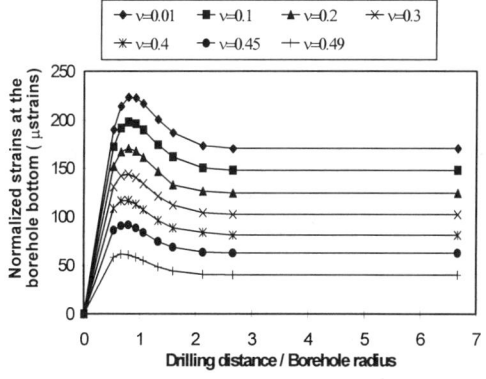

Figure 1 – Normalized strains induced by a water pressure of 5 MPa during stress relief drilling.

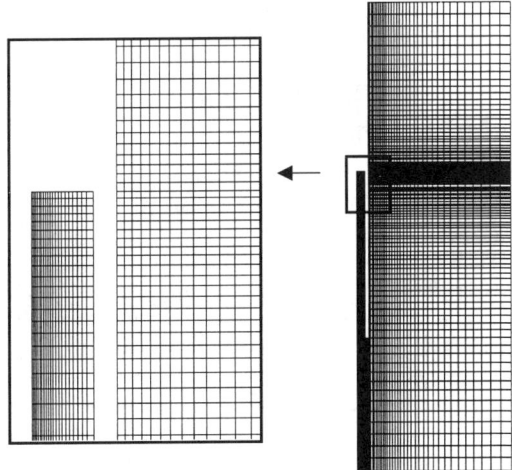

Figure 2 - Grid used for the analyses – excavation after complete stress relief.

Stress-strain relationships for linear elastic materials are formulated in FLAC in terms of the shear and bulk moduli, G and K, defined respectively as:

$$G = \frac{E}{2(1+\nu)} \quad (7)$$

$$K = \frac{E}{3(1-2\nu)} \quad (8)$$

where E is the Young's modulus of the material and ν is the Poisson's ratio of the material.

Four linear elastic analyses are presented, with two different values of Young's modulus. For each value, the elastic moduli K and G were calculated for two values of Poisson's ratio, namely, 0.1 and 0.3, as shown in Table I.

Table I
Tangent elastic moduli for the linear elastic analyses

ν	Elastic modulus #1 (GPa)		Elastic modulus #2 (GPa)	
	K	G	K	G
0.1	5.824	6.354	13.530	14.760
0.3	9.060	4.181	21.047	9.714

The non linear elastic behavior was implemented in the analyses through the use of a programming language called FISH available in FLAC. The elastic tangent moduli K and G were introduced in the code as functions of the mean stress σ_m and of the maximum absolute value of the stress deviators, S_{max}, respectively.

In the following, the procedure leading to these functions is described. The biaxial loading of a recovered core (TD-238.9), considered to be representative of the non linear behavior shown by the recovered cores (Leite et al., 1996), has been chosen as the basis for the definition of the functions relating the tangent elastic moduli K and G to the stress level. For each load level, the values of the mean and deviatoric stresses are calculated. The corresponding mean and deviatoric strains are also calculated from the average strain under the rosette for a certain value of Poisson's ratio. From these values, second-order polynomial regressions are calculated between the mean stress and the mean strain (ε_m) and between the maximum deviatoric stress and the maximum deviatoric strain (e_{max}).

These regressions are of the type:

$$\varepsilon_m = k_o + k_1 \sigma_m + k_2 \sigma_m^2 \quad (9)$$

and

$$e_{max} = g_o + g_1 S_{max} + g_2 S_{max}^2 \quad (10)$$

where k_o, k_1, k_2, g_o, g_1 and g_2 depend in part on the Poisson's ratio assumed for the material.

Table II shows the two sets of constants obtained from the polynomial regressions with Poisson's ratio of 0.1 and 0.3.

Table II
Constants of the polynomial regressions of the ε_m - σ_m and e_{max} - S_{max} relationships

Regression constants	$\nu = 0.1$	$\nu = 0.3$
K_o	-2.894E-12	-2.053E-12
K_1	58.948	37.895
k_2	-1.287	-8.272E-01
g_o	-6.240E-12	-6.3571E-12
g_1	81.054	123.160
g_2	-1.769	-2.688

In the above equations stresses are given in MPa and strains in microstrains.

For each element of the grid, the tangent elastic moduli G and K are calculated using the polynomial regressions by the following functions:

$$G = \frac{1}{2 \frac{\partial}{\partial S_{max}}(g_o + g_1 S_{max} + g_2 S_{max}^2)} \quad (11)$$

$$K = \frac{1}{3 \frac{\partial}{\partial \sigma_m}(k_o + k_1 \sigma_m + k_2 \sigma_m^2)} \quad (12)$$

As stress relief drilling proceeds, the mean stress and the stress deviators are periodically calculated at the center of each element of the grid and the tangent elastic moduli K and G are recalculated according to the functions described above. A record of the recalculated values is kept so that the evolution of the tangent elastic moduli at the measuring point (borehole bottom) can be followed. The two sets of elastic moduli (#1 and #2) used for the linear elastic analyses correspond to the tangent initial and final moduli of the non linear analyses.

Table III presents the cases studied in the present paper.

Table III
Cases studied in the present paper

Case	Stress-strain Relationship	Water pressure (MPa)	ν
1	Linear, modulus #1	0	0.1
2	Linear, modulus #1	5	
3	Linear, modulus #2	5	
4	Non linear	5	
5	Linear, modulus #1	0	0.3
6	Linear, modulus #1	5	
7	Linear, modulus #2	5	
8	Non linear	5	
9	Non linear	0	

Figure 3 illustrates the strain recovery curves for both the linear elastic and non linear elastic analyses for a Poisson's ratio of 0.3.

The strain recovery curves obtained from the numerical analyses can be used to calculate the RPR values for both the linear and non linear elastic analyses. These values are presented in Table IV.

The results of the numerical analyses performed can be used to make a preliminary evaluation of the influence of the non linearity of the stress-strain relationships on the stress concentration factors at the borehole bottom. A complete investigation on this subject requires a considerably higher number of numerical analyses with a 3D version of the code so that the influence of each far-field stress component on the stresses at the borehole bottom can be isolated. However, the comparison of the stress components at the borehole bottom for both linear and non linear analyses can give some insight on this problem.

Table IV
RPR values calculated from the numerical analyses

Elastic behavior	RPR	
	ν=0.1	ν=0.3
Linear modulus #1, no water	0.771	0.762
Linear modulus #1	0.774	0.767
Linear modulus #2	0.776	0.766
Non linear	0.806	0.791

Four numerical analyses are chosen to evaluate the influence of non linearity on the stress concentration factors. They correspond to linear and non linear tangent moduli calculated for Poisson's ratios of 0.1 and 0.3, considered to be representative of the recovered cores from the stress measurements performed in the deep boreholes. No water pressure is applied to the borehole walls. Table V presents the values of the stress component in the plane of measurement, at the centre of the borehole, obtained from the numerical analyses as well as the value of this stress component calculated with the stress concentration factors proposed by Rahn (1984) for linear elastic materials.

Table V
Stress component at the borehole bottom

ν	Elastic behavior	σ_{NUM} (MPa)	σ_{RAHN} (MPa)	$\frac{\sigma_{LINEAR}}{\sigma_{RAHN}}$	$\frac{\sigma_{NON\ LINEAR}}{\sigma_{LINEAR}}$
0.1	Linear	75.32	75.08	1.003	-
	Non linear	76.76	-	-	1.019
0.3	Linear	71.80	71.79	1.000	-
	Non linear	77.55	-	-	1.079

4 DISCUSSION AND CONCLUSIONS

A complete non linear elastic stress calculation model should include the influence of non linear elasticity at three levels: on the calculation of stresses present at the borehole bottom from the recovered strains and the stress-strain relationships,

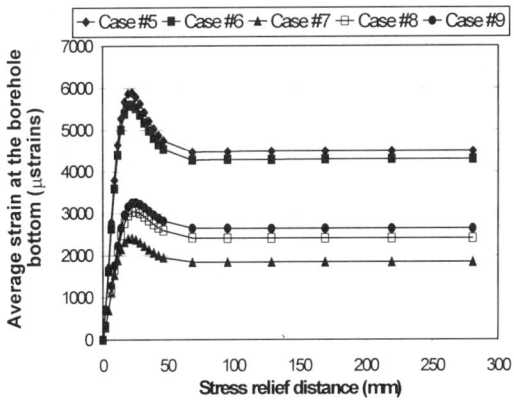

Figure 3 – Average strain at the borehole bottom form the numerical analyses (Cases #5 to 9).

on the stress concentration factors at the borehole bottom and on the RPR values. Although the first step can be done with a reasonable effort (Corthésy et al., 1993), the second two are very time consuming. This can only be accomplished through 3D numerical analyses where non linear elastic behavior of the of rock under study is modelled. Moreover, the response of a numerical analysis depends on the stress state applied to the model which is not known *a priori*. An iterative procedure has to be adopted and a great number of analyses performed to evaluate the influence of a given degree of non linearity on the stress concentration factors and RPR values. This is also true for the magnitude of the recovered strains induced by the water pressure.

Therefore it seems appropriate to estimate the error associated by neglecting the influence of non linearity on both the RPR values and stress concentration factors on the calculated stresses. From the results shown in Tables IV and V, it seems that for the degree of non linearity observed on the Lac du Bonnet granite, RPR values and stress concentration factors obtained from linear analyses do not differ significantly from the non linear cases. In the following, the recovered strains obtained from the numerical analysis corresponding to case #9 are used as an in situ strain recovery curve to calculate the stresses applied to the model. The non linear elastic behavior is incorporated in the calculations only at the first level which again is the calculation of the stresses at the borehole bottom form the recovered strains. Then, RPR values and stress concentration factors for a linear material are used to calculate the far-field stress components.

Table VI
Calculated stresses

Calculation model for the stresses at the borehole bottom	Stress component (MPa)	
	$\sigma_x = \sigma_y$	σ_z
Applied	80.00	50.00
Non linear elasticity	80.52	53.88
Linear elasticity	44.61	29.85

Also included in Table VI are the stresses calculated assuming a linear elastic behavior of the rock for all the calculation process, including the calculation of the stresses at the borehole bottom. When compared to the applied stresses, it becomes evident that the linear elastic approach is not suitable. On the other hand, maximum errors of 10.8% are found when non linearity is considered for the calculation of stresses at the borehole bottom even though the RPR values and stress concentration factors for linear rocks are considered in the calculation.

This simple example shows that the non linear elastic behavior cannot be neglected on the calculation of the stresses at the borehole bottom. However, depending on the degree of non linearity, stress concentration factors and RPR values obtained for linear materials can be used. Once a preliminary stress state is obtained in this way, numerical analyses can be performed to evaluate the influence of non linear elasticity on the stress concentration factors, on the RPR and on the recovered strains induced by water pressure.

ACKNOWLEDGMENTS

The senior author thanks FCAR from the Québec governement for the research grant 98-NC-1567.

REFERENCES

Chandler, N.A., Read, R.S., Martin, C.D. 1996 In situ stress measurement for nuclear fuel waste repository design, *NARMS'96*, Vol.1: 929-936.

Corthésy, R., Gill, D.E., Leite, M.H., Thompson, P.M. 1993 Stress measurements in high stress zones using the modified doorstopper cell, Can. Geotech. J., Vol. 30: 991-1002.

Leite, M.H., Corthésy, R., Gill, D.E., St-Onge, M., Nguyen, D. 1996 The IAM - A down the hole conditioner-data logger for the modified doorstopper technique, *NARMS'96*, Vol.1: 897-904.

Rahn, W. 1984 Stress concentration factors for the interpretation of doorstopper measurements in anisotropic rocks, *Int. J. Rock Mech.*, Vol. 21:313-326.

Thompson, P.M., Corthésy, R., Leite, M.H. 1997 Overcoring rock stress determinations at great depth using the doorstopper gauge, *Proc. RS Kumamoto'97*.

Use of the modified doorstopper-IAM combination as a stress-meter

Robert Corthésy, Maria Helena Leite & Denis E. Gill
Department of Civil, Geological and Mining Engineering, Ecole Polytechnique, Montréal, Qué., Canada

Don Nguyen
Service Géologie, Géotechnique et Accès, Hydro-Québec, Montréal, Qué., Canada

ABSTRACT: The modified doorstopper stress-meter developped jointly by École Polytechnique and Hydro-Québec, was designed for the monitoring of the very low stress variations found in civil engineering concrete construction such as dams. The sensor uses a double modified doorstopper half-bridge cell encapsulated in a water resistant aluminium chamber. It is linked to the IAM, a high precision conditionner-data logger, specifically designed to work in conjunction with the modified doorstopper. Results from both laboratory and field tests show the stability and sensitivity that can be attained with the new stress-meter.

1 INTRODUCTION

Stress monitoring has become part of the design methodology in rock mechanics as it allows to check the validity of the models, parameters, assumptions and hypotheses on which this design is based. The purpose of stress-meters is to measure relative stresses (stress variations in time). These instruments are usually installed in boreholes where they monitor strain or displacement variations at borehole walls. They can be divided into three categories depending on their stiffness when compared to that of the rock being monitored. They can be classified as stiff, semi-stiff or soft stress-meters.

In order to be considered stiff, the instrument must have a stiffness two to four times greater than that of the host material. The principles of stiff inclusions are presented and discussed in detail by Peleg (1968). The advantage of the stiff inclusion is that only the Poisson's ratio of the host rock must be known in order to calculate the stress variations. These stiff inclusions are photoelastic discs, bronze cylinders, steel cylinders. Due to the incompressibility of the fluids, hydraulic cells can also be considered as stiff inclusions. The problem associated with this category of stress-meter is the fact that due to their relatively high stiffness, they are not very sensitive since they will not deform much. The other problem is that when they are bonded to the hole wall, expansion of the hole will eventually break the contact with the sensor.

In the second category of stress-meters, the semi-stiff meters require the knowledge of both the rock deformability properties and the inclusion properties. Initially developed by Hawkes and Hooker (1974), these instruments are usually steel rings instrumented with vibrating wire gauges. These rings are pressed fit in a borehole and will deform along a diameter. One of the problems associated with these instruments is the difficulty to calculate correctly the stress variations since the formulas require the knowledge of many parameters, some of which are difficult to estimate. Moreover, due to the relatively high contact pressure between the rings and the borehole walls, creep may occur in softer rocks. Another type of stress-meter which can be associated to the semi-stiff category is the solid inclusion which is made of the same material as the host material. This concept has been adopted more recently by Bois et al. (1994) to monitor stress changes in concrete dams using a concrete cylinder instrumented with differently oriented vibrating wire strain gauges. Although no experimental data is presented, this device has the potential (in theory) to monitor three dimensionnal stress changes. The problem is that the interpretation of the measurements is quite complex and very much affected by the boundary conditions between the cylinder and the borehole wall, which again, are difficult to control and evaluate. Moreover, the concrete and grout used to bond the cylinder to the hole wall are not stable in time due to curing effects. Consequently, semi-stiff instruments although a little more sensitive than the stiff inclusions, present very few advantages over the latter.

The last category of stress-meters is the soft stress-meter which does not interfere with the deformation of the host material. The advantages are a higher sensitivity and simpler interpretation models since there is no interaction between the stress meter and the borehole. Although special instruments have been developped for this purpose like the CSIRO yoke gauge (Walton & Worotnicki, 1986), these soft stress-meters are mostly conventionnal stress measurement cells like the CSIRO hollow inclusion cell or CSIR triaxial cells and CSIR biaxial cells or doorstoppers (Myrvang & Hansen, 1990).

From this very brief review of stress-meters, we have at one end the stiff instruments giving results which are relatively simple to interpret but which lack sensitivity. At the other end, there are the soft inclusions which are sensitive, yield easily interpretable results but which suffer from stability problems. In between, the semi-stiff instruments yield results that are complex to interpret, show drift problems and a low sensitivity.

2 DESIGN OF THE MODIFIED DOORSTOPPER STRESS-METER

As mentioned in the previous section, the only instrument category which has the potential to measure low stress variations and which minimizes the complexity involved in the stress calculations are the soft inclusions. Another advantage with this category of instruments is the possibility to recover them by overcoring, which allows the calculation of absolute stresses at the measurement point, so the measured stress variations can be linked to an absolute stress tensor. If the stability problems reported in the literature can be overcome with soft stress-meters, they constitute, in the authors view, the best approach to stress variation monitoring. Moreover, if the stress-meter allows the measurement of low stress variations over long periods of time, it will become a universal instrument as it will certainly allow to monitor higher stress variations on shorter periods of time as found, for instance, in some mining applications.

2.1 Design considerations

The objective was to develop a stress meter with an accuracy of ±0.1 MPa for monitoring time spans of over 1 year. Because of the intrinsic advantages of the biaxial CSIR cell (doorstopper cell), it was decided to use it as the basis of the sensor used to monitor stress variations. This instrument comprises a four element strain gauge rosette encapsulated in a rubber casing. This rosette is bonded at the flattened bottom of a borehole. The advantage of using the doorstopper is that very closely spaced measurements can be performed in the same hole.

The measurement sequence requires the modified doorstopper stress-meter to be installed at the point of interest. Following the monitoring period, the stress-meter is recovered by stress relief drilling, allowing an evaluation of the absolute stress tensor. The stress components in the plane perpendicular to the hole axis and the normal component parallel to it can be calculated with the RPR method (Corthésy et al., 1994). With this sequence, the stress variations can be monitored in absolute terms.

An alternate measurement sequence which requires the stress field to be homogeneous near the measurement point, would consist in performing an absolute stress measurement a few cm before the monitoring point. This would allow a second estimation of the stress variation which would be calculated as the difference between the two measured absolute stress tensors.

The modified doorstopper stress-meter which will now be described, can be divided into three subsystems. One is the sensor which includes the sensing elements for strains and temperature, the second comprises the conditioning system and the third is the data logger. Detail on these last two items can be found in Leite et al. (1996).

2.2 Sensor head

Because Hydro-Québec was interested in monitoring stress variations of both mechanical and thermal origin in its concrete dams, the sensor had to be designed accordingly. This requires to measure strains from all origins but to exclude thermoelectrical effects or resistance variations due to a change in the resistivity ρ of the strain gauge material and conductors. This is achieved by bonding a dummy doorstopper to an Invar disk and using it as the compensator arm in a half bridge connection scheme. Since the Invar disk will show very low dilation or contraction under temperature variations (the thermal coefficient of expansion is approximately 1.5 µstrains /°C), the compensating arm will eliminate all electric induced drifts. In Myrvang & Hansen's (1990) design, the

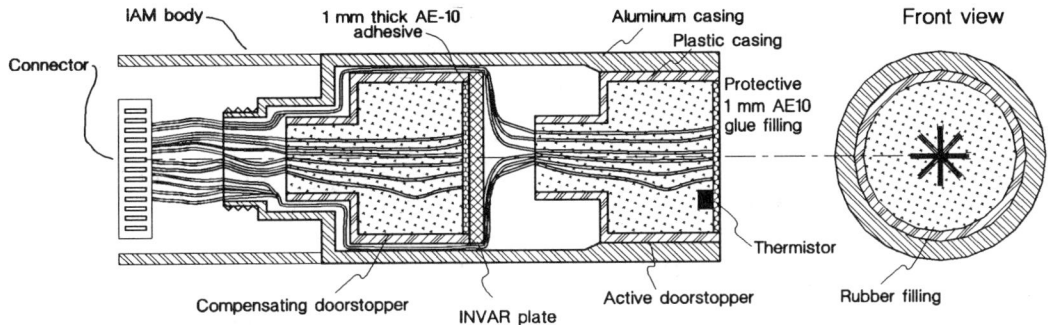

Figure 1: Cross sectional view of the modified doorstopper stress-meter sensor head.

compensating doorstopper is bonded on a piece of rock core. With this scheme, correct thermoelectrical compensation is obtained but thermomechanical effects will only be eliminated if the active and compensating gauges are bonded on rock showing exactly the same thermal expansion coefficients, which is difficult to achieve on heterogeneous materials such as rocks. The modified doorstopper also includes a thermistor in contact with the borehole bottom that allows to monitor temperature variations at the measurement point. The active gauges are covered by a 1 mm thick protective film made of AE-10 adhesive from Micro-Measurement Corp.

Finite element analyses have shown that the loss of sensitivity (strains lost between the rock and the strain gauges) due to a 1 mm thick protective film is negligible. The active and compensating modified doorstoppers are sealed in a protective aluminium housing which is also used to mount the sensor head to the data logger-conditioner. Figure 1 illustrates a cut through the sensor head showing all its components. The back end of the sensor head is connected directly to the IAM conditioner-data logger, which limits the lead wire length to a few centimetres.

3 LABORATORY TESTING OF THE MODIFIED DOORSTOPPER STRESS-METER

Prior to trial testing of the modified doorstopper stress-meter in the field, it was submitted to adverse conditions in the laboratory for a two month period. Stress-meters were bonded to aluminium and concrete cores and submitted to a highly humid environment (100% relative humidity) in a soil storage chamber whith no temperature control. Figure 2 shows the measured strains and

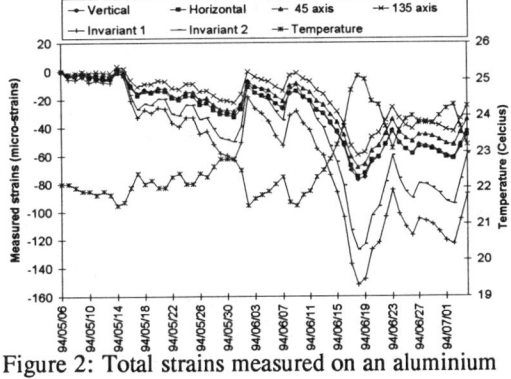

Figure 2: Total strains measured on an aluminium core.

temperature on the aluminium core during the two months period covered by the lab tests.

The strain readings show important fluctuations and as will be shown, this is caused by the temperature variations in the chamber which dilate and contract the aluminium. It must be remembered that the sensor is designed to monitor these thermal strains. Figure 3 shows the relationship between the strain gauge readings and the temperature.

Theoretically, the linear regressions should give the thermal expansion factor α of the aluminium. Since the Invar compensator reduces the measured strains by 1.5 μ strain per °C, this value must be added to the regression slopes. The mean α is thus equal to 18.2 μ strains per °C, which compares very well with published α values comprised between 19.9 to 23.2 μ strains per °C for aluminium. Knowing the α parameter for each strain gauge, it is possible to subtract from the measured strains the thermomechanical effects in order to evaluate the stability of the stress-meter. These corrected curves are shown in figure 4.

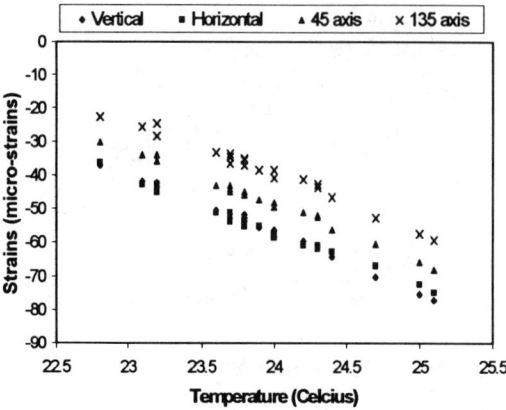

Figure 3 : Temperature-strain relationships on aluminium core.

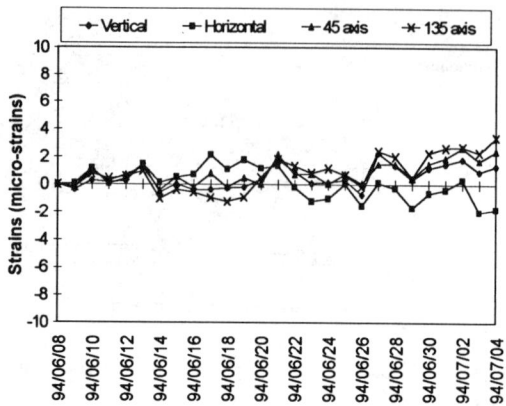

Figure 5: Removal of temperature effects and adhesive curing period.

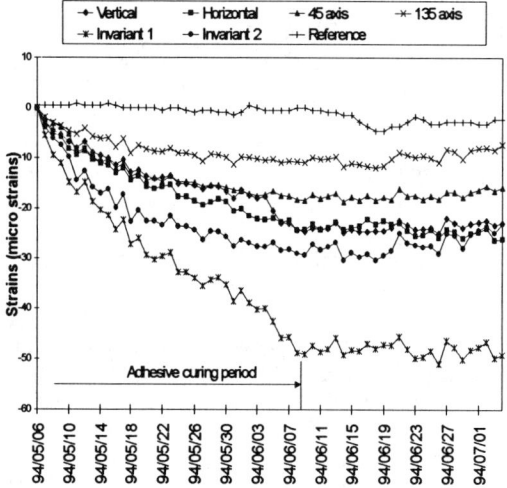

Figure 4 : Temperature effects removed from the total strains.

What comes out from these curves is that during the first month, there is a drift which we believe to be related to the curing of the adhesive. If this first month of readings is eliminated, we end up with figure 5 where, over a one month period, extreme values of strains are comprised between -2 and +3.4 μ strains (average of 0.1 μ strains per day).

A stress meter was also bonded to a concrete core and stored in the same conditions as the aluminium core. The magnitude of the strain readings was much greater than what was observed on the aluminium core and no stabilization occurred after the adhesive curing period. Since the concrete core was initially dry, it is believed that the monitored strains were caused by the absorption of water that caused the core to dilate. This was confirmed by putting the instrumented core in a dry environment which caused the strains to show a contraction of the concrete. This test showed the importance of maintaining a constant humidity in the borehole where the stress-meter is to be installed.

4 FIELD APPLICATION OF THE MODIFIED DOORSTOPPER STRESS-METER

After successfully testing the modified doorstopper stress-meter in the laboratory, three instruments were installed in a multiple arch dam in north-eastern Québec in May 1996. The holes were drilled from a permanent shelter which maintains a relatively constant temperature at the base of the arches. This made the site ideal for a field validation as the stress variations should be very low and the stress-meter should not monitor high stress variations. In the authors view, demonstrating the performance of a stress-meter should not be done next to an underground mine stope being exploited, as is often done, since this will not allow to verify the stability of the instrument which is an essential requirement for a stress-meter.

Figure 6 shows the setup used to maintain the instrument in a stable position for long periods of time so the weight of the stress-meter does not cause creep at the measurement point. The spring loaded stabilizing cylinder is kept in position as

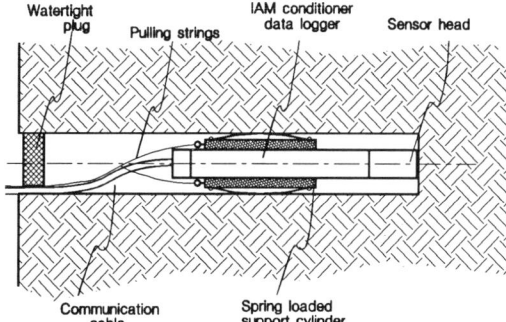

Figure 6: Field setup used to maintain stress-meter in a stable position in the borehole.

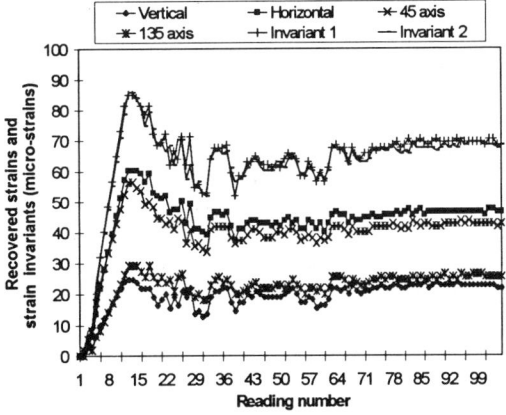

Figure 8 : Strain recovery curves for absolute stress measurement using the stress-meter.

long as the stress variations are monitored. When comes the time to recover the modified doorstopper stress-meter by performing an absolute stress measurement, the stabilizing cylinder is retrieved by pulling on the strings attached to it. Retrieving the cylinder allows the drill bit to pass freely around the stress-meter. To avoid having changes in relative humidity inside the borehole during the monitoring period, the collar is plugged and sealed with caulking. The plug is removed when the absolute measurement is performed. Figure 7 shows the strain and temperature variations monitored during a six months period with stress-meter #3 installed in the multiple arch dam.

As already mentioned, the first month of readings is not considered because of the initial adhesive related drift. As expected, this figure shows that no significant strain variations has occurred. The reference gauge shows a maximum drift of 2.7 µ strains while the temperature changed less than 0.6 °C. It is interesting to note that during the monitoring period, the temperature outside the shelter varied from over 30 °C to less that -40 °C, which shows the effectiveness of the thermal shelter. In December 1996, the three modified doorstopper stress-meters were recovered, allowing the calculation of the absolute stress tensor at the monitoring points using the RPR method (Corthésy et al., 1994). Figure 8 shows the strain recovery curves obtained from stress-meter #3.

Although some vibrations are sensed during the stress relief drilling, the quality of the measurement can be assessed by the perfect match of the strain invariants and the overall aspect of the curves.

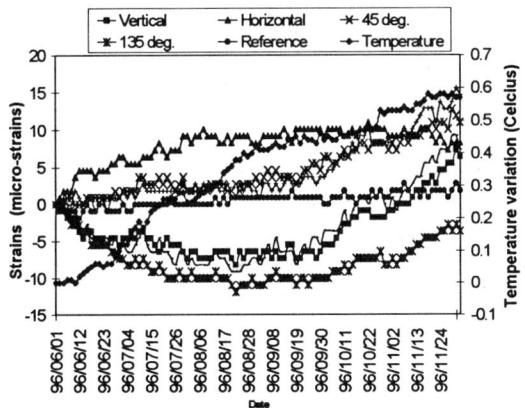

Figure 7: Total strain variations measured in multiple arch dam.

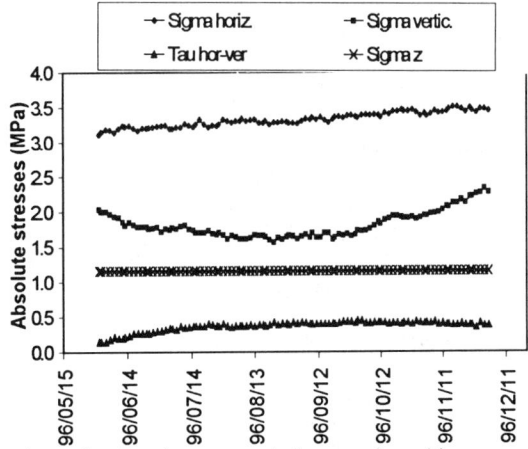

Figure 9 : Total stress variation monitored in a multiple arch dam.

Starting from these known stress values, and working our way back with the measured strain variations, allows to plot the total stress variations in the measurement plane as shown in Figure 9.

This figure confirms that the stress variations in the monitored zone are relatively small (0.5 MPa being the maximum variation monitored for σ_{vert}). It can be noted that the stress component σ_z, parallel to the hole axis calculated with the RPR method, has been considered constant throughout the monitoring period.

5 DISCUSSION AND CONCLUSIONS

As is the case with most stress-meters, the calculation of the stress variations presented in Figure 9 using the modified doorstopper stress-meter in a single hole requires the assumption that the stress component along the hole axis is constant throughout the monitoring period. If initial and final absolute stresses are measured, it is possible to avoid using this assumption by considering the difference between the initial and final stress component parallel to the hole axis as being distributed in time following a certain pattern. One such pattern is a linear distribution in time, although there is no way to verify it. Working with three converging boreholes is the only way to determine the stress variation in 3D without any assumption regarding the behaviour of certain stress components.

However, the stress-meter offers the possibility of bonding at a free surface instead of a borehole bottom. This greatly simplifies the stress calculation since plane stress conditions prevail and no unverified assumption is required.

As mentioned previously, one problem encountered with most stress-meters is to convert the measured strains or displacements variations into stress variations. One reason for that is the difficulty of knowing the correct deformability parameters at the measurement point. With the modified doorstopper stress-meter, reloading the recovered core following a procedure developed by Corthésy et al. (1993), not only can these parameters be obtained simply but the transformation of strains into stresses can be done by considering the heterogeneity (Leite et al., 1993) and the anisotropy (Corthésy et al., 1993) found at the measurement point. This advantage is unique to the modified doorstopper stress-meter.

The modified doorstopper stress-meter presented in this paper has various advantages, the most important being its sensitivity and stability, as confirmed by both laboratory and field tests once the initial curing period is eliminated. The initial drift we noted in the lab is also present in Myrvang & Hansen's 1990 paper, but these authors relate it to actual stress variations.

The laboratory tests on an aluminium cylinder have shown that the stress-meter allows the correct estimation of the thermal coefficient of deformability α.

Moreover, this instrument has the advantage of allowing the measurement of the absolute stresses, so the stress variations can be expressed in terms of total variations.

Finally, these stresses are accurately determined since the heterogeneity and anisotropy of the rock or concrete at the measurement point can be accounted for. Such an advantage is not available with other stress monitoring instruments.

REFERENCES

Bois, A.P., Ballivy, G., Saleh, K., 1994 Monitoring stress changes in three dimensions using a solid cylindrical cell. *Int. J. of Rock Mech. Min. Sci. and Geomech. Abstr.* vol. 31, no 6, pp. 707-718.

Corthésy, R., Gill, D.E., Leite, M.H. 1993 An integrated approach to rock stress measurement in anisotropic non linear elastic rock. *Int.J. Rock Mech. Min. Sci.*, Vol. 30, no. 3, pp. 395-411.

Corthésy, R., Leite, M.H., He, G., Gill, D.E. 1994. The RPR method for the doorstopper technique; Four or six stress components from one or two boreholes", *Int.J.Rock Mech .Min. Sci.*, Vol. 31, no. 5., pp. 507-516.

Hawkes, I., Hooker, V.E. 1974. The vibrating wire stressmeter", *Proc. 3rd ISRM Cong, Denver.* Vol. 2, part A, pp. 439-444.

Leite M.H., Corthésy, R., Gill, D.E. 1993 Stress and strain measurement scales Influence of micro-heterogeneity, *Proc. 24th APCOM*, pp. 277-284.

Leite, M.H., Corthésy, R., Gill, D.E., St-Onge, M., Nguyen, D. 1996. The IAM - A down-the-hole data logger conditionner for the modified doorstopper technique. *2nd North American Rock Mechanics Symposium, Montréal*, pp. 897-904.

Myrvang A.M., Hansen, S.E. 1990. Use of modified doorstoppers for rock stress change monitoring. *Proc. 31st U.S. Rock Mech. Symp.*, pp.999-1004.

Peleg, N. 1968. The use of high modulus inclusions for in situ stress determination in viscoelastic rocks", *Tech. Rept, 22-268, Misouri River Division, Corps of Eng., Nebraska*, 68012, p.114.

Improvement in accuracy of the conical-ended borehole technique

Y. Obara & K. Sugawara
Department of Civil Engineering and Architecture, Kumamoto University, Japan

ABSTRACT: The conical-ended borehole technique with 16-element conical shaped strain cell is modified and refined to improve the accuracy in rock stress measurement, increasing the number of strain measured on the conical bottom surface of the borehole from 16 to 24 with a rosette typed strain gauge. It is shown that the proposed method is effective for measuring rock stress with a high accuracy.

1 INTRODUCTION

Knowledge of the rock stress is one of keys to design and construct rock structures. The *in-situ* stresses, therefore, have to be accurately measured. Since rock stress measurement is generally time consuming task, the new technique development is being expected to determine the complete stress state from a measurement in a single borehole. Thus, the stress relief method should be improved to meet its demand.

Many stress relief methods to determine the complete state of stress have been proposed and developed (Mohr 1956, Leeman et al. 1966, Obert et al. 1962, Oka et al. 1968). Among these methods, the CSIRO hollow inclusion stress cell (Warotnicki 1993) has been most popular in the world, since it enables us to accurately measure *in-situ* stresses. The 8-element strain gauge (Kanagawa et al. 1986), the hemispherical shaped strain cell (Sugawara & Obara 1986) and the conical shaped strain cell (Sakaguchi et al. 1992) have been used in Japan. In these three methods, the conical-ended borehole technique with 16-element conical shaped strain cell has an advantage to reduce the time, effort and cost for a series of rock stress measurements, combining the compact overcoring, the diameter of which equals to that of the pilot borehole.

In the present paper, the conical-shaped strain cell is modified and refined to improve the accuracy in rock stress measurement, increasing the number of strain measured on the conical bottom surface of the borehole from 16 to 24 with a rosette typed strain gauge. This paper, firstly, shows how the stress tensor can be determined from the strains on a conical bottom surface of a single borehole. Then the accuracy of the proposed method is compared with that of existing method. Secondly, demonstrating an *in-situ* rock stress measurement by the proposed method and process simulation of the strains and stresses on the conical bottom surface during the stress relieving, it is shown that the proposed method is reliable for *in-situ* rock stress measurements.

2 STRESS TENSOR DETERMINATION

As illustrated in Figure 1, the diameter of the pilot borehole $2R$ is 76mm. The strain measuring points on the conical bottom surface are arranged axisymmetrically along the strain measuring circle of radius 19mm by rotating 45° at a step. The strains ε_θ, ε_ρ and ε_φ on the measuring points, which number is 24, are measured to determine the stress tensor during the compact overcoring, the diameter of which equals to the pilot borehole. The angles between ε_θ, ε_ρ and ε_φ equal to 45°.

For the analysis of the relation between the strains and the stress tensor, the cylindrical coordinates (ρ, θ, z), the spherical coordinates (ρ, θ, ϕ) and the Cartesian coordinates (x, y, z) are defined respectively, making the z-axis coincident with the axis of a borehole. The difference between the z coordinate of the plane including the strain measuring circle and the head of the compact overcoring is defined by L.

The stress tensor, i.e. the original stress, at a certain point within a rock mass, existing prior to boring, can be represented as

$$\{\sigma\} = \{\sigma_x, \sigma_y, \sigma_z, \tau_{yz}, \tau_{zx}, \tau_{xy}\}^T \qquad (1)$$

in the Cartesian coordinates. The strains ε_θ, ε_ρ and ε_φ on a measuring point represent ε_1, ε_2 and ε_3. Since

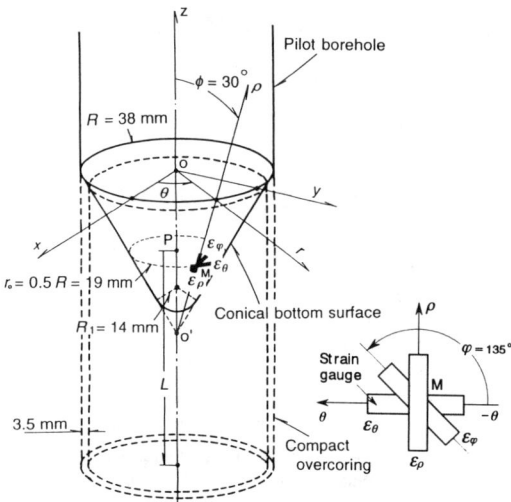

Figure 1 Coordinate system and strains to be measured on a conical bottom surface, compact overcoring, and three components of strain at a measuring point M in the left figure.

these depend on the distance L and the coordinate θ, ε_j can be written as $\varepsilon_j(L,\theta)$, and represents as $\varepsilon_j(-\infty,\theta)$ at the commencement of the compact overcoring in the case that L equals to -33mm, and as $\varepsilon_j(-\infty,\theta)$ at the completion of the compact overcoring. In the latter case, $\varepsilon_j(-\infty,\theta)$ equals to zero.

The measured strains represent as $\varepsilon^*_j(L,\theta)$ in the same manner. These are expressed in the value relative to the strains at the commencement of the compact overcoring. Accordingly,

$$\varepsilon^*_j(-\infty,\theta) = 0$$
$$\varepsilon^*_j(+\infty,\theta) = -\varepsilon_j(-\infty,\theta) \quad, \quad j = 1, 2, 3 \quad (2)$$

The measured strains are the value of the strain recovered by means of the stress relief. The strains are written as follows:

$$\varepsilon_j(L,\theta) = \varepsilon^*_j(L,\theta) - \varepsilon^*_j(+\infty,\theta), \quad j = 1, 2, 3 \quad (3)$$

Substituting eqn.(3) into eqn.(2), we obtain eqn.(4).

$$\varepsilon^*_j(L,\theta) = \varepsilon_j(L,\theta) - \varepsilon_j(-\infty,\theta), \quad j = 1, 2, 3 \quad (4)$$

Assuming that the rock mass follows linear elasticity, the relation between the strains and the original stress is written as follows:

$$\varepsilon_j(L,\theta) = F_j(L,\theta) \cdot \{\sigma\}/E, \quad j = 1, 2, 3 \quad (5)$$

where E is the Young's modulus. $F_j(L,\theta)$ is a coefficient matrix and can be represented by eqn.(6).

$$F_j(L,\theta) = \{ A_{j1}(L) + A_{j2}(L)\cos 2\theta,$$
$$A_{j1}(L) - A_{j2}(L)\cos 2\theta, \ C_j(L), \ D_j(L)\sin\theta,$$
$$D_j(L)\cos\theta, \ 2A_{j2}(L)\sin 2\theta \ \}, j = 1, 2, 3 \quad (6)$$

where $A_{j1}(L)$, $A_{j2}(L)$, $C_j(L)$ and $D_j(L)$ are the strain coefficients and functions of L and the Poisson's ratio ν.

By substituting eqn.(5) into eqn.(4), the measured strains are written as follows:

$$\varepsilon^*_j(L,\theta) = H_j(L,\theta) \cdot \{\sigma\}/E$$
$$H_j(L,\theta) = F_j(L,\theta) - F_j(-\infty,\theta), \quad j = 1, 2, 3 \quad (7)$$

Eqn.(7) is the relation between the measured strain and the original stress at a certain stage of the stress relief.

The original stress is also determined from a set of the measured strains at the completion of the compact overcoring. The observation equation is obtained as follows in the case that $L = +\infty$ and $F_j(-\infty,\theta) = 0$.

$$\varepsilon^*_j(+\infty,\theta) = -F_j(-\infty,\theta) \cdot \{\sigma\}/E, \quad j = 1, 2, 3 \quad (8)$$

When the measured strains at the completion of the compact overcoring, number of 24, are denoted by

$$\{\beta(+\infty)\} = \{\beta_1, \beta_2, \ldots, \beta_{24}\}^T \quad (9)$$

the observation equation (8), i.e. the relation between $\{\sigma\}$ and $\{\beta(+\infty)\}$, is rewritten as the following matrix equation.

$$[A(+\infty)]\{\sigma\} = E\{\beta(+\infty)\} \quad (10)$$

where $[A(+\infty)]$ is a 24 by 6 coefficient matrix, elements of which are calculated according to eqn.(6). The normalized version of eqn. (10) is

$$[B(+\infty)]\{\sigma\} = E\{\beta^*(+\infty)\} \quad (11)$$

where $[B(+\infty)] = [A(+\infty)]^T[A(+\infty)]$ and $\{\beta^*(+\infty)\} = [A(+\infty)]^T\{\beta(+\infty)\}$. The most probable values of stress $\{\sigma^*\}$ is determined as follows

$$\{\sigma^*\} = E[C(+\infty)]\{\beta^*(+\infty)\} \quad (12)$$

where $[C(+\infty)]$ is the inverse matrix of $[B(+\infty)]$. The measured strain during the compact overcoring process can be analyzed by substituting the most probable stress, i.e. the original stress, into eqn.(7).

This determination procedure of the original stress, using a set of the measured strains at the completion of the compact overcoring is special case. The original stress can be also determined from a set of the measured strains at a certain stage of the stress relief, evaluating the strain coefficients during the compact overcoring process.

The value of the variances of $\{\sigma^*\}$, represented by

$\{\xi_i^2\} = \{\xi_1^2, \xi_2^2, ..., \xi_6^2\}^T$, can be evaluated as follows:

$$\xi_i^2 = c_{ii} E^2 \xi_m^2 \quad (13)$$

where ξ_m^2 is the variance of the measured strains as follows:

$$\xi_m^2 = S/(n-6), \quad S = \sum_{i=1}^{24} e_i \quad (14)$$

where n is the number of measured strains and equals to 24, and e_i is the residual error of the measured strain. The variance of the measured strains is assumed to be a constant, and c_{ii} is the value of the diagonal elements of $[C(+\infty)]$.

The value of the variance of the stress component is proportional to the magnitude of the c_{ii}. Therefore, the theoretical accuracy of the stress tensor determination can be evaluated by c_{ii}. This means that the high accuracy in the stress tensor determination can be obtained by minimizing the magnitude of the maximum value c_{max} of the diagonal elements c_{ii}.

3 STRAIN COEFFICIENTS

Since no closed-form solutions for the determination of the strain coefficients are available, they have to be evaluated by numerical analysis. In this paper, the Boundary Element Method (BEM) is used to calculate the strain coefficients in eqn.(6). Firstly, the displacements are analyzed by BEM (Mayr et al. 1980), then the strain coefficients have been evaluated for each strain components.

Figure 2 shows the changes of the strain coefficients with the compact overcoring in the case of $v = 0.2$. The lateral axis is the progress of the compact overcoring. The strain coefficients are calculated every 5mm in progress of the compact overcoring. All strain coefficients are changed when the compact overcoring approaches the bottom. After the compact overcoring reaches the bottom section,

Table 1 Starin coefficients on Poisson's ratio : v.

v	A_{11}	A_{13}	A_{21}	A_{23}	A_{31}	A_{32}	A_{33}
1/6	1.015	-1.790	0.052	0.361	0.533	-0.814	-0.715
1/4	1.014	-1.762	-0.021	0.377	0.496	-0.821	-0.693
1/3	1.012	-1.708	-0.095	0.388	0.458	-0.816	-0.660

v	C_1	C_2	C_3	D_{11}	D_{21}	D_{31}	D_{32}
1/6	-0.232	0.642	0.205	0.089	1.593	0.841	-1.816
1/4	-0.323	0.634	0.155	0.100	1.672	0.886	-1.923
1/3	-0.415	0.630	0.108	0.111	1.740	0.926	-2.021

Remarks : $A_{12} = A_{22} = D_{12} = D_{22} = 0$

their changes become small. Then all stain coefficients almost converge to zero more than $L = 50$mm. It is concluded that the stress relief may be achieved in a short progress of the compact overcoring. In addition, the strain coefficients at the completion of the compact overcoring, i.e. $L = +\infty$, are summarized in Table 1.

4 COMPARISON OF ACCURACY

The value of c_{max} are summarized in Table 2, when the stresses around borehole for measurement are relived completely. It is clear that the value of c_{max} decreases with increasing the number of measured strains in the conical-ended borehole techniques. The accuracy of the proposed method is slightly inferior to that of the hemispherical-ended borehole technique. However, the overcoring in the hemispherical-ended borehole technique is adopted a larger diameter one, since the radius of the measuring circle is larger than that of the others. On the other hand, combining the compact overcoring, the conical-ended borehole technique can reduce the time, effort and cost for measurements. Consequently, it is concluded that the 24-element conical-ended borehole technique can be more effectively used for rock stress measurements than the existing one.

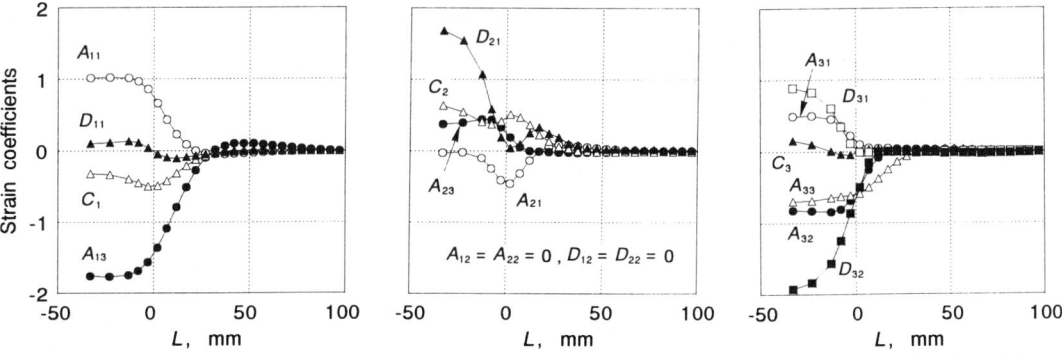

Figure 2 Changes of strain coefficients with the progress of the compact overcoring in the case of $v = 0.2$.

Table 2 Comparison of c_{max}.

Method	Radius of measuring circle: r/R	Number of measured strains: n	Poisson's ratio of rock: v	Maximum value of c_{ii}: c_{max}	Remarks
Conical-ended borehole technique	0.5	24	1/6 1/4 1/3	0.248 0.262 0.289	Proposed
	0.5	16	1/6 1/4 1/3	0.291 0.316 0.360	Sakaguchi et al 1992
	0.589	12	1/6 1/3	0.387 0.467	Kobayashi et al. 1987
Hemispherical-ended borehole technique	0.766	16	1/6 1/4 1/3	0.127 0.133 0.148	Sugawara et al. 1986

5 IN-SITU ROCK STRESS MEASUREMENT

The *in-situ* measurement procedure of the proposed method is almost the same as that of the conventional conical-ended borehole technique. The difference is the strain cell used. The 24-element conical shaped strain cell with rosette typed strain gauges is shown in Figure 3. The 8 rosette gauges, which length is 5mm and width is 1.4mm, are set on the surface of the strain cell. Then the dimensions of the strain cell are the same as those used in the conventional one.

The three times stress measurements were carried out within granodiorite. The borehole for measurement was drilled horizontally from a gallery wall at a depth of 730m. The granodiorite in this field is almost homogeneous and isotropic.

Figure 4 shows an example of changes in strain during the compact overcoring. The lateral axis represents the distance between the measuring circle on the conical bottom and the head of the compact overcoring. The plots are the results of the measurement. The stress relief is achieved at a distance of 70mm, then the strains converge certain constant values each other.

In the case that the rock mass is almost homogeneous and isotopic, it is considered that the most probable stress by the proposed method, represented in the coordinates fixed at the borehole bottom as shown in Figure 1, are almost the same as those by the conventional one and that the standard deviation by the former is smaller than that by the latter. The most probable stress and the standard deviation determined from 24 and 16 strains measured at the completion of the compact overcoring by the procedure of eqn.(9) to (12) with the strain coefficients in Table 1 are summarized in Table 3. It came true as expected results, then it is concluded that the proposed method is more precise than the conventional method.

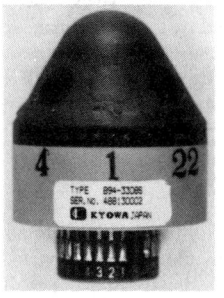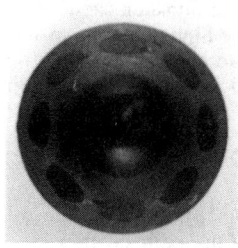

Figure 3 A 24-element conical shaped strain cell.

Theoretical distribution of strain on the bottom surface, corresponding to the most probable stress, are shown in Figure 5 by solid curves. These curves agree well with the measured strains plotted. This means that the measurement was carried out successfully.

6 PROCESS SIMULATION

The process simulation of strain and stress during the compact overcoring can be achieved by means of the strain coefficients shown in Figure 2. Furthermore, the reliability of the measurement can be certified by the process simulation.

The strains of the process simulation during compact overcoring by means of eqn.(8) are shown in Figure 4 as the solid curves. The influence of stress concentration appears when the overcoring approaches the bottom, but the changes in strain are rapid, in all cases, after the overcoring reaches the bottom section. Consequently, the strains are converged to a stable terminal value. The results of the measured strain are good agreement with those of the process simulation. This means that the

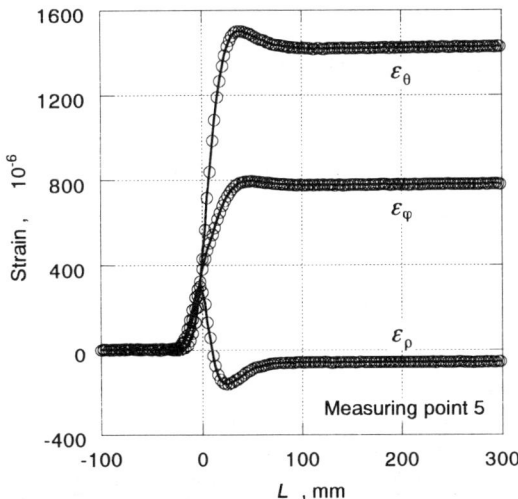

Figure 4 An example of the strain changes measured during compact overcoring operation at the measuring point No.5 and the theoretical strains calculated on the process simulation.

Table 3 Rock stress determined.

Number of strains		24	16
Stress components, standard deviations in the xyz co-ordinates in MPa	σ_x	-41.9±0.4	-42.5±0.6
	σ_y	-14.5±0.4	-14.8±0.6
	σ_z	-25.8±1.1	-26.0±1.4
	τ_{yz}	4.9±0.4	6.2±0.7
	τ_{zx}	2.9±0.4	3.0±0.7
	τ_{xy}	0.2±0.3	0.2±0.4
Principal stresses in MPa, principal direction in degrees (dip direction form the y-axis / dip)	σ_1	-12.6 (182/21)	-12.0 (183/24)
	σ_2	-27.1 (334/67)	-28.3 (336/63)
	σ_3	-42.4 (89/10)	-43.1 (88/11)

Remarks : Young's modulus and Poisson's ratio in the rock stress determination are 68GPa and 0.23.

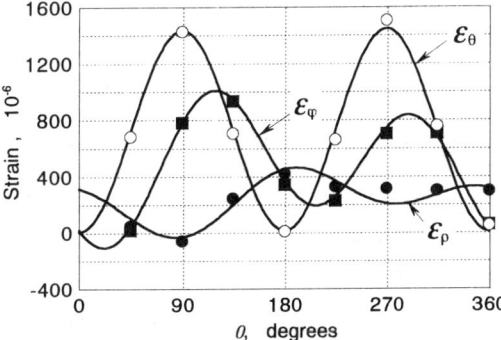

Figure 5 Comparison of the measured strains with the theoretical ones on the measuring circle on the conical bottom surface.

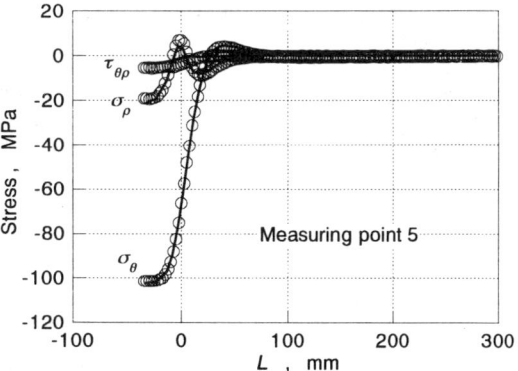

Figure 6 Comparison of the stress components at the measuring point No.5 calculated from the measured strains with those from the theoretical ones on the process simulation, based on the theory of the rosette gauge.

measurement was successfully performed with a high accuracy.

If the results of the process simulation are different from those of the measured strain, the anomalous strain data is rejected, then another process simulation is performed by remained strain data again. The accurate rock stress can be determined by the repetition of this procedure. It is concluded that the measured strains in progress of the compact overcoring offer important information to determine the original stress, and the anomalous data rejection based on the process simulation is indispensable for the minimization of error in rock stress determination

The three components of strain in independent directions one another are measured at a measuring point on the borehole bottom. Therefore, the stresses at the point on the surface during the compact overcoring can be evaluated according to the theory of the rosette gauge. Figure 6 shows the comparison of the stress components at a measuring point calculated from the measured strains with those from the theoretical ones in the process simulation. The plots represent the results from the measured strains, the curves are those of theoretical ones in the figure. Both results are good agreement each other. The stresses are rapidly changed when the overcoring approaches the bottom, then the stresses around the borehole is completely relieved at a distance of 70mm of the overcoring. Since the shear stress is almost zero, the normal stresses can be seemed to be principal stresses. The maximum tensile stress induced during the overcoring is about 10MPa at L=0mm. It is considered that the strain diverges and

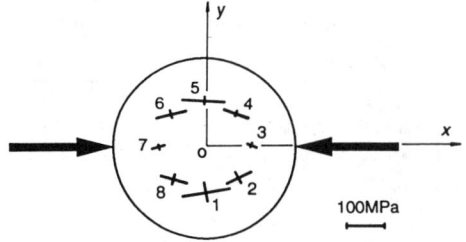

Figure 7 The principal stresses and their direction at the 8 measuring points on the conical bottom surface and the direction of the maximum principal stress in the plane perpendicular to the borehole axis.

the core discing occurs due to the tensile stress.

The trend of changes and values of stresses at a measuring point which is symmetric with respect to the measuring point No.5 is almost the same. Therefore the two components in three principal stresses may exist in the plane perpendicular to the borehole axis. Figure 7 shows the comparison of the principal stress state induced on the borehole bottom surface before the overcoring with the direction of maximum principal stress in the plane perpendicular to the borehole axis prior to boring. The figure is drawn as the borehole bottom looked from the mouth of the borehole. The eight crosses in the circle represent the magnitude and direction of the principal stresses at the measuring points on the borehole bottom, and the arrows out of the circle are the direction of the maximum principal stress in the plane perpendicular to the borehole axis prior to boring. All of stresses induced on the borehole surface are compressive, their magnitudes and directions are symmetric with respect to the plane including the direction of the maximum principal stress in the plane perpendicular to the borehole axis. The magnitudes of maximum stress at the measuring points No.1 and No.5 are greater than the others and the their directions are in harmony with that of maximum principal stress as the arrows. These results indicate that the 24-element conical-ended borehole technique with rosette gauge is reliable for *in-situ* rock stress measurements.

7 CONCLUSIONS

In order to improve the accuracy of the conventional conical-ended borehole technique with cross typed strain gauges, it was modified using rosette typed strain gauges, so-called 24-element conical-ended borehole technique.

Firstly, the theory of the rock stress determination was shown from 24 strain components measured on a conical bottom surface of a single borehole. Then comparing of the accuracy of the proposed method with that of existing method, it was confirmed that the proposed method gives us more accurate results. Secondly, based on *in-situ* rock stress measurement, it was clarified that the proposed method can be more effectively used for *in-situ* rock stress measurements than the existing one. Also, showing that the process simulation of the strains and stresses on the conical bottom surface during the stress relieving gave well consistent results with measured data, it was concluded that the proposed method is reliable for *in-situ* rock stress measurements.

REFERENCES

Kanagawa, T., S. Hibino & T. Ishida 1986. In-situ stress measurements by overcoring method. Development of 8-element gauge for three-dimensional estimation, *CRIPEI Rep. E385033*.

Kobayashi, S., N. Nishimura & K. Matsumoto 1987. Displacements and strains around anon-flat-end borehole. *Proc. of 2nd Int. Symp. on Field Measurements in Geomech.* 12:1079-460.

Leeman, R.E. & D.J.Hayes 1996. A technique for determining the complete state of stress in rock using a single borehole. *Proc. of 1st Cong. on Rock Mechanics.* 17-24.

Mayr, M., W. Dexler & G. Kuhn 1977. A semianalytical boundary integral approach for axisymmetric elastic bodies with arbitrary boundary conditions. *Int. J. Solid & Struct.* 445-451.

Mohr, H.F. 1956. Measurement of rock pressure. *Mine and Quarry Engineering.* 178-189.

Obert, L., R.H. Merril & T.A. Morgan 1962. Borehole deformation gauge for determination of the stress in mine rock. *U.S Bureau of Mines R.I. 5978*.

Oka., Y., Y. Hiramatsu, Y. Saito & K. Sugawara 1976. The observation equations obtained from three-dimensional stress analysis and some examples of stress determination. *J. Min. Metall. Ins. Jpn.* 92:94-99.

Sakaguchi, K, Y. Obara, T. Nakayama & K. Sugawara 1992. Accuracy of rock stress measurement by means of conical-ended borehole technique. *J. Min .Metall. Ins. Jpn.* 108:455-460.

Sugawara, K. & Y. Obara 1986. Measurement of in situ rock stress by hemispherical-ended borehole technique. *J. Min. Sci. Technol.* 3:287-300.

Warotnicki, G. 1993. CSIRO triaxial stress measurement cell. *Comprehensive Rock Engineering,* Ed. J.A.Hudson. 3:329-394.

Applicability of the compact overcoring method for initial stress measurement in highly cracked bedrock

N. Demboya & A. Fukuhara
Electric Power Development Co., Ltd, Kanagawa, Japan

Y. Obara & K. Sugawara
Faculty of Engineering, Kumamoto University, Japan

ABSTRACT: Case examples of the initial rock stress measurements for design of underground pumped-storage power generation plants are presented, which have been conducted in three sites using the compact overcoring method, the borehole deformation method and the sleeve fracturing method, as well as by the hydraulic fracturing method. Analyzing the in situ rock stresses measured, it is clarified that the compact overcoring method is the most promising tool presently available for determining the three-dimensional state of in situ rock stress in highly jointed rock formations under complicated geological conditions. Its strong and weak points are discussed, as well as the importance of combining the other methods based on the different principles to obtain a more reliable assessment of the in situ stress field.

1 INTRODUCTION

Knowledge of rock stress is of importance for the construction of rock structures, such as underground powerhouse caverns, since the mechanical response of surrounding rock mass is mainly dominated by rock stress. Rock stress measurement is, therefore, considered to be a significant field measurement in rock engineering. In Particular, recent developments in rock engineering in Japan have indicated the need for reliable in situ stress measurements in highly jointed rock formations under complicated geological conditions.

In order to determine the complete state of stress at a certain point within a rock mass, the deformation of a borehole, which is a function of the rock stress, needs to be measured by applying the stress relief method. Various types of device have been proposed to measure the changes in length of one or more diameters of the borehole, or to measure the changes in strain on the cylindrical wall or bottom surface of the borehole. For the stress measurement in highly jointed rock formations, it is desired that the stress tensor can be computed from the measurement in a single borehole. For this purpose, Sugawara et al.(1992) proposed the compact overcoring method.

In the present paper, case examples of the three-dimensional in situ stress measurement by means of the compact overcoring method will be presented to make clear its applicability in highly cracked rock formations. Moreover, its strong and weak points are discussed as well as the importance of combining the other methods based on the different principles to obtain a more reliable assessment of the in situ stress field.

Case examples presented here are the initial rock stress measurements at Sites A, B and C in Figure 1, which are carried out to provide the fundamental data required for design of underground pumped-storage power generation plants, which are now planing at those sites.

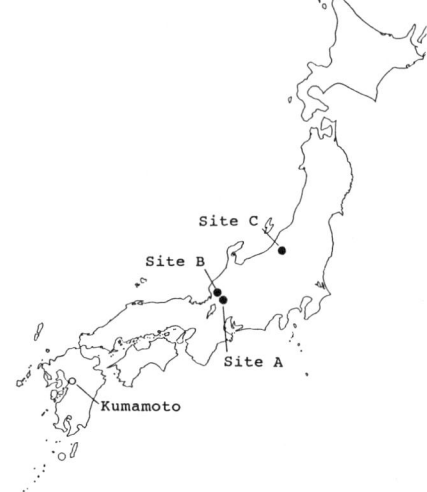

Figure 1 Location of Sites A, B and C.

2 COMPACT OVERCORING METHOD

The compact overcoring method is considered to be the latest version of the stress relief method using the conical-ended borehole technique. This method was developed by modifying the doorstopper system (Leeman, 1969) and the hemispherical-ended borehole technique (Sugawara et al., 1985), and by improving the conical-ended borehole technique (Kobayashi et al., 1987). The theory and practice of the compact overcoring method can be found in Sakaguchi et al. (1994).

The compact overcoring method is based on a principle much similar to the doorstopper system, apart from the shape of the borehole bottom. By measuring the 16-element of induced strain on the conical bottom surface, the stress tensor is back-analyzed by the theory of elasticity. As illustrated in Figure 2, the relief of the stresses acting on the conical surface of a pilot borehole is conducted using a thin-wall diamond bit of special make having a diameter of 76mm, which is equal to the diameter of the pilot borehole. This results in reducing the time, effort and cost for the in situ measurement.

3 CASE EXAMPLE - SITE A

Site A has a rugged topography featured by narrow V-shaped valleys and flattened ridges, which is unique to the Paleozoic region in Japan. The rock stress measurement has been conducted in the center part of the region where an underground powerhouse cavern is planed, at the depth of about 240m below the surface. Geology consists of schalstein having a mean joint spacing less than 10cm. The schalstein can be divided into the two of a part which is coarse-grained, massive, and hard, and a part which is fine-grained and slightly weak. Numerous calcite veins are interspersed, with smooth surfaces to be frequently found at joint planes. Faults in the vicinity are mostly of E-W character and NE-SW to N-S character, and the majority has sheared widths less than several tens of centimeters. Adits do not have severe springing of water, but dripping is seen here and there along faults and joints.

In situ stress state at Site A has been investigated firstly by the two-dimensional stress measurements using the borehole deformation method, and then by the three-dimensional stress measurement applying the compact over coring method. An example of the two-dimensional measurements in a single borehole is given in Table 1, which have been carried out using two types of gauge, the borehole deformation gauge (BDG) proposed by Suzuki & Ishijima (1968) and the plugged 5-element strain gauge (PSG) developed by the Central Research Institute Electric Power Industry, Japan (Kanagawa et al., 1979).

Both can provide the maximum and minimum stresses: σ_{max} and σ_{min} in the plane perpendicular to the borehole axis and their directions, but require the large-diameter overcoring. The direction of σ_{max} is given by θ, in Table 1, which is a counterclockwise angle from the rightward horizon.

It is noteworthy that the values of σ_{min} are small, since this means that the minimum principal stress is nearly zero. A large amount of scattering can be found in the direction of in situ stresses determined. Such a fluctuation of direction may be associated with the presence of joints with small spacings.

An example of the three-dimensional stress measurement in a single borehole is given in Table 2 and Figure 3. From the values of the principal stresses in

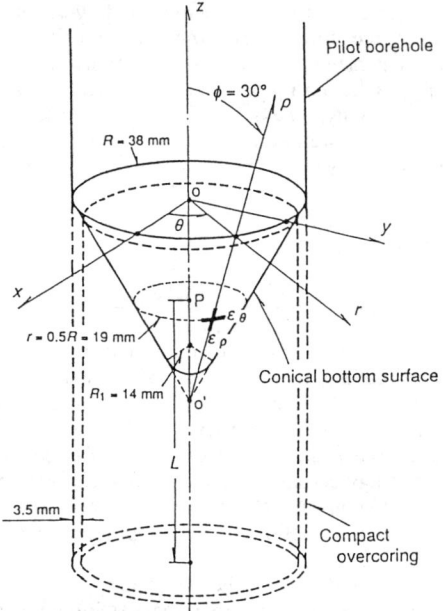

Figure 2 Conical-ended borehole and the Compact overcoring operation.

Table 1 The two-dimensional stress measurement at Site A, by the borehole deformation method.

Gauge	Distance z, m	Rock type	Stress & orientation		
			σ_{max}	σ_{min}	θ
BDG	1.9	Schalstein	7.5	0.1	73
BDG	5.3	Schalstein	10.3	0.4	78
PSG	6.8	Schalstein	17.8	0.0	−48
PSG	8.0	Schalstein	6.3	0.5	−47
BDG	11.8	Schalstein	3.6	0.6	−70

Remarks: z : distance from adit wall; stresses in MPa, and compression is positive; θ in degrees.

Table 2 The three-dimensional stress measurement at Site A, by the compact overcoring method.

No.	Distance z, m	Rock type	Principal stresses, MPa		
			σ_1	σ_2	σ_3
1	13.1	Schalstein	16.5	4.5	1.2
2	13.6	Schalstein	21.8	9.2	6.5
3	21.9	Schalstein	9.6	4.9	0.8
4	24.2	Schalstein	12.0	6.5	0.2

Remarks: measurement in a borehole; z is distance from adit wall; compressive stress is positive.

Table 2, it can be reconfirmed that the in situ stress state is characterized by a small value of σ_3. In Figure 3, it must be emphasized that the pole of the maximum principal stress σ_1 is comparatively concentrated, though the poles of the intermediate and minimum principal stresses migrate. This migration may be concluded to be deeply related to the sliding and/or local opening of adjacent joint systems, and it proves that many measurements need to be carried out in highly jointed rock formations to present more reliable information on the in situ stress state.

Case example presented here clearly indicates that the compact overcoring method is more effective. However, a problem is brought forward, that is how many measurements need to be carried out in a highly jointed formation by the compact overcoring method, and in what directions to accurately evaluate the magnitude and orientation of the intermediate and minimum principal stresses. The combination with several methods may provide a solution, since the limitation and disadvantages of the compact overcoring method may be covered by the methods based on the different principles. The benefits of the combination will be discussed in the following.

4 CASE EXAMPLE - SITE B

Site B is located below a valley which runs down from southeast to northwest, and the overburden is ranging from 300 to 350m. Geology consists of the Mesozoic sedimentary rocks, mainly coarse grained sandstone (css) and partially intercalated with medium grained sandstone (mss) and fine grained sandstone (fss). The strikes of these strata are ENE-WSW. The coarse grained sandstone is generally massive with distinct bedding planes not indicated, being hard and dense with many parts having joint spacings of about 5 to 30cm, while at places patches of shale several millimeters to several centimeters in diameter are contained. Where there are numerous patches shear planes of very small displacements are developed along rows of patches, and there are discontinuity planes of slickenside accompanied by thin film-like intercalated matter. The rock is easily exfoliated at these planes, so that the rock mass is often brittle as a whole. In general, there is little springing of water. A prominent fault in the vicinity is one with a strike of ENE-WSW, which is sharply dipped. Also, faults of sheared widths 10cm or more are found at a rate of about 3 per every 10m within the coarse grained sandstone. Most of these have slickenside-like smooth planes and those parallel to the bedding planes of the coarse grained sandstone with ENE-WSW strikes, and dipping south at high angles, are predominant.

In situ stress state at Site B has been investigated by the three-dimensional stress measurement using the compact overcoring method, and subsequently at the same location by the sleeve fracturing method. The former has been conducted in two boreholes, B-1 and B-2, by selecting a formation convenient for the measurement, that is continuous, homogeneous and elastic. The dip directions of B-1 and B-2 were fixed to 216 degrees, and the dipping angles were arranged to 2.0 and 13.0 degrees, respectively. The magnitudes of the principal stresses and the stress components refer to the Cartesian co-ordinate (X, Y, Z) are given in Table 3, and the poles of the principal axes of stress are illustrated in Figure 4. The two-dimensional stress measurement by means of the sleeve fracturing method has been performed in a borehole, of which the dip direction is 36 degrees and the dipping angle is 34 degrees. The results obtained are shown in Table 4, comparing with the stresses computed from the stress tensor determined by the compact overcoring method. Theory used in

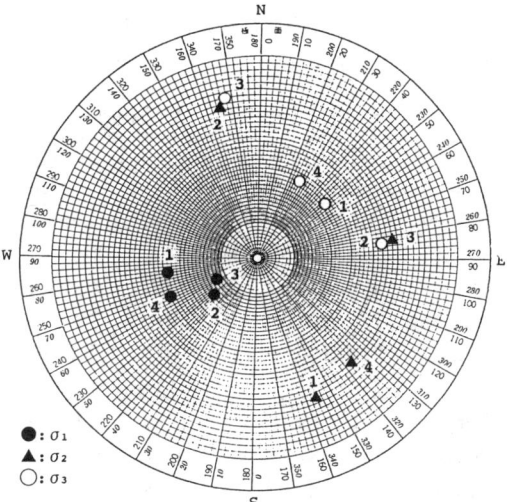

Figure 3 Poles of the principal axes of stress determined by the compact overcoring method at Site A, lower hemisphere of Schmidt net.

Table 3 The three-dimensional stress measurement at Site B, by the compact overcoring method.

Bore-hole	No.	Distance z, m	Rock type	Principal stresses, MPa			Stresses of the Cartesian co-ordinates (X, Y, Z)					
				σ_1	σ_2	σ_3	σ_X	σ_Y	σ_Z	τ_{YZ}	τ_{ZX}	τ_{XY}
B-1	1	11.7	css	6.0	3.2	0.2	1.3	3.2	4.9	0.1	2.2	0.6
	2	15.6	css	20.0	11.7	7.7	13.3	1.8	3.8	2.5	5.4	0.5
B-2	1	6.2	fss	18.0	11.0	6.8	13.0	6.8	16.0	−0.2	3.1	−0.2
	2	7.3	fss	17.7	3.8	1.2	3.5	2.9	16.3	1.2	4.1	1.7

Remarks: Measurement in two boreholes; z : distance from adit wall; stresses in MPa, compression is positive; X-axis: east direction, Y-axis: north direction, Z-axis: upward direction.

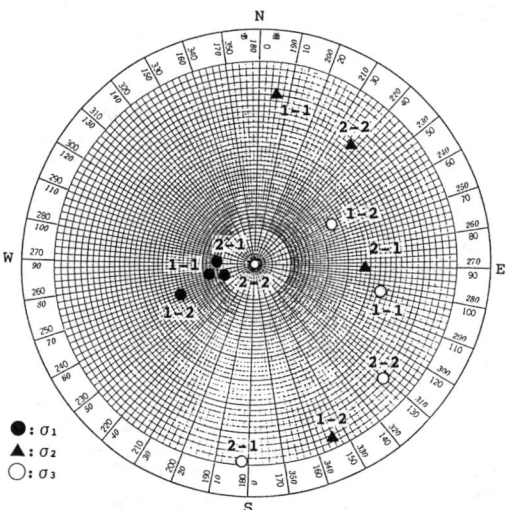

Figure 4 Poles of the principal axes of stress determined by the compact overcoring method at Site B, lower hemisphere of Schmidt net.

Table 4 The two-dimensional stress measurements at Site B, by the sleeve fracturing method, compared to stresses computed from the stress tensor obtained by the compact overcoring method.

Method	No.	Rock type	Distance z, m	Stress & orientation		
				σ_{max}	σ_{min}	θ
Sleeve fracturing method	1	css	9.2	10.7	8.8	62
	2	css	10.5	10.2	7.9	46
	3	mss	17.9	10.3	8.3	54
	4	fss	46.0	10.9	7.6	90
Compact overcoring method	B-1-1	css	-	5.9	1.1	14
	2	css	-	14.7	3.6	44
	B-2-1	fss	-	17.5	8.8	30
	2	fss	-	16.3	1.2	10

Remarks: z is distance from adit wall; stresses are in MPa, and compression is positive; θ is in degrees.

the sleeve fracturing method are based from Sakuma et al. (1987, 1989).

The stresses in Table 3 have a large amount of scattering in value, but the stresses in Table 4 evaluated by the sleeve fracturing method have little dispersion. This discrepancy of the trends is great. The reason can not be explained clearly. Saying by force, it may be associated with the volume of rock involved in the method of rock stress measurement, or the length concerned. If the effect of the volume or the length is significant, the sleeve fracturing method is considered to be more suitable to highly jointed rock formations.

In Figure 4, it is noteworthy that the pole of the maximum principal stress σ_1 is well concentrated, and that the poles of the intermediate and minimum principal stresses migrate on a great circle. A similar migration has been found in Figure 3, then this may be concluded to be a significant characteristic of the in situ stress state in highly jointed rock formations. As described previously, such a migration must be related to the sliding and/or local opening of adjacent joint systems.

5 CASE EXAMPLE - SITE C

Site C is located just below the tip of a rugged ridge extending northwest in a straight line sandwiched two valleys. The bottom elevations of these valleys are ranging from 350 to 400m, while the elevations of the ridges line are ranging from 600 to 800m, and the mountain body of the vicinity presents a rugged topography of maturity where gullies of V-shape reaching 50m in depth are developed. The rock mass consists of medium grained granite having aplite veins at parts of thickness several centimeters and porphyrite intruding the granite and aplite. On the geological time scale this is considered to have been formed from the Cretaceous Period to the Paleocene Epoch. The medium grained granite is comparatively fresh and is mostly a hardrock mass with joint spacings of 10 to 40cm. There is a fault about 300m southeast of this site, called the K-Fault, having a strike in the NE-SW direction, and this fault forms a

Table 5 The three-dimensional stress measurement at Site C, by the compact overcoring method.

No.	Distance z, m	Rock type	Principal stresses, MPa			Stresses of the Cartesian co-ordinates (X, Y, Z)					
			σ_1	σ_2	σ_3	σ_X	σ_Y	σ_Z	τ_{YZ}	τ_{ZX}	τ_{XY}
1	9.4	Granite	13.1	2.6	0.4	6.6	6.6	3.0	−3.0	1.6	−5.5
2	13.6	Granite	9.5	3.1	0.4	3.8	6.2	3.0	−3.7	0.6	−2.3
3	15.1	Granite	13.9	2.5	0.2	5.4	9.4	1.7	−3.8	1.9	−4.6
4	15.5	Granite	17.1	6.4	3.1	8.5	13.7	4.4	−3.6	1.9	−3.9
5	27.6	Granite	19.1	2.7	2.1	5.0	15.7	3.2	−2.9	1.0	−6.0

Remarks: z is distance from adit wall; stresses are in MPa and compression is positive; X-axis: east direction, Y-axis: north direction, Z-axis: upward direction.

boundary in distribution of hornfels and granites. Major faults in the vicinity of this site consist of three faults of strikes E-W and dipping north with 60 to 70degrees, parts of which have sheared zones of about 120cm at maximum. Water springs are about 8 liters per minute from these three faults, while much dripping is found in the surroundings. A number of joint systems has been found. In Particular, the joint system parallel to the K-Fault and a joint system of orthogonal to the K-Fault are conspicuous and continuous. The latter joint system is frequently subject to displacements of several centimeters due to other joint systems, then is considered to be the oldest of all the joint systems.

In-situ stress measurements have been conducted at the depth of about 180m by the compact overcoring method and the hydraulic fracturing method, at a different location and in a different direction. According to the hydraulic fracturing method, the re-opening pressure has been detected by overlying of pressure transient curve based on Haimson et al. (1980) and Lee & Haimson (1989), and the shut-in pressure has been detected by the bilinear pressure-decay-rate method (Lee & Haimson, 1989).

Results of measurements by the compact overcoring method are given in Table 5 and Figure 5, and the results of the hydraulic fracturing method are summarized in Table 6, comparing the stresses computed from the results of the compact overcoring method. By comparing with the significant stress fluctuation which has been observed previously at Sites A and B, it can be pointed out that the variation of stresses is comparatively smaller, and that the migration of the poles of σ_2 and σ_3 is limited in a part on a great circle. This means that the disturbance due to joints is comparatively small, and suggests that the joint systems have a high frictional resistance or high frictional coefficients. As discussed previously by Sugawara (1993), the shear stress and the normal stress acting on the adjacent joint surface can be estimated from the stress tensor in Table 5, based on the stress transformation law, and may provide the vital information for the characterization of joints in granite.

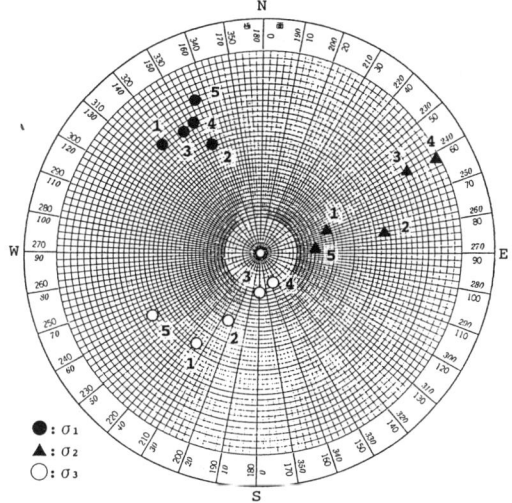

Figure 5 Poles of the principal axes of stress determined by the compact overcoring method at Site C, lower hemisphere of Schmidt net.

In relation to σ_{min} in Table 6, a clear difference can be found between the two methods. Similar discrepancy can be found concerning the value of θ. These may be considered to be related with the variation of in situ stresses from region to region, since the distance between the two boreholes for measurement is ranging from 100 to 130m.

This case example indicates that the compact overcoring method is promising, and that the combination with the hydraulic fracturing method provides a measure of consistency and reliability. Then, it can be concluded that, in highly jointed rock formations, stresses can be determined firstly by applying the compact overcoring method. When it is done, the formation more convenient for the measurement by means of the stress relief technique must be carefully selected. For this purpose, it is emphasized that the geological condition and environmental aspects must

Table 6 The two-dimensional stress measurement at Site C, by the hydraulic fracturing method, comparing to stresses computed from the stress tensor obtained by compact overcoring method.

Method	No.	Distance z, m	Stresses & orientation		
			σ_{max}	σ_{min}	θ
Hydraulic fracturing method in granite	1	8.4	12.9	5.2	44
	2	9.4	10.2	4.2	46
	3	12.8	23.5	9.8	51
	4	13.3	18.3	8.3	35
	5	15.5	17.3	7.3	56
	6	18.6	12.9	6.7	29
	7	20.1	11.3	5.1	49
Compact overcoring method	1	-	13.1	2.0	18
	2	-	9.1	1.4	28
	3	-	13.6	3.3	19
	4	-	16.6	3.1	18
	5	-	17.5	2.7	12

Remarks: z is distance from adit wall; stresses are in MPa and compression is positive; θ is in degrees.

be identified including topography, rock type, joint systems, the mechanical properties of them, other geological structures, anisotropy, heterogeneities and so on. These factors are important also in the interpretation of the measurements themselves. Subsequently, combining several methods have to be conducted by taking the purpose of the project into considerations. This approach is recommended since it will provide more rigorous constants on the in situ stresses.

6 CONCLUDING REMARKS

Presenting the successful case examples of initial rock stress measurement for design of underground pumped-storage power generation plants, it has been concluded that the compact overcoring method is the most promising tool presently available for determining the three-dimensional state of in situ rock stress within highly jointed rock formations under complicated geological conditions. Additionally, the results of the two-dimensional stress measurements by means of the borehole deformation method, the sleeve fracturing method and the hydraulic fracturing method have been compared with the results of the compact overcoring method, and the combination of the compact overcoring method and several methods based on the difference principles has been recommended to obtain a more reliable assessment of the in situ stress field.

REFERENCES

Haimson, B. 1980. Near surface and deep hydrofracturing stress measurements in Waterloo quartzite. *Int. Rock Mech. Min. Sci. & Geomech. Abstr.* 17: 81-88.

Kanagawa, T., M. Hayashi and Y. Kitahara 1979. Measuring method and application in-situ rock stress. *Elec. Pwr. Civil. Eng. Jpn.* 163: 31-42.

Kobayashi, S., N. Nishimura and K. Matsumoto 1987. Displacements and strains around a non-flat-end borehole, *Proc. 2nd Int. Symp. on Field Measurements in Geomech.*, Kobe, Vol.2, pp.1079-1084.

Lee, M. & B. Haimson 1989. Statistical evaluation of hydraulic fracturing stress measurement parameter. *Int. Rock Mech. Min. Sci. & Geomech. Abstr.* 26: 447-456.

Leeman, E. R. 1969. The doorstopper and triaxial rock stress measuring instruments developed by the CSIR, *J. S. Afr. Inst. Min. Metall.*, 69: 305-339.

Sakaguchi, K., T. Takehara, Y. Obara, T. Nakayama and K. Sugawara 1994. Rock stress measurement by means of the compact overcoring method. *J. Min. Mater. Inst. Jpn.* 110: 331-336.

Sakuma, S., S. Kikuchi, T. Nakamura and Y. Mizuta 1987. A study on fracture initiation and re-opening conditions in double fracturing method. *Proc. 7th Jpn. Symp. Rock Mechanics.* pp.187-192.

Sakuma, S., S. Kikuchi, Y. Mizuta and S. Serata 1989. In-situ stress measurement by double fracturing. *Proc. Jpn. Soc. Civil Eng.* 406:87-96.

Sugawara, K., Y. Obara, H. Okamura and Y. Wang 1985. The determination of the complete state of stress in rock by the measurement of strains on a hemispherical borehole-bottom. *J. Min. Metall. Inst. Jpn.* 101: 277-282.

Sugawara, K., K. Sakaguchi, Y. Obara, T. Nakayama and H. Jang 1992. Rock Stress Measurement and Numerical Approach for Cavern Designing. *J. Korean Rock Mechanics Society.* 2, 1, 164-176.

Sugawara, K. 1993. Initial Stress. *Rock Mechanics*: 357-383, Tokyo: Maruzen.

Suzuki, K. & Y. Ishijima 1968. Theory and practice of rock stress measurement by borehole deformation method. *J. Soc. Mater. Sci. Jpn.* 17, 856-862.

Improvement on hollow inclusion technique and its application to in situ stress measurement in four Chinese metal mines

M.Cai, L.Qiao, C.Li, B.Yu & S.Wang
University of Science and Technology, Beijing, People's Republic of China

ABSTRACT: Effective temperature compensation is critical to reliability and accuracy of in situ stress measurement with the hollow inclusion cells. Traditional compensation method using a dummy gauge is not valid for hollow inclusion cell and other devices which are bonded to rock during overcoring. To solve this problem, a new temperature compensation system was developed and the measuring procedure as well as structure of the hollow inclusion cell was accordingly improved. With the improved hollow inclusion technique in situ stress measurements in four Chinese metal mines have been completed and satisfactory results were obtained.

1 INTRODUCTION

CSIRO type hollow inclusion cells with borehole overcoring technique are widely used for *in situ* stress measurement in the world (Worotnicki and Walton, 1976). Like most overcoring measurement instruments, the hollow inclusion cells use strain gauges as the sensing elements and measure the values of strain sensed by every strain gauge through Wheatstone bridges. Since strain gauges are susceptive to temperature changes, temperature compensation is critical to reliability and accuracy of the measurement with the hollow inclusion cells. The traditional temperature compensation method is to use a dummy gauge in the bridge. Based on the principle of Wheatstone bridge, for effective compensation, the dummy gauge should sense the same strain as the working gauges during the same temperature change. However, during overcoring, the working gauges are indirectly bonded to rock and their deformation behaviour is mainly controlled by the rock, but the dummy gauge cannot be bonded to the rock; otherwise, it will not be stress free. So the dummy gauge cannot sense the same strain as the working gauges at the same temperature change during overcoring and therefore is not effective for temperature compensation. Furthermore, while the cell is bonded to borehole, every strain gauge in it is not in the same condition due to discontinuity, nonhomogeneity and anisotropy of the rock, therefore each working gauge should have its own dummy gauge, but there is only one common dummy gauge inside the cell. Some inclusion cells even use a dummy gauge inside the strain indicator which is far from the measuring point and is not in the same environmental and temperature condition as the working strain gauge, so the compensation is obviously invalid. To solve this problem, a new temperature compensation technique was developed (Cai et al., 1995). Subsequently, the structure and measuring procedure of the traditional hollow inclusion cells were accordingly improved.

2 IMPROVEMENTS ON HOLLOW INCLUSION TECHNIQUE

2.1 *New temperature compensation system*

The new temperature compensation system is basically composed of the following steps:

1) A strain-resistance-voltage transforming unit was made whose function is similar to a strain indicator, i.e. to connect each working strain gauge and other three resistors to form a Wheatstone bridge for changing strain value of each strain gauge to voltage value output from the bridge. In the unit there are 12 bridge circuits used for 12 strain gauges. All resistors in the unit have a low temperature coefficient of 1 ppm/°C, which means each resistor in a bridge could cause a thermal strain of only $0.5\mu\varepsilon$/°C that is negligible. It eliminated the temperature effect caused by the three resistance elements other than the working strain gauge in the bridge.

2) Lead wires of the strain gauge can also induce remarkable thermal strain. For example, the cable between the hollow inclusion and the transforming unit used by us in the field is approximately 20m long.

Each strain gauge has two lead wires, i.e. the total length of lead wire for a strain gauge is about 40m long whose resistance is about 4Ω. When the temperature changes by 1 ℃, the lead wire could cause a thermal strain about 60 με. It is very remarkable because the total strain value measured by a strain gauge during overcoring is usually only a few hundred microstrains. To compensate for the effect, the same long additional lead wire coming from the measuring point is connected to the neighbouring arm of the strain gauge in every bridge.

3) During overcoring, temperature change at the measuring point is continuously monitored by a thermistor, which is embedded in the inclusion.

4) After completion of each overcoring test, the overcore with the inclusion cell inside it is put into an adjustable thermal tank with constant humidity to conduct a temperature calibration test. Based on the test results, the relation between induced strains and temperature changes could be determined for each strain gauge.

5) From the calibration results and the recorded temperature changes during overcoring, the additional thermal strain values for all strain gauges were obtained. After eliminating them from the total strain values recorded during overcoring, correct strain values actually induced by stress relief could be determined for calculation of *in situ* stresses.

2.2 *Modification of hollow inclusion cell*

To use the new temperature compensation system, structure of the traditional hollow inclusion cell is accordingly modified.

1) To monitor temperature changes at the strain gauge position, a thermistor is embedded in the hollow inclusion between two strain gauge rosettes.

2) To compensate for the thermal effect of lead wires, two additional lead wires with no strain gauge connected are welded together at the strain gauge position and exited through the cable with the other lead wires.

3 APPLICATION TO FIELD STRESS MEASUREMENTS

The improved hollow inclusion technique has been used for *in situ* stress measurement in four Chinese metal mines. During the measurement, boreholes were horizontally drilled from underground opening walls about 8-12m deep, i.e. 3-4 times the opening's width to ensure that the stress state in the measuring position was not disturbed. The measuring data were automatically recorded by a programmed datalogger.

3.1 *in Xincheng gold mine*

Xincheng gold mine is the second largest gold mine in China with a gold production of 2.2 tons per year. The orebodies are located in a large fracture zone which is about 80-200m wide, 70-80km long and strikes NE40-50°. The main orebody is 360m long along its strike, stretches down to 600m with a dip angle of 29°.

The *in situ* stress measurement was carried out from September 1991 to October 1992 at 11 points on three levels, i.e. -175m, -205m and -280m levels. The rock types at most measuring points were porphyrite granodioritiod or sericitized granodiorite. The values of RQD calculated from the drilled cores at the measuring points were 52-95%. The 3-D stress state measured at 11 points is shown in Table 1.

Table 1. *In situ* stress measurement results in Xincheng gold mine

Measuring point No.	Depth (m)	σ_1			σ_2			σ_3		
		Value (MPa)	Bearing (°)	Dip (°)	Value (MPa)	Bearing (°)	Dip (°)	Value (MPa)	Bearing (°)	Dip (°)
1	205	11.45	307.1	-17.6	5.69	286.3	71.3	4.03	35.1	6.2
2	205	11.54	270.0	4.3	6.77	181.5	-19.0	5.72	347.8	-70.4
3	205	11.27	218.9	10.2	5.68	220.2	-79.8	3.98	129.0	-0.2
4	235	14.62	237.6	9.2	10.17	329.9	13.9	5.63	295.1	-73.2
5	235	13.69	129.7	-7.8	6.93	131.1	82.2	5.06	38.8	0.3
6	235	12.99	301.9	-0.6	6.14	208.2	-81.3	5.00	212.0	8.7
7	235	13.60	311.0	-1.4	8.93	220.7	-10.4	6.85	228.8	79.5
8	235	12.58	280.0	-13.2	7.85	187.3	-11.1	6.92	238.5	72.6
9	235	12.80	127.1	-7.2	7.41	35.7	-9.7	5.89	72.4	78.0
10	310	17.63	119.0	-2.1	11.65	209.2	-4.7	10.73	185.6	84.8
11	310	18.50	285.5	-17.7	8.89	80.8	-70.6	7.05	13.0	7.6

3.2 In Ekou iron mine

The Ekou mine is an open pit mine with an ore production of five million tons per year. The mine is situated in Shanxi plateau which is basically 1500m above the sea level. The mine area is composed of a series of folded structures which are close each other. Synclinorium, anticlinorium and fracture structures are very developed. They totally shaped a multiple overturned synclince. The orebody of the mine is a down fold structure and is 2100m long along its strike with a dip angle of 50°. It is buried between 2485m and 1420m levels with a thickness varied from 18m to 300m. The top wall of the orebody is mainly composed of bornblende schist and the bottom wall is composed of chlorite schist. The vertical height of the final slope designed is 720m and it is 450m high at the moment.

In situ stress measurement was completed by both borehole overcoring technique with hollow inclusion cells and hydraulic fracturing technique.

Borehole overcoring stress measurement was performed in a ventilation tunnel which is in service to the belt conveyer adit. It was the only place for the borehole overcoring test to be conducted. Four overcoring boreholes were distributed with an interval of 100m and they were approximately located in the center of the open pit. The measured results are listed in the lines of measuring points No.1-No.4 in Table 2.

The hydraulic fracturing test was carried out in four vertical boreholes during September to November 1992. The four boreholes were located close to the final mining boundary of the mine which were also used for investigating hydrogeological and rock mass conditions in the deep bottom of the slope.

The hydraulic fracturing equipment was mainly composed of two 120cm long sealing packers, an impressing packer, oil pump, water pump, chart recorder and flow meter. While the flow of high pressure oil between the oil pump and the sealing packers was via a pressure resistant hose, the flow between the water pump and the isolated test section of the borehole was via drilling rods which enabled the packers to be hoisted easily. The test was completed at two points in one borehole, and only one point in the other three boreholes due to breakage of the sealing packer during transfer form the lower point to the upper point. The measured results are listed in the lines of measuring points No5-No.9 in Table 2.

It should be noted that the value of σ_v for measuring points No5-No.9 was estimated from the weight of the overburden while it was calculated from the actually measured borehole strains for measuring points No1-No.4.

3.3 *In Meishan iron mine*

Meishan iron mine is the largest underground iron mine in China with an ore reserve of 334 million tons. It is located near the Yangtze River and is 25km south-west to Nanjing city, the Capital of Jiangsu Province.

The lanticular orebody is flatly inclined and strikes NE. It is very thick with an average thickness of 134m. Its level projection presents a rough oval shape which is 1370m long and 824m wide. The top wall of the orebody is mainly composed of andesite and the bottom wall is mainly composed of porphyrite.

The overcoring stress measurements were carried out at eight points in three levels from November 1993 to January 1994. The values of RQD at eight measuring points were 42-90%. The measured results are shown in Table 3.

3.4 *In Jinchuan nickel mine*

Jinchuan nickel mine is situated in the middle of Hexi

Table 2. *In situ* stress measurement results in Ekou iron mine

Measuring point No.	Depth (m)	σ_1 Value (MPa)	σ_1 Bearing (°)	σ_1 Dip (°)	σ_2 Value (MPa)	σ_2 Bearing (°)	σ_2 Dip (°)	σ_3 Value (MPa)	σ_3 Bearing (°)	σ_3 Dip (°)
1	310	23.10	359.9	-2.0	7.64	89.9	1.1	9.41	331.4	87.7
2	310	23.11	170.0	-0.5	8.25	258.1	74.5	10.72	260.2	-15.5
3	310	22.96	183.2	0.8	8.85	93.4	-15.6	10.97	90.5	74.3
4	310	19.34	153.1	-0.3	8.57	64.6	78.0	8.99	63.0	-12.0
5	118.0	13.30	140.0		6.40	50.0		3.10		
6	99.1	13.30	102.0		6.50	12.0		2.60		
7	133.5	14.00	118.0		7.20	28.0		3.50		
8	151.3	18.50	97.0		9.10	7.0		4.00		
9	110.9	13.20	112.0		6.80	22.0		2.10		

Table 3. *In situ* stress measurement results in Meishan iron mine

Measuring point No.	Depth (m)	σ₁ Value (MPa)	σ₁ Bearing (°)	σ₁ Dip (°)	σ₂ Value (MPa)	σ₂ Bearing (°)	σ₂ Dip (°)	σ₃ Value (MPa)	σ₃ Bearing (°)	σ₃ Dip (°)
1	342	20.19	107.3	-3.1	9.79	114.7	86.9	7.48	17.3	0.4
2	355	16.16	345.5	-0.3	10.28	211.3	-89.5	7.59	255.5	0.3
3	355	20.32	195.9	12.6	11.79	287.3	6.2	9.57	43.0	76.0
4	350	18.37	335.1	-4.5	9.57	307.2	85.2	6.92	64.9	2.4
5	218	9.46	228.1	2.0	4.36	318.5	11.7	3.04	308.6	-78.1
6	218	11.47	359.5	-4.5	5.61	270.3	9.9	4.80	65.2	79.1
7	210	11.79	140.2	-5.7	5.86	48.9	-13.1	5.03	73.2	75.7
8	420	21.50	313.7	-3.3	12.32	193.3	-83.5	11.56	224.1	5.6

Table 4. *In situ* stress measurement results in Jinchuan nickel mine

Measuring point No.	Depth (m)	σ₁ Value (MPa)	σ₁ Bearing (°)	σ₁ Dip (°)	σ₂ Value (MPa)	σ₂ Bearing (°)	σ₂ Dip (°)	σ₃ Value (MPa)	σ₃ Bearing (°)	σ₃ Dip (°)
1	580	31.18	33.8	6.3	13.74	280.9	74.1	10.88	305.4	-14.5
2	580	24.88	1.9	15.5	13.59	271.3	2.1	12.96	353.6	-74.4
3	580	28.08	35.2	5.0	14.28	88.7	-82.7	11.59	305.8	-6.7
4	580	28.44	36.6	2.2	13.34	299.4	72.9	9.44	307.2	-16.9
5	730	36.95	176.7	-8.8	17.55	2.6	-81.1	13.09	86.8	0.9
6	730	37.86	18.2	1.4	16.79	130.6	86.2	12.22	108.2	-3.5
7	730	34.68	348.0	-5.1	17.34	238.6	-74.9	13.48	259.2	14.2
8	730	31.64	13.2	3.8	18.68	79.9	-80.5	11.59	283.8	-8.7
9	790	40.55	160.6	-1.9	20.55	0.3	-84.3	16.75	70.6	0.7
10	790	37.26	226.0	14.6	18.19	204.2	-74.5	17.66	314.6	-5.6

Corridor and the edge of Gobi Desert. It is the second largest nickel deposit in the world with a nickel metal production of 40000 tons per year. The nickel ore was borne in ultrabasic rock mass. The main orebody zone strikes NW 50-70° and has a dip angle of 50-70°. It is tens to 500m wide, 6500m long and more than 1000m deep. Most rich ore is reserved in the middle area of the orebody zone where the mining operation has been down to 800m under the ground level.

In situ stress measurement at shallow depth (20-480m) was completed at 8 points by Beijing Institute of Geomechanics in late 1970's (Liao et al., 1983). A nickel stress cell of Hast type with overcoring technique was used at that time. Among 8 points, 3-D stress state was determined at 4 points and only a planar stress state was obtained at the other 4 points. To obtain more accurate and more detailed information on stress state in deep position, stress measurement at 10 points between depths of 580-790m was carried out by the authors in 1995. All the 10 measuring points were distributed in the middle area of the mine. The rock mass around the measuring points was mainly composed of marble (in 1150m level) and granite (in 1000m and 940m levels). The measured results are shown in Table 4.

4 ANALYSES OF THE MEASURED RESULTS

Measuring results obtained in the four Chinese metal mines, as shown in Tables 1-4, showed similar regularities of *in situ* stress state:

1) There are two principal stresses which are almost horizontal and the third one is almost vertical. This regularity is more rigorous in plain areas than in mountain areas.

2) The maximum horizontal stress is about two times that expected from gravity. The specific number is: 2.1-2.3 times in Xincheng mine, 1.6-2.4 times in Meishan mine, 2.1-5.1 times in Ekou mine and 1.7-2.3 times in Jinchuan mine. The number in Ekou mine is obviously larger than that in the other three mines. It was caused by that the values of horizontal stresses

measured by hydraulic fracturing technique were little over large. Direction of maximum horizontal stress is NWW-SEE in Xincheng mine, NW-SE in Meishan mine, NNW-SSE in Ekou mine and NEE-SWW in Jinchuan mine, which is close to the direction of the tectonic stress field in the corresponding areas. These show that the horizontal tectonic stress field plays a dominant role in stress field in Chinese mainland.

3) The difference between two horizontal principal stresses is quite large which is about 1.5-2.8 times in Xincheng mine, 1.7-2.7 times in Meishan mine, 1.9-3.1 times in Ekou mine and in Jinchuan mine. This fact is an important reason to cause failure of underground openings and stopping areas.

4) The vertical stress is about equal to or, strictly speaking, is little greater than the weight of overburden in Xincheng mine, Meishan mine and Ekou mine, and little smaller than that in Jinchuan mine.

5) The maximum horizontal principal stress ($\sigma_{h.max}$) and vertical principal stress (σ_v) in all the four mines were approximately increased with depth. The minimum horizontal principal stress also showed the similar trend, but the regularity was not as strong as $\sigma_{h.max}$ and σ_v. Linear regression equations of $\sigma_{h.max}$, $\sigma_{h.min}$ and σ_v versus depth (H, unit is m) are as follows:

In Xincheng gold mine:
$\sigma_{h.max} = -0.44 + 0.0592H$ (MPa)
$\sigma_{h.min} = 0.44 + 0.0314H$ (MPa)
$\sigma_v = -0.07 + 0.0281H$ (Mpa)

In Meishan iron mine:
$\sigma_{h.max} = 0.14 + 0.0511H$ (MPa)
$\sigma_{h.Min} = -0.19 + 0.0253H$ (MPa)
$\sigma_v = -0.09 + 0.0282H$ (Mpa)

In Jinchuan nickel mine:
$\sigma_{h.max} = 0.10 + 0.0507H$ (MPa)
$\sigma_{h.min} = -0.02 + 0.0200H$ (MPa)
$\sigma_v = -0.21 + 0.0254H$ (Mpa)

In Ekou iron mine:
$\sigma_{h.max} = 5.61 + 0.0565H$ (MPa)
$\sigma_{h.min} = 3.55 + 0.0198H$ (MPa)
$\sigma_v = 0.45 + 0.0312H$ (MPa)

Two over large constant items, i.e. 5.61 and 3.55 in the above equations were also caused by some values of horizontal stresses measured by hydraulic fracturing technique in Ekou mine.

REFERENCES

Cai, M., Qiao, L. and Yu, J. 1995. Study and tests of techniques for increasing overcoring stress measurement accuracy. *Int. J. Rock Mech. Min. Sci. & Geomech. Abstr.*, 32: 375-384.

Liao, C. and Shi, Z. 1983. *In situ* stress measurements and their application to engineering design in the Jinchuan mine. *Proc. Fifth ISRM Congr.*, Mel-bourne, pp. D.87-89.

Worotnicki, G. and Walton, R. 1976. Triaxial "hollow" inclusion gauges for determination of rock stress *in situ*. *Proceedings of International Symposium on Investigation of Stress in Rock-Advances in Stress Measurement*. Sydney, pp. 1-8 (supplement).

Comparison of the results of stress measurements determined by various methods at the Kamaishi mine

Hiroya Matsui, Toshinori Sato & Kozo Sugihara
Power Reactor and Nuclear Fuel Development Corporation, Kamaishi, Japan

Naoaki Nakamura
Nittetsu Mining Co., Ltd, Tokyo, Japan

ABSTRACT: PNC(Power Reactor and Nuclear Fuel Development Corporation) has carried out several kinds of in-situ experiments to understand the deep underground geological environment at the Kamaishi mine. As a part of these experiments, the authors have performed a number of in-situ stress measurements with different measurement methods to assess the applicability of each method to determine the three dimensional in-situ stress state. The study site is located in granodiorite. Three laboratory stress measurement methods using core samples, AE, DSCA and DRA, and two field stress measurement methods, overcoring and hydraulic fracturing, were selected as representative of the methods currently used in Japan. In-situ stress measurements by each method have been carried out in the same boreholes in a drift about 260m below the surface and a drift about 730m below the surface.

1. INTRODUCTION

It is important for reliable design and underground construction to assess in-situ stress conditions exactly. Many kinds of methods for in-situ stress measurement have been proposed to date, but the applicability and accuracy of these methods in real field situations is still not clear.

The authors have carried out in-situ stress measurements by various methods at two locations in crystalline rock. In-situ stress conditions in the Kamaishi mine are discussed based on these results and the data from shallow earthquakes. Then, the applicability of each method is examined.

2. SITE LOCATIONS AND LOCAL GEOLOGY

Fig.1 shows the locations of the study sites in the Kamaishi mine. In-situ stress measurements were performed in the end of a drift about 260m below the surface(EL. 550m drift) and about 730m below the surface (EL. 250m drift). At EL. 250m, a new drift was excavated for the study of excavation disturbance. In addition to the stress measurements in the EL. 550m and EL. 250m drifts, stress measurement with the conventional hydraulic fracturing method was carried out in a 500m deep borehole drilled from the EL. 550m drift, KH-1(Fig 1). The rock type in both study sites and KH-1 borehole is granodiorite. The average rock properties of this granodiorite are shown in Table-1.The fracture frequencies around the sites at EL. 550m and EL. 250m are 1.1, 1.8/m, respectively. The dominant fracture orientation has an almost EW strike and a dip of 80~85 degrees. The axis of the EL. 550m drift is oriented about 130 degree from the dominant fracture orientation and that of the EL.250m drift is oriented about 90 degree from the dominant fracture orientation.

Table 1. Rock properties for Kurihashi granodiorite

	Density (gf/cm^3)	Porosity (%)	P-wave velocity (km/s)	Elastic modulus (GPa)	Uniaxial compression strength (MPa)
EL. 550m	2.74	0.5~0.8	5.1	58~67	115~160
EL. 250m	2.79	0.4~0.7	5.8	60~69	115~150

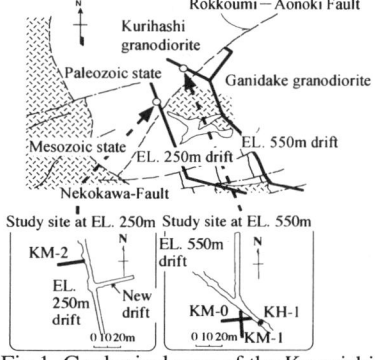

Fig 1. Geological map of the Kamaishi mine, locations of the study sites and the layout of boreholes

3. METHODS FOR STRESS MEASUREMENT

The measurement methods used in this study are shown in Table-2. These methods are representative of the stress measurement methods used currently in Japan. The conical-ended borehole and the 16-element conical strain cell technique(Fig. 2) was used, which is a type of overcoring method, and it is possible to calculate the stress tensor from a set of strain measurements made at any point in a single borehole with this cell[1]. The hydraulic fracturing method used can determine three dimensional stress by opening existing fractures and producing new fractures which have different orientations [2]. AE[3], DRA[4] and DSCA methods[5] are laboratory methods to determine the stress tensor. These stress measurement methods are able to determine the stress tensor in three dimensions.

All measurements were performed in the same boreholes or on cores of the same boreholes to facilitate comparisons. In the EL. 250m drift, overcoring, AE, DRA and DSCA methods were performed at 3~4 points in borehole KM-2(Fig.1) or on its core samples and stress measurements by hydraulic fracturing were also performed at 9 points in the same borehole. In the EL. 550m drift, overcoring, AE, DRA and DSCA methods were performed at 3~5 points in two boreholes KM-0,1(Fig.1) or on those core samples and stress measurements by hydraulic fracturing method were also carried out at 10 points in these boreholes. The locations of each stress measurement in each borehole are shown in Table-3.

As only the ratios between three principal stresses can be determined by DSCA method, these were converted into three dimensional principal stresses by assuming the vertical component of the stress tensor to be equal to the overburden pressure.

4. RESULTS

The results of each stress measurement are summarized in Table-4 and Table-5, which gives the average value for magnitude, azimuth and dip of principal stresses and directions of the principal stresses in the horizontal plane. Fig.3 shows the directions of three dimensional principal stresses with each stress measurement method in the EL. 250m and the EL. 550m drifts. The principal stress values calculated are shown in Fig.4. The ratios of measured vertical stress, σv, and estimated overburden pressure, $\sigma vcal$, are plotted in Fig.5.

In addition, the principal horizontal stresses measured in the KH-1 borehole by hydraulic fracturing and the calculated horizontal principal stresses based on each stress measurement method are plotted in Fig. 6,7.

Table 2. Major stress measurement methods used in Japan

In-situ measurements
Overcoring method
Hydraulic fracturing method
Sleeve fracturing method
Laboratory measurements
AE(Acoustic Emission) method
DRA(Deformatiion Rate Analysis) method
DSCA(Differential Strain Curve Analysis) method
ASR(Anelastic Strain Recovery) method

Remarks : Under lines show the methods used in this study

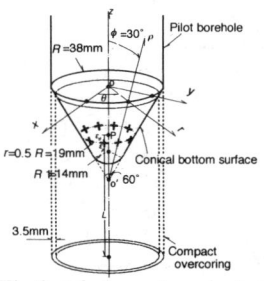

Fig 2. 16 element conical strain cell

Table 3. Location of each stress measurement
KM-2 (Inclination is 1° up)

	Overcoring	Hydraulic fracturing	AE,DRA,DSCA
Depth(m)	10.92~18.64	3.8~20.56	10.95~20.71

KM-0,1 (Inclinations are 1° up)

	Overcoring	Hydraulic fracturing	AE,DRA	DSCA
Depth(m)	10.1~19.6	5.0~18.8	14.12~20.52	14.01~21.00

* Width of EL.550m and EL.250m drifts are 3m

Table 4. Results of each stress measurement in the EL. 250m drift
250m level(Overburden : 730m)

	Overcoring	Hydraulic fracturing	AE/DRA methods	DSCA methods
σ1(MPa)	43.8	26	21.2	1*
Azimuth (degree)	181	359	79	124
Dip(degree)	26	52	56	49
σ2(MPa)	26.8	15.1	16.6	0.69*
Azimuth (degree)	348	237	207	22
Dip(degree)	64	23	23	11
σ3(MPa)	17.8	11.4	5.8	0.45*
Azimuth (degree)	89	133	308	283
Dip(degree)	5	29	24	39
σv(MPa)	29.9	21	18	
σvcal(MPa)	19.7	19.7	19.7	19.7
σH1(MPa)	40.7	18.3	17.5	
σH2(MPa)	17.9	13.2	8.1	
Direction of σH1 (degree)	NS	N16W	N42E	
K	0.98	0.75	0.71	

Remarks
σv: Measured vertical stress
σvcal:calculated overburden pressure, σvcal=27kN/m3×Depth(m)
σH1, σH2: Major and minimum principal stress in horizontal plane
K:Lateral pressure ratio. Where, K=σHave/σv,
σHave= (σH1+σH2)/2

Table 5. Reslults of each stress measurement in the EL. 550m

550m level(Overburden : 260m)

	Overcoring	Hydraulic fracturing	AE method	DRA method	DSCA method
σ1(MPa)	29.3	17.4	15.6	15.5	1*
Azimuth (degree)	342	332	356	345	204
Dip(degree)	13	4	20	14	33
σ2(MPa)	7.6	8.7	7.5	7.7	0.77*
Azimuth (degree)	248	237	257	191	294
Dip(degree)	17	49	23	75	1
σ3(MPa)	2.9	4.5	5.6	6.3	0.52*
Azimuth (degree)	107	64	122	77	25
Dip(degree)	68	40	59	6	57
σv(MPa)	4.7	7	7	8.1	8.1
σvcal(MPa)	7	7	7	7	7
σH1(MPa)	28	17.3	14	15	
σH2(MPa)	7.2	6.2	7.2	6.4	
Direction of σH1 (degree)	N17W	N28W	N3W	N14W	
K	3.77	1.77	1.51	1.32	

Remarks
σv, σvcal, σH1, σH2,K: See Table-3

4.1 Overcoring method

The direction of maximum principal stress, σ1, determined by the overcoring method is almost NS in the vicinity of the EL. 550m and EL. 250m drifts. The magnitude of σ1 is about 1.5 times larger than that estimated with the other stress measurement methods. The magnitude of σv at the EL. 550m drift is about 60% of σvcal, lower than the σv estimated with the other stress measurements. The magnitude of the horizontal maximum principal stress is also somewhat higher than that estimated with the other stress measurement methods and hydraulic fracturing method performed in KH-1.

4.2 Hydraulic fracturing method

The azimuth of σ1 determined by hydraulic fracturing method is almost NS in the EL. 550m and EL. 250m drifts, but dip is comparatively higher than that of the overcoring method in the EL. 250m drift. σv is almost equal to the overburden pressure at the EL. 550m and EL. 250m drifts. The magnitude of the horizontal principal stress in the EL. 250m drift is lower than the magnitude of principal stress determined by the hydraulic fracturing method at the same depth in KH-1.

4.3 AE and DRA methods

The azimuth of σ1 obtained by AE/DRA methods is almost EW in the EL. 250m drift, NS in the EL. 550m drift.

The principal stress magnitudes determined by AE and DRA methods are almost equal to that determined by the hydraulic fracturing method in the EL. 250m drift. The magnitudes of the horizontal principal stresses, σH1, σH2 in the EL. 250m drift are extremely low compared to the results from the hydraulic fracturing method in KH-1 and the other measurement methods. In the EL. 550m drift, the difference between the intermediate and minimum principal stresses is small compared to the results of the overcoring and hydraulic fracturing methods.

4.4 DSCA method

The azimuth of σ1 estimated by the DSCA method is almost EW in the EL. 250m drift, however the azimuth of σ1 in EL. 550m drift is nearly NS.

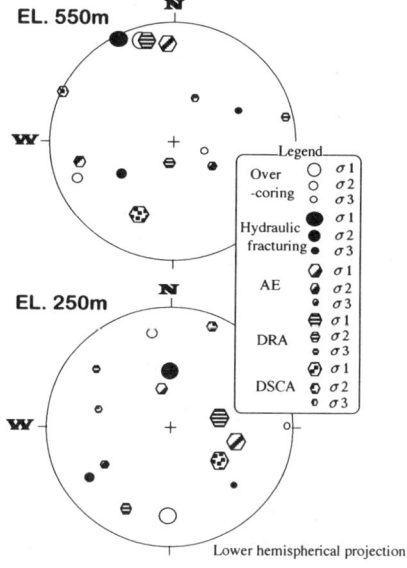

Fig 3. Directions of the principal stresses estimated with each stress measurement method

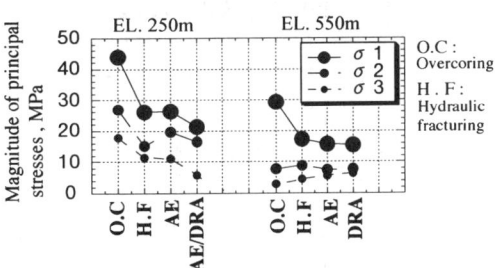

Fig 4. Magnitude of principal stresses estimated with each method

5. DISCUSSION

5.1 In-situ stress condition around the study sites

Fig. 8 shows the estimated direction of maximum stress based on the analysis of earthquake seismic waves [6]. Almost all of the earthquakes occurred at a shallow depth in the Tohoku area, northern Japan. The Tohoku area is in a state of EW compression because of the subduction zone along the coast of Tohoku area. However, in the area near the Kamaishi mine, several earthquakes show a nearly NS compression state.

Moreover, all of the results with conventional hydraulic fracturing method in KH-1 indicate that the direction of maximum horizontal stress is NS. Therefore, it is strongly suggested that the direction of maximum principal stress around the study site is almost NS.

Fig.9 shows the variation of the average lateral stress ratio K, $(\sigma H1 + \sigma H2)/2$ to σv, with depth in Japan and overseas. The overseas results are plotted between the two solid lines forming upper(K=0.1/Z+0.3) and lower (K=1.5/Z+0.5) limits. The results in Japan are distributed near the lower limit. K values calculated from stress measurements in this study are higher than the average values in Japan. This indicates that a high differential stress state exists around the study sites relative to the average stress state in Japan.

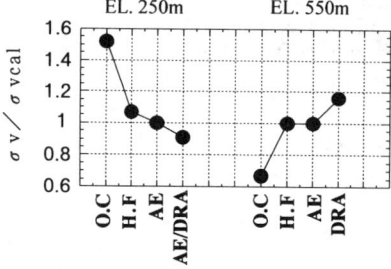

Fig 5. $\sigma v / \sigma$ vcal estimated with each method

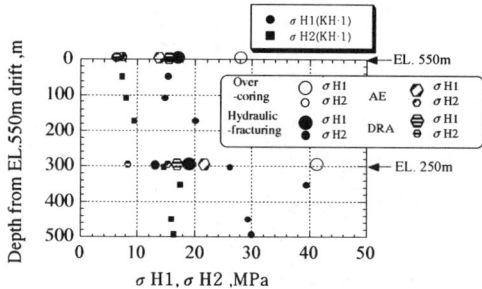

Fig 6. Relationship between depth and major and minor horizontal principal stresses, σ H1 and σ H2 with each method

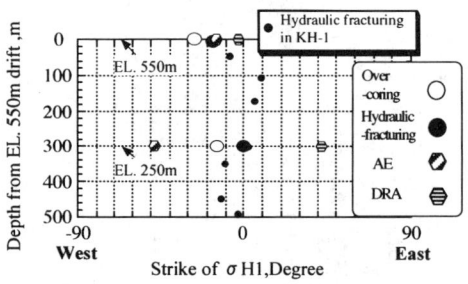

Fig 7. Relationship between depth and strike of σ H1 with each method

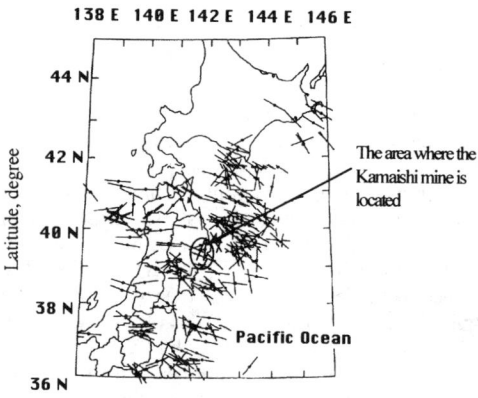

Fig 8. Direction of the major compression axis estimaeted by analysis of earthquake seismic waves from 1926 to 1993 (6)

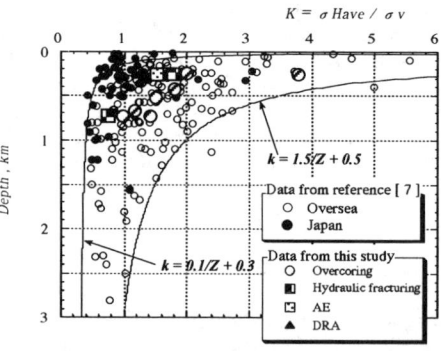

Fig 9. Variation of the lateral stress ratio, K with depth

5.2 Accuracy of the stress measurement methods

5.2.1 Stress measurement methods using core samples (AE, DRA and DSCA methods)

The strikes of the maximum principal stress determined by the AE and DRA methods in EL. 250m drift are N40E, and the strike determined by DSCA method is almost EW. The magnitudes of the horizontal principal stresses determined by these methods are quite low. These results differ from those of overcoring and hydraulic fracturing methods in the EL. 250m drift. It is considered that this difference is due to the period between drilling and laboratory testing, as these laboratory tests were carried out later than 60 days after drilling. Fig. 10 shows an example of the time dependency of measured stress magnitude by the DRA method [8]. In this experiment, a pre-stress of 30~40MPa was applied to cylindrical specimens in an uniaxial compression state by either cyclic loading or static loading. Then, the remaining stresses in the specimens were measured by the DRA method at different time periods after loading. The rock type of specimens is Inada granite, which is a standard granitic rock for laboratory tests in Japan. Similar results were obtained for the AE method as well[9].

On the other hand, in the EL. 550m drift, laboratory tests were carried out within 5 days after drilling and the results are in good agreement with those of the overcoring and hydraulic fracturing methods. It is important to shorten the time between testing and core retrieval as much as possible to improve the accuracy of stress measurements using core samples.

5.2.2 Stress measurement methods in the field

In the EL. 250m drift, the principal stress directions estimated by overcoring and hydraulic fracturing methods in the vertical plane perpendicular to a new drift axis are different as shown in Fig.11.

The distribution of the shear stress around a new drift by 2-D FEM analysis in the case of these stress conditions are shown in Fig. 12. In addition, Fig. 13 shows the results of drift shape measurements performed in a new drift.

Overcoring

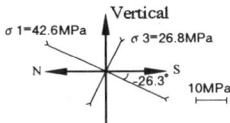

Hydraulic fracturing

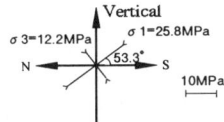

Fig 11. Measured Stresses in the vertical plane to a new drift at EL. 250m

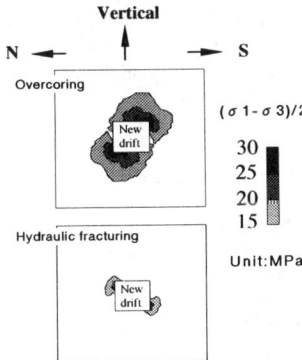

Fig 12. Shear stress distribution around a excavated new drift at EL. 250m (2-D FEM)

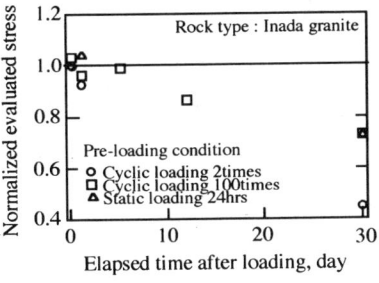

Fig 10. Time dependency of measured stress by DRA method (8)

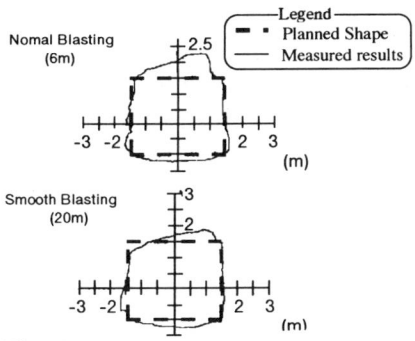

Fig 13. Results of drift shape measurement in a new drift

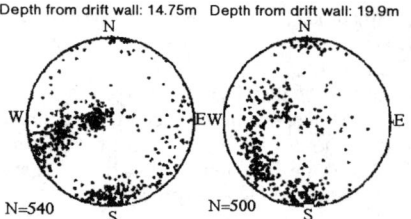

Fig 14. Distribution of poles to microcrack planes (Borehole KM-2 in EL. 250m drift)

The results of drift shape measurement, indicate that the excavated new drift was peeled off the rock at right upper part of the drift and small rock burst was also observed at the same part (Fig. 13). Comparing the shear stress distribution by FEM analysis and the measured drift shape, the result by FEM analysis in the case of the results with overcoring method suggest that the concentration part of shear stress corresponds to the part where rock burst was observed. Therefore , the principal stress direction by overcoring method is considered to be more accurate.

On the other hand , the direction of maximum principal stress measured by the overcoring and hydraulic fracturing methods in the EL.550m drift agree well with each other. The dip and strike of existing fractures used for hydraulic fracturing method in EL. 250m drift are not sufficiently different from each other so that the estimated stress parallel to these existing fractures is likely to be less accurate.

The magnitude of the maximum principal stress estimated with the overcoring method is considered to be overestimated because of the assumptions of measurement method. Namely, the factors which are not taken into account in the theory ,such as scale dependence, anisotropy of elastic modulus due to existing microcracks (Fig.14) and inhomogeneities in the local area, possibly affect the stress magnitude estimated with this method.

CONCLUSION

The results of this study are summarized as follows:

1) Maximum principal stress direction around the study site is found to be almost NS and horizontal . The average lateral stress ratio, K, around the study site is relatively high compared to the average values in Japan.
2) For the stress measurement methods using core samples ,the period between core sampling and testing should be kept short to improve the accuracy of the stress measurement.
3) The principal stress directions determined by overcoring are more accurate than those of the other methods tried in this study.

However, the magnitude of the maximum principal stress by the overcoring method is possibly overestimated due to the combined effect of the scale dependence and anisotropy of the rock's elastic modulus due to existing microcracks, local inhomogeneities and anisotropy of the rock mass.

ACKNOWLEDGMENT

The authors thank Dr. Yoshida and Dr. Steven Carlson of the Tono Geoscience Center of PNC for valuable comments and manuscript revision.

REFERENCE

1) Obara Y., Sugawara K., and Takehara T. :Rock stress measurement by stress relieving in Japan. AusIMM Joint Symposium' 94 Ube(1994)
2) Mizuta Y., Sano O., Ogino S., Katoh H. : Three dimensional stress determination by hydraulic fracturing for underground excavation design. Int. J. Rock Mech. Sci. Geomech. Abstr. Vol 24, No. 1 pp. 15-29 (1987)
3) Michihoro. K.,Hata K., Yoshioka H. and Fujiwara T. : Determination of the initial stresses on rock mass using acoustic emission method, J. of Acoustic Emission, s63-76(1992)
4) Yamamoto K. et al.:Tohoku Geophysical Journal , Vol.33, pp.127~147(1990)
5) Ren N.K and Rogiers J.C. : Differential strain curve analysis - a new method for determining the pre-existing in-situ stress state from rock core measurements., 5th Int. Congr. ISRM ,pp.117~127(1983)
6) Geographical survey institute ministry of construction of Japan : Microearthquake Activity in and around the Tohoku District (May-October,1993), Report of the coordinating committee for earthquake prediction , vol 51 pp. 152~164
7) Japan Society of Materials : Iwa-no-rikigaku ,pp.359
8) Kojima K., Nishiyama T. and Matsuki K. : A fundamental study of three-dimensional in-situ stress measurement by deformation rate analysis(DRA) , J. of Sigen-to-Sozai Vol.110 pp.143~148(1994)
9) Kojima T., Matsuki K. : A fundamental study on the kaiser effect of rocks under low stress conditions , J. of Sigen-to-Sozai Vol.110 pp.435~440(1994)

Numerical simulations of overcoring stress measurements in elastoplastic rocks

A. Giraud, F. Homand & A. Nechnech
LEGO, Ecole Nationale Supérieure de Géologie, Vandoeuvre-lès-Nancy, France

J. F. Shao
LML URA-CNRS, Université de Lille, France

ABSTRACT: The influence of the rock mass constitutive law and *in situ* stress on the response to overcoring is studied. Numerical simulations of the direct problem show that the response of the rock depends on the hardening law. A plastic zone can develop first during coring phase and this has an effect on strains even at the beginning of overcoring. The strain variations are different from those predicted by a linear elastic model. Mainly due to tensile mean stress variation during coring and overcoring, plasticity can develop again at the end of the overcoring phase. Residual mean stresses of tension can be observed for Drucker-Prager model.

1 INTRODUCTION

In situ stress measurements are an important part of the design and monitoring of underground rock structures. A large variety of overcoring techniques have been developed and refined over the years: doorstopper, USBM, CSIR or CSIRO cells (Amadei & Stephansson, 1996). In contrast, the theoretical aspects concerning the interpretations are essentially limited to anisotropy (Amadei, 1983 & 1996) and recently Corthésy et al.(1993) take into account the non-isotropic non-linear elastic behavior of rocks. Amadei's results clearly indicate the errors in both *in situ* stress magnitude and orientation, obtained by neglecting rock anisotropy. But the *in situ* stress determination by overcoring is inferred from strains or displacements; the constitutive law has a first effect. To be able to calculate the *in situ* stress field, a disturbing of the stress equilibrium is necessary and the stress-strain relationship has a second effect, without taking in consideration the dependence of the loading path associated with the local disturbance of the stress field. Finally, if the rock mass has a plastic behavior, the results as a whole will depend on the initial unknown natural stress. But it is common practice to use the equations derived from the theory of linear elasticity.

This paper outlines the results of the direct problem study by fixing the natural stresses and taking into account the constitutive behavior of the considered rock. The coring and overcoring phases are simulated in order to calculate displacements, strains and stresses. The basic idea is that we shall be able to find the main factors influencing the behavior of the borehole during the overcoring. One of the interest of our approach is to take into account the total loading history. Indeed, the detailed analysis of the coring stage holds the key to understand the behavior of the borehole near area during the overcoring.

The approach to solve the overcoring problem is in a first stage only 2D, and plane strain hypothesis is assumed. Consequently for a CSIRO cell, the strain gages placed in an orthogonal plane to the borehole axis are only considered. Then the problem is simulated by an axisymmétrical model, whose the main objective is to study the extension of plastic area during the coring and overcoring stages and the response of the axial strain gages. The final phase will be 3D modeling in order to consider a borehole out of the principal axis of anisotropy. An other way of the methodology is to invert the equation system to calculate stresses from registered strains (Shao et al., 1997). From a general point of view, this methodology can be used for any elastoplastic constitutive laws (Drucker-Prager without hardening, Khan, modified Cam-Clay). In this paper, Drucker-Prager model is only considered and the results will be compared with those obtained for elastic models. Furthermore, only the 2D computation results will be explained.

2. CONSTITUTIVE LAW FOR THE MARL

The considered rock is a deep marl whose laboratory behavior is well known and in which *in situ* stress measurements have been carried out (Ben Slimane et al. 1996). Its elastic behavior is transversely isotropic due to bedding planes. However, if the borehole is perpendicular to this plane, anisotropy can be neglected. The analysis of triaxial tests showed that:
- the behavior is globally elastoplastic, without

damage, in the sense of the elastic parameters decreasing is not significant,
- the volume dilatancy is observed only for triaxial tests under low confining pressures,
- the anisotropy is highly reduced when confining pressure increases,
- the Young's modulus perpendicular to the bedding plane increases with confining pressure, whereas the Young's modulus in this plane and the Poisson's ratios do not vary.

Considering these experimental observations the elastoplastic Drucker-Prager model (1952) and Khan's model (1991) were chosen. The parameters were calibrated from triaxial tests carried out with loading -unloading paths (cores in the bedding plane) and at confining pressures 0, 3, 10, 25 and 40 MPa.

The elastoplastic Drucker-Prager model just considered in this paper, has 5 parameters: 2 characterizing the elastic behavior (E=21 000 MPa; ν = 0,29) and 3 characterizing the plastic behavior. These parameters are α and k characterizing the yield function $f(\underline{\sigma}, k)$, and β the flow rule. The α and k values can be expressed with respect to cohesion C and internal friction angle ϕ (Mohr - Coulomb model) by using the following relationships:

$$\alpha = \frac{3 \, tg[\phi]}{\sqrt{9 + 12 \, tg^2[\phi]}} \quad k = \frac{3 \, C}{\sqrt{9 + 12 \, tg^2[\phi]}}$$

These two equations square with the case where the Drucker - Prager cone passes through the inner corners of the Mohr - Coulomb pyramid. The α and k fitting gives the values

$\alpha = 0.454 \qquad k = 7.17$ MPa
corresponding to:
$\phi \approx 28° \qquad C \approx 8.4$ MPa

The dilatancy angle ψ is assumed equal to 0, and by consequence $\beta=0$; accordingly, the plastic deformations are purely deviatoric. The material behavior is assumed elastic perfectly plastic with hardening.

3. OVERCORING MODELING

3.1 CSIRO HI cell

The considered CSIRO HI cell is a three four-component strain rosette version of the Hi cell containing twelve strain gages instead of nine (Amadei & Stephansson, 1996). Two strain gages are parallel to the axis of the cell, five gages measure circumferential strains and five gages measure strains at ± 45°. The three additional strain gages (two circumferential and one at 45°) provide additional strain measurement redundancy.

A 2D-model will allow to analyze the strains corresponding to the circumferential strain gages and an axisymmetrical model will take moreover into account the axial strain gages.

3.2 The 2D model

The coring and overcoring stages were simulated by using CESAR-LCPC finite element code. The drill advance is simulated by using λ parameter (deconfinement rate); λ is connected to the drill location or lining placement by this equation:

$$\lambda(z) = \frac{1}{2}\left(1 - th\left[\frac{1}{3} - \frac{z}{D}\right]\right)$$

where : th is the hyperbolic tangent, z: drill location with regard to the standard drillhole end; D: hole diameter. For the plots as illustrated in Fig.4, the values of λ are:

$0 \leq \lambda \leq 1$:coring stage,

$1 \leq \lambda \leq 2$:overcoring stage.

Assuming strain plane condition and transversely isotropy, a quarter of section is considered where the strain gages are located. The finite elements mesh is composed of 1060 Q8 elements. The loading history is simulated with 3 steps :
- the first step is intended to initiate stresses in rock mass by means of a constant initial stress field loading,
- the second step is the coring by using 10 increments and the stresses are decreased up to 0 at the borehole wall,
- the third step is the overcoring simulation from results of the second stage. A mechanical unloading is done by decreasing (10 increments) of the stress in the external area of the overcoring rock.

The overcoring problem under plane strain condition is a hollow cylinder subjected to a pressure on the inner radius and to a pressure and a circumferential load on the external radius. During the overcoring the tensile stress variations are imposed on the external radius of the hollow cylinder.

The results concern essentially four points of the borehole wall, corresponding to the five strain gages A90, B90, C90, E90 & F90, A & C points being confounded (Fig. 1). Point B is the direction associated with the major principal stress and point F is the direction associated to the minor principal stress. The results analysis has required the total strain calculations at the nodes of the considered points and the transformation of the Cartesian components ($\varepsilon_{xx}, \varepsilon_{xy}, \varepsilon_{yy}$) in cylindrical components ($\varepsilon_{rr}, \varepsilon_{r\theta}, \varepsilon_{\theta\theta}$).

If the coring stage is classical, on the contrary the numerical procedure used to simulate the overcoring is original, leading to validate the numerical simulations by using an analytical solution of the coring and overcoring problem (Kirsch and Lame solutions for an elastic rock).

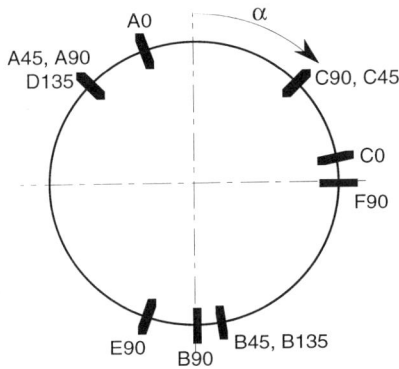

Fig.1 - Orientation of points A, B, C, D, E and F.

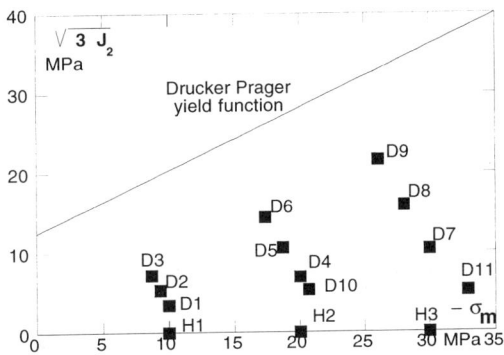

Fig. 2 - Initial stresses in the $|\sigma_m| - \sqrt{3 J_2}$ plane

3.3 - Initial stresses

The initial stress state is characterized by initial principal stresses σ_h and σ_H, whose directions are perpendicular to the coring axis and by σ_z (axial initial stress). This last value is fixed and the parametric study concerns σ_h and σ_H, K being the stress ratio. Four values of K were taken into consideration (K = 1, 1.5, 2 and 3) for three values of σ_H (-12, -24 and -36 MPa). The initial stress states are plotted in Fig. 2, in the first and second stress invariants space, and compared with the yield surface of Drucker-Prager model.

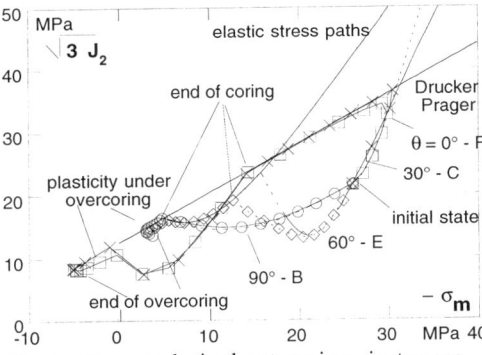

Fig. 3- Stress paths in the stress invariant space.

4. RESULTS OF AN EXAMPLE OF DEVIATORIC STRESS

The analyzed case corresponds to σ_H = -36 MPa, σ_h = -12 MPa, $\sigma_{z.init}$ = -30 MPa (Fig. 3) and plasticity occurs during coring, the first plastic point being F, corresponding to the minor stress direction.

4.1 Stress paths

The stress path interpretation is immediate for the Drucker-Prager model without hardening because the elastic domain is constant. The stress state D9 leads to stress paths quite different in linear elasticity during coring for the four studied points at the borehole wall (Fig. 3). At F and C points during the coring, an increasing of equivalent deviatoric stress and a compressive mean stress variation are observed while at E and B points a tensile mean stress variation is observed.

The overcoring shows an unloading (decompression), i.e. a variation of the tensile mean stress. If the coring phase is entirely elastic, this variation is added to a compressive mean stress variation at F and C points where the deviatoric stress is maximum at the end of the coring. It is clear from the elastoplastic calculations that variations of the tensile mean stress occur when plasticity is reached at point F during coring. The points E and B are located in the area where the elastic stress path during coring is characterized by a tensile mean stress also observed when the behavior is plastic. For these points the plasticity has an influence on deviatoric stress. The deviatoric stress increase at the end of the coring for an elastic behavior is relatively restricted for a plastic behavior.

At the beginning of the overcoring, the four studied points are located in the elasticity domain, by effect of a decrease of the equivalent deviatoric stress. Then during overcoring, the equivalent deviatoric stress increases with a tensile mean stress variation leading the stresses to plasticity at the end of overcoring. The final locations of the stresses in the stress invariant space are different from those obtained in the case of an elastic behavior (Fig.3).

The tensile mean stress variation due to plasticity during coring is crucial for the plastic reloading at the end of overcoring. This plasticity extent is observed at points B and E. It must be emphasized that it is impossible to observe plasticity during overcoring if there is no plasticity during coring.

4.2 - Plasticity influence on circumferential strains during coring

The curves in Fig. 4 show that the plasticity influence is significant and that it is different according to the point location. At the point F ($\alpha=90°$) corresponding to the minor principal stress direction, where the plasticity appears in the first place, the predicted total strain by the elastoplastic model is markedly higher at the end of the coring than the circumferential strain predicted by using the linear elastic model. The elastic-elastoplastic strains gap increases as the plasticity is expanding. For all the considered deviatoric stress states, the total plastic circumferential strain is always higher or equal to the elastic circumferential strain at a given deconfinement rate.

At point C (Figs. 1 and 4) the plasticity influence is more complex, the predicted total strain by the elastoplastic model is smaller at the coring beginning than the one computed by elasticity. This trend reverses at the end of the coring.

At points E and B (Figs. 1 and 4) the plastic strain is always smaller or equal to the elastic circumferential strain for a given deconfinement rate. The gap between plastic and elastic strains markedly increases as a function of confinement decrease.

4.3 - Plasticity influence on circumferential strains during overcoring

The higher strain variations during overcoring are those observed at point F. At the end of the overcoring, the strain variations decrease progressively from point F ($\alpha = 0°$) to point B ($\alpha = 90°$). During overcoring, the elastic strain variation increases regularly. The plastic strain variations at points F, C and E behave similarly. In contrast, this variation is particular for strains at point B, the strain increases up to maximum then it drops at the end of overcoring. This unusual trend is due to an effect of the constitutive behavior on the rock mass response. It is observed in the radial direction corresponding to the major principal stress where the strain variations are however the smallest. This effect depends on the initial stress state.

The comparison between the elastic and plastic total strain variations demonstrates that an elastoplastic constitutive model does not lead necessarily to higher strains than an elastic model. For the last increment, at the points B and F the variation of elastoplastic strains are higher than the elastic strains, but at points C and E the elastic and plastic strain variations are very close to each other. This depends on the initial stress state too.

5. DISCUSSION

The analysis of the overcoring problem in elastoplastic rock provides the undisputed evidence

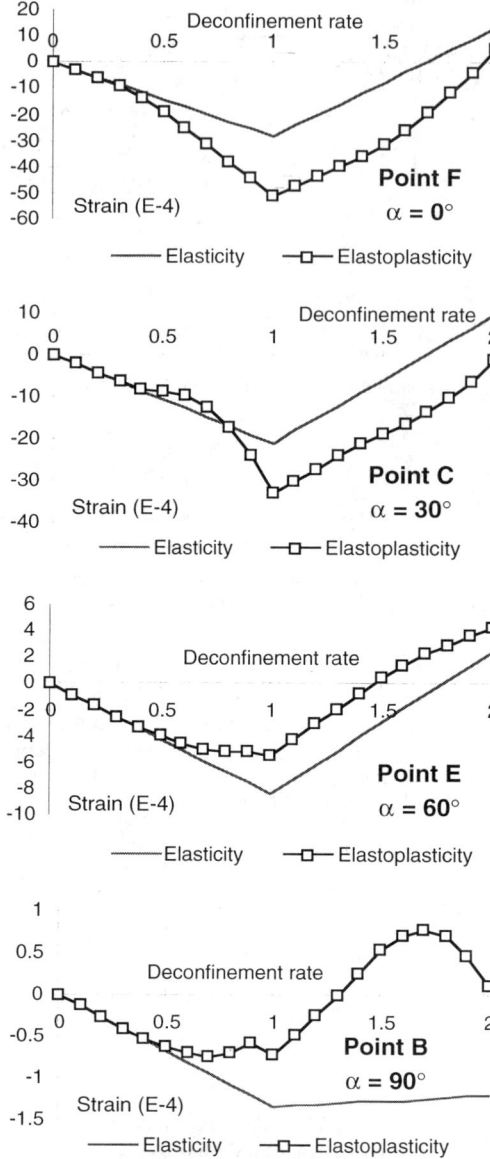

Fig. 4 - Variation of circumferential strains vs deconfinement rate ($\lambda =1$ coring; $\lambda =2$ overcoring) at points F, B, E and C.

that the constitutive law has a strong influence on the rock response. The radial direction relative to the principal stress can be theoretically determined with the circumferential strain variations during the overcoring:
- the maximum variations are obtained at the point corresponding to the minor initial stress and vice versa,

- the maximum diameter is measured along the radial direction corresponding to the major initial stress.

The response of the plastic rock mass during overcoring varies with respect to the previous loading, that is the coring. The mechanical loading history has a strong influence. Our computation have shown that the plasticity during the overcoring occurs always if it is occurred during the coring.

During coring, initial stresses highly deviatoric lead to a localized plasticity around the radial direction corresponding to the minor principal stress. This local plasticity has an influence on the mechanical behavior of the volume around the borehole.

The plasticity classically appears during coring, at the point of the borehole wall where the equivalent deviatoric stress is maximum, that is at point F. The plasticity growth is connected to the initial stress state. Higher is the stress ratio K, more the plasticity is localized during coring in the direction corresponding to the minor principal stress. When K is close to 1 (hydrostatic state) the plasticity is not localized, but "isotropic" around the borehole.

A comprehensive treatment of the influence of initial stress state on the plastic zone shape may be found in a paper by Detournay and Fairhurst (1987), for Mohr-Coulomb model. The authors point out a parameter "m" (obliquity parameter) characterizing the initial stress state whose the influence on the plastic shape is significant. The parameter "m" is the ratio of the deviatoric stress to infinity over the yield function. More "m" is high, more the plasticity is high and localized in the direction corresponding to the minor principal stress, that fits in with what we observed. In our study the obliquity parameter would be connected to K and to the equivalent initial deviatoric stress. In the case of the Drucker-Prager model, relatively similar to Mohr-Coulomb, at the end of the overcoring, the plastic zone does not surround the borehole or initial stress state # D7, D10 and D11 (Fig. 2). For example, the point B can not be plastic, however its evolution will be different from that obtained in an elastic rock. A localized plasticity has an effect on the behavior of the borehole zone, whether the point is plastic or not. An example of the plastic zone extension at the end of coring and overcoring is shown in Figs. 5 & 6.

The influence of plasticity during coring is noticeable at the beginning of the overcoring for many stress states. By example about 30 % of relative difference between elastic and elastoplastic strains at the four points considered are superior to 10 %, for the first increment. This is observed even though the first increment of the stress path is in the elastic field. The reason is that the stress, strain and displacement fields are modified as early as the plasticity appears.

At the beginning of the overcoring, initial hydrostatic stresses lead to an elastic unloading. The plasticity influence is possible only if the initial stress state is deviatoric, that is if plasticity does not occur quite symmetrically to the drill axis.

The influence of the constitutive behavior on circumferential stain variations of the borehole wall is significant for many stress states. By comparing with the elasticity, the plasticity can have an inverse effect. The Drucker-Prager model increases the heterogeneity of the circumferential strain variations. Some computations realized with Khan's model show an opposite trend.

The tensile mean stress variations during the coring phase which are added to tensile mean stress variations due to the overcoring, can induce a plastic reloading of the rock, close to the hole, at the end of the overcoring. Furthermore, final tensile mean stress can be found. The plasticity or plastic reloading of the rock at the end of the overcoring is manifested by non-linear curves of circumferential strain variations.

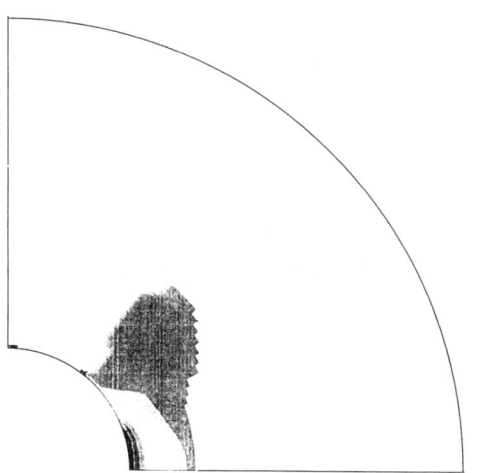

Fig. 5 - Plastic zone extension at the end of coring.

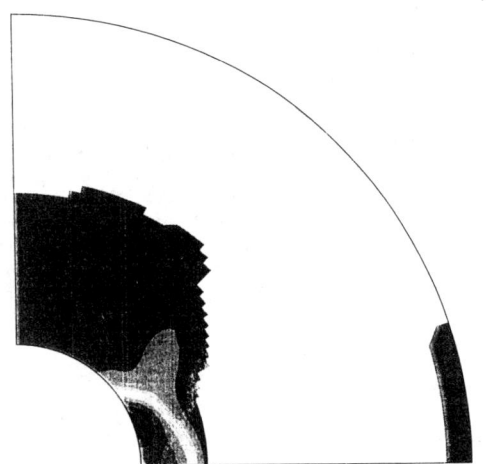

Fig. 6 - Plastic zone extension at the end of overcoring.

In the case of the Drucker-Prager model, the plastic reloading increases the strain variations corresponding to the minor principal stress direction.

Concerning the constitutive model, it is important to quantify by laboratory tests the tensile threshold (plastically admissible tensile stress). In the case of the Drucker-Prager model, the main parameters are cohesion and friction angle. To interpret an overcoring test in deep marls, the knowledge of the constitutive model is necessary:
- the yield function which is connected to the grade of plasticity during coring and overcoring,
- the hardening rule.

In fact, the behavior has to be studied under low confining pressure, with loading-unloading stress paths, simulating the *in situ* stress paths.

6 CONCLUSION

This study demonstrates the importance of constitutive model (elasticity vs. plasticity) for a successful interpretation of overcoring tests.

A serious difficulty is that it is hard to differentiate the effects related to constitutive behavior from those related to the initial stress.

This paper outlines the results of the direct problem by fixing the natural stresses and taking into account the constitutive law of the considered rock. One of the interest of our approach is to take into account the total loading history. A detailed analysis of the coring stage holds the key to understand the behavior of the borehole near area during the overcoring.

By using a Drucker-Prager type model, this 2D parametric study establishes the possibility of unmonotonous evolution of the circumferential strains during overcoring. An elastic model gives only a monotonous increase of the circumferential strains during overcoring.

According to the parametric study, two different reasons can lead to increase the uniformity of the circumferential strains. The first reason is related to the constitutive behavior and the second is related to the stress state. Concerning the constitutive behavior, a low yield stress and a high positive hardening trend to smooth the strains. A null or negative hardening, a low tensile threshold can lead to a major plastic reloading at the end of the overcoring and to an increase of the strains heterogeneity. Concerning the stress level, the circumferential strains are all the more regular because the initial stress are close to a hydrostatic state. On the contrary, these strains are heterogeneous if the anisotropy of initial stress increases.

ACKNOWLEDGMENTS - The authors wish to thank the Agence Nationale pour la Gestion des Déchets Radioactifs (ANDRA) for the financial support for this project.

REFERENCES

Amadei B. 1983. Rock anisotropy and the theory of stress measurements. *Lecture Notes in Engineering Series*. Springer, New York.

Amadei B. 1996. Importance of Anisotropy When Estimating and Measuring *In situ* Stresses in Rock. *Int. J. Rock Mech. Min. Sci. & Geomech. Abstr.*, **33**, No 3, pp. 293-325.

Amadei B. and Stephanson O. 1996. Rock stress and its measurement. Chapman & Hall, 490 p.

Ben Slimane K., Cournut A., Durand-Smet J.-F. and Trentesaux C. 1996. *In situ* study and modeling of the mechanical behavior of a large diameter vertical blind hole in marl. *Int. Conf. on Deep Geological Disposal of Radioactive Waste*, Winnipeg, pp. 6-71-6-80.

Corthésy R., Gill D.E. and Leite M.H. 1993. An Integrated Approach to Rock Stress Measurement in Anisotropic Non-linear Elastic Rock. *Int. J. Rock Mech. Min. Sci. & Geomech. Abstr.*, **30**, No 4, pp. 395-411.

Detournay E. and Fairhurst C. 1987. Two-dimensional Elastoplastic Analysis of a Long, Cylindrical Cavity Under Non-hydrostatic Loading. *Int. J. Rock Mech. Min. Sci. & Geomech. Abstr.*, **24**, No 4, pp. 197-211.

Drucker D.C., Prager W. 1952. Soil mechanics and plastic analysis or limit design. *Quarterly of Applied Mathematics*, **X**, No 2, pp. 157-165.

Khan A.S., Xiang Y., Huang S. 1991. Behavior of Berea Sandstone under confining pressure part I: Yield and Failure surface, and non linear elastic response. *Int. Journ. of Plasticity*, **7(5)**, pp. 607-628.

Khan A.S., Xiang Y., Huang S. 1992. Behavior of Berea Sandstone under confining pressure part II: elastic plastic response. *Int. Journ. of Plasticity*, pp. 209-220.

Quiertant M., Shao J.F. 1997. Application of the inverse problem theory to *in situ* stress determination in elastoplastic rocks. *Proc. NUMOG VI*, Montreal.

Conventional hydrofrac method in arbitrarily oriented stress fields

A. Sato, T. Ito & K. Hayashi
Institute of Fluid Science, Tohoku University, Sendai, Japan

ABSTRACT: The applicability of the conventional hydraulic fracturing method to arbitrarily oriented stress field has been clarified quantitatively, where the method was proposed originally for the 2D stress state. The results show that the applicability depends on the strength of rock, and if the tensile strength of rock is relatively large compared with the mean value of the in-situ stress, the state of stress in the plane perpendicular to the borehole axis can be estimated approximately from the azimuth of the induced longitudinal cracks and their reopening and shut-in pressures independently of borehole inclination.

1 INTRODUCTION

In hydraulic fracturing stress measurements, the state of stress in a plane perpendicular to borehole axis is determined from orientation of induced longitudinal cracks and several pressures, i.e., the breakdown pressure, the reopening pressure and the shut-in pressure (e.g., Bredehoeft et al. 1976, Zoback et al. 1977, Haimson 1978). The procedure for stress determination is simple in the case that one axis of the principal stress is coincident with the borehole axis. On the contrary, in the case that all axes of the principal stress deviate from the borehole axis, the procedure becomes fairly complicated in order to take account of not only the stress components in the plane perpendicular to the borehole axis but also those parallel to the borehole axis (Cornet et al. 1984, Hayashi et al. 1985, 1989). However, even if all axes of the principal stress deviate from the borehole axis, the crack behavior is mainly governed by the state of stress in a plane perpendicular to the borehole axis as inferred from the shapes of the borehole and the cracks. Hence, in many cases independently of the borehole inclination, the state of stress in a plane perpendicular to the borehole axis may be evaluated approximately through the procedure originally developed for the case that one axis of the principal stress is coincident with the borehole axis. In order to verify such a concept, the effects of the stress components parallel to the borehole axis on the crack behavior were clarified theoretically in this work.

2 THEORY OF HYDRAULIC FRACTURING

2.1 Crack behavior

Even if all axes of the in-situ principal stress deviate from a borehole axis, the hydraulic fracturing generally induces longitudinal cracks, i.e., the cracks parallel to a borehole axis, as well known experimentally and theoretically (Daneshy 1973, Hayashi et al. 1985, 1989). The behavior of the longitudinal cracks are related to the in-situ stress as follows.

The hydraulic fracturing is conducted in a borehole drilled into an infinite rock mass which is subjected to the in-situ principal stresses σ_i ($i = 1, 2, 3$; $\sigma_1 \geq \sigma_2 \geq \sigma_3$). The compressive stresses are taken to be positive in this paper. A Cartesian coordinate system (X_i, $i = 1, 2, 3$) is introduced such that the axes of X_1, X_2 and X_3 are aligned with those of σ_1, σ_2 and σ_3 respectively as shown in Figure 1. Another coordinate system (x_i, $i = 1, 2, 3$) is also introduced such that x_3 is the borehole

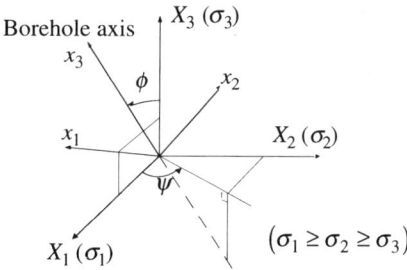

Figure 1. Coordinate systems.

axis and x_1 lies on the X_1-X_3 plane. In Figure 1, the angles ϕ and ψ are the angle between X_3 and x_3 and that between X_1 and the projection of x_3 on the X_1-X_2 plane. We assume the impermeable rock and pore pressure is assumed to be zero. When the borehole is subjected to a hydraulic pressure p, the stress on the borehole surface are given as follows (Daneshy 1973):

$$\left.\begin{array}{l}\sigma_r = p, \\ \sigma_\omega = \tau_{11} + \tau_{22} - 2(\tau_{11} - \tau_{22})\cos 2\omega \\ \qquad - 4\tau_{12}\sin 2\omega - p, \\ \sigma_z = \tau_{33} - v\{2(\tau_{11} - \tau_{22})\cos 2\omega + 4\tau_{12}\sin 2\omega\}, \\ \sigma_{\omega z} = 2(\tau_{23}\cos\omega - \tau_{31}\sin\omega), \quad \sigma_{r\omega} = \sigma_{rz} = 0.\end{array}\right\} \quad (1)$$

where v is Poisson's ratio, σ_r, σ_ω, σ_z, $\sigma_{r\omega}$, σ_{rz} and $\sigma_{\omega z}$ are the stresses referring to a cylindrical coordinate system (r, ω, z) shown in Figure 2, and τ_{ij} ($i, j = 1, 2, 3$) are the in-situ stress components referring to x_i and are related to σ_i by the expression:

$$\tau_{ij} = \sum_{k=1}^{3} l_{ik} l_{jk} \sigma_k \quad (2)$$

where l_{ij} ($i, j = 1, 2, 3$) are direction cosines of (x_1, x_2, x_3) with respect to (X_1, X_2, X_3) and are the functions of ϕ and ψ. The least normal stress at each point on the borehole surface is

$$\sigma_t = \frac{1}{2}\left\{\sigma_\omega + \sigma_z - \sqrt{(\sigma_\omega - \sigma_z)^2 + 4\sigma_{\omega z}^2}\right\}. \quad (3)$$

Along the generating lines of $\omega = \omega_f$ and $\omega_f + \pi$ at which σ_t is least for all points, small cracks are induced as shown in Figure 2, when p reaches p_f and σ_t satisfies the following conditions:

$$\left.\frac{\partial \sigma_t}{\partial \omega}\right|_{\omega=\omega_f, p=p_f} = 0 \quad (4)$$

$$\left.\sigma_t\right|_{\omega=\omega_f, p=p_f} + T = 0 \quad (5)$$

where T is the tensile strength of rock. As p increases, the small cracks grow up to form two macroscopically straight cracks, i.e., the longitudinal cracks. The cracks would grow normally to the least compressive stress acting in the x_1 - x_2 plane as shown in Figure 3. In this figure, σ_{max} and σ_{min} are the maximum and minimum compressive stresses acting in the x_1 - x_2 plane, respectively, and are given by

$$\left.\begin{array}{l}\sigma_{max} \\ \sigma_{min}\end{array}\right\} = \frac{1}{2}\left\{\tau_{11} + \tau_{22} \pm \sqrt{(\tau_{11} - \tau_{22})^2 + 4\tau_{12}^2}\right\} \quad (6)$$

The azimuth of σ_{max}, ω_{max}, is given by

$$\omega_{max} = \frac{1}{2}\tan^{-1}\left(\frac{2\tau_{12}}{\tau_{11} - \tau_{22}}\right) \quad (7)$$

In pressurizing cycle for reopening of the cracks, the cracks begin to open when the hoop stress σ_ω at $\omega = \omega_f$ becomes zero. Therefore, we obtain the following equation from Eq. (1);

$$\tau_{11} + \tau_{22} - 2(\tau_{11} - \tau_{22})\cos 2\omega_f \\ - 4\tau_{12}\sin 2\omega_f - p_r = 0 \quad (8)$$

where p_r is the so-called reopening pressure. When we shut-in the pressurizing circuit, the cracks close. The greater parts of the cracks are considered to be normal to σ_{min}, therefore, the pressure in the cracks just after the shut-in, p_s, would balance with σ_{min}, namely

$$\sigma_{min} - p_s = 0 \quad (9)$$

where p_s is the so-called shut-in pressure.

2.2 *Estimation of in-situ stress*

Now let us consider to estimate the in-situ stress state from the azimuth of the cracks and the pressures of p_r and p_s which are obtained by hydraulic fracturing.

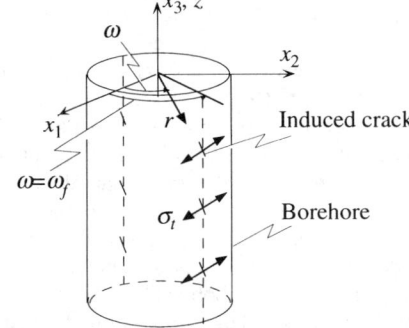

Figure 2. Coordinate system and initiation of small cracks resulting in lomgitudinal cracks.

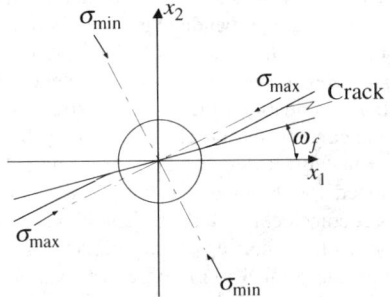

Figure 3. Propagation of longitudinal cracks into the rock-mass.

Then we have two observation equations of Eqs.(8) and (9) for the four unknown quantities of τ_{11}, τ_{22}, τ_{12} and ω_f. The ω_f is unknown, because the azimuth of the cracks is known but the orientation of x_1 is unknown. The number of the unknown quantities are larger than that of the observation equations, hence, we cannot estimate the in-situ stress state except for the magnitude of σ_{min} in this situation. On the other hand, if the cracks are assumed to be induced at $\omega \approx \omega_{max}$, Eq.(8) can be rewritten approximately as

$$3\sigma_{min} - \sigma_{max} - p_r \approx 0 \qquad (10)$$

In this case, we have two observation equations of Eqs. (9) and (10) for the two unknown quantities of σ_{max} and σ_{min}. Hence, the magnitudes of σ_{max} and σ_{min} can be estimated approximately as the solutions which satisfy Eqs. (9) and (10), and ω_{max} can be estimated approximately as the azimuth of the cracks, i.e., ω_f. If the borehole axis is coincident with one of the axes of the in-situ principal stress, Eq.(10) and such approach are valid strictly (Bredehoeft et al. 1976, Zoback et al. 1977).

3 ERROR IN ESTIMATED STRESS STATE

3.1 *Quantification of error*

Next let us examine the amount of error in the magnitude and azimuth of σ_{max} estimated upon the assumption that the azimuth of the cracks is aligned with that of σ_{max} independently of the borehole inclination. The estimated azimuth and magnitude of σ_{max} are denoted by $\omega_{max}'(= \omega_f)$ and σ_{max}' respectively. The indexes e_ω and e_σ are here introduced in order to represent the amount of errors in ω_{max}' and σ_{max}'. They are defined as

$$e_\omega = |\omega_{max} - \omega_{max}'|, \quad e_\sigma = \frac{|\sigma_{max} - \sigma_{max}'|}{\sigma_m} \qquad (11)$$

where σ_m is mean stress, i.e., $\sigma_m = (\sigma_1 + \sigma_2 + \sigma_3)/3$.
 The error of e_ω and e_σ can be evaluated theoretically as functions of T, ϕ, ψ and σ_i from Eq.(1) - (10). We shall consider the boreholes defined by the combinations of every ϕ and ψ at the interval of $\pi/18$ in the range of $0 - \pi$. Furthermore, we shall consider the magnitudes of σ_i as follows. Every state of in-situ stress is limited in the triangle area on the σ_1/σ_m vs σ_2/σ_m diagram as shown in Figure 4 (Hongo et al. 1997). From this fact, as the typical stress states, Hongo et al. have selected the eleven points numbered from 1 to 11 shown in Figure 4 which are distributed uniformly in the triangle area. Following their consideration, we shall also consider these

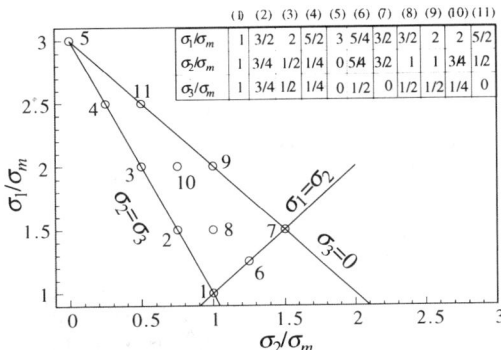

Figure 4. 3-D stress states.

eleven stress states. Furthermore, we shall consider the three types of rock with $\overline{T} = T / \sigma_m = 0.1$, 1 and 10. If T is fixed, those three cases for $\overline{T}$ correspond to the cases that the hydraulic fracturings are conducted at three different depths, i.e., the depth becomes larger as $\overline{T}$ becomes smaller, because σ_m increases with depth in general. Then we can evaluate the error of e_ω and e_σ as the functions of $\overline{T}$, ϕ, ψ and σ_i / σ_m.

3.2 *Results*

The results for e_ω are summarized in Figures 5 (a) - (c). These figures show that the ratio of the cases inducing large error decreases with increasing $\overline{T}$. The reason of this can be drawn as follows. When $\overline{T}$ is larger, the borehole pressure at the crack initiation, p_f, becomes larger and then the stress σ_ω becomes dominant in Eq.(3). It means that the crack initiation is mainly governed by the stress state in the plane normal to the borehole, i.e., σ_{max} and σ_{min}. Hence, the cracks tends to be induced at $\omega = \omega_{max}$, and e_ω becomes small. In the case of $\overline{T} = 0.1$, the ratio of the cases inducing large error becomes large. However, if we permit the error of e_ω less than $\pi/12$, ω_{max} can be estimated from the azimuth of the cracks at probability of 86 %. We excluded here the results for the cases that the stress state around the borehole is nearly all round compression, because e_ω can not be defined in such cases. The results for e_σ are summarized in Figures 6 (a) - (c). Similarly to the results of e_ω, the ratio of the cases inducing large error decreases with increasing $\overline{T}$. However, even if $\overline{T} = 0.1$, σ_{max}' is considered to be correct at probability of 82 % under the condition that we permit the error of e_σ less than 20 %. We excluded here the results for the cases that the cracks are already open without pressurization, because Eq. (8) cannot be applied and the magnitude of σ_{max} must be estimated by a different way in such cases.

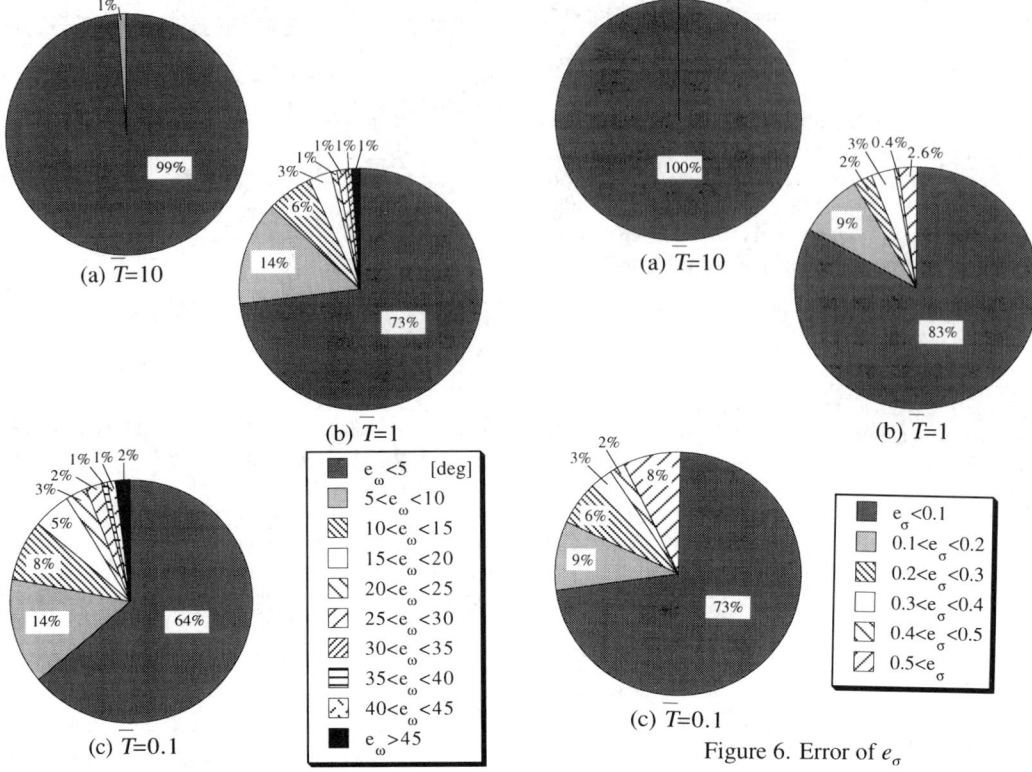

Figure 5. Error of e_ω

Figure 6. Error of e_σ

4 CONCLUSIONS

The results obtained in this study are summarized as follows. In arbitrarily oriented stress field, the state of stress in the plane perpendicular to the borehole axis can be estimated approximately from the azimuth of the hydraulically induced cracks and their reopening and shut-in pressures, if the tensile strength of rock is relatively large compared with the mean value of the in-situ stress. The error in the estimated results increases with decreasing the tensile strength or with increasing the depth where the hydraulic fracturing is conducted. However, with increasing the depth, the overburden is likely one of the in-situ principal stresses. Hence, in such a case, the stress state in the plane normal to the borehole can be estimated basically through the approximate way, if the borehole is nearly vertical.

REFERENCES

Bredehoeft, J.D., R.G.Wolff., W.S.Keys & Eugene Shuter 1976. Hydraulic fracturing to determine the regional in situ stress field. *Geol. Soc. Amer Bull.* 87:250-258. Colorado:Piceance Basinm.

Cornet, F.H. & B.Valette 1984. In situ stress determination from hydraulic injection test data. *J. Geophys. Res.* 89:11527-11537.

Daneshy, A.A. 1973. A study of inclined hydraulic fractures. *Soc. Pet. Engng. J.* 13:61-68.

Haimson, B.C. 1978. Crustal stress in the Michigan basin. *J. Geophys. Res.* 83: 5857-5863.

Hayashi, K., T.Shoji, H.Niitsuma, T.Ito & H.Abé 1985. A new in situ tectonic stress measurements and its application to a geothermal model field. *GRC Trans.* 9:99-104.

Hayashi, K., T.Ito & H.Abé 1989. In situ stress determination by hydraulic fracturing - a method employing an artificial notch. *Int. J. Rock Mech. Min. Sci. & Geomech. Abstr.* 26:197-202.

Hongo, K., K.Matsuki & K.Sakaguchi 1997. A criterion on core disking in the general state of in-situ stresses. *J. Mining and Materials Processing Institute of Japan.* 113:155-161(in Japanese).

Zoback, M.D., J.H.Healy & J.C.Roller 1977. Preliminary stress measurements in central California using the hydraulic fracturing technique. *Pure Appl. Geophys.* 115:135-152.

Material non-linearity and alteration of breakdown pressures in hydraulic fracturing

P.A. Nawrocki & M.B. Dusseault
Department of Earth Sciences, University of Waterloo, Ont., Canada

ABSTRACT: Breakdown pressures obtained from the classic, linear elastic breakdown model developed by Hubbert and Willis (1957) are compared with the corresponding pressures obtained using a non-linear material model. Compression test results obtained on sandstone and siltstone have been used for that purpose together with a previously formulated non-linear model which introduces stress-dependent elasticity functions $C(\sigma')$ (compressibility modulus) and $D(\tau_2)$ (inverted shear modulus). As well as breakdown pressures, linear and non-linear collapse pressures are also contrasted in this paper. It is shown that non-linear material properties have significant effects on both breakdown and collapse pressures.

1 METHOD OF HYDRAULIC FRACTURING

Hydraulic fracturing (HF) is used for fluid injection operations of sealed-off borehole intervals to induce and propagate tensile fractures to enhance either injectivity or recovery in the petroleum and geothermal energy industries. During HF a fluid is pumped into a well at a rate and pressure high enough to overcome the *in situ* confining stress and tensile strength of a formation, causing a fracture to form. In the oil industry it was first applied in 1948 to simulate productivity from low permeability oil-bearing formations (Clark, 1949). Since then, HF has been used for deep gas or water well simulation, for geothermal energy extraction to induce heat exchange surfaces, in coal gasification pilot projects, and for *in situ* stress determination.

Normally, hydraulic fractures will develop in directions perpendicular to the least *in situ* horizontal stress σ_h. As σ_h often is in horizontal direction, the resulting fractures will be vertical. For the case of unequal *in situ* stresses, $\sigma_H > \sigma_h$, two symmetric fracture wings will develop perpendicularly to the least principal stress. If the two horizontal principal stresses are equal, the fracture direction will be indeterminate. Such a case is also considered in this paper.

An idealized pressure-time curve of a HF test is shown in Fig. 1, in which the various parameters recorded during the test are defined. The test procedure is described by Kim and Franklin (1987), and by Haimson (1978); among others, interpretation has been provided by Guo *et al.* (1993)b. The peak pressure observed before the formation fractures and the well starts to take fluid is referred to as the break

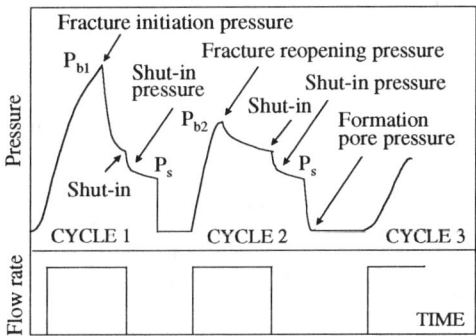

Fig. 1: Idealized HF curve (Kim and Franklin, 1987)

down pressure (BP) and is denoted by P_{b1}. BP is an important parameter obtained during hydraulic fracturing stress measurements. When a vertical fracture is induced, the maximum horizontal stress σ_H can be determined from the BP if the σ_h (obtained as the closure pressure after fracture extension and shut-in) and the properties of rocks such as the tensile strength T_o or the fracture toughness are known. However, breakdown is a complex process affected by many parameters such as the injection rate, the fracture fluid, the wellbore size, the state of stress, and the properties of rocks. As a result, many models have been put forward to analyze breakdown pressures. None of these models are generally accepted because they cannot explain all observed breakdown phenomena. Therefore, the estimation of σ_H is accorded a low level of confidence, and the prediction or analysis of BP is still an open question. In tests where the fractures are clearly vertical, the current method of interpretation (Haimson and Fairhurst 1969) applies, and the results obtained are usually unambiguous and reliable. For cases where the fractures are horizontal, inclined, or mixed mode, appropriate solutions of the problem have been also provided, cf. Ljunggren and Amadei (1989) and Hefny and Lo (1992).

In this paper we will show that non-linear (NL) stress-strain properties of geomaterials can lead to substantial uncertainties in the estimation of σ_H from hydraulic fracturing data. The goal of this paper is to compare breakdown pressures obtained using linear and NL constitutive models. This first step towards introducing more realistic material models into BP analysis will be done for the isotropic *in situ* stress field. This is partly because closed--form NL stress solutions are very hard if not impossible to obtain for circular openings in anisotropic *in situ* stress fields without referring to numerical methods, and we want to remain on the grounds of semi-analytical solutions for now. Once the bounds of uncertainty are quantified, then anisotropic material properties and anisotropic stress fields can be introduced through numerical methods (reserved for a later paper).

2 THE CLASSIC BREAKDOWN MODEL

Existing breakdown models include the classic linear elastic (LE) model by Hubbert and Willis (1957), the model eliminating the tensile strength by Bredehoeft *et al.* (1976), Haimson's poroelastic model (1968), Schmitt and Zoback's model (1989), and many others. The classical treatment of HF is based on Kirsch's solution (Kirsch 1898) for the stress distribution around a circular hole in a homogeneous, isotropic, elastic material subjected to external compression. In this method, the vertical *in situ* stress is considered to be one of the principal stresses in the ground, and the fracture is assumed to develop perpendicular to the least horizontal principal stress. This classical method was used by Hubbert and Willis (1957) who stated that a fracture in the borehole wall will be initiated if the acting fluid pressure in a hole exceeds the minimum tangential stress and the tensile strength of the material. For a vertical hole with an internal pressure P_w drilled from the surface in LE, isotropic, and unfractured rock, the minimum tangential stress is (Obert and Duvall 1967):

$$\sigma_\theta = 3\sigma_h - \sigma_H - P_w \tag{1}$$

As P_w is increased, σ_θ is reduced, finally to a value of the tensile strength T_o of the rock. The injection pressure at this stage is the critical pressure at fracture initiation P_{bl}, and it is denoted as breakdown pressure, Fig. 1. Thus, the condition for formation of the vertical fracture is

$$3\sigma_h - \sigma_H - P_{bl} = T_o \tag{2}$$

where T_o is negative (compressive stresses are assumed to be positive in this paper). To account for the initial pore-water pressure P_o at the test depth, Haimson (1978) applied the effective stress law and presented the following modification of Eqn. (2):

$$\sigma_H = 3\sigma_h - P_{bl} - P_o - T_o \tag{3}$$

The last equation has often been used for stress determination and is typically referred to as the conventional method. Note, that for the specific case $\sigma_H = \sigma_h = \sigma_{ho}$, (3) reduces to

$$P_{bl} = 2\sigma_{ho} - P_o - T_o \tag{4}$$

which predicts fracture initiation in crustal environments characterized by a lithostatic stress field or in internally pressurized thick cylinders subjected to a confining pressure σ.

The fracture, once formed, will continue to propagate as long as the internal pressure is greater than the stress normal to the plane of the fracture. If then the pumps are shut down and the well closed in, the pressure will fall off to a level where it balances the formation stresses trying to close the fracture. This pressure is called the shut-in pressure P_{si}. Since one also assumes that the fracture propagates in the direction of least resistance, the pressure to merely keep an induced vertical fracture open is equal to the least principal horizontal stress σ_h, that is $P_{si}=\sigma_h$. In principle P_{si} should be measured as the fluid pressure within the fracture at the moment the fracture closes, and is then called the closure pressure.

3 METHOD OF ANALYSIS

Existing breakdown models are all based on some form of elastic theory. Borehole stresses more realistic than those obtained from LE analysis have not been used in breakdown models to this point. On the other hand, because of significant differences between borehole stresses predicted by linear and NL methods, it can be expected that the constitutive material model assumed has important consequences on calculated breakdown pressures. There is now general agreement that linear elasticity analyses invariably underpredict opening stability, and that models which are more realistic (and less conservative) in their predictions should be utilised in the analysis. There are other important indicators that such an approach can have merit. For example, abnormally high breakdown pressures were observed in laboratory single-well hydraulic fracture tests, Guo *et al.* (1993)a. Therefore, the discussion in this paper is focused on the classic model, and the results obtained from this model will be compared with the results obtained when NL properties of the material are assumed.

Different predictive models linking rock stresses to rock deformation through experimentally determined elasticity constants of the rock material have been developed in the past for the purpose of borehole stress analysis used in this study. For realistic simulation of rock stresses, such elasticity "constants" have to be considered as elasticity functions, rather then constants. Different NL approaches postulate different mathematical representations for the "elasticity" functions mentioned above. For example, Santarelli (1986) introduced a confining stress dependent Young's modulus, and Nawrocki & Dusseault (1995) used the assumption of stiffness related to damage or radial distance measured from the opening wall.

The NL model used in this study for BP calculations is based on the underlying assumption that state of deformation of geomaterials at any stress level can be represented as a superposition of hydrostatic and deviatoric states of deformation. The model itself has been previously presented in a separate paper (Nawrocki et al. 1996). Let us only briefly summarize: to explicitly introduce material non-linearities into the analysis, our approach assumes that hydrostatic deformation is governed by a mean stress-dependent compressibility modulus $C=C(\sigma')$, whereas deviatoric deformation is governed by an inverted shear modulus D which is both confining stress- and shear stress-dependent, $D=D(\tau_2,\sigma_3)$. Actually, a simplified version of the model, neglecting the effect of σ_3 on material behaviour has been used in BP calculations presented further in this paper. That means that the following constitutive law is used herein:

$$6\varepsilon_1 = 2C(\sigma')\sigma' - 3D(\tau_2)(\sigma' - \sigma'_1)$$
$$6\varepsilon_2 = 2C(\sigma')\sigma' - 3D(\tau_2)(\sigma' - \sigma'_2) \quad (5)$$
$$6\varepsilon_3 = 2C(\sigma')\sigma' - 3D(\tau_2)(\sigma' - \sigma'_3)$$

where σ' is the mean effective stress, $\tau_2=\frac{1}{2}(\sigma_1-\sigma_3)$ is the shear stress ($\sigma_1 > \sigma_2 > \sigma_3$ are principal stresses), and material non-linearities are introduced through stress-dependent functions $C(\sigma')$ and $D(\tau_2)$, which are expressed in the form of power series as:

$$C(\sigma') = C_o + C_1\sigma' + ... + C_n\sigma'^n = \sum_{i=0}^{n} C_i\sigma'^i \quad (6)$$
$$D(\tau_2) = D_o + D_1\tau_2 + ... + D_m\tau_2^m = \sum_{j=0}^{m} D_j\tau_2^j$$

Parameters of the power series must be determined using compression test data. When series (6) are truncated at the first term, that is, when $C(\sigma')=C_o$ and $D(\tau_2)=D_o$, then the linear equations are recovered as a special case for the constitutive law (5).

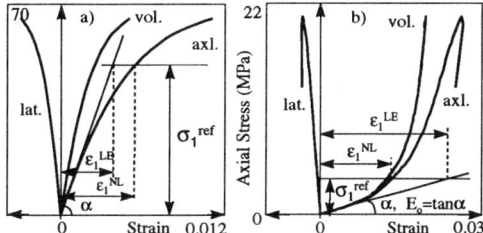

Fig. 2: Compression curves a)sandstone, b)siltstone

Uniaxial compression tests provided means for estimating constitutive parameters used both for linear and NL part of this study. Coefficients C_i (i=0,1,...,n), and D_j (j=0,1,2,...,m) can be determined by uniaxial compression tests where σ_1' is the axial compressive stress and $\sigma_2'=\sigma_3'=0$. The strain measured in the direction of σ_1' is ε_1 and $\varepsilon_2=\varepsilon_3$ are lateral strains. C_i and D_j can be identified by plotting $(\varepsilon_1+2\varepsilon_2)$ versus $\sigma_1'/3$, and $(\varepsilon_1-\varepsilon_2)$ versus $\sigma_1'/2$, respectively. Then C_o is the slope of the ε versus σ' curve at $\sigma'=0$, and D_o is the slope of the $(\varepsilon_1-\varepsilon_2)$ versus $\sigma_1'/2$ curve at $\tau_2=0$. The constants C_o and D_o may be viewed as the compressibility and inverted shear moduli of the NL material behaving linearly for very small stresses and strains. Indeed, for linear materials, the power law is merely a straight line. To track NL material behaviour, those lines have to become curved when the uniaxial compression curve departs from linearity. Thus, the more NL material behaviour is, the more terms must be taken into account in the power series (6).

4 BREAKDOWN PRESSURE CALCULATIONS

Mechanical properties of two rocks have been taken into account in NL breakdown pressure calculations. These are sandstone and siltstone. Cylindrical specimens 121 mm high and 61 mm in diameter made of these two rocks have been tested in uniaxial compression. Obtained results are shown in Fig. 2a (sandstone) and 2b (siltstone). The sandstone compression curve is convex upward, whereas that of the siltstone is convex downward. Thus, at a given reference stress level σ_1^{ref}, linear approximation of a real, NL, compression curve overestimates strains for siltstone ($\varepsilon_1^{LE} > \varepsilon_1^{NL}$), and underestimates strains for sandstone ($\varepsilon_1^{LE} < \varepsilon_1^{NL}$).

Using the power series methodology, compression curves of Figs. 2 have been presented in a format allowing for C_i's and D_j's determination; the coefficients are presented in Table 1. For the sandstone, four C_i and four D_j coefficients reproduce accurately its compressional behaviour; five C_i and five D_j coefficients are needed for siltstone. Figs. 3 and 4 show distributions of normalized σ_θ versus normalized radius for both linear and NL models, using data from Fig. 2. The hollow cylinder geometry has been

Table 1: Power series coefficients

COEFFICIENT	SANDSTONE	SILTSTONE
C_o	0.1093E-04	0.1636E00
C_1	0.4479E-06	-0.6562E-01
C_2	-0.6678E-07	0.1325E-01
C_3	0.3199E-08	-0.1251E-02
C_4	---	0.4261E-04
D_o	0.2041E-04	0.1132E00
D_1	0.5574E-06	-0.2642E-01
D_2	-0.5541E-07	0.3340E-02
D_3	0.1769E-08	-0.1987E-03
D_4	---	0.4423E-05

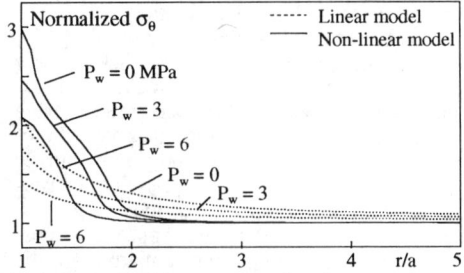

Fig. 4: Normalized hoop stresses for siltstone

used for the purpose of generating the results shown. Here, the borehole radius is a=0.3m, and the external radius is b=2.1m (sandstone), whereas a=0.3m, and b=1.5m for siltstone. For sandstone the far field stress is σ_{ho}=100 MPa, and several different non-penetrating internal pressures, P_w=0 (open hole case), P_w=20, 40, and 60 MPa, have been used for calculations. The respective values for siltstone are: σ_{ho}=15 MPa, and P_w=0, P_w=3, and P_w=6 MPa. Both linear and NL results are presented for comparison. The initial Young's modulus E_o (the modulus determined at zero strain, Fig. 2) and the initial Poisson's ratio v_o have been used for the linear analysis.

Significant differences in σ_θ predictions are apparent: compared to a linear calculation, the NL model gives lower σ_θ stresses for sandstone and higher σ_θ values for siltstone. This difference is most significant for low well pressures. Moreover, hoop stresses obtained using the NL model show $\sigma_{\theta|max}$ not at the cylinder wall, as the LE model predicts, but at some distance in the wall. Hoop stresses obtained using the NL model herein are undoubtedly more realistic than those predicted by linear elasticity.

Obtained results have been used for the purpose of BP calculations. In addition to breakdown pressure, the collapse pressure has been also calculated. The Coulomb failure criterion has been used for calculating the well collapse pressure P_{coll} corresponding to the onset of shear failure:

$$(\sigma_1' - \sigma_3') - (\sigma_1' + \sigma_3')\sin\varphi - 2c_o\cos\varphi = 0 \quad (7)$$

where c_o is cohesion, and φ is the angle of internal friction. Graphical representation of (7) is shown in Fig. 5. The tension cut-off part of the criterion shown in Fig. 5 has been used in BP calculations. Instead of principal stresses σ_1 and σ_3, borehole stresses σ_r and σ_θ are shown in Fig. 5. Two stress regimes can be seen: σ_θ is a major principal stress σ_1 above the hydrostatic line (shear failure criterion CD, and breakdown criterion AC), whereas $\sigma_1=\sigma_r$ below it (shear failure criterion BE, and breakdown criterion AB). Actually, if one assumes that only positive well pressures are admissible (no suction on the wellbore wall), then only FD, BE, and FB represent the active criterion. No stress states corresponding to AC and FB are possible. AB shrinks to FB because σ_{ho} is the minimum value of well pressure for which radial stress can become a major principal stress σ_1.

For the case of two *in situ* horizontal stresses being equal assumed in this paper, the LE borehole stresses are given by the Lame' solution:

$$\sigma_\theta = \frac{b^2(r^2+a^2)}{r^2(b^2-a^2)}\sigma_{ho} - \frac{a^2(r^2+b^2)}{r^2(b^2-a^2)}P_w$$
$$\sigma_r = \frac{b^2(r^2-a^2)}{r^2(b^2-a^2)}\sigma_{ho} - \frac{a^2(r^2-b^2)}{r^2(b^2-a^2)}P_w \quad (8)$$

Eqn. (8) can be readily used with breakdown and collapse criteria to establish the limits of LE solution. Thus, for LE case the following equation for breakdown pressure along FB has been derived:

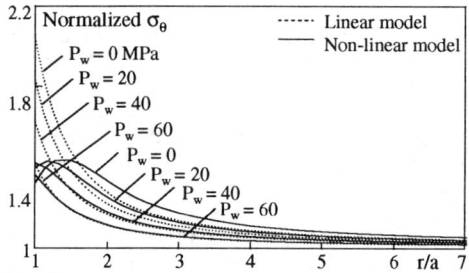

Fig. 3: Normalized hoop stresses for sandstone

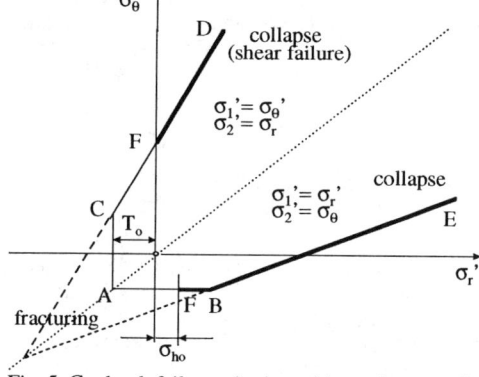

Fig. 5: Coulomb failure criterion with tension cut-off

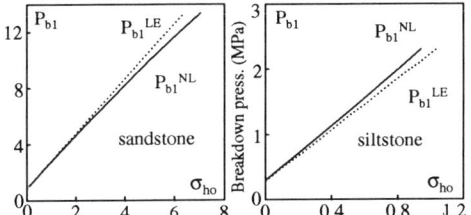

Fig. 6: Linear and non-linear breakdown pressures

$$(P_{b1})^{LE} = \frac{2b^2\sigma_{ho} + (b^2 - a^2)T_o}{a^2 + b^2} \quad (9)$$

and the upper limit for the LE breakdown pressure is:

$$(P_{b1})^{LE}_{max} = \frac{2c_o\cos\varphi - (1+\sin\varphi)T_o}{1-\sin\varphi} \quad (10)$$

Accordingly, the LE collapse pressure corresponding to the FD regime is given by:

$$(P_{coll})^{LE} = \frac{b^2(1-\sin\varphi)\sigma_{ho} - c_o\cos\varphi(b^2-a^2)}{b^2 - a^2\sin\varphi} \quad (11)$$

and the LE collapse pressure corresponding to the BE regime is:

$$(P_{coll})^{LE} = \frac{(b^2-a^2)\cos\varphi + b^2(1+\sin\varphi)\sigma_{ho}}{b^2 + a^2\sin\varphi} \quad (12)$$

The linear and NL breakdown pressures are compared on Fig. 6. On this figure, the breakdown pressure has been presented as a function of σ_{ho}. It can be seen in Fig. 6, that NL breakdown pressures are lower than the linear breakdown pressures for sandstone, and greater than the linear pressures for siltstone. In both cases the discrepancy between LE and NL solutions increases with σ_{ho} increase.

Finally, Figs. 7 and 8 provide the comparison between LE and NL collapse pressures. Actually, Fig. 7 referrs to the failure regime FD, whereas linear and non-linear collapse pressures corresponding to the stress regime BE are shown in Fig. 8. It can be seen in both cases that LE P_{coll} is greater than NL P_{coll} for sandstone, and the opposite statement is

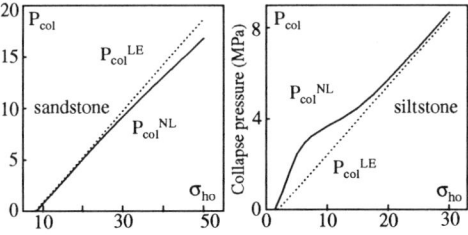

Fig. 7: Collapse pressures for stress regime FD

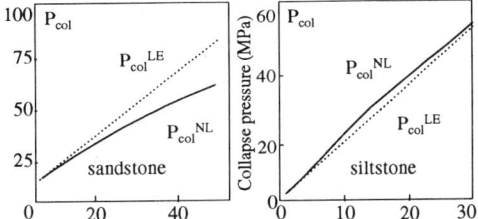

Fig. 8: Collapse pressures for stress regime BE

true for siltstone, where the major differences between those two solutions are visible at low stresses.

5 DISCUSSION AND CONCLUSIONS

It is believed that both the approach and methods of analysis presented in this paper should be effective in more robust and accurate breakdown pressure analysis than provided by the classic model. They can be used for any rock showing NL compressional behaviour. A comparison between the NL and LE breakdown and collapse pressures done in this paper emphasises the importance of a more accurate analysis, such as provided by the NL models. Obtained results show, that NL model predictions are quite different from LE model predictions both in terms of borehole stresses and also in terms of breakdown and collapse pressures.

For the specific case of predicting tangential stresses, which control breakdown pressure around a borehole, the LE model predicts a substantially different tangential stress than the NL model. One interesting conclusion is that, contrary to common assumptions, a LE model does not necessarily over-predict borehole stresses. Over-predictions are common because most geomaterials tested in compression have convex upward compression curves, as for the sandstone. The opposite case can be true, depending on rock type and test interpretation, thus results depend strongly on the constitutive model. Thus, the NL model can give either higher or lower P_{b1} and P_{coll} pressures than the classic, linear model. This means that the estimates of σ_H made using linear models give stress values which are different than the real values in the earth. We carried out a sensitivity analysis using varying but still reasonable degrees of non-linearity in order to estimate the typical percentage errors which may arise in practice if conventional elastic models are used. We conclude that most published data on σ_H are under-estimates of the actual values, and we propose means of improving those estimates, in the case of stress fields that are not too far from isotropic.

Finding the effect of material properties significant for predicted breakdown pressures, it seems worthwhile to develop a numerical model for NL breakdown pressure analysis in anisotropic *in situ* stress field. Unfortunately, the development of analytical or semi-analytical solutions does not seem feasible in that case, and it looks like a model developed will have to be numerical.

ACKNOWLEDGEMENTS

Financial assistance and scientific involvement in this research from the Natural Sciences and Engineering Research Council of Canada and The Waterloo Shale Project, an industry-university research project, is deeply appreciated.

REFERENCES

Bredehoeft J.D., R.G. Wolff, W.S. Keyes & E. Shuter. 1976. Hydraulic fracturing to determine the regional *in situ* stress field, Piceance Basin, Colorado. *Geol. Soc. Am. Bull.* 87: 250-258.

Clark, J.B. 1949. *Trans. AIME* 186: 1-3.

Guo, F., N.R. Morgenstern & J.D. Scott 1993a. An experimental investigation into hydraulic fracture propagation. Part I: An experimental facilities, and Part II: Single well tests. *Int. J. Rock Mech. Min. Sci. & Geomech. Abstr.* 30: 177-202.

Guo, F., N.R. Morgenstern & J.D. Scott 1993b. Interpretation of hydraulic fracturing breakdown pressure. *Int. J. Rock Mech. Min. Sci. & Geomech. Abstr.* 30(6): 617-626.

Haimson, B.C. 1968. Hydraulic fracturing in porous and nonporous rock and its potential for determining *in situ* stresses at great depth. Ph.D. Thesis, University of Minnesota.

Haimson, B.C. & C. Fairhurst 1969. In-situ stress determination at great depth by means of hydraulic fracturing. *Proc. 11th U.S. Symp. on Rock Mech.* Berkeley, pp.559-584.

Haimson, B.C. 1978a The hydrofracturing stress measuring method and recent field results. *Int. J. Rock Mech. Min. Sci. & Geomech. Abstr.* 15: 167-178.

Hefny A. & K.Y. Lo 1992. The interpretation of horizontal and mixed-mode fractures in hydraulic fracturing tests of rocks. *Can. Geotechn. J.* 29: 902-917

Hubbert, K.M. & Willis D.G. 1957. Mechanics of hydraulic fracturing. *Petrol. Trans. AIME* 210: 153-166.

Kim, K. & J.A. Franklin 1987. International Society for Rock Mechanics. Commission on Testing Methods. Suggested methods for rock stress determination. *Int. J. Rock Mech. Min. Sci. & Geomech. Abstr.* 24: 53-73

Kirsch, G. 1898. *Z. Verein Deutscher Ing. (VDI)* 42: 113.

Ljunggren, C. & B. Amadei 1989. Estimation of vargin rock stress from horizontal hydrofractures. *Int. J. Rock Mech. Min. Sci. & Geomech. Abstr.* 26: 69-78

Nawrocki, P.A. & M.B. Dusseault 1995. Modelling of damaged zones around openings using radius-dependent Young's modulus. *Rock Mech. and Rock Engng.* 28 (4): 227-239.

Nawrocki, P.A., M.B.Dusseault & R.K.Bratli 1996. Semi-analytical models for predicting stresses around openings in non-linear geomaterials. Proc. EUROCK'96, A.A. Balkema (G. Barla, Ed.). Torino, Italy, Sept 2-5. pp.785-782.

Obert, L. & W.I. Duvall 1967. *Rock Mechanics and the Design of Structures in Rock.* John Wiley & Sons, Inc. 650pp.

Santarelli F., E.T.Brown E.T. & V.Maury 1986. Anaysis of borehole stresses using pressure-dependent linear elasticity. *Int. J. Rock Mech. Min. Sci & Geomech. Abstr.* 23: 445-449.

Schmitt D.R. & M.D. Zoback 1989. Poroelastic effects in the determination of the maximum horizontal principal stress in hydraulic fracturing tests - a proposed breakdown equation employing a modified effective stress relation for tensile failure. *Int. J. Rock Mech. Min. Sci. & Geomech. Abstr.* 26: 499-506.

Estimation of in-situ stress state by the measurement of the wall displacement during hydraulic fracturing and injection tests at Kamioka mine

T.Takehara, T.Yamaguchi, M.Kuriyagawa & H.Ishihara
National Institute for Resources and Environment, Tsukuba, Japan

M.Yamashita
Mitsui Mineral Development Engineering Co., Ltd, Tokyo, Japan

ABSTRACT: In Kamioka mine, an artificial fracture was made by hydraulic fracturing. After hydraulic fracturing, water was injected into the fracture and movements of wall surface were measured. An analysis was made by a combined Gandi-Lomize model. There was a fair agreement between measured and estimated value by the model. This analysis could be used for not only fracture aperture but also the *in-situ* stress state.

1 INTRODUCTION

An *in-situ* hydraulic fracturing test was conducted at the Kamioka mine in Gifu prefecture, Japan. As is mentioned in following section, the main object of the experiment is to estimate a fracture aperture, which is hard to measure directly. Yamashita et al. (1995) proposed a Gandi-Lomize model to analyze the experimental data and found that the maximum fracture aperture during the hydraulic fracturing test was about $100\mu m$. Using the same data, Mizuta (1995) proposed a combined 3 dimensional BEM-FEM model to predict the surface movement of a wall. Although the main object of this experiment was to estimate the fracture aperture, it was found that the stress concentration around a mine tunnel, which is induced by primary stress, played an important role. In this paper, an analytical procedure is described in detail.

2 EXPERIMENT

2.1 Procedure

The experiment was conducted in Mozumi tunnel in Kamioka mine. A schematic plane view of the test site is shown in Figure 1. The test site is located about 1350-m from the tunnel entrance and the overburden is about 750m. A rock around tunnel consists of gneiss. Mechanical properties of test specimen are summarized in Table 1. As is seen from Figure 1, a horizontal borehole for hydraulic fracturing, which has a diameter of 76-mm, was drilled at first. Because there was no natural joint or fracture nearby the depth of 1.7m, this depth was chosen for hydraulic fracturing operation. In this hydraulic fracturing, the direction of fracture initiation was controlled by disc-shape slot made by abrasive water jet cutting. After hydraulic fracturing, it was found that the fracture had initiated and propagated almost vertical to the borehole.

Movements of the surface of the wall were measured by 24 LVDTs, which has resolving ability of $0.25\mu m$. An arrangement of 24 LVDTs are shown in Figure 2. These LVDTs were attached rigidly to a steel frame that had been constructed on the floor. At the height of the injection borehole, about 1-m

Table 1. Mechanical Properties of Core Samples.
Property	Value
Uni-axial Compressive Strength	79.0 MPa
Tensile Strength (Discs)	4.7 MPa
Young's Modulus	48.4 GPa
Poisson's Ration	0.15

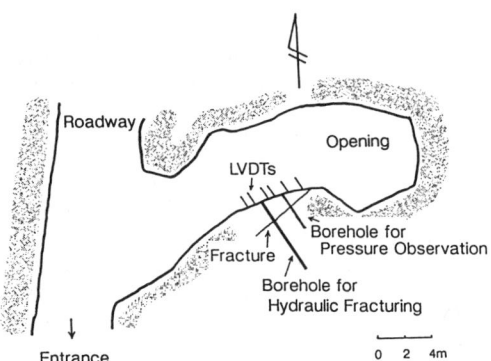

Figure 1. Schematic view of test site.

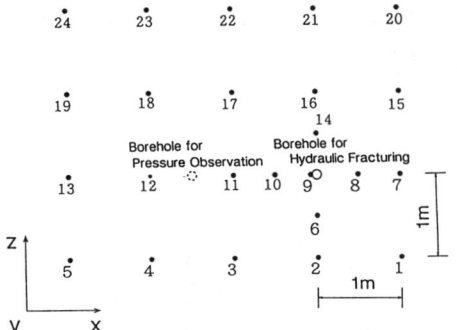

Figure 2. Arrangement of LVDTs against the wall.

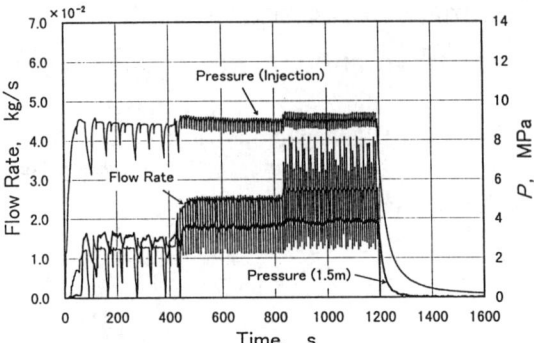

Figure 3. Observed pressures and flow rate during experiment B2.

Table 2. Summary of Fracturing and Injection Tests.

Test I.D.	Date	Injection Fluid
A1	95/12/17	Water
A2	95/12/17	Water
A3	95/12/17	Water with red paint
B1	95/12/22	Water
B2	95/12/22	Water
C1	95/12/23	High viscosity fluid

from the floor, 7 LVDTs were placed in a row. Because the behavior of wall surface was considered to be represented best by this row, observed data from this row was used for the following analysis.

Table 2 summarizes the hydraulic fracturing test and succeeding water injection tests. After the hydraulic fracturing operation (from A1 to A3 in Table 2), the steel flame together with attached LVDTs were removed to drill a pressure observation borehole shown in Figure 1. This pressure observation borehole was drilled to penetrate the artificial fracture.

The steel frame was set again to measure a pressure within the fracture during succeeding water injection tests (from B1 to C1 in Table 2).

2.2 Results

Figure 3 shows injection flow rate, injection pressure, and a pressure measured in an observation borehole in test B2. The object of this test was to observe the surface displacements under step-wisely increasing flow rate. Flow rates were intended to increase 3 steps. Because of a restriction of pumping equipment, flow rate could not be kept at constant value. The averages of flow rates at each step were 1.28×10^{-2}, 2.50×10^{-2} and 2.78×10^{-2} kg/s, respectively. Figure 4 shows the surface displacements observed by 7 LVDTs in the row. In this figure, the location of the injection borehole is taken as origin in horizontal axis. From Figure 4, it is clear that the surface movement did not take its peak at the vicinity of the

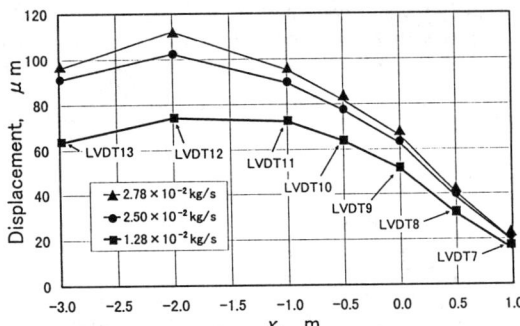

Figure 4. Observed displacements measure by LVDTs during experiment B2.

injection borehole, but about 2-m away from the borehole. This phenomenon was common for all the experiment except for the beginning stage of experiment A1.

3 ANALYSIS

3.1 Numerical model and boundary conditions

Basically, a conventional 2-dimensional FEM model shown in Figure 5 was used to analyze the surface movements during injection tests. Figure 6 is a flow chart of the procedure to match the calculated and measured value. At here, experiment B2 is taken as a sample to explain the procedure.

Measured values in the experiment are as follows.
a. Injection flow rates at 3 flow rate stages.
b. Injection pressure at a flow rate.
c. Surface movements measured by LVDTs.
d. Pressure within the fracture.

On the other hand, unknown values or values to be estimated are as follows.
e. Pressure distribution within a fracture.

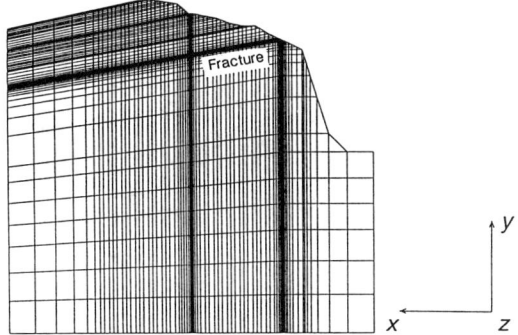

Figure 5. Finite elements for the analysis.

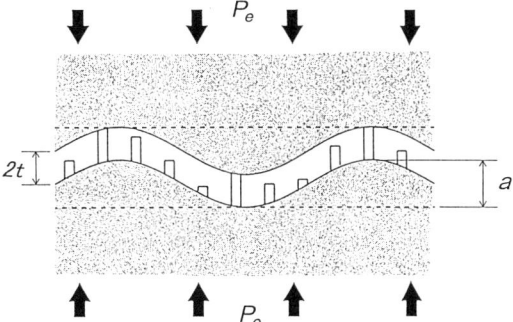

Figure 7. Conceptual view of Lomize-Gandi model.

f. Aperture distribution of the fracture during injection tests.
g. Initial fracture aperture distribution.
h. *In-situ* stress acting on a fracture.

A pressure distribution was calculated from an equation proposed by Lomize(Witherspoon, 1980). A schematic view of this Lomize model is shown in Figure 7. Usually, a pressure drop dP along a flow path x is revealed by a following equation.

$$\frac{dP}{dx} = -\frac{12\mu Q}{(2t)^3 W} \quad (3.1)$$

In this equation, μ is a viscosity of a fluid, Q is a flow rate, and W is a width of a fracture. An average fracture aperture $2t$ in equation (3.1) is shown in Figure 7. This equation is known as a cubic low of fluid flow. Lomize introduce friction factor into this equation. This friction factor is related to an average height of the asperities of a fracture surface shown in Figure 7. The friction factor is given by next equation.

$$f = 1 + 17\left(\frac{a}{4t}\right)^{1.5} \quad (3.2)$$

If an average asperity height a was determined, then a pressure distribution over a fracture is calculated using equations (3.1) and (3.2) as a function of fracture aperture distribution $2t$. Basically, equation (3.1) gives just a relation between fracture aperture and a pressure drop. In practice, a fracture aperture is affected by pressure within a fracture. Thus, another equation, which defines mechanical rigidity of a fracture, must be given. Gandi(1981) proposed a non-linear elastic constitutive equation using Bed-of-Nails model. Original Bed-of-Nails model proposed by Gandi has nails on a flat and smooth plane. The authors combined the Bed-of-Nails model with Lomize model as is shown in Figure 7. A mechanical property of a fracture is expressed by next equation.

$$2t = 2t_0 \left\{ 1 - \left(\frac{P_e}{P_1}\right)^{\frac{1}{n}} \right\} \quad (3.3)$$

In equation (3.3), P_e is a effective stress that acts vertical to a fracture plane as is shown in Figure 7, and t_0 is an aperture of fracture when P_e is zero or the height of longest nail. And P_1 is a constant that is related to a ratio of total area of nails compared to surface area. A density of nails calculated was very small and nails occupied less than 1 % in area. Thus, the substance of modeled nails is considered as debris separated from a fracture surface. In our experiment, the artificial fracture was newly created by the hydraulic fracturing (Experiment A1 in Table 1). Although water pressure had been completely released after hydraulic fracturing operation, measured surface displacements did not return to their initial value. This observed phenomena

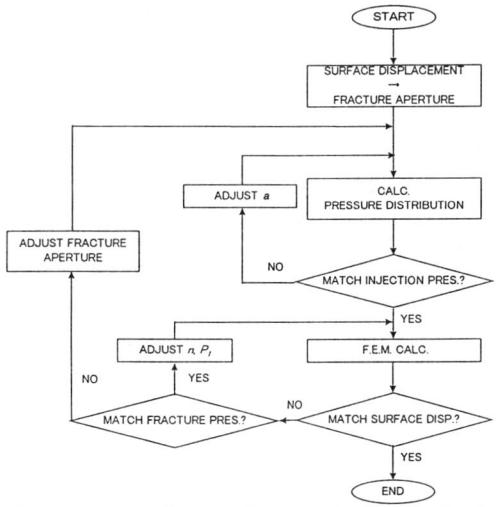

Figure 6. Flow chart used to match calculated values to observed data.

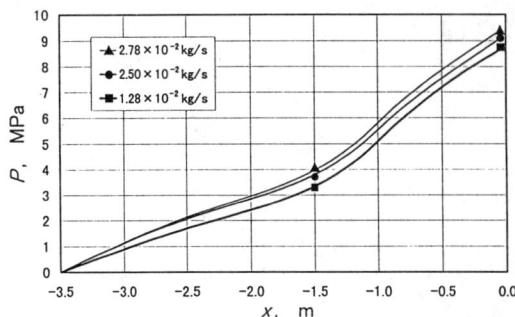

Figure 8. Comparison between observed pressures (triangles, squares, circles) and estimated pressure distribution within the fracture.

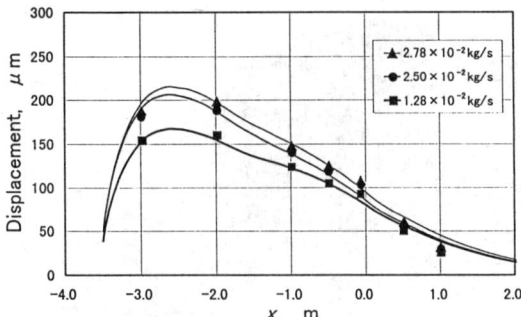

Figure 9. Comparison between observed wall surface displacements (triangles, squares, circles) and estimated displacement distribution.

supports that the fracture could not close completely even if the pressure was released. Before injecting water at the beginning of the experiment B2, there was a residual fracture opening at that time. Because the water pressure within the fracture was zero before injection, *in-situ* stress directly acted on the fracture plane. After the commencement of water injection, the water pressure within a fracture was increasing, and the effective stress P_e was decreasing. Thus the fracture aperture $2t$ was increasing according to the equation (3.3)

Because the steel frame width LVDTs was removed and re-constructed during experiments A3 and B1, zero-points of LVDTs were shifted. This made it difficult to estimate absolute fracture aperture before water injection experiment B3. Consequently, the initial fracture aperture distribution at experiment B1 was treated as parameter to be estimated in the analysis.

In-situ stress acting on the fracture is also unknown value. This stress is caused by stress concentration around the mine tunnel. As is seen from Figure 1, the artificial fracture was not parallel to the wall. Thus the *in-situ* stress acting on the fracture is not uniform but distributed. By making an assumption that far-field principle stresses are 17MPa, 12MPa and 21MPa, the distribution of *in-situ* stress acting on the fracture plane was estimated by F.E.M.

3.2 Estimated fracture behavior

According to the flow chart shown in Figure 6, distributions of fracture aperture and pressure distribution within the fracture were obtained after trial and error. Figures 8 and 9 show estimated distribution of pressure within the fracture, and aperture, respectively. There are fair agreements between measured and calculated value in both Figures 8 and 9. These agreements are considered to certify the validity of the analysis.

4 SUMMARY

In this paper, a combined Gandi-Lomize model is introduced to analyze the wall surface movements during water injection tests into an artificial fracture. The result shows that there is good agreement between measured and calculated value. This method could be used not only to estimate the fracture aperture but also *in-situ* stress state.

REFERENCES

Gandi, A.F. 1981, The variation of mechanical and transport properties of cracked rock with pressure, *Proc. of 22nd U.S. Rock Symp. on Rock Mech.* 91-95.

Mizuta, Y et al. 1995. In-situ measurement and numerical simulation of rock deformation induced by fluid injection into artificial fracture. *Proc of Korea-Japan Joint Symp. on Rock Engg*, 383-388.

Witherspoon, P.A. et al. 1980, Validity of cubic law for fluid flow in a deformable rock fracture, *Water Resources Research*, 16:1016-1024.

Yamashita, M et al. 1995.An estimation of fracture aperture and pressure distribution in a fracture made by in situ hydraulic fracturing test, *J. of the Mining and Materials Processing Inst. Of Japan*, 113:15-21.

Hydrofracturing stress measurement in granitic rock with scarce joints

K. Shin
Central Research Institute of Electric Power Industry, Chiba, Japan

B. Zhang & F. Li
Institute of Crustal Dynamics, SSB, People's Republic of China

S. Okubo
Graduate School of Engineering, The University of Tokyo, Japan

ABSTRACT: Based on an in-situ hydrofracturing experiment for about two month at an intact granitic rock mass, some findings about breakdown pressure, reopening pressure and shut-in pressure are discussed. From the discussion, a procedure for hydrofracturing stress measurement is also suggested.

1. INTRODUCTION

Hydrofracturing technique is a widely used method for rock stress measurement because of its practical advantages like accessibility to deep rock, economy, reliability, and so on. The principle is that characteristic pressures such as breakdown, shut-in and reopening pressures depend on the rock stress. To relate the characteristic pressures to the rock stress precisely, many theoretical and laboratory-based experimental studies have been done to make clear the mechanism of crack initiation, reopening and closing. But apart from the practical application of hydrofracturing, in-situ experiments with research purpose has been rare. In the in-situ experiments, we cannot set the stress condition at will but it has an important advantage; it eliminates the scale effect. To get a clearer understanding about the crack behavior in hydrofracturing, an in-situ experiment with research purpose is very important.

A rock site with very low frequencies of pre-existing discontinuities was selected to make sure the boundary condition. At the test site near Beijing, China, a fracturing borehole of 110mm dia. and 300m long was drilled. And a series of careful experiments were performed. Some of the results were already reported [Shin et al. 1996] and is briefly summarized in this paper. Also this paper deals with the characteristics of pressure curve during reopening and closing in detail. And then the rock stress at the test site is estimated to be compared with previous works. Thus this paper is intended to offer some findings about crack behavior, an example of pressure curves with some quality, and an observation of the rock stress at the site.

2. TEST SITE DESCRIPTION

2.1 *Geology*

The test site is located at a granitic intrusion on the outskirts of Beijing. The age of the granite is about 130 million years. The intrusion is roundly exposed on the surface with $37km^2$ area. The representative grain size of the granite is roughly 2mm.

The number of joints and veins that physically separated the core is only 37 below the weathered zone down to 30m from the surface. The ground water level was in the weathered zone, so the rock for the hydrofracturing experiment was water saturated.

2.2 *Rock mass permeability*

Before the hydraulic fracturing, permeability was measured along the entire length of the borehole with 5m step by pressure pulse test. Initial pressure was set to be 1 MPa and declining pressure was measured after the valve was closed. The permeability was analyzed based on numerical calculation [Bredehoeft et al, 1980].

It was found from the result [Shin et al,1996] that the rock is divided into three regions according to the permeability. At the first region from the depth 30m to 200m, the permeability is about 10^{-18} to 10^{-17} m^2. The second region from 210m to 250m depth has the permeability of about 10^{-17} to 10^{-16} m^2, one order higher than the above region. In the third region below 260m, the permeability is about 10^{-19} to 10^{-18} m^2, two orders lower than the second region. These three regions are referred to as medium, high and low permeability region respectively.

2.3 *Other properties of the rock*

Brazilian strength and P-wave velocity of the core were measured at various depths.

The specimens for the Vp measurement were horizontally taken in 8 directions from the oriented core to check the anisotropy of Vp at four depths. A pair of piezo-electric transducers of 1MHz resonance frequency were used. The anisotropy was not large but clearly observed. The direction with maximum Vp was N50W to N60W. This direction is parallel to the concentric circles of lithofacies at the test site. The average of all Vp data is 5450 m/s.

For the Brazilian test, the oriented specimens at 10 depths were water saturated before the test. The loading direction was set in the same 8 directions as the Vp test to check the anisotropy. But the anisotropy was less than the variation and unrecognizable. The mean of the strength at each depth was almost constant around 8.3MPa, except two depths where pre-existing joints or veins were observed near by.

Other than the P-wave velocity and the Brazilian strength, dry bulk density, uniaxial strength, Young's modulus, and the Poisson's ratio were obtained to be 2.74g/cm^3, 136MPa, 37000MPa, 0.21, respectively.

3. BREAKDOWN PRESSURE

Two criteria of breakdown have been derived theoretically based on the effective stress at the well wall and tensile strength. When no permeation of water into the rock wall occurs, then eq.1 stands [Fairhurst,1964]. On the other hand, when water permeates into the rock, then eq.2 [Haimson et al,1969].

$$P_b = 3S_h - S_H + T - p_0 \quad (1)$$

$$P_b = (3S_h - S_H + T - 2n \cdot p_0) / [2(1-n)] \quad (2)$$

In the equations, S_h, S_H, T, n and p_0 are horizontal minimum and maximum compressional stress, tensile strength, poroelastic coefficient, and far field pore water pressure.

Practically, the both equations have been pointed out to give the maximum and minimum limits of the breakdown pressure [Detournay et al,1988]. But it has not been clarified which equation stands in what condition.

To cope with this problem, two flow rates were used for breaking the rock, about 12 dm^3/min for fast hydrofracturing and 0.2 dm^3/min for slow fracturing. The time from the start of pressurization to breakdown was approximately 4sec for fast and 4min for slow fracturing. The pressure was measured in the hole to avoid the pressure loss in the pipe.

The distribution of the breakdown pressure for fast and slow fracturing revealed that, P_b was the same for the both flow rates at the low permeability region, but that P_b for slow fracturing was 20% to 40% lower than that for fast fracturing at the high permeability region, and that P_b for slow rate pressurization was a little lower than P_b for fast rate at the medium permeability region[Shin et al. 1996].

This experimental results are explained as follows. In the low permeability region, the width of water permeated zone around the well wall just before the breakdown is negligibly small for both fast and slow rate pressurization. Thus both P_b are given by eq.1 which is the maximum limit criterion. On the other hand in the higher permeability regions, the water permeated zone for the slow pressurization is large enough to lower the breakdown pressure, while the zone for fast pressurization remains relatively small.

From the consideration above, we defined the normalized pressurization rate (N.P.R.) which would be a parameter about the size of the water permeated zone around the hole just before the breakdown.

$$N.P.R. \equiv r_s^2/(c \cdot t_c) \quad (3)$$

where r_s is the borehole radius and t_c is the time to breakdown. The diffusivity coefficient c is given by

$$c = 2GB^2(k/\mu)(1-\nu)(1+\nu_u)^2 / [9(\nu_u - \nu)(1-\nu_u)] \quad (4)$$

where G, B, k, μ, ν and ν_u are shear modulus, Skempton's coefficient, permeability, fluid viscosity, drained and undrained Poisson's ratio, respectively.

Applying this normalized pressurization rate to this field result and also to previous laboratory experiments, we roughly got the condition for the two breakdown criteria as follows [Shin et al,1996]. Eq.1 is valid when N.P.R. is larger than 0.1 and eq.2 is valid when N.P.R. is lower than 0.001.

4. REOPENING PRESSURE

The criterion of P_r is often expressed as the following equation, substituting T in eq.1 with zero.

$$P_r = 3S_h - S_H - p_0 \quad (5)$$

But other possibilities of the criterion have been pointed out depending on water permeation into the crack before reopening.

$$P_r = (3S_h - S_H)/2 \quad (6)$$

$$P_r = S_h \quad (7)$$

The criterion of P_r itself is thus ambiguous and there is another problem, reading of P_r on the pressure curve. Usually the maximum pressure or the departure point from the initial tangent line of the reopening curve are taken. So it would be valuable to look into these points through the present data.

Fig.1 shows an example of the interval pressure and injected water volume relation, repeated 5 times at the same depth. The flow rate of each cycle of reopening was usually set to be almost the same as that of fast fracturing. To avoid the subjectiveness of reading, two person read P_r individually. The value had some scatter, but they distributed with good agreement with P_s^{pq}, shut-in pressure by step flow rate test [Shin et al,1996].

In some depths, reopening pressurization were repeated with different levels of flow rate, from a little higher value to a lower value than the standard around 10 dm^3 (Fig.2). The deflection is not clear to read and

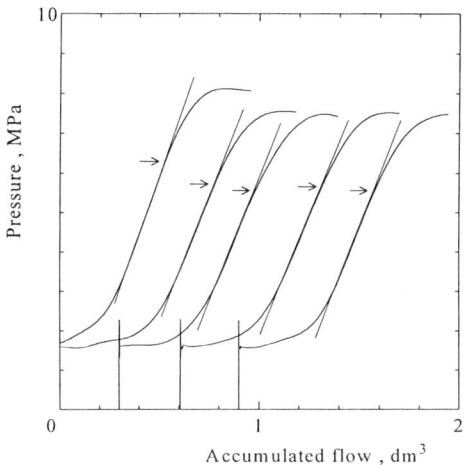

Fig.1 An example of reopening pressure curves

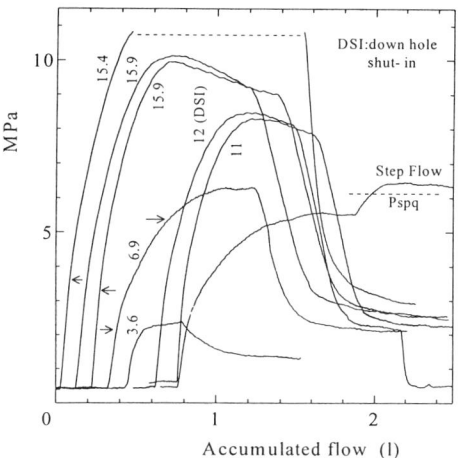

Fig.2 Reopening curves when flow rate is varied

more than one deflection seems existing in some cases. Roughly, one of the deflections seems near the P_s^{pq} level and another near the foot level of the shut-in curve.

In Fig.3, the relation between the maximum pressure P_{max} of reopening curve and the nominal flow rate is shown by solid square. The corresponding shut-in pressure read by the 2-line method is shown by open circle. The order of pressurization is shown under the dots. We may expect that P_{max} has the tendency to decrease with repeating the pressurization, but the flow rate is found to have the dominant effect on P_{max}. It is considered that P_{max} is the stationary pressure corresponding to the flow rate and crack geometry, and that when the crack extension is negligible P_{max} increase with the flow rate.

In the series of the experiment, sleeve fracturing other than fast and slow hydrofracturing was also used to introduce fractures. These sleeve fractured cracks were also used for the reopening and shut-in test. In Fig.4, the distribution of P_{max} of the first reopening is shown with solid circle, open square and open circle for sleeve, fast and slow hydro-fractured crack, respectively. P_{max} for sleeve fractured crack is clearly higher than those for other two hydro-fractured cracks. This is considered that the sleeve fractured crack is not extending as much as the crack by fast or slow hydrofracturing. Small crack gives higher impedance to the flow and hence higher P_{max}. But after this, P_s and P_{max} for subsequent tests at the sleeve fractured crack were identical to those of hydro-fractured crack.

5. SHUT-IN CURVE

Shut-in pressure P_s is read as a deflection point on a shut-in curve. P_s is considered as the water pressure in the crack that balances with S_h.

But the deflection is sometimes not clear and various ways of reading the deflection have been proposed. Hayashi,K et al.(1991) has analyzed the process of crack closing and theoretically proposed two deflection points in the shut-in curve; where the first deflection pressure or the crack tip closing pressure coincides with S_h. Another way of estimating S_h by step flow rate test has been proposed [Aamodt et al,1982], where a deflection pressure P_s^{pq} on a stationary pressure vs. flow rate graph is read.

A series of shut-in tests were performed in this field experiment to look into such shut-in pressures.

Fig.5 shows various patterns of shut-in curves. In these cases, the flow rate for reopening pressurization was set to the standard value of 10 to 20 dm^3/min. Cases (a) and (b) are the typical ones, where the foot of the shut-in curve is decreasing gradually or remains constant when tested repeatedly at the same depth. Type (c) and (d) were observed occasionally, where the foot level decreased step-like at some points of the tests, or the deflection point became clearer gradually. Through observing these shut-in curves, the foot level pressure seems decreasing as the crack extends little by little when tested repeatedly.

Fig.6 shows another example of the shut-in curves at the depth of 122m. In this case, the flow rate for reopening were varied from the standard value of 10 to 20 dm^3/min to a lower value than that. Standard value of flow rate was used for the 1st and 2nd shut-in. In these two cases, P_{ctc}, the crack-tip closing pressure, was observed as the first deflection on the dt/dP - P diagram of the shut-in curve as shown in Fig.7. In the 3rd shut-in test, the flow rate used was a little lower than the standard value and coinciding P_{ctc} was not observed. When the flow rate was further lowered in the 4th shut-in test, the foot level of the curve became lower than before. In the last test, a step flow rate test was conducted and P_s^{pq} level is shown.

Other than P_{ctc} and P_s^{pq} reading, P_s was read by the two tangent lines intersection method (2-line method) for the shut-in tests after standard flow rate reopening

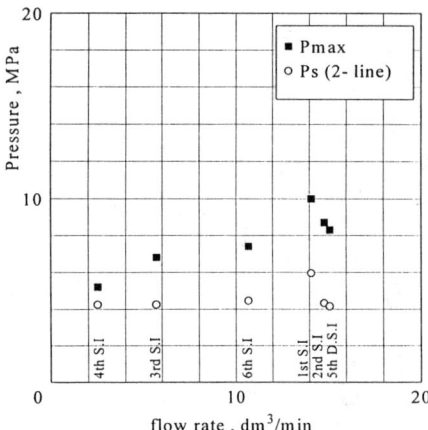

Fig.3 P_{max} and P_{s2} vs. flow rate

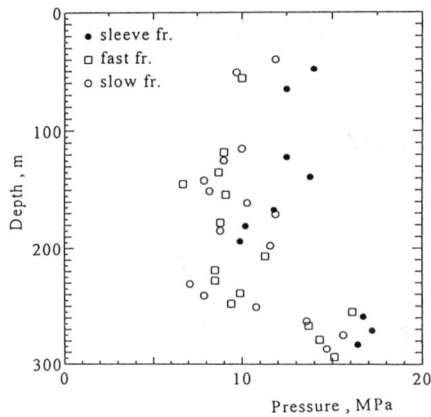

Fig.4 Distribution of P_{max} of first reopening for three kinds of fracture

at every depth tested. The P_s by 2-line method coincides with the onset of the foot of shut-in curve. Fig.8 shows the distribution of P_{ctc}, P_s^{pq}, P_s by the two line method and others. From the figure, it is observed that P_{ctc} and P_s^{pq} are coinciding well with each other through the whole depth, and that P_s reading by 2-line method gives a lower value than them. In the depth range of about 30 to 60m, the difference is large. This seems suggesting that the two levels of deflection on a shut-in curve have different physical meanings, not that the two levels are the result of the difference of just reading method for a conventional shut-in pressure. This test results agrees with the theoretical conclusion by Hayashi,K. et al.(1991) mentioned before that there are two deflections on a shut-in curve. From the theory and additional consideration, following equations stands, where P_{s2} is the second deflection point on a shut-in curve, at this pressure the crack mouth extending past the straddle packer closes.

the first deflection   : $P_{ctc} = S_h$ (8)
the second deflection   : $P_{s2} > (3S_h - S_H)/2$ (9)

The eq.9 may stands when water leak through the crack past the packer is negligible at the latter part of a shut-in curve. If water leak continues, we may not read the valid second deflection.

6. ROCK STRESS ESTIMATION

The direction of one of the principle stress is assumed parallel to the borehole. Almost all the hydrofractured cracks were parallel to the hole axis. The strike is roughly N-S direction in the entire depth. And the anisotropy of the Brazilian tensile strength was unrecognizable. From these, the direction of the maximum compressional stress is in N-S.

6.1 S_h estimation

As discussed in Section 5., the first deflection point on a shut-in curve represents the minimum compressional stress S_h, and P_s^{pq} agreed well with it along the entire length of the borehole. Here P_s^{pq} is adopted because of its stable reading on pressure vs. flow rate diagrams, and its smoother distribution in depth.

$$S_h = P_s^{pq} \; (= P_{ctc}) \tag{10}$$

The distribution of S_h is shown in Fig.9 by solid circle. We observe here that in the depth region from 220m to 250m where joint frequency is higher than other region, S_h distributes lower, that S_h remains high compared to S_v at shallower region in this very intact rock mass, and that S_h at deeper than 250m where rock mass seems highly intact distributes higher than others.

In hydrofracturing stress measurement, it is important to set the flow rate for pressurization properly, when to vent or close the valve, and how to read characteristic pressures on the pressure curve. In this experiment, the valve was operated so that the induced crack does not extend too far, i.e. immediate venting after breakdown and immediate shut-in (closing the valve) after P_{max} of reopening cycle. The flow rate used for reopening is considered large enough to open the crack tip but not so large to extend it too much. The shut-in should be done at this proper condition. And the first deflection on a shut-in curve was considered equal to S_h normal to the crack.

The above concept of hydrofracturing has been applied to an intact rock mass in Japan. At the site, various kinds of overcoring stress measurements have also been done[Ishiguro et al,1997]. The shut-in pressure was read at the first deflection on the shut-in curve and it agreed very well with the overcoring result. Step-flow rate test was also done at the site and it gave very consistent value of P_s^{pq} with P_s. Thus the procedure for hydrofracturing stress measurement described above has been proved very well.

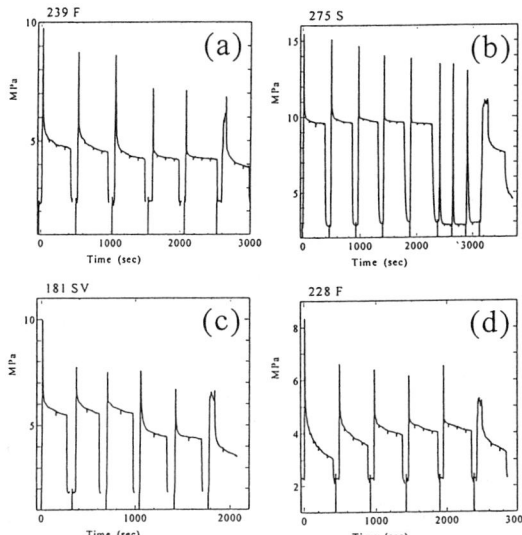

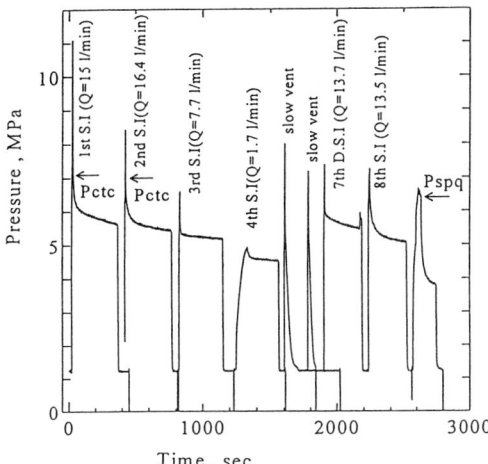

Fig.5 Various patterns of shut-in curves

Fig.6 Example of repeated shut-in curves at 122m depth

6.2 S_H estimation

Breakdown pressures whose N.P.R. larger than 0.1 apply to eq.1. P_b with N.P.R. near to 0.001 apply to eq.2 or specifically the following eq.2'.

$$S_H^f = 3S_h - P_b + T - p_0 \quad (1)$$
$$S_H^s = 3S_h - 1.83P_b + T - 0.172p_0 \quad (2')$$

For the tensile strength T, the Brazilian strength of water saturated specimens were used. The far field pore pressure p_0 was set to the water head pressure at the depth.
 The resultant S_H by eq.1 and eq.2' are dotted by solid square and double circle respectively in Fig.9. Although there are only two points of S_H^s, the results seems agreeing and thus proving the theory of normalized pressurization rate described in section 3.
 New possibilities of estimating S_H from the scatter of crack direction and also from the second deflection pressure P_{s2} on the shut-in curve have been mentioned in the previous report [Shin et al,1996].

6.3 Comparison to previous measurements

Stress measurement at three other sites in the same granitic intrusion have been done and listed in table 1. These three places are 1 to 2 km apart from the present test site. One is by overcoring method and others by hydrofracturing. Although the measurement for each site is not many, the common fact is that the horizontal stress is much larger than the overburden stress calculated from the rock density. This is the same tendency as the present result. The stress direction has some scatter but in NE-SW direction, and

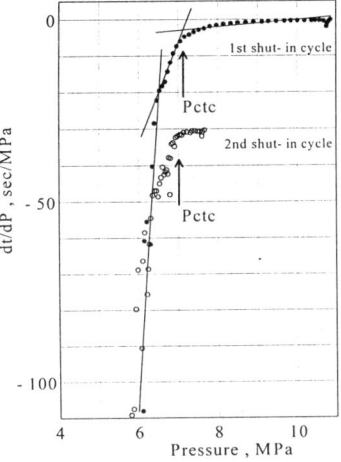

Fig.7 Example of dt/dP-P analysis at 122m depth

this is a little different tendency from the present result of consistent N-S direction along the entire 300m long borehole.
 The small earthquake focal mechanism and structural geological data has revealed that the stress direction in the region around Beijing including the test site is in about NEE-SWW direction[Li et al, 1985][Jin et al,1987]. So the difference of the present result of clear N-S direction is thought to be caused by the stress locality of the intrusion.

7. CONCLUSION

To avoid the scale effect and make clearer the crack behavior during the hydrofracturing stress measurement procedure, an in-situ experiment was

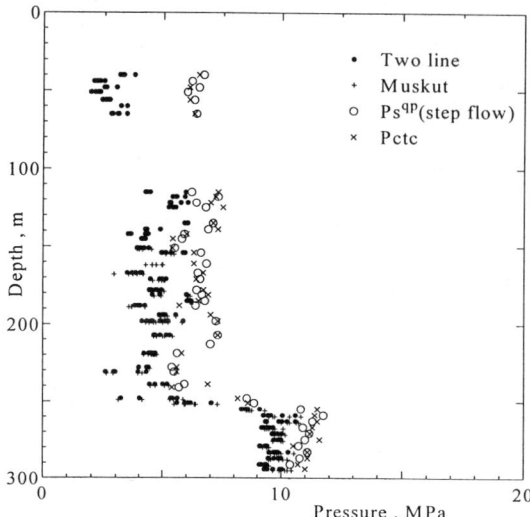

Fig.8 Distribution of various readings of shut-in pressure

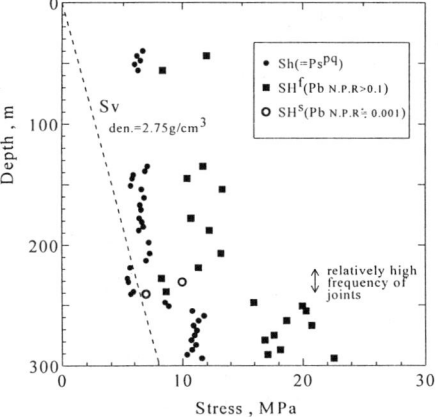

Fig.9 Distribution of S_H and S_h with depth

Table 1 Other stress measurement results at the same granitic intrusion

Site	Depth (m)	SH (MPa)	Direc. (Degree)	Sh (MPa)	Method
D	5 - 17	5.3	N15E	2.6	OC
X	8.7 - 20.9	7.3	N59E	4.2	HF
T	15.5- 18.0	5.8	N22E	4.7	HF
	34.6- 36.6	6.8	N43E	5.9	HF
	51.6- 53.7	9.1	N63E	6.6	HF
	107.6-110.2	11.4	N76E	7.7	HF
	126.5-129.1	13.9	N36E	7.9	HF

done at a very intact rock site. The following main results have been obtained.
1) Breakdown pressure P_b should be related to the rock stress according to the permeation condition. When $N.P.R.>0.1$ eq.1 stands, and when $N.P.R. < 0.001$ eq.2 stands. The pressurization rate should be set in conjunction with this.
2) Reopening pressure P_r, read as the departure point from the initial tangent line of pressurization, distributed agreeably with P_s^{pq}, the shut-in pressure by step-flow rate test. But when the flow rate is decreased, P_r also decreased and so the reading is vague. The maximum pressure in the reopening test increased with the flow rate linearly.
3) The shut-in pressure as the equivalent pressure to S_h was read at the first deflection point on a shut-in curve. This P_{ctc} agreed well with P_s^{pq} by step-flow rate test along the entire borehole. The procedure adopted is, immediate venting after breakdown, flow rate just large enough to open the crack tip, immediate closing of the valve after Pmax of reopening, reading the first deflection on the shut-in curve for Sh, and the step flow rate test at the last.
   In the later hydrofracturing at other site in Japan, in which the similar procedure was adopted, the first deflection also agreed with P_s^{pq} and it coincided with the overcoring result well.
   The second deflection is considered the pressure when the part of the crack mouth extending the packer just closes.
4) The stress at the test site was clearly in N-S direction. And it is different from the regional stress tendency of north China. So we have observed the stress locality caused by the intrusion. Also we observed horizontal stress larger than the overburden pressure in the intact rock mass.

REFERENCES

Shin,K., Li,F. & Okubo,S.: Hydro-fracturing for stress measurement in intact granitic rock, *Eurock'96/Torino*, 1996

Y.Ishiguro, K.Nishino, H.Nishimura & K.Sugawara: Rock stress measurement for design of underground power house and considerations, *RS Kumamoto '97*, 1997

Li,Z., Cao,X., Chen,J., Liu,J. & Zhang,Z.: Some considerations on the recent tectonic stress field of China, *Tectonophysics*, Vol.117, p.161-176, 1985

Jin,Y. & Yu,X.: Dynamic variation of composite fault plane solution of small earthquakes in the north China, *Seismology and Geology*, Vol.9, No.4, Dec. 1987

Fairhurst,C.: Measurement of in situ rock stresses, with particular reference to hydraulic fracturing, *Felsmechanik*, Vol.II/3-4, p.129-147, 1964

Haimson,B.C. & Fairhurst,C.:Hydraulic fracturing in porous-permeable materials, *J. Petroleum Technology*, p.811-817, July 1969

Detournay,E & Cheng,A.H-D.: Poroelastic response of a borehole in a non-hydrostatic stress field, *Int. J. Rock Mech. Min. Sci. & Geomech. Abstr.*, Vol.25, No.3, p.171-182, 1988

Influence of fracture aperture and normal stiffness on the reopening pressure in classical hydraulic fracturing stress measurements

Jonny Rutqvist
Earth Sciences Division, Ernest Orlando Lawrence Berkeley National Laboratory, Calif., USA

Ove Stephansson
Royal Institute of Technology, Division of Engineering Geology, Stockholm, Sweden

ABSTRACT: Reopening tests of a vertical hydraulic fracture intersecting a vertical borehole is simulated by means of coupled hydromechanical modeling. The modeling includes coupled interaction between stress and flow in both the rock matrix and the fracture. The results of the modeling indicate that, after fracturing, the hydraulic fracture itself disturbs the stress field around the borehole. The minimum tangential stress at the intersection of the fracture and borehole is therefore smaller than predicted for a linear elastic, isotropic and homogenous media. During injection, fluid penetrates the fractures which therefore opens gradually as a function of the effective normal stress. The study shows that the initial hydraulic aperture and normal stiffness are very important factors to be considered in the evaluation of the maximum principal stress.

1 INTRODUCTION

In classical hydro-fracturing stress measurements, a vertical hydraulic fracture is induced of a vertical borehole in a direction perpendicular to the minimum compressive horizontal stress. Thereafter, a reopening test is conduced by injecting water at constant flow rate until the fracture is completely open. During the injection, the well pressure increases linearly with time due to the storage effects in the hydraulic hose, as long as the fracture is "closed". Later, when the pressure is high enough to reopen the fracture, the well pressure will stabilize and then drop slightly due to loss of water into the fracture. The pressure at the moment where the pressure versus time curve deviates from the linear relationship is defined as the breakdown or reopening pressure. After a few minutes of injection, the pump is stopped and the hydraulic hose to the test interval kept shut-in.

The minimum principal stress, σ_h is determined from the shut-in pressure and the maximum principal stress, σ_H may be derived using the classical equation:

$$\sigma_H = 3\sigma_h - P_{2b} - P_0 \qquad (1)$$

where P_{2b} is the secondary breakdown pressure and P_0 is the pore pressure in the fracture. This equation is derived from Kirsch solution for a circular hole subjected to an internal pressure in an isotropic, homogeneous and linear elastic medium. It is assumed that the secondary breakdown occurs when the fluid pressure applied on the borehole wall is high enough to cancel out the minimum tangential stress, σ_θ^{min} at the borehole wall:

$$\sigma_\theta^{min} = 3\sigma_h - \sigma_H \qquad (2)$$

In the field it has been shown that the reopening pressure depends on the injection flow rate (Cornet, 1983). This indicates that the fluid is penetrating the fracture and opens it by or with help of internal pressure inside the fracture. If fluid is penetrating the fracture, the use of equation (1) may give a poor estimate of the maximum principal stress and an alternative equation should be used.

In a resent study, Rutqvist and coworkers (1997), conducted pulse injection tests on hydraulic fractures in granitic rocks. The tests showed that the fractures were incompletely closed with a hydraulic aperture of 3 to 5 μm near the borehole and 6 to 15 μm away from the borehole. The study also indicated that the hydraulic fractures had similar properties to tensile fractures induced in core samples, with a normal stiffness of 2000 GPa/m or less.

In this paper, the consequences of incomplete fracture closure on the reopening pressure is studied. Reopening tests are simulated using coupled hydromechanical finite element modeling and important parameters for the reopening pressure are determined in a parameter study.

2 COUPLED NUMERICAL MODELLING OF REOPENING TESTS

The reopening tests are modeled with the coupled hydromechanical finite element program ROCMAS (Noorishad et al. 1992). The code simulates coupled hydromechanical processes of fractures embedded in a porous rock matrix. Coupling of the fluid flow and mechanical deformation is based on Biot's generalized effective stress law (Biot, 1941).

2.1 Model geometry

The reopening tests are simulated with a two-dimensional model in a horizontal plane (Fig. 1). It consists of 1200 elements including special Goodman's joint elements (Goodman, 1974) for the hydraulic fracture. The borehole is 76 mm in diameter and the size of the model is 7 by 7 meters.

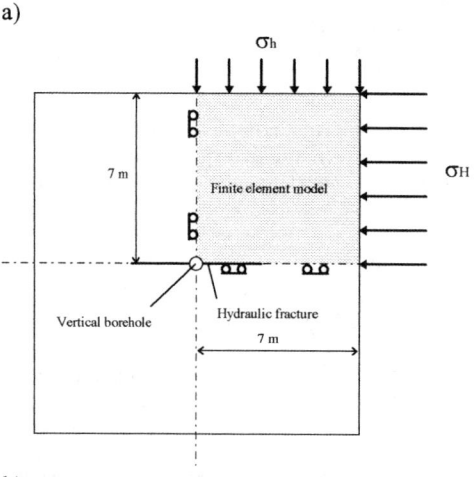

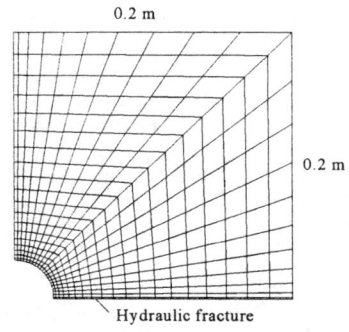

Figure 1. Finite element model of a horizontal section through a vertical borehole and a vertical hydraulic fracture. a) Overview with mechanical boundary conditions. b) Detail of the finite element mesh near the borehole.

2.2 Material properties

Table 1 presents the material properties for the modeling of a base case. The properties of the rock matrix corresponds to intact rock material properties of a competent granite. The fracture is modeled with non-linear normal stress versus normal displacement relation according to (Goodman, 1974). In this study, a mechanical fracture aperture b_m is defined as being equal to the current maximum normal closure which, according to Goodman's model, is related to the effective normal stress, σ'_n as:

$$\sigma'_n = \frac{A_i}{b_m} \qquad (3)$$

where A_i is a constant defined as:

$$A_i = \sigma'_{ni} \cdot b_{mi} \qquad (4)$$

where σ'_{ni} and b_{mi} are the effective normal stress and mechanical aperture, respectively, at an initial or reference state. The normal stiffness, k_n of the fracture is:

$$k_n = \frac{\sigma'_n}{b_m} \qquad (5)$$

The effective stress in the fracture is related to the total stress σ_n and fluid pressure p, according to:

$$\sigma'_n = \sigma_n - \alpha \cdot p \qquad (6)$$

where α is Biot's effective stress parameter (Biot, 1941).

The hydraulic aperture, defined from the "cubic law" (Witherspoon et al. 1980), is assumed to be related to the mechanical aperture according to:

$$b_h = b_{hr} + f \cdot b_m \qquad (7)$$

where b_{hr} is the residual hydraulic aperture when the fracture is mechanically closed and f is a factor that compensates for the deviation of flow in a natural rough fracture from the ideal case of parallel plate type of fracture surfaces (Witherspoon et al. 1980).
The hydraulic aperture and normal stiffness in Table 1 are typical values deduced from pulse tests at Laxemar (Rutqvist et al. 1997).

2.3 Modeling of the base case

The reopening test is modeled by injecting water at constant rate of 3 l/min into the well which has a storage capacity of $S_w = 2.4 \cdot 10^{-6}$ m^2. A constant

Table 1. Material properties of the base case for modeling of a reopening test in granitic rock.

Material	Parameter	Value
Fluid	Mass density, ρ_f	1000 kg/m³
	Compressibility, C_f	4.4×10^{-10} Pa⁻¹
	Dynamic viscosity, μ_f	1×10^{-3} Ns/m²
Rock matrix	Young's modulus, E_r	60 GPa
	Poisson's ratio, ν_r	0.25
	Mass density, ρ_r	2700 kg/m³
	Permeability, k	1×10^{-19} m²
	Biot's constant, α_r	1.0
	Biot's constant, M_r	130 Gpa
Fracture	Goodman's constant, A	125
	Res. Hydraulic aperture, b_{hr}	0
	Factor, f	0.5
	Normal stiffness*, k_{n5}	200 GPa/m
	Hydraulic aperture*, b_{h5}	12.5 μm
	Biot's constant, α	1.0
	Biot's constant, M	2.27×10^{-9}
	Length, l	1 m

*At 5 MPa effective normal stress

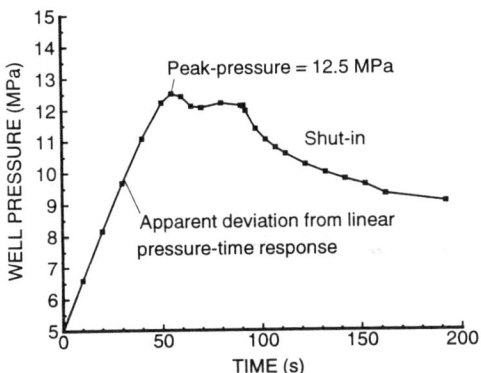

Figure 2. Pressure versus time record as a result of the numerical modeling of the base case.

pressure boundary was assumed at the outer edge of the fracture simulating an intersection to a secondary hydraulic conducting joint. Figure 2 presents the pressure versus time response with reopening and shut-in. In this study we concentrate our effort on the first reopening phase up to the peak-pressure.

Figure 3 presents the results of the modeling at different stages of the reopening test in Figure 2. Before fracturing, the stress distribution follows the classical solution for a circular opening in a linear elastic, homogenous and isotropic medium (Fig. 3a). The least tangential stress at the wall of the borehole can here be calculated from equation (2) to be 20 MPa.

Figure 3c presents the new maximum stress distribution, after the fracturing. This calculation was conducted by using the stresses from before fracturing (Fig. 3a) as an initial condition and thereafter activating a closed fracture. The solution is iterated to equilibrium to obtain the conditions before injection. Figure 3c, shows that the introduction of the fracture disturbs the stress field and the tangential stress at the intersection of the fracture and borehole (fracture mouth) has reduced from 20 MPa to 14 MPa. This reduction in tangential stress imply that equation (2) is no longer valid which may lead to an error in the calculation of the maximum principal horizontal stress. The mechanical aperture varies with the smallest aperture of 7 μm near the borehole where the normal stress is largest. Away from the borehole, the hydraulic aperture is about 10 μm and the normal stiffness is about 300 GPa/m.

At 30 seconds and at a well pressure of 10 MPa, the pressure time curve apparently deviates from the earlier linear response (Fig. 2). This could be interpreted as a reopening pressure. However, in this case the deviation occurs at a pressure much lower than the peak-pressure value. This indicates that our pressurization rate is too low and that faster rate would be recommended.

At 45 seconds, the pressure-time record deviates considerable from the earlier sub-linear response and reaches a peak-value of 12.5 MPa. At this stage, the flow rate into the fracture is balancing with the injection flow rate of 3 l/min and the hydraulic aperture near the well is 48 μm. The effective stresses in the fracture are now low but still positive indicating that the fracture surfaces are in contact. The peak-pressure is 1.5 MPa less than the initial minimum tangential stress of 14 MPa and much less than the theoretical value from equation (2) of 20 MPa.

2.4 Parameter variation

A parameter variation were conducted to determine the most important parameters for the reopening pressure under the given stress field. Table 2 compares the maximum difference in peak-pressure for the range of variation of each parameter. The analysis showed that the most important parameters are:

1) Fracture normal stiffness
2) Fracture residual hydraulic aperture
3) Flow rate (borehole pressurization rate)

The fracture normal stiffness has a dramatic influence on the pressure-time record (Fig. 4). The

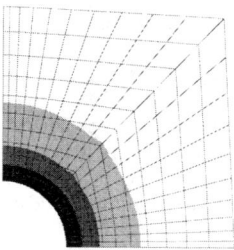
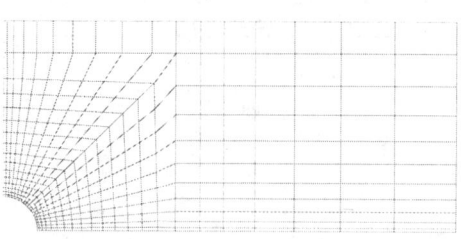

a) Max compressive stress before fracturing. b) Fluid pressure before fracturing.

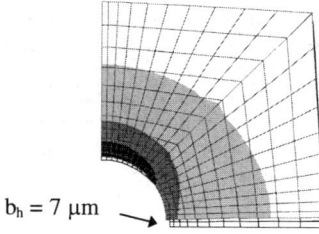
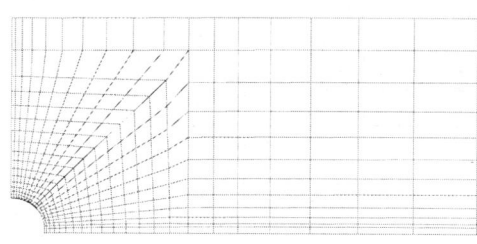

$b_h = 7\ \mu m$

c) Max compressive stress after fracturing. d) Fluid pressure after fracturing.

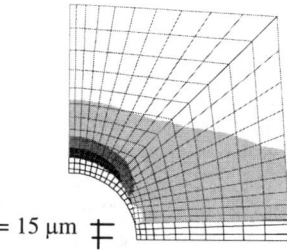
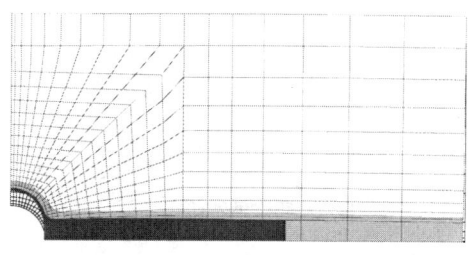

$b_h = 15\ \mu m$

e) Max compressive stress at 30 seconds. f) Fluid pressure at 30 seconds.

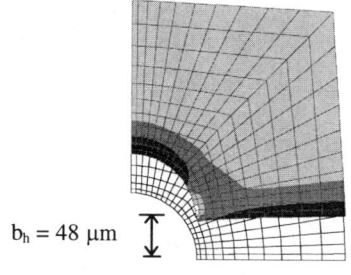
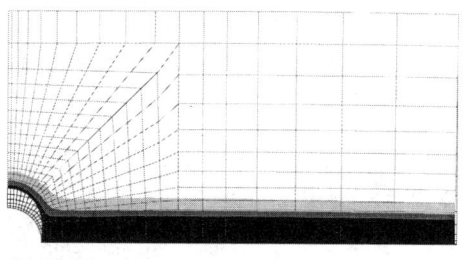

$b_h = 48\ \mu m$

g) Max compressive stress at peak-pressure. h) Fluid pressure at peak-pressure.

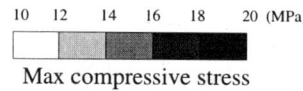

10 12 14 16 18 20 (MPa)

Max compressive stress

13 11 9 7 5 (MPa)

Fluid pressure

Figure 3. Stress, fluid pressure and deformed mesh as a results of modeling of a reopening test with material properties according to Table 1.

normal stiffness is varied only by a factor of 4 but gives completely different responses. The higher stiffness gives a higher initial normal stress at the fracture mouth which is closer to the theoretical value according to equation (2). The higher stiffness do also give a more sharp reopening and peak-pressure. A softer fracture gives a lower normal stress at the fracture mouth and smooth slow pumping type of pressure increase with no distinct reopening pressure or peak.

A small initial aperture gives a more distinct and higher peak-value (Fig. 5). This indicates that the fluid flow penetrates the fracture slowly delaying the fracture opening. At the same time, the critical aperture is reached at a higher effective normal stress. With a larger initial aperture of 11 µm, on the other hand, the fluid pressure can penetrate the entire fracture immediately and the critical hydraulic aperture for reopening is reached earlier.

An increasing fracture length gives a reduced peak-pressure (Fig 6). This is in agreement with field observations which shows a reduced reopening pressure during the first few reopening cycles. This indicates that the fracture is propagating during the first reopening cycles. For a fracture of 0.5 meters length, the stiffness of the rock surrounding the fracture confined its opening. This gave a slightly smaller initial aperture and a higher initial normal stiffness which affects the reopening.

The variation of flow rate showed an increasing re-opening pressure with flow rate (Fig, 7). This is also frequently observed in the field. A low flow rate implies that the fluid pressure have long time to penetrate the fracture and at the same time the critical hydraulic aperture, at which the flow rate into the fracture is equal to the injected flow rate, will be smaller. The modeling of the base case shows that a flow rate of about 20 to 30 l/min would be required for the peak-pressure to reach the magnitude of normal stress across the fracture mouth.

Table 2 Varied parameters and its affect on the reopening pressure.

Parameter	Range of values	Maximum difference in Peak-pressure
Flow rate, Q_w	1.0 - 30 l/min	2.8 MPa
Goodman's parameter, A_i	62.5 - 250	1.8 MPa
Residual hydraulic aperture, b_{hr}	- 5.0 to 5.0 µm ($b_{hi} \approx 1.5$ to 11 µm)	1.8 MPa
Fracture length, l	0.5 - 5 m	1.0 MPa
Biot's effective stress factor, α	0.1 - 1.0	1.0 MPa
Factor f	0.1 - 1.0	0.4 MPa
Well storage capacity	$1.7 - 6.8 \cdot 10^{-6}$ m^2	0.2 MPa

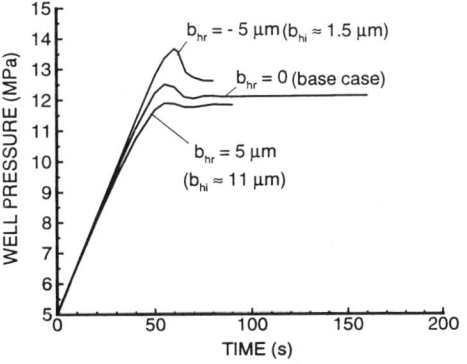

Figure 5. Modeling of a reopening test with variation of residual hydraulic aperture b_{hr}.

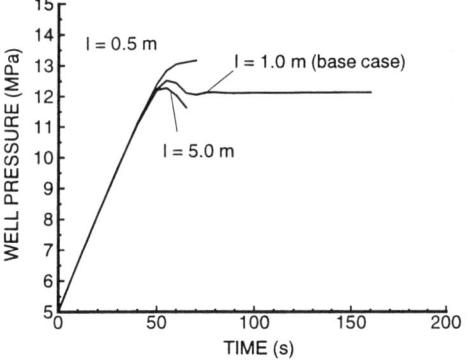

Figure 6. Modeling of a reopening test with variation of fracture length l.

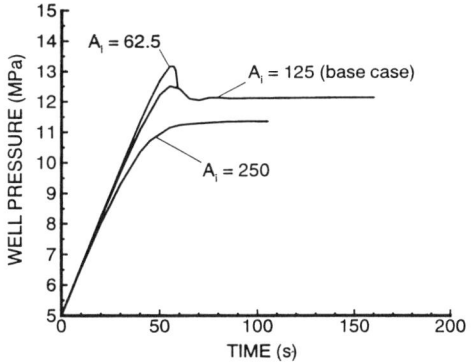

Figure 4. Modeling of a reopening test with variation of Goodman's joint constant A_i.

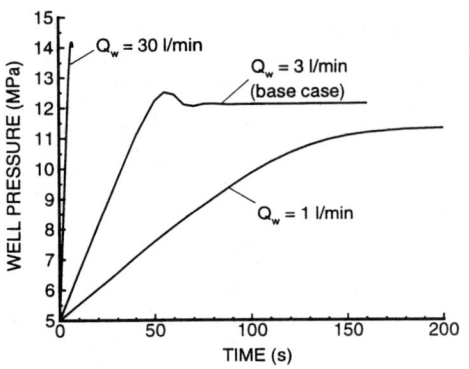

Figure 7. Modeling of a reopening test with variation of flow rate Q_w.

3. CONCLUDING REMARKS

The results in this study should be considered as preliminary and only valid for the material properties assumed. The absolute numbers obtained for the injection rate, cannot be used as an general recommendation. Further model calibration is needed to obtain the most realistic material properties. From these preliminary results it seems that the slightly smaller initial aperture and higher stiffness than the base case would be more realistic. Some improvement of the joint model is also needed. It is likely that the Goodman's one parameter joint model is overestimating the aperture at a low effective normal stress. This is very important for the modeling of the reopening test where reopening occurs at very low effective stress. Bandis' joint normal closure model (Bandis et al. 1983), which is more realistic at low normal stress, should give a more distinct reopening and peak-pressure.

However, regardless of the selected joint model the stress redistribution due to the presence of the fracture would occur (Fig. 3c). This indicates that it is difficult to reach the theoretical values for a homogeneous, linear elastic medium according to equation (2). On the other hand are field test results frequently and consistently showing a reopening pressure slightly less than the first breakdown pressure with a difference corresponding to the tensile strength of the rock. A possible reason to this discrepancy between modeling and field results is that the reopening pressure is affected by the fracture propagation which was not considered in the model. Therefore, a fracture propagation model in combination with a realistic normal stiffness model would be the optimum approach for modeling of reopening tests.

ACKNOWLEDGEMENTS

A grant for post-doctoral studies from the Wenner-Gren Center Foundation in Sweden to the first author is gratefully acknowledged. The field tests where funded by the Swedish Nuclear Fuel and Waste management Company (SKB).

REFERENCES

Bandis, S., A.C. Lunsden & N. R. Barton 1983. Fundamentals of Rock Joint Deformation. *Int. J. Rock. Mech. Min. Sci. & geomech. Abstr.* 29:249-268.

Biot, M. A. 1941. General theory of three dimensional consolidation. *J. Applied Physics*, Vol. 15, 155-164.

Cornet F. H. 1983. Interpretation of hydraulic injection test for in-situ stress determination. *Proc. Int. Workshop on Hydraulic Fracturing Stress Measurements* (Zoback and Haimson, Eds), Monterey, pp 149-158.

Noorishad, J., C.-F. Tsang & P.A. Witherspoon 1992. Theoretical and field studies of coupled behavior of fractured rocks - 1. Development and verification of a numerical simulator. *Int. J. Rock. Mech. Min. Sci. & geomech. Abstr.* 29:401-409.

Witherspoon, P. A., J.S.Y. Wang, K. Iwai & J. E. Gale 1980. Validity of the cubic law for fluid flow in a deformable fracture. *Water Resources Res.* 16:1016-1024.

Goodman, R. E. 1974. The mechanical properties of joints. Proc. 3rd Congr. ISRM. Denver, 1A:127-140.

Rutqvist J., O. Stephansson, & C.-F. Tsang. 1997. Hydraulic field measurements of incompletely closed fractures in granite. *Inj. J. Rock Mech. & Min. Sci.* 34:3-4, Paper No. 267.

Studies on rockmass stress measurement by parallel-borehole-controlled fracturing

Chou Wanxi & Cheng Hua
Huainan Mining Institute, Anhui, People's Republic of China

Sun Jun
Tongji University, Shanghai, People's Republic of China

ABSTRACT: Controlled fracturing technique is developed as a method for in-situ rockmass stress measurement. To confirm the feasibility of such technique, both laboratory and field experiments are conducted for this purpose. The working principales of parallel-borehole-controlled fracturing technique is discussed, and some results obtained by using this technique in the field experiments and their analysis are presented. The plausibility of this technique is thus proved.

1 INTRODUCTION

As yet there is no mothod available for measurement of stresses in in-situ strata as encountered in underground construction and production. This is a frontier in this branch of science, for whether the stability of the rock surrounding the underground constructions and its support is dependent, to a great extent, on the stress state and the mechanic properties of the rockmass. Such traditional ground stres measurement techniques as stress relieving and hydraulic fracturing exhibit shortcomings and drawbacks known to all and, moreover their subject has to be rockmass hard and complete, and with few or no fractures. To seek a technique appropriate for stress measurement in soft and loose strata in coal mines, on the basis of the traditional sleeve-fracturing method is developed a new technique, known as controlled fracturing.

The controlled-fracturing technique is, in essence, to fracture by employing some controlling technique the rockmass twice in the two or three pre-determined directions and calculate, on the accepted dependence between the in-situ rockmass stresses and the pressure peaks (fracturing pressures) measured after each fracturing, the rockmass maximum and the minimum principal stresses and their respective directions.

The controlled-fracturing technique is advantageous over traditional fracturing methods. Sleeve fracturing is limited to measurement in surrouncling rock of a roadway and, worse still, to measurement of planar stresses over the oross-section of the testing borehole. Hydraulic fracturing, though capable of 3-dimensional measurement, demands precision measurement of the direction and the angle of inclination of the fracuring-developed fractures which are governed by natural fractures and stress state of the rockmass. in addition, by using these two traditional methods, the maximum principal stress cannot be calculated until after the shut-in pressure is determined. it is therefore a necessity to develop a new technque for rockmass stress measurement, a technique which is not constrained by natural factors and possess the advantages of both the traditional methods and hence is known as controlled fracturing.

To confirm the feasibility of this new technique, both modelling and field experiments are conducted. As indicated by the experiments, it is practicable to measure rockmass stresses by parallel-borehole-controlled fracturing.

2 PRINCIPLES GOVERNING GONTROLLED FRACTURING FOR ROCKMASS STRESS MEASUREMENT

Similar to controlled fracturing by long-distance parallel boreholes, three pairs of short-distance parallel boreholes are arranged respectively on three straight lines $\theta = \theta_1, \theta_2, \theta_3$ and controlled fracturing experiments are conducted in three directions before the fracturing pressures are measured for the subject boreholes. What remains is to determine the fracturing condition of the bore-

Table 1 Comparison between differently calculated stress effects

L/a	f_x			f_y			f_b	
	herein	Savin	error	herein	Savin	error	herein	BEM
3	−0.630	−0.377	67%	3.074	3.264	5.8%	1.444	
4	−0.773	−0.609	27%	3.023	3.020	0.0%	1.250	1.381
6	−0.894	−0.837	6.8%	3.005	2.992	0.4%	1.111	1.121
10	−0.961	−0.948	1.4%	3.000	2.997	0.1%	1.040	1.000
16	−0.984	−0.981	0.3%	3.000	2.999	0.0%	1.016	1.000
∞	−1.000	−1.000	0.0%	3.000	3.000	0.0%	1.000	1.000

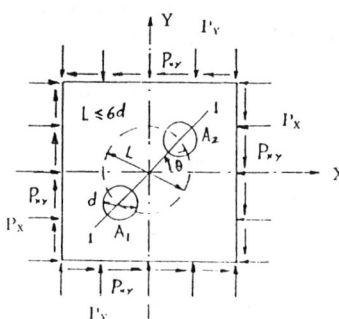

Fig. 1 Arrangement of boreholes

holes in each of the three controlled directions. Theoretically, under the action of the rockmass stresses and the internal pressures of the borehole, the tangential stress on the hole wall is such as can balance the tensile strength of the rockmass. And the tangential stress at the fracturing point on the hole wall

is $\quad \sigma_\theta = f_{x\theta}P_x + f_{y\theta}P_y + f_{xy\theta}P_{xy} + f_b P_{b1}$ (1)

in which $f_{y\theta} = (1 - 2\cos 2\theta) + 2\dfrac{a^2}{L^2}(1 + 2\cos 2\theta)$

$\qquad - 6\dfrac{a^4}{L^4}\cos 2\theta$

$f_{x\theta} = (-4 + 4\dfrac{a^2}{L^2} - 12\dfrac{a^4}{L^4})\sin 2\theta$ (2)

$f_b = 1 + 4\dfrac{a^2}{L^2}$

Where σ_θ is the tangential stress on the hole wall, a is the radius of the borehole and L is the distance between the pair of boreholes.
In the light of the criterion fot the maximum failure due to tensile stress $\sigma_\theta = -T$, we have

$T + f_{x\theta}P_x + f_{y\theta}P_y + f_{xy\theta}P_{xy} = f_b P_{b1}$ (3)

Again similarly, in the experiment on the secondary controlled fracturing, since $T = 0$, the fracturing pressures in the three controlled directions $P'_{b2}, P''_{b2}, P'''_{b2}$ are obtained and thereupon the condition for the secondary fracturing is established:

$f'_{x\theta}P_x + f'_{y\theta}P_y + f'_{xy\theta}P_{xy} + f'_b P'_{b2}$
$f''_{x\theta}P_x + f''_{y\theta}P_y + f''_{xy\theta}P_{xy} + f''_b P''_{b2}$ (4)
$f'''_{x\theta}P_x + f'''_{y\theta}P_y + f'''_{xy\theta}P_{xy} + f'''_b P'''_{b2}$

From the solutions (rockmass stresses) of equation (4) we can determine the maximum and minimum principal stresses and their respective directions.

Incidentally, $f_{x\theta}, f_{y\theta}, f_{xy\theta}, f_b$, the stress affects can also be calculated by such numerical methods as boundary element metod (BEM) and finite element method (FEM). Comparison is made, as shown in Table 1, between the affects calculated by using different methods (with $\theta = 0°$), and it is found that, when $L \geqslant 4a$, adequate accuracy can be attained for the solutions.

3 CASE STUDY: MEASUREMENTS AND ANALYSIS

Experiments on rockmass stress measurement by controlled fracturing are conducted in No. 4 Coal Mine of Pingdingshan, 270m north of the middle panel where the coross-entry in −256m and the surface +450m and the roadway is shotcreted for temporary support and U−arched for permanent support. There is, 20m south of the measurement locality, a fault with a throw of 17m, a strike of NW 30° and a dip angle of 55°. North of the fault zone, the rock surrounding the crossentry is white sandstone, hard and fairly well-jointed, whereas the surrounding rock in the south is broken arnaceous shale. At the measurement locality, two observation points are arranged, 10m apart, both in the west of the cross-entry. At each point, there are 3 boreholes, No.

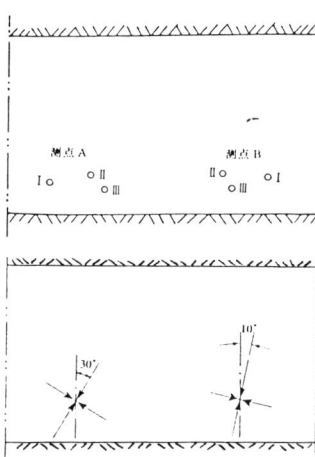

Fig. 2 Arrangement of testing boreholes and directions of principal stresses

Table 2 Rockmass stress measurements by controlled fracturing

Foint BH No.	Point A		Point B	
	BH Ⅰ	BH Ⅱ & Ⅲ	BH Ⅰ	BH Ⅱ & Ⅲ
P_{b1} (MPa)	62.76	65.331	68.88	62.24
T (MPa)	25.63	25.63	25.63	25.63
d (mm)	14	14	14	14
L (mm)		31		32
f_x		2.568		1.096
f_y		−0.364		1.096
f_b		1.204		1.191
θ(°)		70		45
β(°)	30		10	
P_{max} (MPa)	23.5		22.4	
P_{min} (MPa)	20.2		21.9	

Ⅰ for sleeve fracturing while No. Ⅱ and Ⅲ are parallel boreholes for controlled fracturing, with their centre line at a certain angle with the direction of the tensile fracture of No. Ⅰ. At Point A, the distance between Boreholes Ⅱ and Ⅲ is 31mm, whereas that at Point B is 32mm. Other parameters include the diameter of the borehole 14mm and the height from the borehole to the track level of the cross-entry 0.8m.

Table 2 lists the measurements made respectively from sleeve-fracturing tests on Borehole Ⅰ and controlled-fracturing tests on Boreholes Ⅱ and Ⅲ. In the Table, the tensile strength of the rockmass at the locality is obtained from sleeve-fracturing tests of tensile strength on laboratory rock blocks; the stress effects f_x, f_y, f_b are calculated by using the equations in this paper; and the maximum and minimum principal stresses are determined by finding solutions to the coupled equation involving the fracturing condition in the case of Borehole Ⅰ and the contolled-fracturing condition in the case of Boreholes Ⅱ and Ⅲ. The direction of the maximum principal stress at Pont A or at Point B is based on the direction of the tensile fracture of Borehole Ⅰ, notated by β, that is, the angle between the tensile fracture and the vertical axis; and its angle with the controlled fracturing direction is notated by θ.

As indicated by the measurements, the direction of the maximum principal stress at Point A or at Point B is close to the direction of the vertical axis, the angle between them in the former case (30°) being greater than that in the latter (10°) because the former is closer to the fault. The

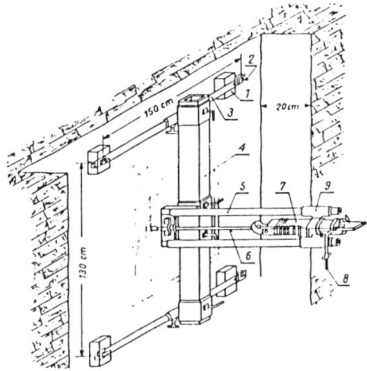

Fig. 3 Drilling process of parallel boreholes
1—wood pad; 2—bolt; 3—round steel rail; 4—mobile guide track; 5—drilling frame; 6—drilling rod; 7—rock drill; 8—comprssed air coupling; 9—buckling device

maximum principal stress P_{max} is greater than the weight vH overlying the cross-entry, indicating that the surrounding rock is still in the state of elastic stress, though the roadway has been rebuilt several times. It can be inferred from the stresses on the peripheries of the roadway at the locality that the horizontal in-situ rockmass stress over the cross-section of the cross-entry is greater its vertical one. --

4 TECHNIQUE FOR ENSURING PARALLELISM

In the case of big difference between the two pruncipal stresses, it is difficult to exert controlled fracturing. This problem can be thoroughly solved by using short-distance parallel boreholes. However, to obtain high-accuracy measurements, it is necessary to work out a technical plan for ensuring the parallelism between a pair of boreholes.

Use can be made of the boring frame of a heavy-duty rock drill to control its drilling direction. Mount the frame on a moble guide track whose two ends slide along two round steel rails which are fixed onto the sides of the roadway with wood-padded bolting rods. In fig. 3, the drill (7) is fixed onto with buckling devices onto the frame (5) which can, prior to the start-up of the dril, move along the guide track (4) which, in turn, slides along round steel rails (3) which are fixed by using bolts (2) with wood pads (1).

5 CONCLUSIONS

As demonstrated by practice, both in the laboratory and on the field, rockmass stress measurement by controlled fracturing is simple in the system, convenient to operate, cheap in cost, and easy to master. It can take representation of average stresses over a large stretch without the necessity to determine the angle of inclination and the direction of the artificial fractures, the module of elasticity of the rockmasss and the shut-in pressure. The controlled fracturing technique by using short-distance paralle boreholes proves applicable and practicable, especially to rockmass stress measurement involving big difference between principal stresses. However, techniques have to be worked out to ensure the parallelism between the boreholes.

REFERENCES

Chou Wanxi and Wei Shanbin. Sleeve-fracturing experiments and studies on stresses and other mechanic properties of roadway countryrock, Journal of Rock Mechanics and Engineering, 1992, No. 2:200—208.

Chou Wanxi and Li Wei. Modelling experiments and studies on rockmass stress measurement by controlled fracturing, Journal of Northeast University, 1995, extraissue :308—315

B. H. Brady and E. T. Brown. Rock Mechanics for Underground Mining, George Allen & Unwin. , London, 1985

G. N. Savin. Stress Concentration Around Holes, Oxford, Pergamon, 1961,134—139

ced fracturing technique is developed as a method for in-situ rockmass stress measurement with an advantage of unnecessary to measure the direction and angle of inclination of artificial fractures and the shut-in pressure. The working principles and the methodology of the modelling experiments of the controlled fracturing technique are described, and results obtained from modelling experiments, with short- or long-distance paralled boreholes, are presented and analysed. The plausibility of this technique is thus confirmed.

Modelling experiments on rockmass stress measurement by controlled fracturing

Chou Wanxi & Cheng Hua
Huainan Mining Institute, Anhui, People's Republic of China

Sun Jun
Tongji University, Shanghai, People's Republic of China

ABSTRACT: Controlled fracturing technique is developed as a method for in-situ rockmass stress measurement with an advantage of unnecessary to measure the direction and angle of inclination of artificial fractures and the shut-in pressure. The working principles and the methodology of the modelling experiments of the controlled fracturing technique are described, and results obtained from modelling experiments, with short- or long-distance paralled boreholes, are presented and analysed. The plausibility of this technique is thus confirmed.

1 INTRODUCTION

A technique for rockmass measurement, controlled fracturing is developed upon the basis of hydraulic fracturing in thermal energy utilization which produces fractures running through a pair of boreholes. The Report on Controlled Fracturing for Rockmass Stress Measurement is supported by China Association of Rock Mechanics and Engineering. In May 1995, researchers of geotechnical engineering from Huainan Mining Institute worked together with technical personnel from No. 4 Coal Mine of Pingdingshan in experiments on controlled fracturing for measurement of stresses in the surrounding rock of a cross-entry in this Mine. The experimentation is a success and provides data about rockmass stresses as basic for experiments on new-type supports. Meanwhile, in order to seek a method of controlled fracturing that is the optimum and most applicable to high-stress areas, a series of experiments in simulation of controlled fracturing are conducted such as on short-distance parallel boreholes, long-distance paralled boreholes, and single borehole with cutting grooves. The technique of controlled fracturing is thus theoretically confirmed and hence its applications in measurement of rockmass stresses and stresses existed in underground structure is with basic.

2 MODELLING EXPERIMENT METHODOLOGY

2.1 Methodology for modelling experiments

The models used in experiments are 200 × 200 × 200mm cement-sand mortar blocks. In order to simulate the stress state of the rockmass, loadings, vertical and horizontal, are exerted on the blocks by a loading system which consists of WY300—ⅢA hydraulic stabilizer, loading frame and 2 hydraulic jacks. Another system is the testing system consisting of oil pump, oil pipe, pressure meter, pressure sensor, XT function grapher, and cylindrical jack.

2.2 Methodology for controlled fractruing

In order to confirm the feasibility of the technique as well as to investigate uncertainties in the experiments, both cement-sand mortar blocks and paraffin-sand blocks are used. As indicated by the experiments, as long as there is no loading on the block surface, and the pair of boreholes are 10~100 diameters apart, every experiment is a success on controlled fracturing. However, fractures will not run through the two boreholes unless, when the block surface is under the action of bi-directional loadings and there is a small difference between the principal stress ($\sigma_1/\sigma_3 = 1.5$ or so), the angle β between the direction of the centre line and that of the maximum principal stress σ_1 is kept less than 60°, or unless, when the difference between the principal stresses is rather great ($\sigma_1/\sigma_2 = 2$ or so), the angle β is kept less than 30°.

To overcome the difficulty of controlled fracturing in the case of great difference between the principal stresses, such methods are proposed as by using short-distance parallel boreholes, by long-distance ones, by single borehole with cutting grooves. Although all these methods for controlled fracturing prove to be practicable, only the method of using parallel boreholes is of significance in the practice of engineering. there should be technical measures for ensuring the parallelism.

3 PRINCIPLES GOVERNING CONTROLLED FRACTURING

3.1 Controlled fracturing by long-distance paralel boreholes

If a pair of parallel boreholes are $L \geqq 6d$ (d is the diameter of the borehole) apart, they are known as long-distance parallel boreholes; if not, they are short-distance ones. Suppose, as shown in Fig. 1, that there are a pair of long-distance parallel boreholes on a circle of diameter L, the centre line at an angle of θ with the holizontal axis. On the (remote) infinite, the initial stresses are taken as Px, Py and Pxy. Then, when the boreholes are simultaneously subjected to internal pressure which are increased to a certain limit, tensile fracture will emerge running through the central point between the pair, provided that there is a small difference between the principal stresses or that th angle between the centre line of the boreholes and the direction of the maximum principal stress is kept less than 60 degrees. This pressure limit is known as P_{b1}, the primary breakdown pressure. The necessary condition for the emergence of tensile fractrue is that P_{b1} has to overcome both the tangential stress on the periphery of the borehole due to initial rock stresses. and the tensile strenght T of the rockmass. That is, the condition for fracturing as given below has to met:

$$P_{b1} = P_x + P_y - 2(P_x - P_y)\cos 2\theta - 4P_{xy}\sin 2\theta + T \quad (1)$$

If repedition is made of the controlled fracturing described above, since there is tensile fracture present, then there is no need to overcome the tensile strength, that is $T = 0$, and obviously the condition for a secondary controlled fracturing is

$$P_{b2} = P_x + P_y - (P_x - P_y)\cos 2\theta - 4P_{xy}\sin 2\theta \quad (2)$$

in which P_{b2} is the pressure for secondary fracturing. Minus equation (2) from (1), it can obtained

$$P_{b1} - P_{b2} = T \quad (3)$$

In order to determine the three stress components of the rockmass in equation (2), it is necessary to conduct controlled fracturing experiments in three directions $\theta = \theta_1$, $\theta = \theta_2$, $\theta = \theta_3$ befor the corresponding three pressures for the secondary fracturing P'_{b2}, P''_{b2}, P'''_{b2} are constituted into a coupled linear equation with the in-situ rockmass stresses P_x, P_y and P_{xy} as the unknown:

$$f_{11}P_X + f_{21}P_Y + f_{31}P_{XY} = P'_{62}$$
$$f_{12}P_X + f_{22}P_Y + f_{32}P_{XY} = P''_{62} \quad (4)$$
$$f_{13}P_X + f_{23}P_Y + f_{33}P_{XY} = P'''_{62}$$

where $f_{1i} = 1 - 2\cos 2\theta i$; $f_{2i} = 1 + 2\cos 2\theta i$; $f_{3i} = -4\sin 2\theta i$; $i = 1, 2, 3$. After the in-situ rockmass stresses P_X, P_Y and P_{XY} are determined by equation (4), the maximum and minimum principal stresses and their respective directions can be obtained by using the following equation:

$$P_{max} = \frac{1}{2}(P_X + P_Y) + \frac{1}{2}\sqrt{(P_X - P_Y)^2 + 4P_{XY}}$$
$$P_{min} = \frac{1}{2}(P_X + P_Y) - \frac{1}{2}\sqrt{(P_X - P_Y)^2 + 4P_{XY}} \quad (5)$$
$$\alpha = \frac{1}{2}\arctan \frac{2P_{XY}}{P_X - P_Y}$$

As indicated above, the key to rockmass stress measurement by controlled fracturing is to determine the fracturing pressure on the subject boreholes and establish and solve a coupled linear equation concerning the fracturing condition, saving measurement of the artificial fracture inclination and determination of the shut-in pressure.

3.2 Controlled fracturing by short-distance parallel boreholes

Similar to what is described above regarding controlled fracturing by long-distance parallel boreholes, three pairs of short-distance parallel boreholes are arranged respectively on three straight lines $\theta = \theta_1$, θ_2, θ_3 and controlled fracturing experiments are conducted in three directions befor the fracturing pressure are measured for the subject boreholes. What remains is to determine the fracturing condition of the boreholes in each of the three controlled fracturing direction. Theoretically, under the action of the rockmass stresses and the internal pressure of the borehole, the tangential stress in the surface is such as can balance the tensile strength of the rockmass. And the tangential stress at the failure point in the surface is

$$\sigma_\theta = f_{X\theta}P_X + f_{Y\theta}P_Y + f_{XY\theta}P_{XY} - f_b P_{b1} \quad (6)$$

in which $f_{Y\theta} = (1 - 2\cos 2\theta) + \frac{2a^2}{L^2}(1 + 2\cos 2\theta) - \frac{6a^4}{L^4}\cos 2\theta$

$f_{Y\theta} = (1 + 2\cos 2\theta) + \frac{2a^2}{L^2}(1 - 2\cos 2\theta) + \frac{6a^4}{L^4}\cos 2\theta$

$$f_{XY\theta}=(-4+4\frac{2a^2}{L^2}-12\frac{2a^4}{L^4})\sin2\theta \qquad (7)$$

$$f_b=1+4\frac{2a^2}{L^2}$$

where σ_θ is the tangential stress in the surface, a is the radius of the borehole and L is the distance between the pair of boreholes.

In the light of the criterion for the maximum failure due to tensile stress $\sigma_\theta=-T$, we have

$$T+f_{X\theta}P_X+f_{Y\theta}P_Y+f_{XY\theta}P_{XY}=f_b P_{b1} \qquad (8)$$

Again similary, in the experiment on the experiment on the secondary controlled fracturing, since $T=0$, the three secondary breakdown pressure P'_{b2}, P''_{b2}, P'''_{b2} are obtained and thereupon the condition for the secondary controlled fracturing is established

$$f'_{X\theta}P_X+f'_{Y\theta}P_Y+f'_{XY\theta}P_{XY}=f'_b P'_{b1}$$
$$f''_{X\theta}P_X+f''_{Y\theta}P_Y+f''_{XY\theta}P_{XY}=f''_b P''_{b1} \qquad (9)$$
$$f'''_{X\theta}P_X+f'''_{Y\theta}P_Y+f'''_{XY\theta}P_{XY}=f'''_b P'''_{b1}$$

Substituting the solutions (rockmass stresses) of equation (9) in eqution (5), we can determine the maximum and minimum principal stresses and their respective directions.

Incidentally, $f_{X\theta}$, $f_{Y\theta}$, $f_{XY\theta}$, f_b, the stress effects can also be calculated by such numerical methods as boundary element method (BEM) and finite element method (FEM). And it is found that, when $L\geq 4a$, adequate accuracy can be attained for the solutions.

4 MEASUREMENT AND ANALYSIS

4.1 Experiments on long-distance parallel boreholes

Experiments on rockmass stress measurement by controlled fracturing are conducted with 13 cement-sand mortar blocks ($200\times200\times200mm$), coded as 6D01, 6D02, ..., 6D03. Of them, 6D01 and 6D02 are used for determination of their normal tensile strength by the technique of sleeve fracturing, which is 10MPa, as shown in Table1. The rest are for controlled fracturing experiments. See Fig. 4 and Fig. 5 for the state of failure of each block. Refer to Table 1 for external loadings, fracturing pressures and other geometrical parameters of the blocks and the tensile strength T obtained by using equation (1) with the previously-mentioned parameters as the known. As revealed through comparison, the T value as obtained by using equation (1) is quited approximate to the normal T value as measured in the experiment on sleeve fracturing. It can thus be concluded that equation (1) is applicable to determination of the tensile strength and further to rockmass stress measurement by controlled fracturing, whereas the theoretical calculation equations are not effective here as they are concerned with hydraulic fracturing and sleeve fracturing.

As indicated by the experiments, when there is only very slight difference between principal stresses ($P_Y/P_X\approx1$), the direction of the centre line between the pair of parallel boreholes may vary and the tensile fractures in the boreholes develop independently of the stress state, when the said difference is bigger ($P_Y/P_X\geq1.5$), the angle betwwen the centre line and maximum principle stress will become bigger and hence great difficulty in the controlled fracturing. When the said angle is greater than 60°, the tensile fractures will not run through the centres of the two boreholes, as occurs in blocks 6D10, 6D11, 6D12 and 6D13 where the fractures do not develop in the direction of the maximum principal stress, a phenomenon contrary to the one deduced by the theory on hydraulic fracturing, probably affected by the empty boreholes in the vicinity. In the light of the failure state of the blocks, it is found that the tensile fractures between the pair of parallel boreholes tend to develop in the direction of the centre line whereas those outside tend to start at the borehole surface and approach gradually towards the direction of the maximum principal stress.

4.2 Experiments on short-distance parallel boreholes

12 cement-sand mortar blocks, $200\times200\times200mm$, are used for the experiments. Of them, 4 are used for determination of the tensile strength by sleeve fracturing, with results respectively 11.0, 12.5, 10.0, and 12.5 MPa, averaging 11.4MPa. The rest are for controlled fracturing, in each of which two parallel boreholes are arranged, 24 – 38mm apart, with the centre line inclined between 0 – 60°. Table 2 lists the loadings on the blocks, the stress effects $f_{X\theta}$, $f_{Y\theta}$, f_b, the breakdown pressure P_{b1}, ete. Typical states of failure are plotted in Fig. 6.

It should be noted that the T values as listed in Table 2 are, after the stress effects are obtained upon the basis of experiment data P_X, P_Y, P_{b1} and by employing equation (7) or BEM, calculated by using equation (8). The said T values are quite approximate to the measurements obtained from the sleeve-fracturing experiments. This approximation indicates that equation (8) is applicable here for determination of the tensile strength and that the theoretical equations as presented in this paper for

Table 1 Results from experiments on long-distance parallel borehole-fracturing

No.	1	2	3	4	5	6	7	8	9	10	11	12	13
P_X, MPa	0	0	0	0.5	0	0.5	1.5	1.5	1.4	1.5	0	0.8	0.8
P_Y, MPa	0	0	1.5	1.5	1.0	1.5	2.7	2.4	1.5	2.4	1.5	1.5	1.5
$\theta°1.2$	75	75	60	60	75	75	60	60	15				
$\theta°3.4$	90	90	90	90		90	90	90	90	90 pred. 30	90 pr. 45	90 pr. 30	90 pr. 15
$P_{bl}, 1.2$	10.5	9.8	9.8	11.0	9.0	11.0	14.0	13.5	13	13.0	8.0	12.0	11.5
$P_{bl}, 3.4$	10.0	9.5	9.0	9.5		10.5	13.0	13.0	12.5				
T, 1.2	10.5	9.8	9.8	10.0	9.7	10.7	11.0	10.5	10.0	10.9	9.5	11.7	10.6
T, 3.4	10.0	9.5	10.5	9.5		10.5	10.2	10.9	9.5				

Note: 1,2,3,4—borehole No.

rockmass stress measurement are correct. As demonstrated by the experiments, even when the centre line is perpendicular to the maximum principal stress or when there is big difference between the principal stresses, the tensile fractures

Table 2 Results of experiments on short-distance parallel boreholes-fracturing

Sample No.	1	2	3	4	5	6
L, mm	32	32	32	36	34	30
Borehole dia. mm	10	10	14	14	14	14
Direction of P_{max}, $\theta°$	0	30	45	60	0	40
P_X, MPa	2.4	2.0	1.2	1.2	1.2	2.9
P_Y, MPa	2.9	3.0	2.0	2.0	2.0	
P_{XY}, MPa	16.5	14.5	11.5	11.5	14.5	13.3
From Eg. (6), $f_{X\theta}$	−0.906	0.071	1.096	2.04	−0.84	0.774
From BEM, $f_{X\theta}$	0.879	0.08	1.113	2.03	−0.75	0.84
From Eg. (6), $f_{Y\theta}$	3.00	2.021	1.09	0.16	3.01	1.44
From BEM, $f_{Y\theta}$	2.96	2.02	1.11	0.18	2.96	1.45
From Eg. (6), f_{bl}	1.09	1.098	1.191	1.151	1.17	1.213
From BEM, f_{bl}	1.09	1.092	1.213	1.220	1.23	1.313
From Eg. (6), TMa	11.5	9.7	10.21	10.6	11.4	11.1
From BEM, TMa	11.6	9.7	11.2	11.2	12.2	12.1

Note: Pmax—maximum principal stress.

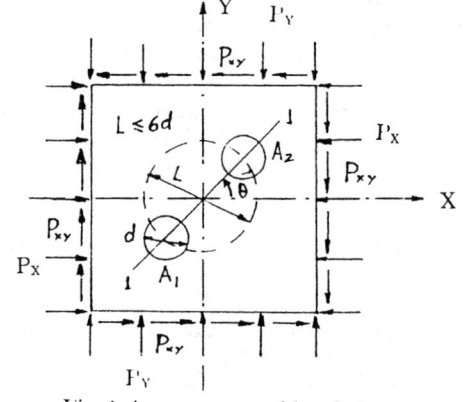

Fig. 1 Arrangement of boreholes

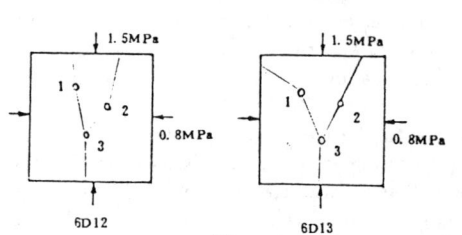

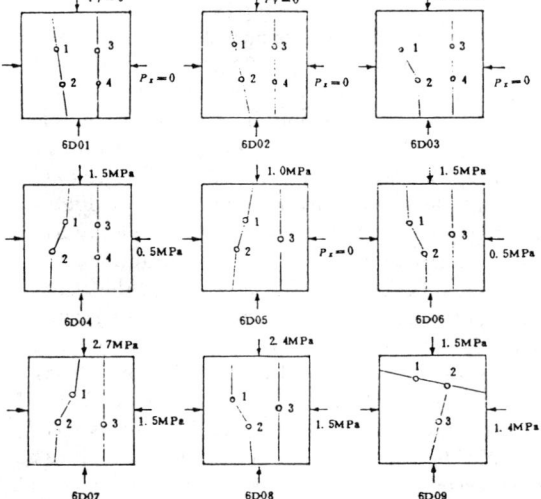

Fig. 2 Experiments on long-distance parallel borehole-fracturing

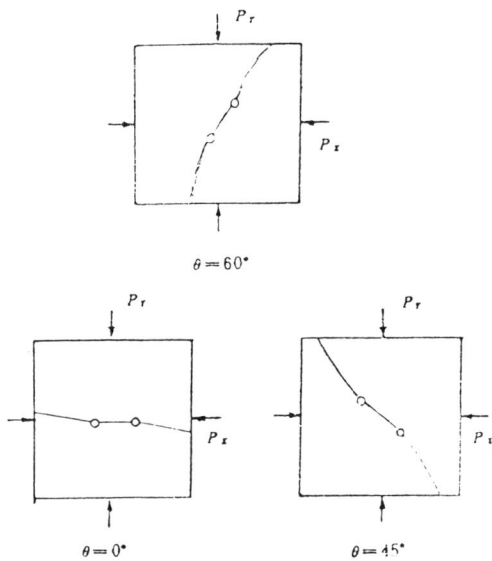

Fig. 3 Experiments on short-distance paralled borehole-fracturing

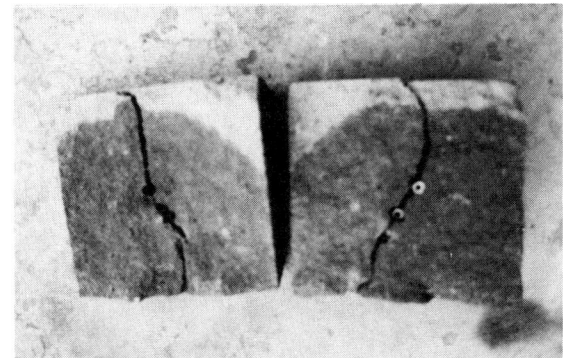

Fig. 4 Developed tendency of tensile fracture of test-boreholes

run through the centres of the two boreholes. It can thus be concluded that controlled fracturing by using short-distance parallel boreholes is independent of the effects of the maximum principal stress, capable of being steered in any direction and therefore applicalbe to cases with comparatively big difference between the principal stresses.

5 CONCLUSIONS

As demonstrated by practice, both in the laboratory and on the field, rockmass stress measurement by controlled fracturing is simple in the system, convenient to operate, cheap in cost, and easy to master. It can take representation of average stress over a large stretch and it is not necessary to measure the angle of inclination and the direction of the artificial fractures, the module of elasticity of the rockmass and the shut-in pressure. The fracturing condition developed in cach case, in conformity with the failure criterion of the maximum tensile strength, is verified by experiments both in the laboratory and on the field. And hence the theory on rockmass stress measurement by controlled fracturing proves correct. The controlled fracturing technique by using long-or short-distance parallel boreholes proves applicable and practicable. However, the former is appropriate for cases involving comparatively small difference between the principal stresses, whereas the latter is practicable in case involving comparatively great such difference and hence in more cases, provided that technical measures have to be worked out to ensure the parallelism between the boreholes.

REFERENCES

GUO A. et. al. An experimental investigation into hydraulic fracture propagation -Part 2; Single well test, Int. J. Rock Mech. Min. Sci., Vol. 30, No. 3. 1993, 189—202

Brady B. H. G., Brown P. T., Rock Mechanics for Underground Mining, Greorge Allen & Unwin, 1985, 153—228.

Chou Wanxi, Controlled fracturing for measurement of rockmass stress. Journal of China Coal Society, Vol. 20 No. 3, 1995 241—244.

Chou Wanxi, Cardinal principle of rockmass stress measurement by controlled fracturing technique, Journal of China University of Mining & Technology, Vol. 25 No. 1. 1996, 40—45.

A proposal of geo-stress measurement technique by plate fracturing

T.Yokoyama & A.Nakanishi
Oyo Corporation, Ohmiya, Japan

ABSTRACT: We propose "Plate Fracturing Technique" to measure geo-stresses. The theory of this technique is similar to that of hydraulic fracturing method and sleeve fracturing method. By using this technique, we can create the fracture in controlled direction. We can, then skip the procedure for checking the direction of the fracture. The assumed conditions of stress analysis are also simplified. Therefore, we can improve the precision of measurements by using this technique. This paper describes outline of this technique, demonstrates state of stress around the fracture by Finite Element Method (FEM) and results of an experiment in laboratory with a simple model.

1 INTRODUCTION

Geo-stress has no influence of the physical properties and mechanical properties of rock mass. But geo-stress is one of the most important parameter that the rock exhibits in-situ circumstance. For example, in the field of the civil engineering, it is necessary to determine initial stresses in case of designing the underground excavation. And when we evaluate the stability on the cavity particularly by elasto-plastic model, initial stresses becomes a very important parameter. Also, in the field of the earth science, it is very important to find the state of stress at the underground while estimating the crustal stress condition with in wide area. Further, continuous observation of crustal stress charge is important for the earthquake prediction and the measures of the protection against disasters.

We propose a new technique of geo-stress measurement, which use a borehole. Theoretically this technique is similar to hydraulic fracturing method and sleeve fracturing method. The main characteristic of this technique lies in the fact that it can control the direction of fracture artificially generated in the borehole. If it is possible to generate fractures in more than 3 differential directions at any depth, this technique can determine the state of 2 dimensional stress in the horizontal plane which is crossed with the borehole axis. In the conventional techniques, the direction of the fracture in the borehole must be checked in some way, but this technique can omit that aspect. Therefore, we can measure geo-stress more efficiently.

This paper describes the principle of measurement in this technique, results of the laboratory experiment with a simple model and calculating the state of stress around the fracture by FEM.

Finally we refer to the prospect to make this technique in practice, investigate its merits and demerits.

2 MEASUREMENT METHOD

2.1 Conventional Method

As the technique of using the fracture in rock mass for geo-stress measurements, hydraulic fracturing method and sleeve fracturing method are made practicable at present. To generate the tensile fracture in the rock, a stress larger than the sum of the tensile strength and the initial stress should be applied perpendicularly to the fracture plane. In any techniques, the procedure of propagation of tensile fracture in borehole wall are similar with the method of pressuring the inside of the borehole. Then, we can determine the state of stress.

Hydraulic fracturing method was first employed around 1984 because of the purpose to take out petroleum, stimulating a drying up oil well. Later, Scheidegger[1] suggested the possibility of measuring geo-stress using this method. At a latter time, many scholars like Kehle[2] Fairhurst[3] Haimson[4] performed research and development experimentally.

Sleeve fracturing method[5] and double fracturing

method[6] came in the way of pressurizing a borehole wall through the flexible rubber sleeve. As a result, these methods can prevent pressure from decreasing when the fracture is opening.

Therefore, it is possible to measure geo-stress preciously by generating 1_{st} fracture to and 2_{nd} fracture to occur separately. These methods can determine the principle stresses even if the direction of the fracture which has occurred in the borehole wall can not be observed. Because those method can directly measure the deformation of borehole wall by using the displacement transducer in the 4 independent directions.

2.2 Measurement Principle

The main characteristic of the plate fracturing technique is that the direction of fracture can be controlled artificially. A couple of the stiff plate applies load to the borehole wall and generate fractures perpendicular to the loading axis. The direction of the stiff plate can be controlled and we can measure geo-stress efficiently at the deep point without confirming the direction of the fracture.

According to De la Cruz[7], tangential stress $\sigma_{\theta\theta}$ ($\beta \leq \theta \leq \pi/2$) in the borehole wall by the load of the stiff plate is given by the following equation (Figure-1).

$$\sigma_{\theta\theta} = K(\kappa, \beta, \theta) \ (F/R) \qquad (1)$$

where K =function of κ, β, θ; β =load per unit length; R =the radius of a borehole.

κ value of eqn. (1) is the coefficient expressing the non-uniformity of the load distribution due to the difference of the curvature between the stiff plate and the borehole wall. K becomes a constant value without the influence of κ when $\theta = \pi/2$ and $\beta = \pi/4$. In this case, tangential stress in the borehole wall is given by the following equation.

$$\sigma_{\theta(\pi/2)} = K(\kappa, \beta, \theta) \cdot F/R \qquad (2)$$

In eqn. (2), tangential stress in the borehole wall depends only on load of the stiff plate. Since load is applied by hydraulic pressure, the relation of hydraulic pressure to the stiff plate load is given by the following equation.

$$F = (\gamma \cdot 2R \cdot \sin \beta) \cdot P \qquad (3)$$

where P =jack pressure on the stiff plate (= hydraulic pressure) ; γ =the effective area ratio of the jack cylinder.

It is, then possible to design the cylinder of the jack and the stiff plate so that $\sigma_{\theta(\pi/2)}$ because equal to P.

$$\sigma_{\theta(\pi/2)} = P \qquad (4)$$

(The shape having the relation $K \cdot \gamma \cdot 2R \cdot \sin \beta / R = 1$)

That is, it is possible to generate the tensile stress which is equal to the jack pressure P at the borehole wall of $\theta = \pi/2$.

In case that geo-stress of σ_1, σ_2 is existing around this borehole wall, tangential stress in borehole wall is given by the following equation (Figure-2).

$$\sigma'_{\theta\theta}{}^* = -\sigma_1 - \sigma_2 + 2\cos 2(\theta^* - \alpha) \cdot (\sigma_1 - \sigma_2) \qquad (5)$$

where α =angle of σ_1 with the load axis.

Therefore, the tangential stress at the point 'a'

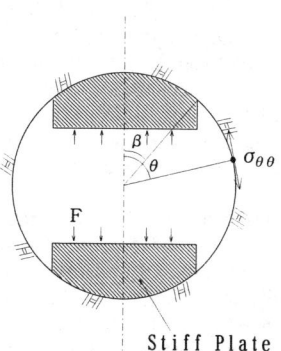

Figure-1. Tangential stress by the load of stiff plate.

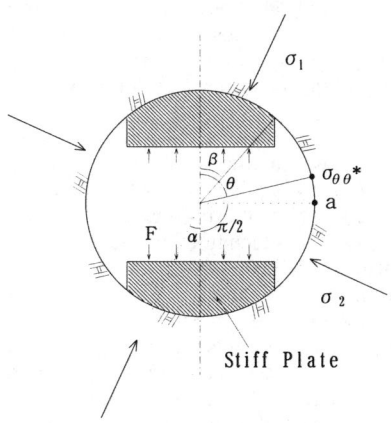

Figure-2. Tangential stress of borehole wall in geo-stress field.

($\theta^* = \pi/2$) of Figure-2 equals to the sum of eqn.(4) and eqn.(5). This is given by the following equation.

$$\sigma_{\theta(\pi/2)} = P + \sigma'_{\theta(\pi/2)}$$
$$= -\sigma_1 - \sigma_2 + 2\cos 2(\pi/2 - \alpha) \cdot (\sigma_1 - \sigma_2) + P \quad (6)$$

If the tensile strength of rock is σ_t, the condition to generate the tensile fracture occurred at the point 'a' is given by the following equation.

$$\sigma_t = \sigma_{\theta(\pi/2)}$$
$$= -\sigma_1 - \sigma_2 + 2\cos 2(\pi/2 - \alpha) \cdot (\alpha_1 - \alpha_2) + P \quad (7)$$

Pressure-displacement curve as shown in Figure-3 is expected when cyclic load is applied to the borehole wall without fracture. By the same view of interpretation as the hydraulic fracturing method, P_0 is the opening pressure at the 'a' point and P' is the re-opening pressure. Therefore eqn. (7) can be changed into the following equation.

$$\sigma_t = -\sigma_1 - \sigma_2 + 2\cos 2\alpha \cdot (\alpha_1 - \alpha_2) + P_0$$
$$0 = -\sigma_1 - \sigma_2 + 2\cos 2\alpha \cdot (\alpha_1 - \alpha_2) + P' \quad (8)$$

By checking more than three P' by changing load directions, the value and the directions of principal stresses in plane can be determined.

3. MODEL EXPERIMENT

3.1 *Procedure of Experiment*

A model experiment of the artificial material was performed to confirm both the displacement behavior of the stiff plate and the strain distribution in the borehole wall with the propagation of the fracture. In this experiment, we used the most simple procedures, since there was limitation in the model size and the examination equipment.

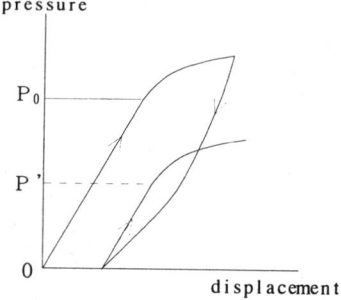

Figure-3. Pressure-Displacement Curve

The shape of the specimen used for the experiment is shown in Figure-4. The specimen is a rectangular which is 40 cm in width, 40 cm in height and 20 cm in thickness. The hole with the diameter of 76 mm is opened at the center of the specimen. Strain distribution of the specimen surface was measured by 16 sets of rosette gauges affixed to the specimen surface.

The mixing ratio of the materials for the specimen and its properties are shown in Table-1.

The specimen was set in the stiff servo examination machine, and the Good-Man Jack was inserted into the hole and constant stress was applied in vertical direction. Main specifications of the Good-Man Jack are shown in Table-2. It is possible to consider that the oil pressure is equal to the tangential stress at borehole wall at the point 'a' of 90 degree to loading axis. It is because the Good-Man Jack is designed as eqn. (4) to stand up.

In this experiment, under the constant stress of 0.5 MPa on the specimen, 1.0MPa, 2.0MPa, 3.9MPa, 5.9MPa and 3.9MPa cyclic loading was applied by Good-Man Jack. Then strain of the specimen, displacement of the stiff plate and hydraulic pressure of Good-Man Jack was observed. Sampling interval was every 0.2 MPa.

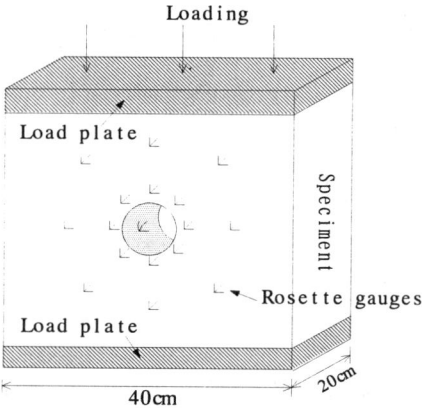

Figure-4. Specimen of model experiment

Table-1. The mixing ratio of the materials for the specimen and its properties

mixing ratio (weight ratio)	high-early-strength cement:non-contractile material :water reducing material:water=95:5:1:45	
material properties	density	uni-axial strength	tensile strength
	19g/cm^3	30MPa	3.5MPa
	Young's modulus	Poisson's ratio	
	10GPa	0.25	
	P wave velocity	S wave velocity	
	3400m/sec	1700m/sec	

Table-2. Main specifications of Good-Man Jack

maximum pressure	63.7MPa
borehole diameter	NX(ϕ 76.2mm)
jack stroke	12.7mm(69.9〜82.6mm)
displacement meter	±3.81mm resolution 1/1000mm
stiff plate	length:204mm angle of an arc:90 degree

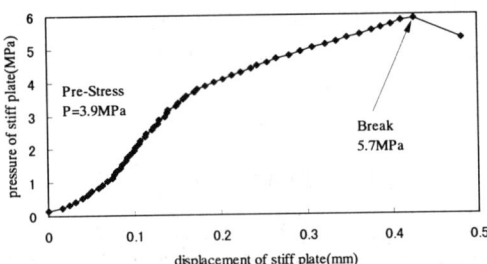

Figure-6. Pressure-Displacement curve of the Stiff Plate

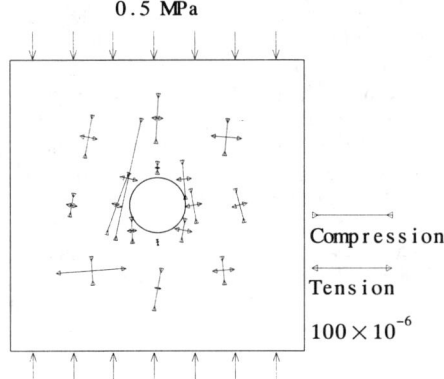

Figure-5. Distribution of the principal strains by uni-axial loading

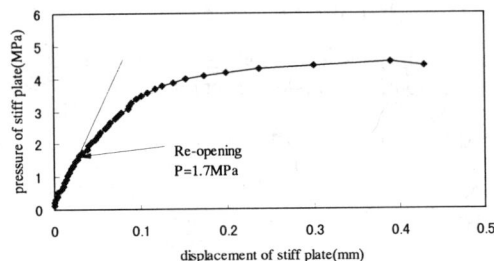

Figure-7. Pressure-Displacement Curve of the Stiff Plate

3.2 Experimental Results

The distribution of the principal strains on the surface of the specimen by vertical uni-axial loading is shown in Figure-5. From eqn. (5), the value of the 'a' point ($\theta = \pi/2$) of Figure-2 is given by the following equation.

$$\sigma'_{\theta(\pi/2)} = -\sigma_1 - \sigma_2 + 2\cos2(\pi/2 - \alpha)\cdot(\sigma_1 - \sigma_2) \quad (9)$$

At the time of $\alpha = 0$ degree, $\sigma_2 = 0$MPa, it is given by the following equation.

$$\sigma'_{\theta(\pi/2)} = -3\sigma_1 \quad (10)$$

The average magnitude of the strain in the direction of the loading axis is about 50×10^{-6}, and the tangential strain at the 'a' point is about 150×10^{-6}, it shows that the experimental values are consistent with the theoretical value.

The relation between the pressure and the displacement of the stiff plate is shown in Figure-6 and Figure-7. The deviation in the slope of the curve at about 3.9MPa as shown in Figure-6 presents the influence of the previous stress of 3.9MPa which was loaded just before the test.

And the fracture of the borehole wall seems to occurred at the pressure of the stiff plate of 5.7 MPa.

The relation between the pressure and the displacement of the stiff plate at re-loading to 3.9 MPa behind unloading is shown in Figure-7. The deviation at the slope of the curve which indicates the re-opening of the fracture as shown Figure-3 was seen at 1.7MPa. This pressure is equivalent to about 3 times of the uni-axial stress as expressed in eqn. (10).

4. NUMERICAL ANALYSIS

4.1 Numerical Modeling

In the plate fracturing technique, the assumption that the direction of the fracture on the borehole wall is perpendicular to the loading axis of the stiff plate. Generally, the direction of principle stresses does not consist agree with the loading axis of the stiff plate. Therefore, in the state of anisotropic stress, the above premise become a subject of discussion.

Here, we perform the simple checking by FEM in the condition limited to the above subject. An analysis model is shown in Figure-8 and the properties of the material are shown in Table-3. In the model a thin rubber plate (1mm thickness) is placed in the surface of the stiff plate. The geo-

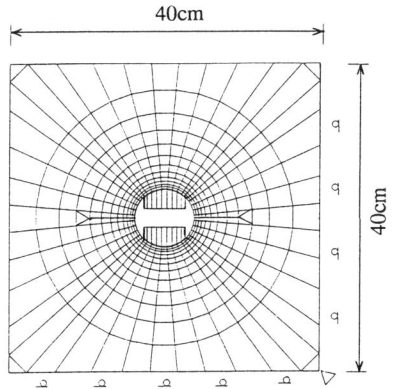

(diameter of a borehole:7.6mm)
Figure-8.   Finite element mesh

Table-3.   Material Properties

material	Young's modulus (GPa)	Poisson's ratio
rock	29	0.20
stiff plate	206	0.17
rubber	0.1	0.49

stress is assumed as σ_1=9.8MPa σ_2=4.9MPa, the pressure of the stiff plate is given P=34.3MPa and 5 cases are calculated by changing the direction of the loading against the direction of the principle stresses.

4.2 Numerical Results

The distributions of each tensile stress in case of α =0°, 20°, 45°, 70° and 90° is shown in Figure-9. Then α is a crossing angle of the loading axis of the stiff plate to the direction of σ_2. When α =0°, it is possible to expect that it generate fracture at the position of $\theta = \pi/2$. Because tensile stress concentration area by being geo-stress is consistent with one by the loading with the stiff plate. However, the stress concentration area shift to the direction of α_1 axis as α value increasing.
Therefore it causes an error to assume that the fracture occurred at the position of $\theta = \pi/2$.

5 DISCUSSION

In the plate fracturing technique, we propose a method to determine the state of 2-dimensional stress by measuring the pressures at more than three fractures re-opening.
The model experiment was done under the uni-

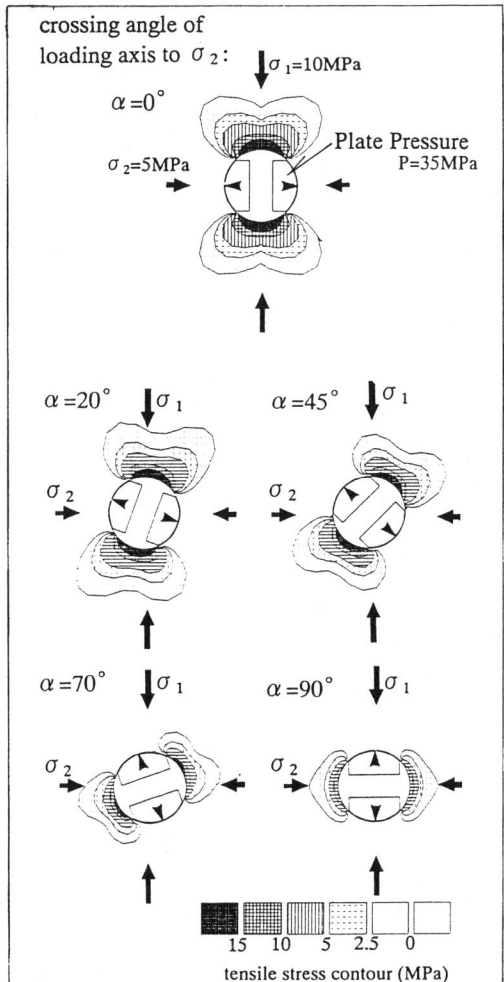

Figure-9.   Distribution of tensile stress concentration area with α changing

(σ_1=9.8MPa, σ_2=4.9MPa, P=34.3MPa)

axial compressive stress of 0.5MPa. A specimen has a borehole in its center. We generated new fractures by loading pressure to the borehole wall through the stiff plate to the compressional direction. In this case, the stiff plate pressure, which measured during fractures occurring was 5.7MPa. Also, the deviating was seen to pressure and displacement curve at about 1.7MPa, during the re-loading pressure after unloading pressure. This phenomena is explained as follows: Assuming that the fracture occurs on the borehole wall, when the stiff plate pressure reaches to the sum magnitude of tensile strength of the specimen and tangential stress of borehole wall, the tensile strength is estimated to be

4.5MPa. Because tangential stress is 3 times of uni-axial stress ($\sigma_1 = 0.5$MPa), i.e. 1.5MPa. Also, assuming that the tensile strength is 0MPa in this case, re-opening pressure of the fracture is estimated to be 1.5MPa. The estimated tensile strength (4.5MPa) is nearly equal to the experimental value (3.4MPa). Moreover, the re-opening pressure of 1.5MPa, which is theoretical value, is consistent with 1.7MPa, which was measured during the model experiment. And also, we were able to measure the pressure at the fracture re-opening by the behavior of the stiff plate.

The result of the numerical analysis shows that in the case that the loading direction of the stiff plate slightly differs from the direction of principal stress, position of generated fracture was nearly consisted with the theoretical position. Since the condition of calculation is fairly limited, the result of above numerical analysis can not be discussed strictly. But if anisotropic stress is not so remarkable like $\sigma_1/\sigma_2 \leq 2$, the geo-stress measurement by this technique will be able to be practically use.

6 CONCLUSIONS

The geo-stress measurement method by the plate fracturing is theoretically simple. As the results of the model experiment, it is possible to find both the fracture occurring and the behavior of re-opening in the borehole wall by using the relation between displacement and the pressure of the stiff plate. Also, this technique can be available to measuring the geo-stress under the anisotropic stress states due to the result of the numerical analysis.

However the following problem must be solved in order to make a practical use of this method in the future.

There is a possibility that the fracture might occur in the contact part at the corner of the stiff plate. To solve this problem, it is necessary to examine the surface treatment and the shape of the stiff plate. It is necessary to grasp the position of the fracture in the various geo-stress conditions.

The plate fracturing technique leaves a few problems as mentioned above. We intend to do more research to come out with the practical use including the development of the measurement technique and the equipment.

7 REFERENCE

Scheidegger,A.E. 1962. Stress in the earth crust as determined from hydraulic fracturing data, Geologie und Bauwesen, Vol.27.

Kehle, R.O. 1964. The determination of tectonic stresses through analysis of hydraulic well fracturing, J.Geophys. Res., Vol. 69, No.2, pp.259~274

Fairhurst, C. 1964. Measurement of in situ rock stresses with particular reference to hydraulic fracturing, Rock Mechanics and Engineering Geol., Vol.2.

Haimson,B.C. 1978. The hydrofracturing stress measurement technique method and recent field results. Int. J.Rock Mech.Min.Sci.&Geomech. Abstr., Vol,15, pp.167~178

K. Sugawara, Y. Obara, H. Arali, Y. Ariga 1987. Sleeve fracturing for Determining Rock Stresses. Proceeding of the 7th Japan Symposium on Rock Mechanics. pp.181~pp.186

S. Serata, S. Sakuma, S.Kikuchi and Y Mizuta 1992-1993. Double Fracturing Method of In Situ Stress Measurement in Brittle Rock. Selected Research of Yamaguchi Rock Engineering Society. 1992-1993

De La Crus 1978. Modified Borehole Jack Method for Elastic Property Determination in Rocks. Rock Mechanics.,10,pp221~239

In situ stress measurement using the ANZI stress cell

K.W. Mills
Strata Control Technology Pty Ltd, Wollongong, N.S.W., Australia

ABSTRACT: This paper describes the operation of the ANZI (Australia, New Zealand Inflatable) stress cell. Laboratory and field measurements are used to illustrate the instrument's operation. The ANZI stress cell has a pressuremeter design that enables 18 electrical resistance strain gauges to be pressure bonded directly to the rock of a borehole wall. The strain gauges are monitored during overcoring to obtain stress relief strains. An up hole pressure test is undertaken prior to overcoring to obtain the elastic properties of the rock in situ and to confirm the correct operation of all the strain gauges. The elastic properties of the rock are also obtained after overcoring in a biaxial test. The ANZI stress cell is widely used for routine three dimensional stress measurement in underground coal operations in Australia. It is being increasingly used in the United Kingdom, China, Japan and Vietnam in coal mining, civil and hard rock applications.

1 INTRODUCTION

The original ANZSI cell (Mills & Pender 1986) was developed in the early 1980's to allow measurement of three dimensional in situ stresses in coal. The instrument was primarily designed to overcome the tensile stresses generated in soft rocks at the borehole wall by more rigid hollow inclusion type cells.

The very soft pressuremeter design of the ANZSI cell provided various practical advantages that have since justified further development for use in a wide range of rock types. This further development was accompanied by a change of name to ANZI (Australia New Zealand Inflatable) stress cell reflecting the instruments combined development history and essential mode of operation.

This paper describes the operation of the ANZI stress cell with examples of laboratory and field test results that illustrate the instruments operation in a range of applications.

2 DESCRIPTION

The ANZI cell is a strain measuring instrument that uses the overcoring method of stress relief to determine in situ stress. The 56 mm diameter version of the instrument is shown in Figure 1. The instrument is essentially an inflatable membrane of low modulus polyurethane material with strain gauges on its outer surface.

Eighteen electrical resistance strain gauges of various orientations are mounted flush on the outside surface of the membrane. When the membrane is pneumatically inflated during installation, the electrical resistance strain gauges become cemented directly to the borehole wall allowing direct measurement of strain changes in the rock. The wiring of the strain gauges is embedded in the membrane so that the instrument is waterproof.

The mechanics of stress measurement are similar to other types of overcoring operations except that an additional in situ pressure test is conducted prior to overcoring to confirm the correct operation of the strain gauges, and to measure in situ modulus.

In situ stresses are determined from the measured strains using the technique described by Leeman & Hayes (1966). A minor correction can be made during analysis to include the effect of the 0.3-0.5 mm epoxy cement layer formed between the membrane and the rock using the analysis described by Duncan-Fama and Pender (1980).

The membrane material has a modulus of elasticity of less than 0.002 GPa and is therefore soft enough to be ignored in the analysis of the strains measured during overcoring. As a result of the low modulus, tensile stresses generated at the rock/instrument interface during overcoring are also low.

The pressurised length of the ANZI cell membrane is designed to be four times the diameter of the borehole in which the instrument is installed so as to generate near plane strain conditions during the up hole pressure test (Laier et al 1975). The increased

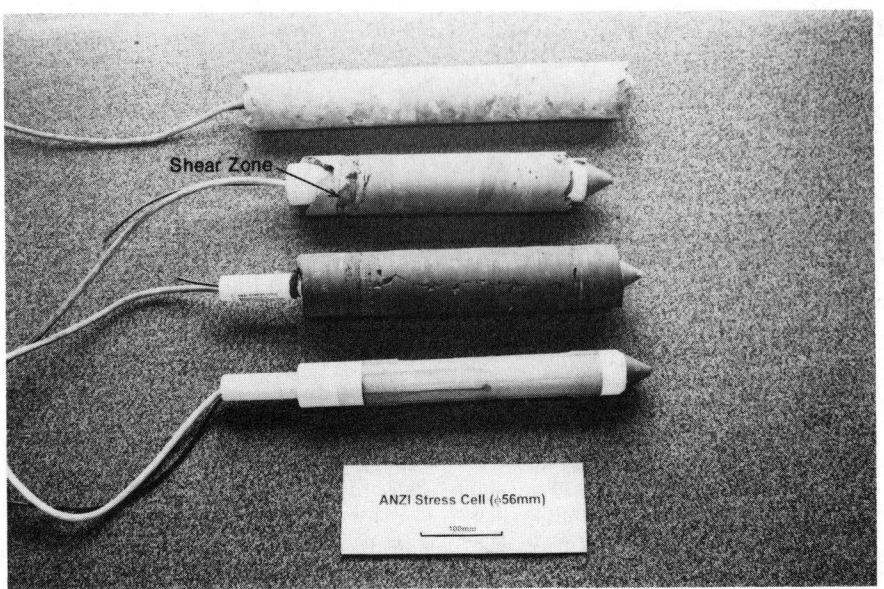

Figure 1. 56 mm diameter ANZI stress cell showing (from top to bottom) overcored instruments in conglomerate, mudstone and coal.

length of the instrument also improves the length of overcore recovered in weak rock.

2.1 Strain gauge configuration

The configuration of strain gauges carried on the instrument can be varied to suit rock conditions. Typically, 5 mm long gauges oriented in rosettes of three gauges each (0°, 45° and 90° to the axis of the borehole) are used. The 5 mm long gauges minimise the strain averaging effect of longer gauges that can affect results in some stress fields. The gauges at 0° and 90° orientations facilitate field interpretation of results.

The six rosettes of three gauges each are oriented at 60° intervals around the circumference of the cell to improve statistical confidence in the in situ stress measured (Gray & Toews 1974). Each rosette has one gauge oriented in a circumferential direction. Every second rosette has one gauge oriented in an axial direction. This combination gives a high degree of redundancy and two or more independent measurements of many individual strain components. For instance, there are three gauges that independently measure the one value of axial strain, three sets of directly opposite circumferential gauges and three sets of directly opposite 45° gauges.

The advantages of having a large number of independent strain measurements include:

1. The consistency of the independent strain measurements provides a strong indication of the confidence that can be placed in the result.
2. Completely independent measurements of the stress field can be determined from the one overcore test if required.
3. If rock conditions are such that some rosettes are damaged during overcoring, strain readings from these rosettes can be ignored while still allowing redundancy in the result determined.

2.2 Instrument configurations

The ANZI cell is currently produced in two different sizes, a 56 mm diameter version (Figure 1) and a more recently developed 29 mm diameter version (Figure 2). The same strain gauges and rosette combinations are used on both sizes of instrument.

The 56 mm instrument is installed in an oversize TT56 diamond drilled hole and is typically overcored using an 82 mm internal diameter thin wall bit. Larger overcore diameters have also been used where there have been particular requirements for larger size drilling gear. The 56 mm instrument is now routinely used for stress measurements in the coal industry in Australia and has also been used in the United Kingdom, Japan, China and Vietnam.

A double cell configuration of the 56 mm instrument is shown in Figure 3 together with

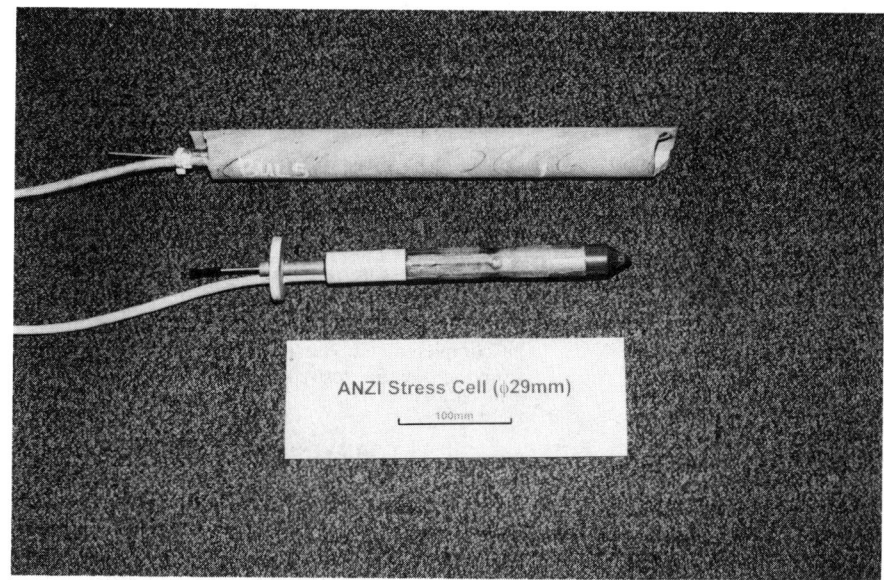

Figure 2. Double ANZI configuration showing instrument and overcores in various coal measure strata.

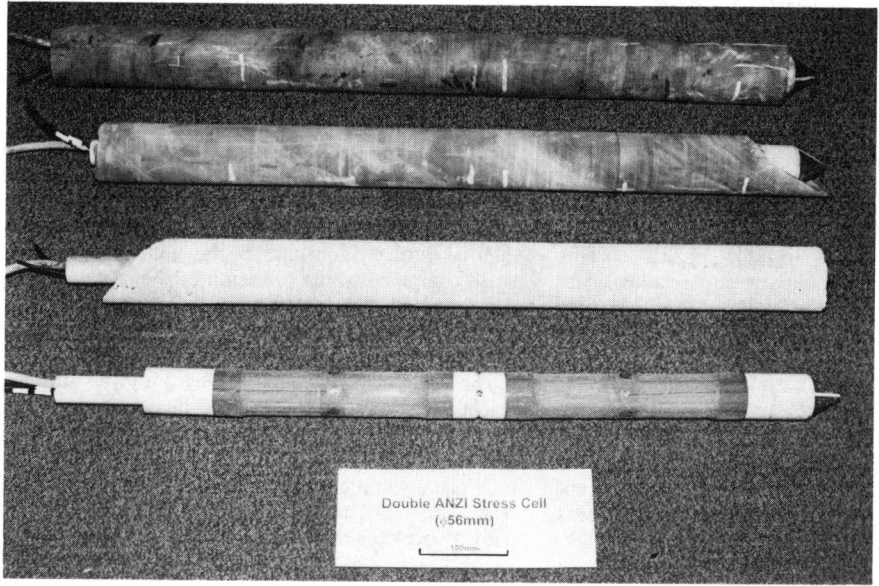

Figure 3. 29 mm diameter version of the ANZI with a 42 mm diameter overcore in sandstone.

several overcores in various coal measure rocks. The two instruments share the same cable but can be independently inflated.

The double cell configuration allows two tests to be conducted in only slightly longer time than it would normally take to conduct a single test. The first instrument is monitored until it is completely overcored. The second instrument is then monitored as drilling continues until it too is completely overcored.

The 29 mm version of the ANZI cell is still being fully developed. The smaller instrument has been used to successfully measure in situ stresses in a range of rock types. It is quicker to install than the

56 mm instrument and requires lighter weight drilling equipment. An installation at 10-15 m from an underground roadway typically takes less than 2 hours from the start of drilling the hole.

3 OPERATION

There are four stages in the ANZI cell test procedure: installation, in situ pressure test, overcoring stress relief and biaxial pressure test. The overcoring and biaxial tests are essentially similar to procedures used for other types of stress relief instrument.

3.1 *Installation*

To install the ANZI cell, the access hole and pilot hole are drilled to the location of the test. The instrument is coated with low slump epoxy cement and installed into the pilot hole to the required depth. There is no requirement for the instrument to be installed near the end of the pilot hole as it can be inflated at any location. The pilot hole is typically drilled well beyond the measurement site and a suitable target horizon chosen on the basis of the core recovered.

When the cement has cured, typically 8-36 hours depending on temperature, the strain gauges are bonded directly to the rock.

In coal mine investigations, tests are typically conducted in holes 10-15 m long drilled up at an angle from underground roadways. There has been no additional difficulty in installing instruments at depths in excess of 40 m or in down holes when required.

3.2 *Pressure test*

Once the cement has cured, a pressure test is conducted using the ANZI cell as a pressuremeter or dilatometer. The pressures used in this test are kept relatively low to avoid disturbing the in situ stress field. The strain changes measured (typically 50-200 µS) are sufficient to confirm the correct operation of all the gauges and provide a measure of the in situ properties of the host rock before it is disturbed by overcoring.

3.3 *Overcoring*

The ANZI cell overcoring operation is conducted in much the same way as for other instruments that use the overcoring stress relief method. Direct bonding of the strain gauges onto the surface of the borehole means that the diameter of the overcore need only be slightly greater (10-20 mm) than the diameter of the instrument and the overcore does not need to remain intact for a valid result to be obtained. These characteristics extend the range of rock types and drilling environments in which the instrument can be used.

3.4 *Biaxial pressure test*

A biaxial pressure test is conducted after the core is recovered to measure elastic modulus and Poisson's ratio. If the core is damaged and a biaxial test cannot be completed, the elastic modulus can be estimated from the pressure test conducted prior to overcoring.

4 LABORATORY CALIBRATION TESTS

Figure 4 shows the results of laboratory calibration tests conducted on an ANZI cell installed in an aluminium cylinder of known elastic properties (Elastic modulus 71 GPa and Poisson's ratio 0.34).

4.1 *Internal pressure test*

The internal pressure of the ANZI cell was incremented to simulate an up hole pressure test. The strain changes observed are shown in Figure 4a together with the strain changes that would be expected for the geometry and elastic properties of the cylinder.

The strain changes observed for a 2000 kPa internal pressure change in the cell are relatively small compared to the precision of the strain reading system. The results are nevertheless sufficient to determine the elastic properties of the aluminium and confirm the correct operation of the gauges.

The strain changes registered by the three different orientations of strain gauge can be seen. The circumferential gauges register the largest strains. The axial gauges register very little strain, confirming near plane strain conditions exist during the pressure test. The 45° and 135° gauges register strains midway between the circumferential and axial strains.

4.2 *Biaxial pressure test*

A second calibration test was conducted by applying pressure to the outside of the aluminium cylinder. This test is effectively a post-overcoring biaxial pressure test. The measured strains are shown in Figure 4b.

The strain changes registered in this test form three groups representing each of the three gauge orientations. The strain changes are linear and hysteresis if negligible.

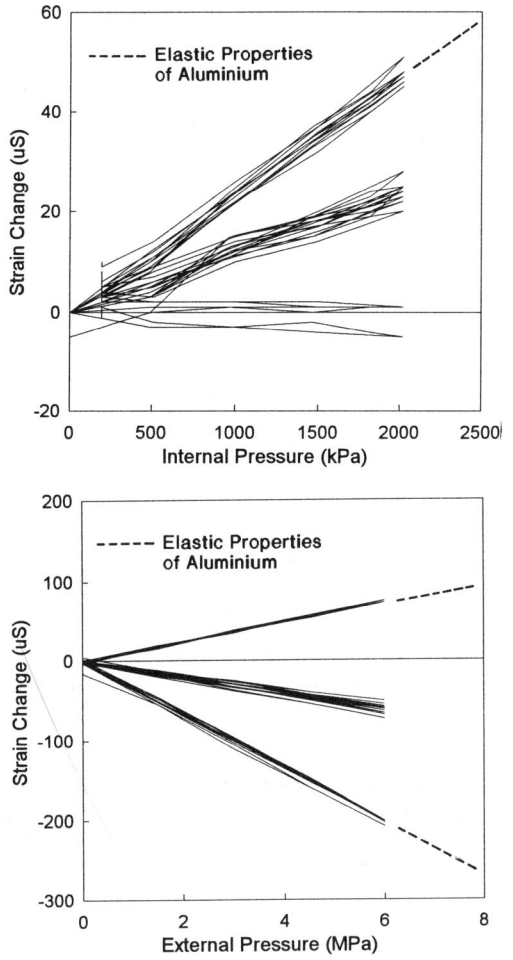

Figure 4. Calibration pressure tests in aluminium cylinder: a) internal and b) external pressure tests.

The elastic modulus and Poisson's ratio of the aluminium determined from the biaxial test equal the known modulus of the material. The 45° gauges register strains midway between strains registered on the circumferential and axial gauges.

This biaxial calibration test confirms the correct operation of the instrument. Furthermore it indicates that useful strain levels can be measured in a stiff material.

5 FIELD MEASUREMENTS

Figure 5 shows the results from a stress measurement test in coal measure strata using the ANZI stress cell. For clarity, the strains measured on the nine 45° gauges are not shown.

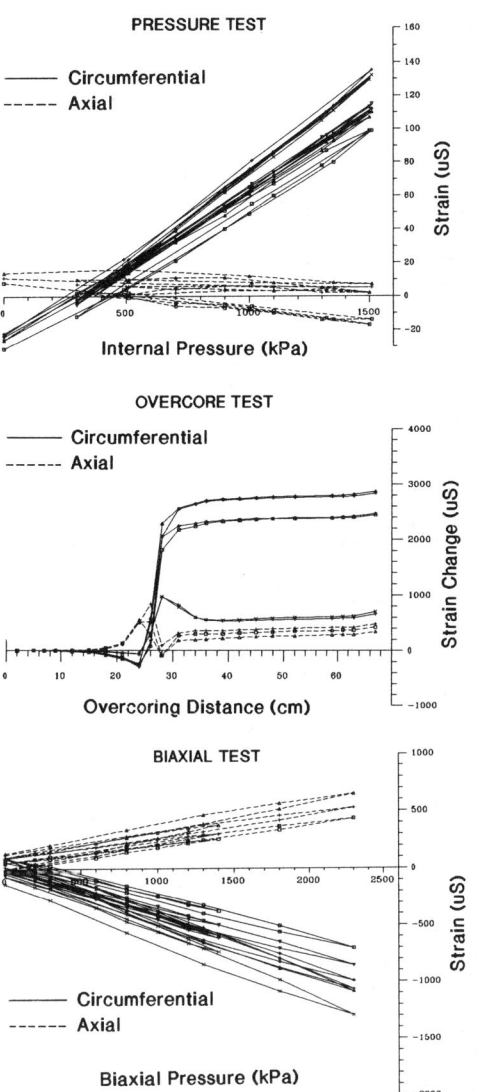

Figure 5. Typical overcoring test in coal measure strata using the ANZI stress cell. a) up hole pressure test b) overcoring test c) biaxial test.

The pressure test indicates the gauges are operating correctly prior to overcoring and the elastic modulus of the sandstone material in situ is approximately 16 GPa.

The overcoring test indicates that the instrument has registered the stress relief correctly. The form of the stress relief is smooth and consistent with expected behaviour. Independent strain gauges on opposite sides of the instrument register almost identical strain changes giving confidence in the result. The three axial gauges also indicate similar strain magnitudes.

The biaxial test shows generally linear behaviour and indicates an elastic modulus of 8 GPa and a Poisson's ratio of 0.43. The variation in the modulus indicated by the biaxial test is partly associated with eccentricity of the pilot hole and partly with drilling induced microfracturing.

The ratio of the elastic modulus determined in the up hole pressure test and that determined in the biaxial test typically ranges 1.8 to 2.0 for coal measure strata. This difference is attributed to stress-relief microfracturing that occurs during drilling.

5.1 *Other field measurement experience*

The ANZI cell has been used to successfully measure in situ stresses in a wide range of strata types. Figure 1 shows some typical overcore specimens recovered from tests in conglomerate, mudstone and coal.

The top core shows an example of a test in conglomerate strata. A large number of redundant gauges is necessary to establish the validity of the measurement because of the obvious inhomogeneous nature of the conglomerate material.

Overcore tests conducted in a mass concrete footing below a loaded column have indicated 1 MPa stresses can be resolved to better than 0.2 MPa in concrete given sufficient gauge redundancy.

The mudstone core in Figure 1 shows an example of a 2 cm wide semi-open shear zone preserved intact in the core. Open fractures have also been "captured" in this way during tests in other heavily deformed strata.

The lower core shows an example of an overcore measurement obtained in a jointed coal material. Individual gauges are often affected by jointing and/or drilling damage, but, with a sufficiently large number of gauges, enough usually remain cemented to intact material and allow the stresses to be determined.

6 CONCLUSIONS

The ANZI stress cell has various analytical and operational advantages that have enabled in situ stresses to be successfully determined in a wide range of rock types and conditions.

Laboratory calibration tests in an aluminium cylinder confirm that the instrument correctly measures the elastic properties of a stiff material in both the pressure test and biaxial test.

Direct bonding of the strain gauges to the rock simplifies analysis and reduces tensile bond stresses at the rock/instrument interface.

The large number of redundant strain measurements on the instrument provides a strong indication of the confidence that can be placed in the result.

The double version of the instrument enables two tests to be conducted in only slightly longer than it normally takes to complete one.

The 29mm diameter version of the instrument allows quicker installation using lighter weight drilling equipment.

REFERENCES

Duncan-Fama, M.E. & M.J. Pender 1980. Analysis of the hollow inclusion technique for measuring in situ rock stress. *Int. J. Rock Mech. & Min. Sci* 17:137-146.

Gray, W.M. & N.A. Toews 1974. Optimisation of the design and use of a triaxial strain cell for stress determination. *STP 554 ASTIM Field Testing and Instrumentation of Rock*:116-134.

Laier, J.E., J.H. Schmertmann, & J.H. Schaub 1975. Effect of finite pressuremeter length in dry sand. *Proc. Conf. on In Situ Measurement of Soil Properties, Rayleigh, North Carolina.*

Leeman, E.R. & D.J. Hayes 1966. A technique for determining the complete state of stress in rock using a single borehole. *Proc. 1st Congress of Int. Soc. of Rock Mechanics* 2:17-24.

Mills, K.W. & M.J. Pender 1986. A soft inclusion instrument for in situ stress measurement in coal. *Proceedings of Int. Symposium on Rock Stress and Rock Stress Measurement, Stockholm, 1-3 September 1986*:247-251. Centek.

A case study of pressuremeter tests for measurement of stresses in sedimentary soft rock ground

Kazuo Tani
Central Research Institute of Electric Power Industry, Chiba, Japan

Yasuo Yoshida
Central Research Service, Ltd, Chiba, Japan

ABSTRACT : Two series of pressuremeter tests were conducted separately at a decade's interval in the same ground of sedimentary soft rocks. In order to keep up with the ever-developing pressuremeter technology, the most advanced pressuremeter probe available at the time of field application was used accordingly for each test series. Attempts were also made of different probe installation methods, namely pre-boring as well as self-boring techniques. Based on this intensive test program, the applicability of pressuremeter tests for measurement of *in-situ* stresses in sedimentary soft rock ground was examined.

1 INTRODUCTION

At a site of sedimentary soft rocks, two series of pressuremeter tests, hereafter denoted as Series I and II, were carried out in 1985 and 1995 respectively. During this interval of a decade, considerable progress had been made in the pressuremeter technology. Central Research Institute of Electric Power Industry (CRIEPI) has been involved in the research project on pressuremeter testing, and three types of pressuremeter probes, Mark I ~ III, have been developed so far in the last two decades. Since the latest apparatus was selected for field application, different pressuremeter probes were used for the separate test series. Although comparisons were made on various rock properties evaluated from the test results in two series, the scope of this paper is directed to the *in-situ* stresses, i.e. the initial stresses in the plane perpendicular to the pressuremeter axis.

2 PRESSUREMETER TESTS

2.1 Site specification

Both series of pressuremeter tests were conducted in the same sedimentary soft rock ground of thick late Miocene series, called the Sagara group in Shizuoka prefecture, Japan (Miyaike et al., 1993). This deposit is typically characterized as alternating layers of sandstone and mudstone. The scarcely jointed mudstone layers appear to be 10~40 centimeters thick, while the sandstone layers of continuous nature are generally thinner, some 5~20 centimeters. Their material properties obtained by laboratory tests on cored samples are summarized in Table 1. The bedding is generally found to have the strikes of N77° E and the dips of 17° to the northwest. All the tests were conducted in the boreholes drilled perpendicular to the bedding planes.

Table 1. Material properties of the alternating strata

Layer		Mudstone	Sandstone
Unit weight	γ_t (kN/m^3)	19.4	20.8
Water content	w (%)	25.2	16.8
Elastic wave velocity[*1]	V_s / V_p (m/s)	930 / 2090	910 / 1930
Undrained shear strength[*2]	q_f (MPa)	10.1	4.57
Secant Young's modulus[*2]	E_{50} (MPa)	1050	———
Poisson's ratio[*2]	v	0.21	0.31
Tensile strength[*3]	σ_t (MPa)	0.8~1.2 / 0.8~1.1	0.2~0.1 / 0.2~0.3

[*1] : Ultrasonic wave velocity measurement under no confining pressure
[*2] : Triaxial compression (CU) test under the confining pressure of effective overburden pressure, $E_{50} = E_{sec}$ at $q/q_f = 0.5$
[*3] : Brazilian test / Triaxial extension (CU) test under the confining pressure of effective overburden pressure

Table 2. Comparison of the CRIEPI pressuremeters

Features	Mark IIb for Series I	Mark IIIa for Series II
Diameter / Length of the pressurizing probe	120mm / 600mm	140mm / 1120mm
Maximum loading pressure	10MPa	40MPa
Thickness of the rubber membrane	5.0mm	2.0mm
Thickness / Width of the metal sheaths	0.5mm / 10mm	0.5mm / 12mm
Drilling bit / Reamer	Tricone roller bit / No reamer	Multi-step impregnated diamond bit / Surface diamond reaming shell
Measurement of cavity wall displacements	Indirect measurement by volume expansion	Direct measurement by proximeter system
Loading system	Two separate servo-controlled hydraulic systems for monotonic and cyclic loading	Servo-controlled hydraulic system

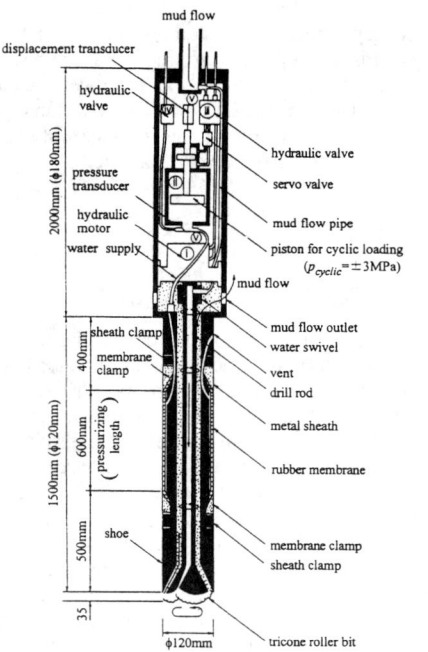
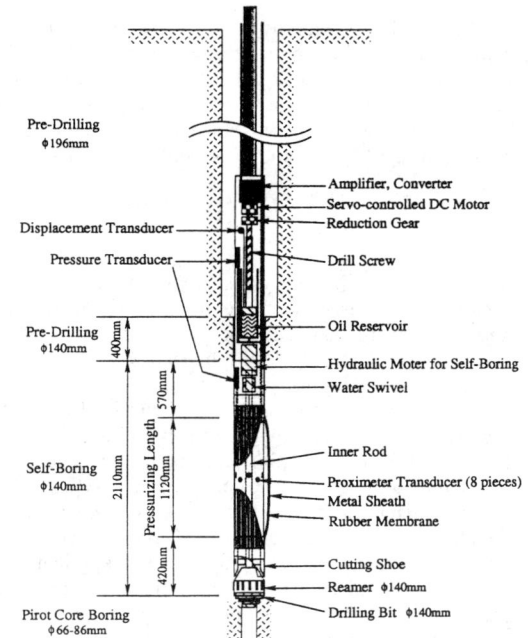

Figure 1. CRIEPI pressuremeters (Left) Mark IIb (Right) Mark IIIa

2.2 *Pressuremeter probes*

Two pressuremeter probes were used of different designs, hereafter denoted as Mark IIb and IIIa for Series I and II respectively. Table 2 and Figure 1 compare their features.

Mark IIb was specifically designed for gravelly soils (Yoshida et al., 1990). To evaluate not only stiffness values but damping ratios, cyclic loading of a sinusoidal waveform was made applicable up to the maximum frequency of 0.5Hz. Moreover, to evaluate the reasonable properties representing the mass behavior of coarse-grained ground, the probe dimension was made to be as large as 120mm in diameter. Cavity wall displacements were calculated from the measured volume expansion of the pressurizing length assuming the axisymmetry.

The due corrections should be made for the system compliance and the bedding errors, which requires the calibration in a thick-walled steel cylinder.

On the other hand, Mark IIIa was later developed specifically for rock ground (Tani et al., 1995). Utmost attention was paid to accurate measurements of cavity wall displacements which were considered as very small in quantity for stiff ground and could be non-uniform if the ground was anisotropic or jointed in nature, or if tensile cracking took place during the course of expansion tests (Mair & Wood, 1987). A total of 8 proximeter transducers were mounted 45° apart in the middle cross-section of the pressurizing length whose diameter was 140mm; to the authors' knowledge, this probe is currently the largest in the world. This proximeter system can monitor the metal sheaths through the rubber membrane, thus measures the movements of the outermost elements of the probe which are directly in contact with the pressurized cavity wall. As a consequence, the measured results are expected as most representative and reliable compared to other available techniques such as the strain arms system. Another feature is that detailed examination of individual transducer's record provides valuable information about the possible onset of tensile failures on the cavity wall.

2.3 Test procedure

4 tests at depths of 17~23m in Series I and 2 tests at depths of 12.0m and 13.9m in Series II are presented for comparison. Each pressuremeter test was preceded by the core drilling by using a 66mm double-core-tube sampler through the expected depths for the test. Continuous measurements of various drilling parameters were carried out including the drilling rate, the thrust, the rotational torque, and the drilling mud pressure. Additionally, the drilled borehole was examined by a borehole TV camera in Series II. The exact depth of the test was then determined based on the drilled core inspection, the records of drilling parameters, and borehole TV observation (Tani et al., 1995).

The insertion of the pressuremeter probe was made by self-boring technique enlarging the 66mm pre-drilled borehole except the test conducted at the depth of 12.0m in Series II. For pressuremeter expansion tests, during the course of the conventional monotonic loading at a rate of 0.2MPa/min, several unload-reload cycles were included at different levels of cavity pressures.

3 TEST RESULTS AND DISCUSSION

The test results are shown in Figure 2 as pressuremeter curves. For the case of Series II using Mark IIIa, the cavity strains ε_c represent the average values measured by the 8 proximeter transducers.

Although all the tests in Series I were self-boring tests, the pressuremeter curves exhibit noticeably convex downward demonstrating significantly overestimated cavity strains in the initial stages, particularly below the pressure 0.5MPa. Since these results are similar to that of the pre-boring test in Series II conducted at the depth 12.0m, the selection of the tricone roller bit used for Mark IIb might be inappropriate for stiff fine-grained ground resulting in oversized test boreholes. For this reason, multi-step diamond bit accompanied by a diamond reaming shell was adopted later for Mark IIIa. The self-boring test results conducted at the depth 13.9m demonstrate considerable improvement in reducing the excessive cavity displacements in the initial stages of the loading.

The *in-situ* stresses in the plane perpendicular to the pressuremeter axis were estimated by the following three-fold methods; i.e. (1) lift-off method, (2) double-tangent method, and (3) crack detection method. The lift-off method and the double-tangent method are illustrated in Figure 3. In the crack detection method, the *in-situ* stresses, p_o, were estimated from the cavity pressure to cause tensile failure on the cavity wall, p_c^*, and the known values of tensile strengths of the ground, σ_t, assuming the theory of elasticity.

$$p_o = (p_c^* - \sigma_t) / 2$$

p_c^* was determined by close examination of the individual proximeter's record trying to detect any telltale signs of tricky response, thus only available for the tests using Mark IIIa in Series II. Since the mid-section of the pressuring length was placed in the mudstone layer, the tensile strengths of 0.8 and 1.2MPa were used as the bounding extreme values (see Table 1).

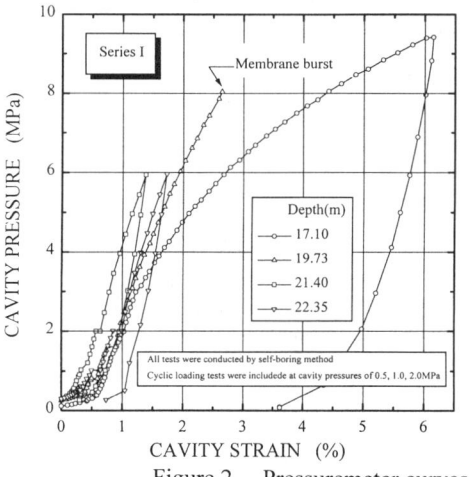
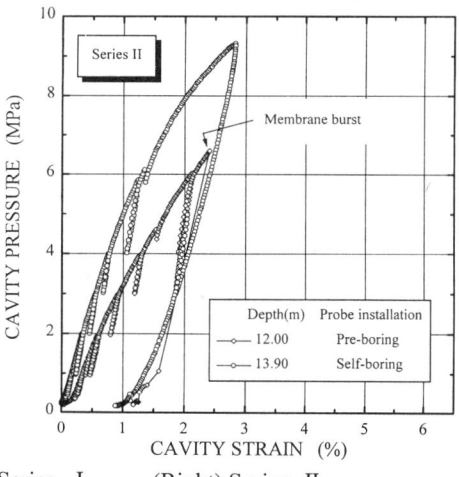

Figure 2. Pressuremeter curves (Left) Series I (Right) Series II

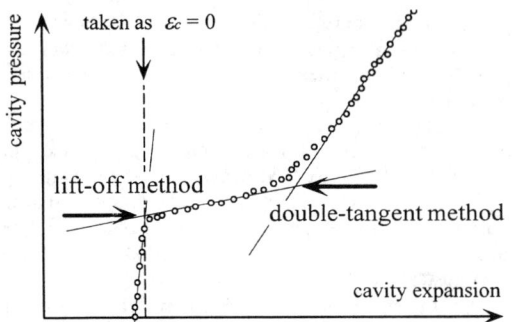

Figure 3. Lift-off method and double tangent method

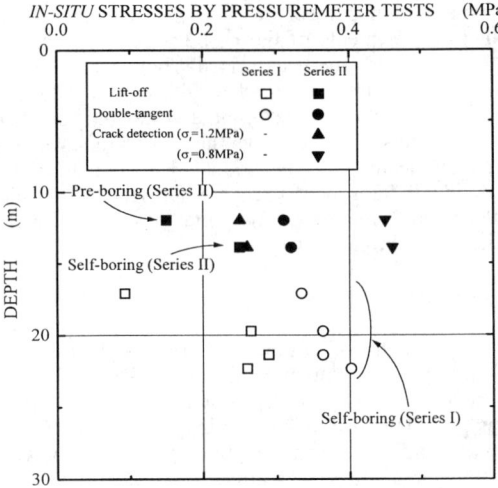

Figure 4. *In-situ* stresses by pressuremeter tests

Figure 4 compares the *in-situ* stresses evaluated by the three methods. Since there are no independent and reliable measurements of the *in-situ* stresses in soft rocks, it cannot be justified to state that any single technique can provide the best estimate. Reasonable speculation, however, may lead to the following discussion;
(1) Unlike soft clays, the popular lift-off method is rather unreliable for stiff ground. It is because the initial stages of the tests are rather sensitive to the surface preparation of the cavity wall:
(2) Although there is no theoretical justification, the double-tangent method may provide fairly consistent estimate without respect to drilling, installation, nor instrumentation techniques:
(3) The estimates by the crack detection method are strongly dependent on the tensile strengths of the ground that should be evaluated separately. Although intensive research has been carried out to identify this sensitive value by triaxial extension tests (Tani, 1997), the results have demonstrated too scattering for the authors to specify any single reliable value:
(4) The double-tangent method and the crack detection method appear to provide consistent estimates of the *in-situ* stresses, while the results by the lift-off method are found to be significantly lower.

4 SUMMARY

Although the lift-off method has been considered as the most reliable analysis to evaluate the *in-situ* stresses from pressuremeter test results particularly for soft ground (Mair & Wood, 1987), the question if the same interpretation holds good for stiff ground is still to be examined carefully. It is because that, in stiff ground, the initial stages of the pressuremeter loading, which are definitely important for most of the *in-situ* stress interpretations, are very sensitive to (1) drilling / preparation of the borehole, (2) installation of the probe, and (3) instrumentation to measure the cavity expansion. The ideal pressuremeter tests require that the probe be inserted into the intact ground without causing any disturbance and that the cavity expansion can be measured with absolute accuracy which is free from bedding errors. Unfortunately, this can not be met even with the current state-of-the-art for the pressuremeter technology.

In this study, comparisons are made among the three different analyses of the *in-situ* stresses from pressuremeter tests; i.e. the lift-off method, the double-tangent method, and crack detection method. At a site of sedimentary soft rock ground, the tests were curried out in two series using different probes. The results demonstrated that the lift-off method was rather unreliable whereas the double-tangent method seemed to be promising in providing consistent estimates. Moreover, reasonable estimates may be obtained by the crack detection method, on condition that the tensile strengths of the ground be evaluated accurately. Further research is needed to establish some reliable test methods to evaluate the *in-situ* stresses in soft rocks.

REFERENCES

Mair, R.J. & Wood, D.M. 1987. *Pressuremeter testing: methods and interpretation*, CIRIA Ground Engineering Report: Butterworths.
Miyaike, Y., Mizuno, N., Momose, Y. & Nakamura, J. 1993. Experimental and analytical studies on mechanical properties of layered soft rock mass, *Proc. 2nd Workshop on Scale Effects in Rock Masses*: 125-132.
Tani, K., Nishi, K. & Okamoto, T. 1995. A new measuring method of borehole wall displacements for pressuremeter tests, *Proc. 4th*

Int. Sym. on Pressuremeters: 373-377.

Tani, K. 1997. Triaxial extension tests of cemented soils and soft rocks *Proc. 1st Asian Rock Mechanics Sym.*, (to be published).

Yoshida, Y., Ikemi, M. & Kokusho, K. 1990. Development of self-boring type pressuremeter and proposal of empirical formula to estimate mechanical properties of gravely soil, *CRIEPI Report*, No. U89048 (in Japanese).

Initial stress estimation in rock using ultrasonic

S. Kobayashi & T. Yamaguchi
Department of Global Environment Engineering, Kyoto University, Japan

T. Yoshikawa
Technical Research Center, The Kansai Electric Power Co., Inc., Hyogo, Japan

ABSTRACT: The objective of the present paper is to develop a new method for estimating initial stress state in rock mass by measuring phase velocities of ultrasonic (elastic) waves traveling in a specimen bored and shaped from the rock mass. The test carried out for several rocks as andesite, granite and sandstone revealed that the phase velocities of longitudinal and shear waves traveling in the diametrical direction of a cylindrical specimen subject to uniaxial compressive loading-unloading cycles change considerably at the maximum stress previously experienced mainly due to hysteresis behavior, although the degree of the change varies according to rocks and the stress level of the previous maximum. From this fact, we can estimate the maximum stress experienced in the specimen and thus the initial stress state in the rock mass from which the specimen is bored and shaped.

1 INTRODUCTION

It is widely known that stress-strain relations of rocks are non-linear in general and that they show hysteresis behavior under loading-unloading cycles. The fact implies that the current elastic modulus varies according to the current stress state. On the other hand, we know that the phase velocity of elastic waves, for example longitudinal wave, is proportional to the square root of the elastic modulus divided by the density of the medium.

Therefore, we may expect that the phase velocities of elastic waves traveling in rocks vary as a function of stress. Moreover, the fact that hysteresis behavior is rather dominant in rocks for loading-unloading cycles suggests that the phase velocity may change considerably at the maximum stress ever experienced. Noting this characteristic behavior of elastic waves in rocks, we can expect to estimate the maximum stress ever experienced in the specimen by measuring the changes in phase velocity under monotoniously increasing load. Therefore, we may estimate the stress state in rock mass by measuring the phase velocities of elastic waves in the specimen bored and shaped from it.

In what follows, first we will briefly review the experiment: testing equipment, measuring technique, specimens and test procedure. Then we will discuss the test results and applicability of the method to estimate the maximum stress ever experienced and thus the initial stress state in rock mass.

In this paper we will confine our attention to the test made using ultrasonic longitudinal and shear waves traveling only in the diametrical direction of the cylindrical specimen made of several kinds of rocks, since the phase velocity does not change much in the axial loading direction as experimentally verified by Kobayashi(1995).

2 EXPERIMENT

In order to estimate stress state accurately by experiment, the key is the precise measurement of phase velocities of the elastic waves. We paid a special attention for it, specifically for the time measurement, and carried out the following experiment.

2.1 *Testing equipment*

The block diagram of the experimental system is shown in Figure 1. In order to measure the time precisely, we use a sing-around equipment (Denpa Kogyo Co., UV-2) in which an ultrasonic pulse generator, an auto-gain amplifier and a period measuring apparatus (electronic counter) are installed altogether in one unit. The measuring principle is as follows;

1. Generate a high-voltage (350V) ultrasonic

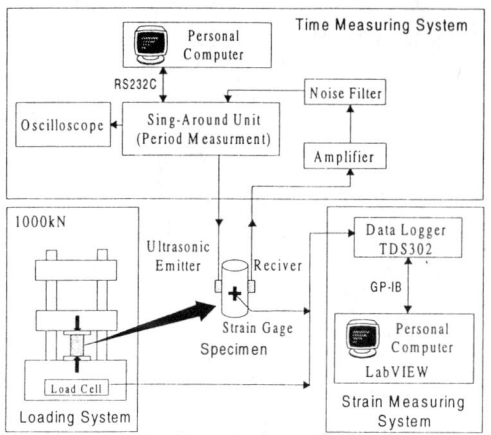

Figure 1. Experimental system.

pulse by the pulse generator and supply it to drive an emitter transducer which generates an elastic (longitudinal or shear) wave and emits it into the specimen. The transducer is made of piezoelectric ceramic (PZT-7) with 10mm circular and 8mm square discs for the longitudinal and shear waves, respectively.

2. The elastic wave traveled across the diameter of the specimen, i.e. perpendicular to the loading direction, is received by a similar transducer and converted to electric voltage signal.

3. The wave signal is supplied and amplified by an auto-gain amplifier in order to keep the amplitude of the wave being constant and to hold the same trigger level.

4. The wave signal is normalized by the auto-gain amplifier and used to trigger to generate the next pulse after a certain delay time elapsed.

5. Repeat this sing-around process, for example, 10,000 times and measure the total time elapsed by the electronic counter and divide it by the number of repeat, say 10,000.

In the sing-around process the time measurement is made by starting at the zero-cross (zero voltage) after the first peak of the first received wave signal (trigger is set at mid-height of the peak) and ending at the same zero-cross of the last wave (after say, 10,000 cycles).

The accuracy of the sing-around period measurement by the system can be expected within 0.2ns by 10,000 times of measurements. The waves are monitored by an oscilloscope, and the gate-width (the gate is used for excluding unfavorable signals) and the trigger level is determined by monitoring. The loads and both axial and circumferential strains are measured during the loading-unloading cycles. All these data are recorded by a data acquisition system controlled by personal computers.

3 SPECIMENS AND MEASUREMENTS

We prepared cylindrical specimens with the diameter 50mm and the height 100mm shaped from blocks of

a) high-strength fine grain andesite from Hakone volcano rim (uniaxial compressive strength σ_c = 214MPa, Young' modulus E=32GPa),

b) two types of biotite granite of fine grain from Oshima (σ_c=121MPa, E=46GPa) and of fine grain from Inada (σ_c=117MPa, E=60Gpa) and

c) two types of sandstone of fine grain from the Tertial sediment at Shirahama (Tanabe) (σ_c=53MPa, E=13GPa) and of medium grain from Izumi (σ_c=186 MPa, E=36GPa), respectively.

These are chosen as typical rocks of volcanic and sedimentary origin. We fixed piezoelectric ceramic devices (elements) on the each side of the diametrical position at the mid-height of the specimen for generating and receiving waves. Piezoelectric ceramic elements of eigenfrequencies of 1MHz and 500kHz are used respectively for the andesite, biotite granite and sandstone specimens. In order to measure the axial and radial strains a cross strain gage is placed on the each side of the diametrical position at the mid-height of the specimen.

In the tests we first initialize the sing-around period and strains both in axial and circumferential directions of the specimen at compressive stress level about 0.5MPa (at nearly zero stress level) and send these data with load (stress) data to the data acquisition system, then we measure these quantities at appropriate stress levels during the several gradually increasing axial compressive (vertical) loading-unloading cycles. All the data of the load, sing-around period and strain are stored in the data acquisition system controlled by personal computers..

4 TEST RESULTS AND DISCUSSIONS

4.1 *Phase velocity*

The tests were carried out for several rocks. In what follows we show some typical results and discuss them.

1. Andesite: Figure 2 shows a typical result of the sing-around period (SAP) of the longitudinal wave

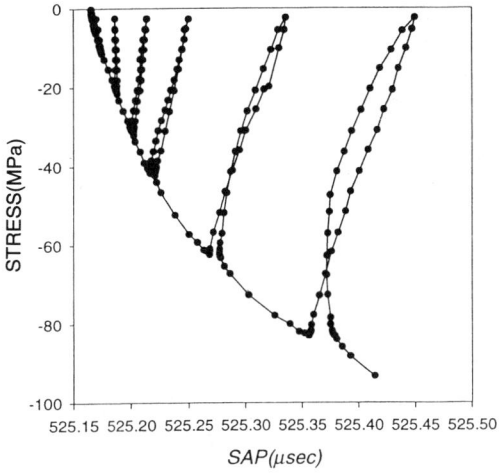

Figure 2. Sing-around period vs. stress in Hakone andesite for longitudinal waves.

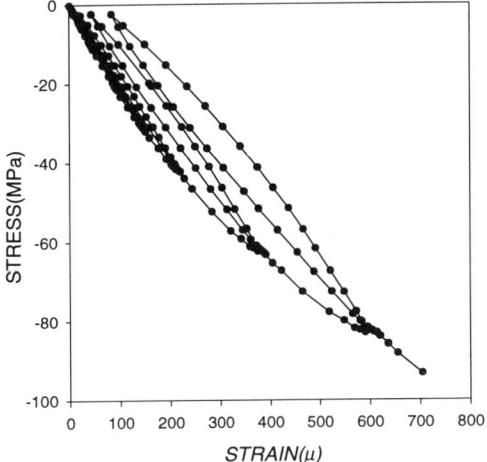

Figure 3. Circumferential strain vs. stress in Hakone andesite for longitudinal wave.

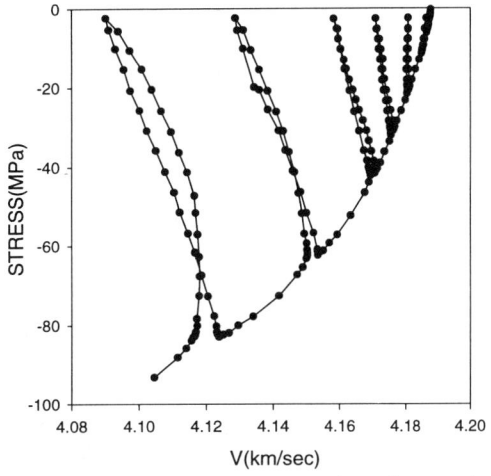

Figure 4. Phase velocity vs. stress in Hakone andesite for longitudinal wave.

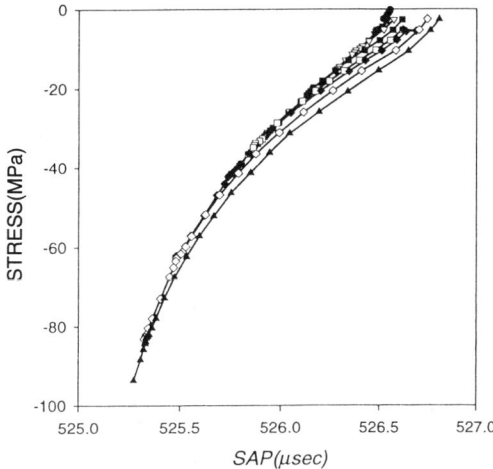

Figure 5. Sing-around period vs. stress in Oshima granite for longitudinal wave.

traveled across the diameter of the specimen versus compressive stress in Hakone andesite specimen. As the compressive stress increases, the sing-around period, *i.e.* the traveling time, increases. The figure also shows dominant hysteresis and that the gradient of the loading curve changes remarkably at the previous maximum stress. The fact suggests that we may estimate the maximum stress existed previously in the specimen by applying the continuously increasing axial compressive load.

Figure 3 shows circumferemtial (radial) strain-stress relation. Although it shows the expansion of the radius of the specimen and hysteresis behavior, we can not observe any remarkable change in the gradient in the loading curves at the previous maximum stress. Therefore, circumferential (radial) strain-stress curve may not be very useful for estimating the maximum stress ever experienced.

The phase velocity versus stress is also shown in Figure 4, which clearly demonstrates the sudden change in the gradient at the previous maximum stress. This figure is quite similar as Figure 2, since the effect of the radial expansion of the specimen is very small (roughly nano-second increase in sing-around period per 100 micro-strains). Figure 4 is also useful as Figure 2 for estimating the maximum stress ever experienced. However, Figure 2 may be more preferable, because the direct readings of the measurements can be plotted in the figure.

2. Granite: Figure 5 shows a typical result of the sing-around period of the longitudinal wave versus compressive stress in Oshima granite specimen. As the curves corresponding to cyclic loadings overlapped, only curves under loading are shown in the figure. A part of the figure for lower stress is expanded and shown in Figure 6. It shows some change in the gradient of the curve near the previous maximum, although it is not so clear as that in the andesite specimen. Anyway we may estimate the previous maximum stress in the specimen by carefully applying the increasing compressive load.

Figure 7 shows the similar results in Inada granite specimen, which may also indicates, but not very clearly, the previous maximum stress existed in the specimen.

Figure 8 shows the sing-around period of the horizontally polarized shear wave versus compressive stress in Inada granite subject to the vertical loading-

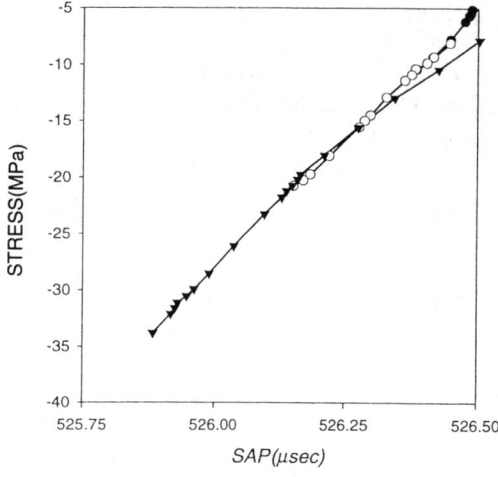

Figure 6. Sing-around period vs. stress in Oshima granite in lower stress level for longitudinal wave.

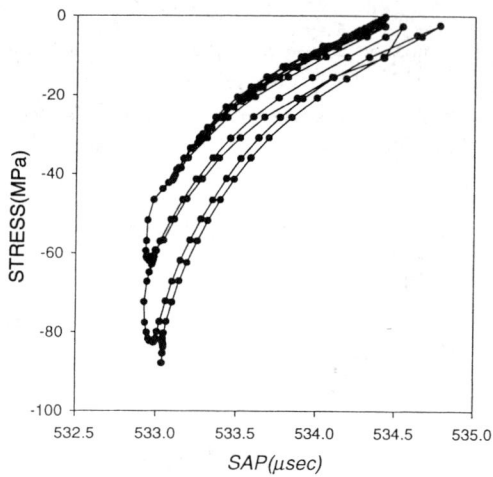

Figure 8. Sing-around period vs. stress in Inada granite for horizontally polarized shear wave.

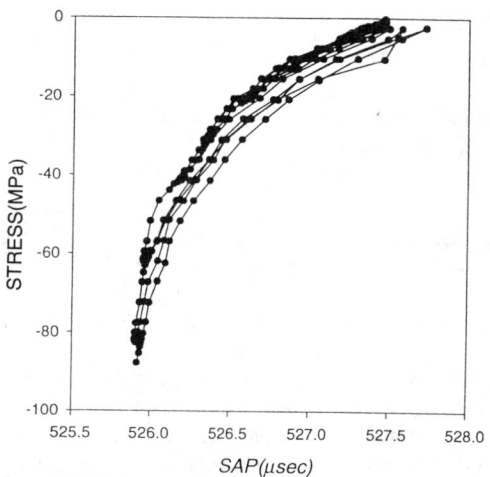

Figure 7. Sing-around period vs. stress in Inada granite for longitudinal wave.

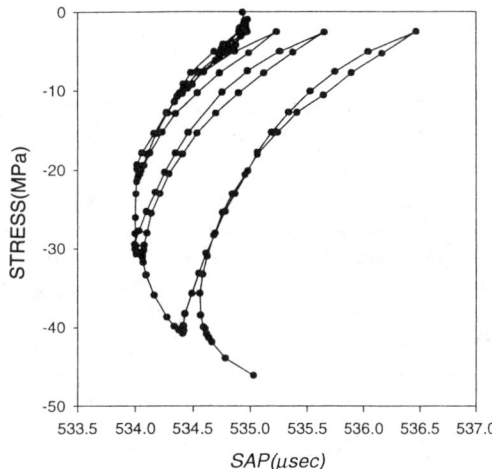

Figure 9. Sing-around period vs. stress in Shirahama sandstone for longitudinal wave.

unloading cycles. This figure shows slightly more distinguishable hysteresis behavior than that due to the longitudinal wave.

3. Sandstone: Typical results of the sing-around period of the longitudinal wave versus stress in the Shirahama and Izumi sandstones are shown respectively in Figures 9 and 10. We may be able to estimate the previously experienced maximum stress rather easily in lower stress level, but not in higher stress level. However, when we use the horizontally polarized shear wave instead of the longitudinal wave as shown in Figure 11 for Izumi sandstone, we can more

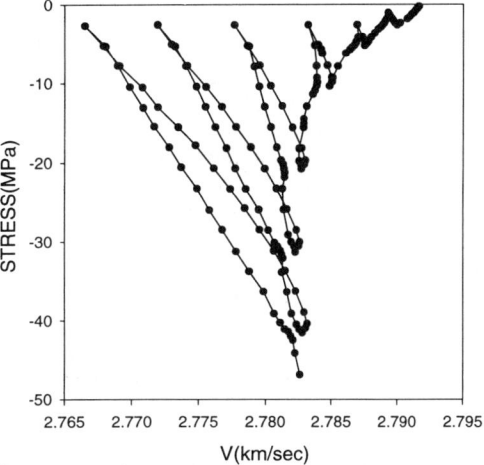

Figure 12. Phase velocity vs. stress in Izumi sandstone for horizontally polarized shear wave.

easily estimate the previous maximum stress. Figure 12 shows the same results for phase velocity vs. stress, which also serves to estimate the maximum stress experienced previously. However, Figure 11 may be preferable to Figure 12, because the former is obtained by the direct readings of the period measurement when the sing-around apparatus is used.

In general, velocity change in the shear wave due to stress variation is more sensitive than that in the longitudinal wave and thus the use of the shear wave is more preferable for the purpose of estimating the previous maximum stress.

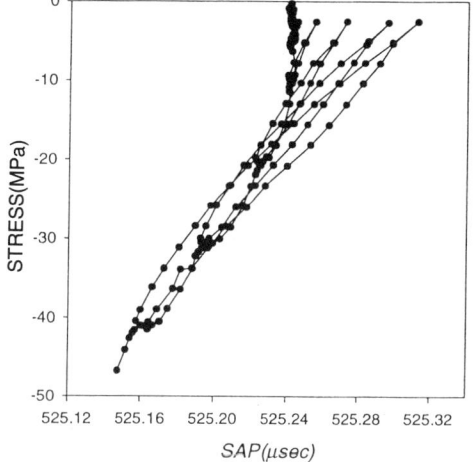

Figure 10. Sing-around period vs. stress in Izumi sandstone for longitudinal wave.

5 CONCLUDING REMARKS

Although more intensive investigation in details may be required for estimating the initial stress state using elastic waves, it my be concluded the following from the present preliminary test:

1. We can use the sing-around period measuring equipment for the accurate time measurement. The accuracy of the time measurement using the sing-around equipment is 0.2ns by 10,000 times of measurements.

2. Phase velocities of longitudinal and shear waves traveling in the diametrical direction of the specimen subject to the uniaxial compressive loading-unloading cycles change remarkably at the maximum stress ever experienced, although the velocity change depends on the stress level of the previous maximum and the kind of rocks.

3. The phase velocity change due to stress varia-

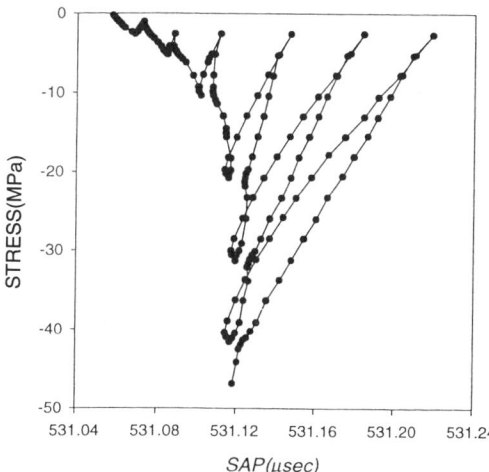

Figure 11. Sing-around period vs. stress in Izumi sandstone for horizontally polarized shear wave.

tion is more clearly observed in general in the horizontally polarized shear wave than that in the longitudinal wave.

4. From the fact that the phase velocity traveling in the direction perpendicular to the loading direction changes remarkably at the previous maximum stress level, we may be able to estimate the maximum stress ever experienced in the rock specimen by measuring the phase velocity under the uniaxial continuously increasing compressive load.

5. The change of the phase velocity at the previous maximum stress is more dominant in horizontally polarized shear wave than that in the longitudinal wave. Therefore, the use of shear wave may be preferable for the purpose of estimating the maximum stress ever experienced.

6. The lower limits of estimating the maximum stress ever experienced may be about 5MPa, 7-8Mpa and 2.5MPa, respectively, for the andesite, granite and sandstone. We can reasonably expect to lower the limit, although more accurate and careful experiment is required.

We have developed a new technique for estimating the maximum stress ever experienced in a rock specimen. It is directly applicable for estimating initial stresses in rock mass by using specimens shaped from the bored core taken out from the rock mass, specifically in the deep level. This method can be used in combination with the method using the Kaiser effect in acoustic-emission technique. The proposed method may provide another candidate for estimating the initial stresses in rock.

AKNOWLEDGMENT

The authors express their gratitude to Messrs. S. Nakao and K. Ueno for their assistance in the experiment. The research was partly supported by Grant-in-Aid for Scientific Research, The Ministry of Education, Japan.

REFERENCES

Kobayashi, S. 1995. Stress Measurement in Rock using Ultrasonic. In C.-P.Hu, T.T.Wu & J.-L.Horng (eds), *Proceedings of the Eighth Asia-Pacific Conference on Nondestructive Testing (8th PCNDT)*, 275-280, Taipei, Taiwan.

Residual stress in rock core samples and stress state at great depths

T. Ito, K. Watanabe & K. Hayashi
Institute of Fluid Science, Tohoku University, Japan

ABSTACT: A new type of core-based methods is proposed to estimate the stress state at great depths. The method is based on a hypothesis on the stress in the core sample: when the core sample is under the same stress conditions as it was when under the in-situ stress, the direction of the principal stress is aligned in the same direction at all points within the core sample. Thus, the magnitudes of the in-situ stresses can be evaluated as those of the applied stresses in a laboratory experiment at which the uniformity of stress distribution in the core sample is maximized.

1 INTRODUCTION

Knowledge of the state of stress at great depths in the lithosphere is an important constraint on our understanding of the forces both driving and resisting plate motions, the mechanics of seismic and aseismic faulting, and the rheology of the crust and upper mantle. The hydraulic fracturing method and the over coring method are widely used for stress measurements. However, the former method costs a great deal and the latter one is not appropriate basically to be applied to great depths.

The core-based method has been proposed in an attempt to develop an inexpensive and simple method for measuring the stress state at great depths. There are several types of the method which are based on different principles, e.g., the Anelastic Strain Recovery method (Teufel 1981, Matsuki & Takeuchi 1993), the Differential Strain Curve Analysis (Simmons et al. 1974), the Deformation Rate Analysis (Yamamoto et al. 1995) and the Acoustic Emission method (Shin & Kanagawa 1995). The ASR method is available for the case that the rock is "soft" in the engineering sense as the anelastic strain recovery is easily seen after retrieving from depths and is considered to be reliable. However, the other methods are still under development, and the core-based method which is appropriate for a "hard" rock such as granite remains unclear.

From these circumstances, we will present a core-based method which is appropriate for the "hard" rock. The method is originated from a principle different from those of the above mentioned methods. The new concept and the results of numerical simulation conducted for verification of it will be shown.

2 NEW CONCEPT

2.1 *Residual stress*

Rock at depths have been subjected to in-situ stress for a long time in a geological scale. Accordingly to the stress, the structure in the rock is deformed as to be stabilized. If core drilling is conducted and the rock is unloaded by coring, a residual stress is induced in the core sample, where the residual stress is defined as the stress at a point in a body subjected to zero external loads and zero temperature gradient (Holzhausen & Johnson 1979). The residual stress is considered to be non-uniform in the core sample, because the rock is composed of several materials with different elastic constants.

The residual stress in the core sample may be expressed analytically as follows. At first, the following assumptions are made.
(a) The individual grains that comprise the core sample are fitted together perfectly without a space such as a crack.
(b) This condition is held independently of stress relief due to coring.
(c) The stress relief occurs immediately at the coring in the manner of the linear theory of elasticity.
(d) Effect of the thermal stress can be ignored.

Then, we have

$$\Delta\sigma_{ij} = \sum_{m,n=1}^{3} k_{ij}^{(mn)} \Delta S_{mn} \quad (1)$$

where $\Delta\sigma_{ij}$ ($i,j=1,2,3$) is the change of the stress component in the core sample, σ_{ij} ($i,j=1,2,3$), referred to the rectangular coordinate system x_i ($i=1,2,3$), ΔS_{ij} ($i,j=1,2,3$) is the change of the stress externally applied on the surface of the core sample, S_{ij} ($i,j=1,2,3$), and

$$k_{ij}^{(mn)} = \partial\sigma_{ij}/\partial S_{mn} \quad (2)$$

The compressive stress is taken to be positive in this paper. When the stress in the core sample is relived due to coring and retrieving from depths, the stress S_{ij} is changed from the in-situ stress S_{ij}^{*} ($i,j=1,2,3$) to zero, i.e., $\Delta S_{ij} = -S_{ij}^{*}$. Here we shall introduce a hypothesis on the stress in the core sample following Yamamoto et al. (1995) : when the core sample is under the in-situ stress S_{ij}^{*} ($i,j=1,2,3$), the stress state is uniform at all points within the core sample, i.e., $\sigma_{ij} = S_{ij}^{*}$. Thus, the residual stress $\sigma_{ij}^{(0)}$ ($i,j=1,2,3$), i.e., the stress in the core sample after retrieving from depths, is given by

$$\sigma_{ij}^{(0)} = S_{ij}^{*} - \sum_{m,n=1}^{3} k_{ij}^{(mn)} S_{mn}^{*} \quad (3)$$

The coefficient $k_{ij}^{(mn)}$ is a function of elastic constants and arrangement of mineral grains composing the core sample. In general, the elastic constants are different for each material of the mineral grains and the arrangement is irregular, therefore, the coefficient $k_{ij}^{(mn)}$ may take different values at each point in the core sample. Hence, the residual stress $\sigma_{ij}^{(0)}$ may be non-uniform in the core sample.

2.2 A new method for estimating in-situ stress

On the other hand, when the external stress S_{ij} is applied artificially on the core sample after retrieving from depths, the stress in the core sample is given by

$$\sigma_{ij} = \sigma_{ij}^{(0)} + \sum_{m,n=1}^{3} k_{ij}^{(mn)} S_{mn} \quad (4)$$

If S_{ij} is equal to S_{ij}^{*}, then σ_{ij} becomes equal to S_{ij}^{*}. Such a relationship is held independently of the position in the core sample. This result suggests that the magnitudes of the in-situ stresses S_{ij}^{*} may be evaluated as those of the applied stresses S_{ij} in a laboratory experiment at which the stresses σ_{ij} are uniform in the core sample.

Now let us consider an algorithm to estimate S_{ij}^{*}, i.e., the magnitudes of the applied stresses S_{ij} which satisfy the condition of the uniformity of σ_{ij}. However, the consideration is limited for the case of 2D stress state in this paper. At first, the condition of the uniformity of σ_{ij} is simplified as a condition that the direction of the principal stress is aligned in the same direction at several points on the surface of the core sample. The angle between the direction of the principal stress and x_1 axis, θ, is given by

$$\tan 2\theta = 2\eta \quad (5)$$

where

$$\eta = \sigma_{12}/(\sigma_{11} - \sigma_{22}) \quad (6)$$

Substituting Eq.(4) into Eq.(6) yields

$$\left\{\eta\left(k_{11}^{(11)} - k_{22}^{(11)}\right) - k_{12}^{(11)}\right\} S_{11}$$
$$+ \left\{\eta\left(k_{11}^{(22)} - k_{22}^{(22)}\right) - k_{12}^{(22)}\right\} S_{22}$$
$$+ \left\{\eta\left(k_{11}^{(12)} - k_{22}^{(12)}\right) - k_{12}^{(12)}\right\} S_{12}$$
$$= \sigma_{12}^{(0)} - \eta\left(\sigma_{11}^{(0)} - \sigma_{22}^{(0)}\right) \quad (7)$$

The $\sigma_{ij}^{(0)}$ and $k_{ij}^{(mn)}$ take different values at different points on the core sample, therefore, we have Eq.(7) independently for each point on the core sample. We can measure $\sigma_{ij}^{(0)}$ and $k_{ij}^{(mn)}$, if we apply the X-ray method (Friedman 1972) for instance. Let N be the total number of the points on the core sample at which $\sigma_{ij}^{(0)}$ and $k_{ij}^{(mn)}$ are measured, then we have N equations for four unknown quantities, i.e., S_{11}, S_{22}, S_{12} and η. Thus, the four unknown quantities are determined as the solution which optimally satisfies the N equations, where N is taken as equal to or larger than four. Finally S_{ij}^{*} and η^{*} can be obtained as the solutions of S_{ij} and η, where η^{*} is η in the case of $\sigma_{ij} = S_{ij}^{*}$. The point at which we have Eq.(7) is hereafter referred as the reference point of stress.

3 NUMERICAL EXPERIMENT

3.1 Model

In order to verify the present method, the residual stress $\sigma_{ij}^{(0)}$ and the coefficient $k_{ij}^{(mn)}$ were estimated for a 2D numerical model of the core sample by using FEM. The present method was applied to these results, and the estimated values of the in-situ

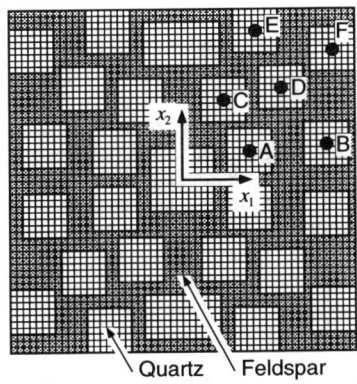

Figure 1. A numerical model of rock sample.

Table 1. The coefficient $k_{ij}^{(mn)}$ for the point A in the rock sample with the content of quartz 50 %.

$k_{11}^{(11)}$	0.9376	$k_{11}^{(22)}$	-0.04142	$k_{11}^{(12)}$	-0.06112		
$k_{22}^{(11)}$	-0.01789	$k_{22}^{(22)}$	0.8626	$k_{22}^{(12)}$	0.02350		
$k_{12}^{(11)}$	-0.02976	$k_{12}^{(22)}$	0.01611	$k_{12}^{(12)}$	0.8632		

Table 2. The residual stress $\sigma_{ij}^{(0)}$ in the rock sample with the content of quartz 50 %.

Location	Residual stress, MPa					
A	$\sigma_{11}^{(0)}$	14.56	$\sigma_{22}^{(0)}$	17.41	$\sigma_{12}^{(0)}$	5.241
B	$\sigma_{11}^{(0)}$	17.73	$\sigma_{22}^{(0)}$	15.45	$\sigma_{12}^{(0)}$	3.392
C	$\sigma_{11}^{(0)}$	15.90	$\sigma_{22}^{(0)}$	15.85	$\sigma_{12}^{(0)}$	3.932
D	$\sigma_{11}^{(0)}$	19.08	$\sigma_{22}^{(0)}$	15.42	$\sigma_{12}^{(0)}$	8.352
E	$\sigma_{11}^{(0)}$	22.88	$\sigma_{22}^{(0)}$	16.40	$\sigma_{12}^{(0)}$	8.925
F	$\sigma_{11}^{(0)}$	20.00	$\sigma_{22}^{(0)}$	15.11	$\sigma_{12}^{(0)}$	5.565

stresses were compared with the given stresses for several cases.

Granite is considered here and is assumed to be composed of quartz and feldspar. Young's moduli for quartz and feldspar are assumed to be 50 GPa and 80 GPa respectively, and Poisson's ratio for both materials is assumed to be 0.2 (Lama & Vutukuri 1978). Taking into account the fact that the content of quartz variates in a range of 10 - 50 % depending on fields, we suppose three types of granite which are composed of quartz 10 %, 25 % and 50 % respectively. The present method described above for estimating the in-situ stresses is independent of the shape of the rock sample in principle. Hence, the shape of the rock sample retrieving from depths is assumed to be square in order for ease of analysis. The FEM model of the rock sample for the case of quartz 50 % is shown in Figure 1, where the white and gray parts correspond to quartz and feldspar respectively. Quartz grain is assumed to be also squre shape. The quartz grain is distributed uniformly keeping its center coincident with each other for the three types of granite with different contents of quartz. The coordinate system x_i ($i=1,2$) is taken as shown in Figure 1.

3.2 Results

Under the above mentioned conditions, the coefficients $k_{ij}^{(mn)}$ at the reference point of stress were evaluated, e.g., the magnitude of $k_{11}^{(11)}$ is obtained as that of σ_{11} at the point obtained by FEM for the case when $S_{11}=1$, $S_{22}=S_{12}=0$ are applied on the boundary of the model (e.g., Figure 1). The six points denoted as A - F in Figure 1 are taken at the center of quartz grain as the reference point of stress in this paper, although the reference point of stress can be selected anywhere in the present method. The coefficient $k_{ij}^{(mn)}$ of the point A are shown in Table 1 for instance. Table 2 shows the residual stresses $\sigma_{ij}^{(0)}$ obtained by Eq.(3) for the case that the content

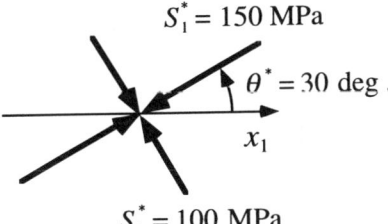

Figure 2. Assumed state of in-situ stress.

of quartz is 50 % and the state of the in-situ stress is assumed as shown in Figure 2, where S_i^* ($i=1,2$; $S_1^* \geq S_2^*$) are the in-situ principal stresses and θ^* is the angle between S_1^* and x_1 axes. The stress state shown in Figure 2 is also expressed as $S_{11}^*=137.5$ MPa, $S_{22}^*=112.5$ MPa and $S_{12}^*=21.65$ MPa. As can be seen from Table 2, the average values of $\sigma_{ij}^{(0)}$ is about 10 % of that of S_i^* in this case.

From the values of $k_{ij}^{(mn)}$ and $\sigma_{ij}^{(0)}$ for the six points A - F summarized in Tables 1 and 2, we have six equations of Eq.(7). Thus, we estimated the in-situ stresses as the optimum solutions which satisfy those equations. The solutions are $S_1^*=150.0$ MPa, $S_2^*=100.0$, MPa and $\theta^*=30.00$ deg, however, the values of $k_{ij}^{(mn)}$ and $\sigma_{ij}^{(0)}$ in the 5 significant digits were used. The estimated values of the in-situ stress are perfectly coincident with the actual ones (Figure 2) in this case.

Next we examined the effect of the number of the reference point of stress, N, and the number of the significant digit of the values of $k_{ij}^{(mn)}$ and $\sigma_{ij}^{(0)}$, M, on the accuracy of the estimated state of the in-situ stress. Thus, the in-situ stresses were estimated for the cases defined by each combination of $N=4, 5, 6$ and $M=2, 3, 4$ and compared with the actual in-situ stresses. The results for the case of $M=2$ are summarized in Figure 3 (a). In this figure, "(yy p)" and "yyy %" correspond to the cases of $N=$yy and the content of quartz yyy % respectively, and the vertical axis is the error in the estimated values of the in-situ principal stresses which is defined as [the difference between the estimated and actual values] / [the actual value]. The results for the cases of $M=3$ and 4 are also summarized in Figures 3(b) and (c).

From these results (Figures 3(a) - (c)), we can understood that the error decreases with increasing N, M and the content of quartz, and that the in-situ stresses can be estimated accurately, if $N>4$ and $M>2$. Even if $M=2$, the in-situ stresses can be estimated within the error of 25 % for the magnitude and the error of $\pi / 12$ for the direction.

4 CONCLUSION

We have theoretically examined a physical background behind a residual stress in a core sample, i.e., the stress in the core sample after retrieving from depths. From this result, we have proposed a core-based method for estimating in-situ stress. In this method, state of the in-situ stress is estimated from stress states at the several points on the core sample which is subjected to artificial external loads. Finally, the present method was verified through numerical experiments using a 2D FEM model of the core sample.

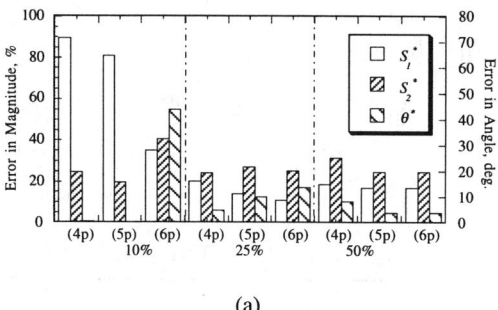

(a)

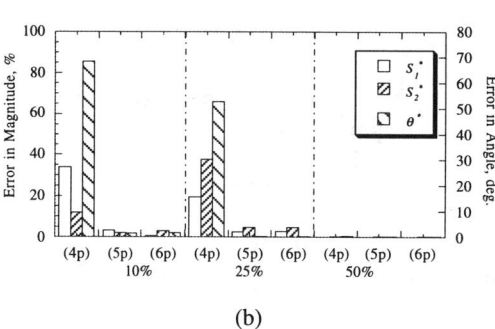

(b)

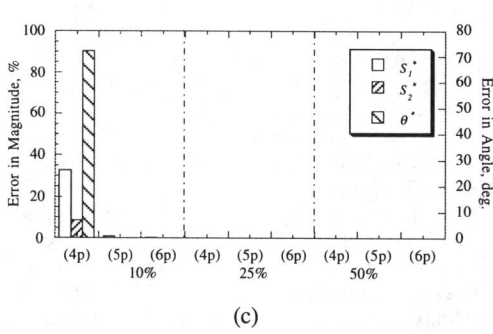

(c)

Figure 3. Effect of the values of N and M on the estimated state of the in-situ principal stresses; (a) $M=2$, (b) $M=3$, (c) $M=4$.

REFERENCES

Friedman, M. 1972. Residual elastic strain in rocks. *Tectonophysics*. 15: 297-330.

Holzhausen, G.R. & A.M. Johnson 1979. The concept of residual stress in rock. *Tectonophysics*, 58: 237-267.

Lama, R.D. & V.S. Vutukuri 1978. *Handbook of Mechanical Properties of Rock - Testing Techniques and Results*, II: Trans Tech Pub..

Matsuki, K. & K. Takeuchi 1993. Three dimensional in-situ stress determination by anelastic strain recovery of a rock core. *Int. J. Rock Mech. Mins. Sci. & Geomech. Abstr.*, 30: 1019-1022.

Shin, K. & T. Kanagawa 1995. Kaiser effect of rock in acousto-elasticity, AE & DR. *in AE/MS in Geological Structures and Materials*. H.R. Hardy, Jr. (ed.): 197-204: Trans Tech Pub.

Simmons, G., R.W. Siegfried & M.L. Feves 1974. Differential strain analysis: A new method for examining cracks in rocks. *J. Geophys. Res.*, 79: 4383-4385.

Teufel, L.W. 1981. Strain relaxation method for predicting hydraulic fracture azimuth from oriented core. Presented at *SPE/DOE Symposium on Low Permeability Rock* SPE/DOE Paper 9836.

Yamamoto, K.1995. The rock properties of in-situ stress memory: Discussion on its mechanism. *Proc. of Int. Wkshp on Rock Stress Meas. at Great Depth*, Tokyo: 46-51.

Estimation of stress state in the deep portion of the Osaka plane

Y. Fujiwara & M. Horie
The Kansai Electric Power Co., Inc., Osaka, Japan

Y. Ito & Y. Hirakawa
NEWJEC Inc., Osaka, Japan

Z. Xue
Kiso-Jiban Consultants Co., Ltd, Nara, Japan

K. Sugawara
Kumamoto University, Japan

ABSTRACT: The DSCA (Differential Strain Curve Analysis) method is applied to estimate the stress state in the deep portion of the Osaka plane, Japan. The principle and practice of the DSCA method are briefly presented and discussed, as well as the reliability analysis using the P-wave velocity of cores which depends on pressure. Subsequently, the increases of in situ horizontal stresses with the depth and the stress jumps of the horizontal stresses in the deep portion of the Osaka plane due to changes in rock stiffness are discussed by comparing the DSCA data at the depth of 1640m to the hydraulic fracturing data at the depth ranging from 70m to 1240m.

1. INTRODUCTION

It is very important to estimate the in situ stress state for designing underground structures, such as an underground powerhouse cavern. Generally, the overcoring method utilizing a borehole drilled from a test adit has been applied to the estimation in Japan. However, if the in situ stress state can be estimated with high accuracy by a method utilizing a drill core, the cost and time for the estimation will be saved. Moreover, for the estimation, it will be able to use a drill core collected from a vertical borehole for geological survey drilled from the ground surface.

Hereafter, the results of the estimation of the in situ stress state using a drill core collected from a deep and vertical borehole at the Osaka plane are described.

The Osaka plane is located in the inner zone on the Central Japan, and the near-surface in situ stress measurements in this zone have been complied by Tanaka (1992). Figure 1 shows the in situ horizontal stresses measured and the standard stress gradients with the depth set out by Tanaka, basing on the in situ stress measurements at less than 600m from the surface. After the Great Hanshin Earthquake occurred in the early morning of 17th January 1995, several borehole survey projects are carried out in the Osaka area as shown in Figure 2, to investigate the geological structures and the in situ stress state in the deep portion. In situ stress measurements associated with these projects can be found in Sato (1997), Ito et al. (1996), Ikeda et al.(1997), among many others.

In the present paper, the differential strain curve analysis (DSCA) method, Strickland & Ren (1980), is applied as well as the P-wave velocity analysis to estimate the in situ stresses in the deep portion of the Osaka plane. The drill core was collected at 1640m depth from the surface in summer 1996.

Subsequently, by compiling the results of in situ stress measurement by means of the hydraulic fracturing methods and comparing them to the stress estimation by the DSCA method, the stress jumps characteristics of the horizontal stresses due to changes in rock stiffness will be discussed.

2. STRESS ESTIMATION BY DSCA

The DSCA method is based on the concept that careful monitoring of the strain behavior of a rock

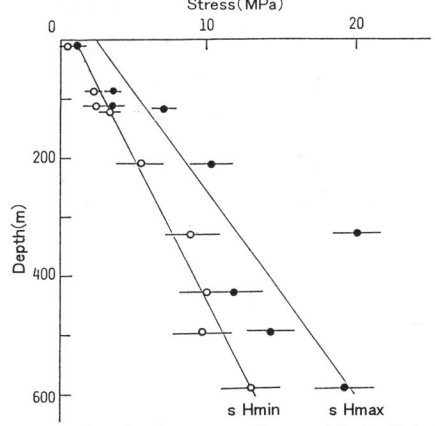

Figure 1   Standard stress gradients with depth in inner zone of central Japan (Tanaka, 1992).

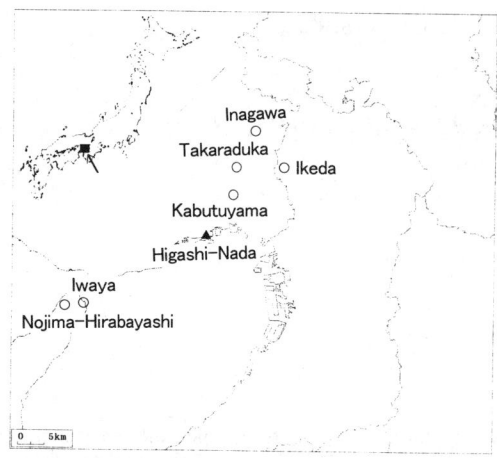

Figure 2   Location of Higashi-Nada.

specimen upon reloading can reflect its past stress history. Generally, it consists of applying a hydrostatic pressure to a cubic sample cut from an oriented drill core, following its removal from the ground. Microcracks which developed during drill core removal and its expansion are closed under pressure. The response of the cubic sample to hydrostatic loading is monitored using strain gauges previously attached to its surface, as shown in Figure 3. Using an 18 strain gauges, the principal strains due to microcrack closure and their orientation can be determined. The principal directions of the in situ stress field and ratios between the three principal in situ stresses can be determined assuming (1) that most of the microcracks in the core samples are due to the relief of the current in situ stress field, (2) that the in situ stress tensor has the same orientation as the strain tensor due to crack closure, (3) that the cracks are proportional volumetrically to the in situ stress magnitude in any direction, and (4) that under hydrostatic loading, contraction of the rock in any specific direction is analogous to the original strain in that direction. Specific stress values can be assigned, in the present paper, by assuming that the vertical stress coincides with the weight of the overlying rock.

Rock samples for the present DSCA experiment have been collected from a deep borehole at Higashi-Nada of Kobe city, of which the location is represented by a black triangle in Figure 2. They are non-oriented core samples of granodiorite. Geology is as follows. In the upper part down to 1550m in depth, geology consists of sand and marine clay, and those soft strata are overlying on a rigid basis which consists of fine granodiorite. Cubical rock samples for the DSCA experiment are cut from a continuous core of granodiorite, 20cm long, collected at 1640m from the surface, within the basis.

Four samples have been tested, which are hereafter called A, B, C and D. They have 37mm on a side respectively, and three strain gauges of 10mm in length are glued on each face, as shown in Figure 3. The number of gauges employed for each sample is 18 in total. The Z-axis coincides with the vertical boring axis, but the orientations of the X- and Y-axes are unknown, since the samples are non-oriented as described previously. The entire assembly covered by a flexible silicon rubber has been placed in a pressure vessel together with a sample of fused quartz, prior to the hydrostatic loading up to 150MPa. Loading has been carried out with steps of 1MPa from 1MPa to 10MPa, 2.5MPa from 10MPa to 40MPa, and 5MPa from 40MPa to 150MPa.

Pressure versus principal strain curves are demonstrated in Figure 4, and the principal strain ratios and the principal stresses determined are summarized in Table 1. The orientation of the principal stress is shown in Figure 5, that is an upper hemisphere stereonet. For the present strain tensor analysis, the gap method proposed by Dey & Brown (1986) has successfully been applied, as well as the optimizing procedure for pressure-strain relationships proposed by Noro (1989), and the results in Table 1 have been calculated from the strains at the pressure of approximately 10MPa. The vertical stress, which is assumed from the weight of the overburden, is 33MPa.

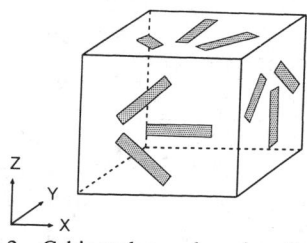

Figure 3   Cubic rock sample and configuration of strain gauges for DSCA.

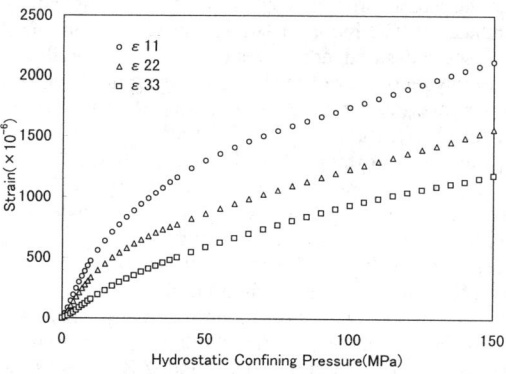

Figure 4   Example of pressure versus strain curve.

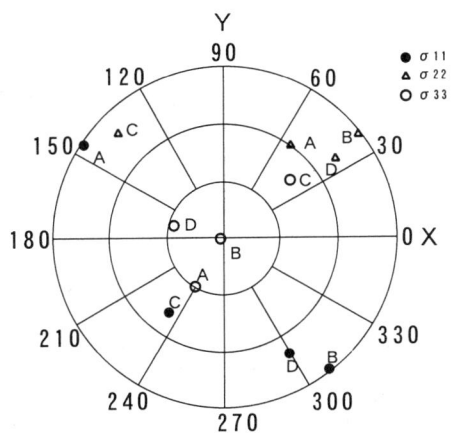

Figure 5   Orientation of principal stresses by DSCA.
(upper hemisphere stereonet)

Table 1   In situ stress state estimated by DSCA

Sample	s1 : s2 : s3	s1	s2	s3	sHmax	sHmin
A	1 : 0.72 : 0.34	77	55	26	76	48
B	1 : 0.49 : 0.41	80	39	33	80	39
C	1 : 0.45 : 0.38	46	21	17	31	21
D	1 : 0.42 : 0.21	103	43	22	94	41

(Stresses in MPa, The vertical stress is 33MPa)

It is noteworthy that the principal stress ratios are almost similar to each other. However, the magnitude and orientations of the principal stresses estimated from Sample C are obviously different from the others, respectively. Then it can be concluded that the results of Samples A, B and D are significant to estimate the in situ stress field. The maximum horizontal stress sHmax is considered to be about 2.5 times greater than the overburden pressure, and the minimum horizontal stress sHmin is nearly equal to the overburden pressure. This stress state is equivalent to a stress mode which results in a reverse faulting as the mechanism of the Great Hanshin Earthquake. These results will be compared to the stress measurement at a shallow depth by means of the hydraulic fracturing method.

3. P-WAVE VELOCITY ANALYSIS

The concept of DSCA suggests that the pressure dependent characteristics of the P-wave velocity of rock also present a valuable information to determine the in situ stress field at great depths. Since the microcracks closure due to the hydrostatic loading to a rock sample results in the increase of the P-wave velocity, it is expected that the P-wave velocity increases with increasing of pressure, and

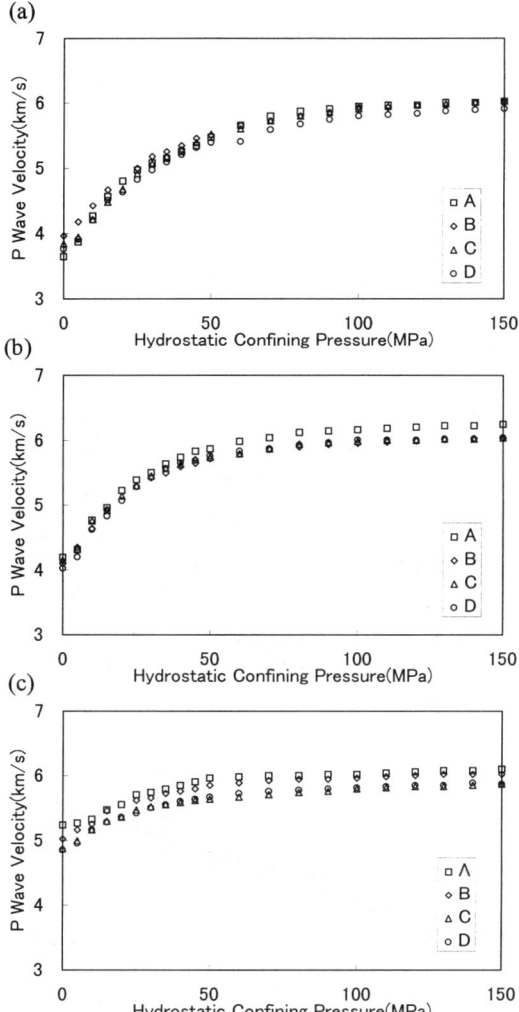

Figure 6   P-wave velocity versus pressure curves,
(a)X-direction; (b)Y-direction; (c)Z-direction.

consequently it reaches to an original constant value of rock.

The changes of the P-wave velocity due to the hydrostatic loading are demonstrated in Figure 6. These have simultaneously been measured with the DSCA experiment within a pressure vessel. The terminal velocity is clearly read as about 6km/s, and the velocity increases monotonously with increasing of pressure. At the commencement stage of hydrostatic loading, the P-wave velocity in Z-direction is greater than those of X- and Y-directions. This suggests that the horizontal in situ stresses are greater than the vertical in situ stress.

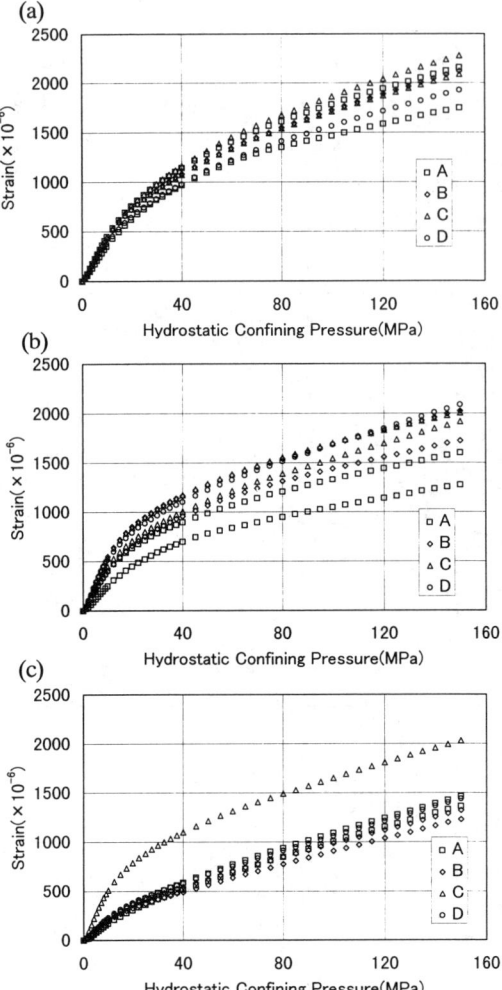

Figure 7 Strain versus pressure curves,
(a) X-direction; (b) Y-direction; (c) Z-direction.

Comparing the P-wave velocity versus pressure curves in Figure 6 to the strain versus pressure curves in Figure 7, it is noteworthy that the amount of scattering of velocity is much smaller. This suggests that the careful measurement of the P-wave velocity using a core collected from great depths can present directly the data to determine the orientation of the maximum horizontal in situ stress. The measurement in the atmosphere is considered to be sufficient in determining the orientation, but the measurements in many directions will be required to assess the distribution of the P-wave velocity in the horizontal plane.

4. DISCUSSION

In order to discuss the in situ stress field in the deep portion of the Osaka plane, the results of the DSCA experiments and the P-wave velocity analysis are compared to the in situ stress measurements performed by means of the hydraulic fracturing method. The data plotted in Figure 8, at the depth ranging from 70m to 1250m, are the maximum and minimum horizontal in-situ stresses measured using the hydraulic fracturing method in Osaka area after the Great Hanshin Earthquake. The solid lines in the figure correspond with the standard horizontal stresses set out by Tanaka (1992), and the broken lines represent the vertical stress calculated from the weight of overlying rock. The stresses previously estimated by means of the DSCA experiments on Samples A, B and D at the Higashi-Nada site are plotted by solid circles in the figure, respectively.

Most of plots locate near the standard horizontal stress lines. However, the in situ stresses measured at the Inagawa site at the depth of 950m and at the Nojima-Hirabayashi site at the depth of 850m are larger than the standard horizontal stresses, respectively. At Inagawa site, earthquake swarms have been observed at the depth of 1km to 5km from the surface in 1995, having a magnitude of 0 to 3. At the Nojima-Hirabayashi site, a fault is found at 1000m from the surface.

At the Higashi-Nada site, the maximum horizontal stress is estimated to be approximately 1.7 times greater than the standard stress set out by Tanaka(1992). Such a clear discrepancy of the maximum horizontal in situ stress from the standard, which is set out from the near-surface measurements, suggests that there is a stress jump in the deeper area. It is considered to be mainly due to changes in rock mass stiffness. The horizontal stress in the Osaka plane can vary from one layer to the next in stratified rock formations, which is common in sedimentary as well as volcanic rock masses, due to changes in rock stiffness. And the magnitude of the in situ stress can increase with increasing of the depth. Moreover, it can be pointed out that the in situ stress state in the deep portion of the Osaka plane is equivalent to a stress mode which results in a reverse faulting, since the horizontal stress is greater than the vertical stress, described previously.

5. CONCLUDING REMARKS

The in situ stress state was estimated by DSCA method utilizing a drill core collected in a rigid basis consists of fine granodiorite at the depth of 1640m in the Osaka plane. The estimated in situ stress state was equivalent to a stress mode in a reverse faulting, and the maximum horizontal stress was approximately 1.7

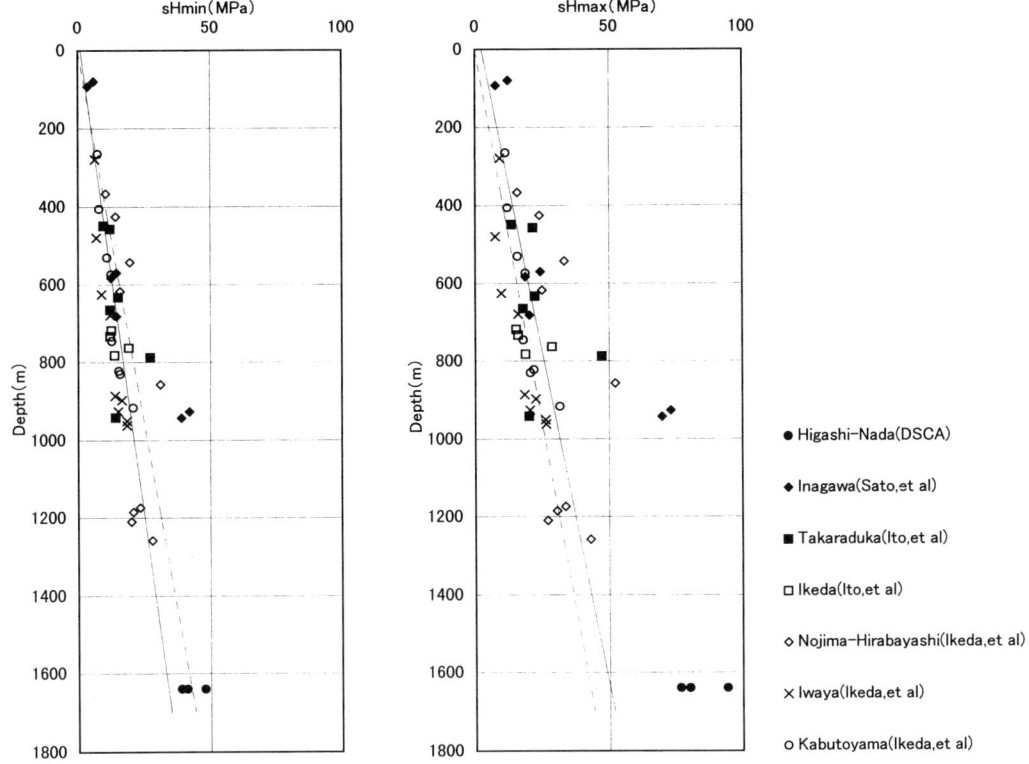

Figure 8   Horizontal in-situ stresses measured in the Osaka plane.

times greater than the stress estimated by the standard maximum horizontal stress gradients. Considering that the rock formation is covered with the sedimentary of approximately 1550m thick, it is supposed that the changes of stiffness of geological formation in the vertical direction cause a stress jump in the deeper area. Therefore, it is considered that the horizontal stress gradients depend on the changes of stiffness of formation in the vertical direction as well as the depth.

Moreover, it is suggested that careful measurement of P-wave velocity in horizontal plane for a drill core under the atmosphere is sufficient to determine the orientation of the maximum horizontal stress.

REFERENCES

Dey, T.N. & D.W. Brown 1986. Stress measurements in a deep granitic rock mass using hydraulic fracturing and differential strain curve analysis. *Proc. Int. Symp. on Rock Stress and Rock Stress Measurements*, Stockholm, pp.351-357.

Ikeda,R.,Y,Iio and K.Omura 1997. Stress state of the Arima-Takatsuki-Rokko fault zone. Japan Earth and Planetary Science Joint Meeting, p.16. (in Japanese)

Ito,H., O.Nishizawa, Y.Kuwahara, K.Yamamoto, O.Sano and Y.Kobayashi 1996. 11th Materials meeting of The Geological Survey of Japan, pp.69-73. (in Japanese)

Noro,H. 1989. A method was concluded trend of unidimensional data, using ABIC. *Jyoho-Chishitsu*, pp.1-10. (in Japanese)

Sato,R., K.Kusunose, A.Cho, T.Kiyama, F.Yamada and T.Aizawa 1997. A crustal stress measurement just above the focal region of Inagawa earthquake swarm. Zisin, Second Series, 50, pp.57-65. (in Japanese)

Strickland, F.G. & N.K. Ren 1980. Use of differential strain curve analysis in predicting the in-situ stress state for deep wells. *Proc. 21st US Symp. Rock Mech.*, Rolla. pp.523-532.

Tanaka,Y. 1992. Estimation of some fracture events in the shallow parts of the crust by in situ stress measurements. *Butsuri-Tansa*, 45, pp.484-502. (in Japanese)

Differential strain curve analysis to estimate stress state around Soultz EPS-1 well

Y. Oikawa & I. Matsunaga
National Institute for Resources and Environment, Tsukuba, Ibaraki, Japan

S. Miyazaki
Tokyo Engineering University, Hachiouji, Japan

ABSTRACT: Differential strain curve analysis (DSCA) of oriented rock cores, was applied to estimate a stress state at Soultz-sous-Forêts, test site of the European hot dry rock, in the upper Rhine graven. Four sets of cores had been chosen from different depths, 1477 m, 1589 m, 1844 m and 2191 m, in well EPS1. Shallower specimens, 1477 m and 1589 m, show a good agreement but deeper specimens show varied results. Only the direction of the maximum principal stress generally agrees with the assumed high vertical stress state, but shallower results of DSCA in the horizontal plane are not agreed well with the other investigations. The direction of N60E is high from DSCA. The ratio of the maximum horizontal stress to the minimum horizontal stress of DSCA result at 2191m depth is 1 to 0.70. This is lower than that of hydraulic fracturing method but higher than the ASR method.

1 INTRODUCTION

The in-situ stress state controls behavior of underground fractures. Hence stress measurements are useful to characterize fractured geothermal reservoirs or to design an artificial fracture system.

Methods using a drilled rock core are considered to be convenient, especially for stress measurements at great depth. For example, Rummel and Baumgärtner (1991) conducted a hydraulic fracturing stress measurement at Soultz and encountered several technical problems.

Differential strain curve analysis (DSCA) uses a drilled core specimen. In this paper, we describe DSCA result at Soultz.

2 SOULTZ TEST SITE

European hot dry rock test site is located at Soultz-sous-Forêts (Soultz) in the upper Rhine graben. There are two circulation wells GPK1 and GPK2 and an observation well EPS1.

Soultz test site is situated inside the Rhine graben that runs to NE-SW. At shallower depth, the stress parallel to the direction of E-W is low and the vertical stress is higher relatively because the earth crust is spreading to the direction of E-W in the Rhine graben.

Granite core of 810m length was recovered from 1420-2230 m in EPS1. Genter et al. (1995) conducted a detailed fracture analysis on the EPS1 cores. The stress parallel to the direction of N-S is higher in the horizontal plane according to their analysis because they observed that most drilling-induced fracture had N-S strike. Results are shown in Table 1.

Dezayes et al. (1995) conducted a fracture analysis by using the slip directions on EPS1 cores. According to their analysis, four stress states that correspond to the paleostress are deduced and the latest one shows that the maximum compression direction is N120E in the horizontal plane.

Tenzer et al. (1992) conducted a fracture analysis that is based on a borehole televiewer observation in EPS1. According to their vertical fracture analysis, from 1700-1840 m, strikes of NW-SE direction were observed most frequently and at 1840-2150 m depth, strikes of NNE-SSW direction were observed most frequently.

Rummel and Baumgärtner (1991) conducted hydraulic fracturing stress measurements in GPK1 that is 500 m apart from EPS1. They found the NW-SE direction is strongly compressed in the horizontal plane. Klee and Rummel (1992) also conducted stress measurement using the hydraulic fracturing method in deep borehole of EPS1, the direction of the principal stresses was not reported, but only stress values were described.

Lienert et al. (1991) conducted the stress evaluation by anelastic strain recovery (ASR) method using rock core specimen at 2226m depth in EPS1. A vertical stress, a maximum horizontal stress and a minimum horizontal stress were estimated but the directions of

Table 1. Other investigations on stress field conducted in Soultz

Method	Well	Depth (m)	Type of stress field[*2]	Ref.[*3]
Frac. Analy.	GPK1	2000-3600	N-S C.	1)
	EPS1	1410-1905	N-S C.	
	EPS1	1905-2000	NNE-SSW C.*1	
	EPS1	2000-2227	NE-SW C.*1	
Frac. Analy.	EPS1	1410-2227	N-S C., vertical: σ_2	2)
			E-W E., vertical: σ_1	
			NE-SW C., vertical: σ_2	
			NW-SE C., vertical: σ_2	
Frac. Analy.	GPK1	1420-2000	NNW-SSE C.	3)
	EPS1	1700-1840	NW-SE C.	
	EPS1	1840-2150	NNE-SSW C.*1	
Hydrofrac stress measurement	GPK1	1458-2000	NW-SE C. $\sigma_H : \sigma_h = 1 : 0.61$-$0.70$	4)
	EPS1	2200	$\sigma_H : \sigma_h = 1 : 0.51$,$\sigma_v:\sigma_H:\sigma_h = 1:0.94:0.48$	5)
ASR	EPS1	2226	$\sigma_H : \sigma_h = 1 : 0.79$,$\sigma_v:\sigma_H:\sigma_h = 1:0.87:0.69$	6)

*1: EPS1 well is deviated much from vertical below 1830m depth.
*2: C.; compression
E.; extension
σ_1; maximum principal stress
σ_2; intermediate principal stress
σ_H; Maximum horizontal stress
σ_h; Minimum horizontal stress
σ_v; Vertical stress
*3: 1) Genter et al.
2) Dezayes et al.
3) Tenzer et al.
4) Rummel & Baumgärtner
5) Klee & Rummel
6) Lienert et al.

principal stress were not reported.
These investigations are summarized about the stress state in Table 1.

3 EXPERIMENT AND ANALYSIS

3.1 Specimen

Four cores obtained from different depths, 1477 m, 1589 m, 1844 m and 2191 m, in EPS1 were used for the DSCA. The cores were classified as porphyritic granite and grain size varied much. Temperature at the depth where cores were obtained is 110°C-140°C. Specimens from shallower depth, 1477m and 1589m depth, were very altered. Three or four cubic test pieces were obtained from each core.

3.2 Methods

The cubic specimens were been sealed with silicon sealant after gluing four strain gauges on each side, then put into a pressure vessel.

The test cubes were cyclically pressurized up to 100 MPa using a servo-controlled oil booster pump at a loading speed of 0.025MPa/sec, except the 2191 m specimen that were pressurized up to 110 MPa. The strains of the 24 gauges and the pressure in loading path were recorded.

3.3 Analysis

When we apply hydrostatic pressure, cracks in rock specimen tend to close. Effects of closure of the cracks appear as shape of the pressure-strain curve. At low pressure, a deformation rate is large because many cracks are still open. At high pressure, it becomes smaller because of a crack closing effect. Strickland and Ren (1980) attributed the difference of the slopes of the curve at high pressure and low pressure to the strains induced by a stress relief when coring. They also used the Hook's law to estimate the in-situ stress magnitudes. Although Soultz cores are considered to be anisotropic, we assumed isotropic elastic properties because of ease of analysis. We use a Poisson's ratio of 0.2 when determining the ratio of principal stress magnitudes.

4 RESULT

An example of pressure-strain behaviors of a test cube when loading is shown in Fig.1. Pressure-strain curves obtained on EPS1 cores were scattered. EPS1 core showed disturbed pressure-strain relation when loading. This shows that the specimen contains many weak planes and also shows that the deformation characteristics where strain gauges were glued on are varied. In some cases, the whole gauge was glued on a single large grain crystal. Four experiments are eliminated by bad quality.

Directions of the principal stresses from DSCA are shown in Fig.2 (a), (b). Also, principal stress values and principal stress ratios are shown in Table 2. It was assumed that the vertical stress was equal to the

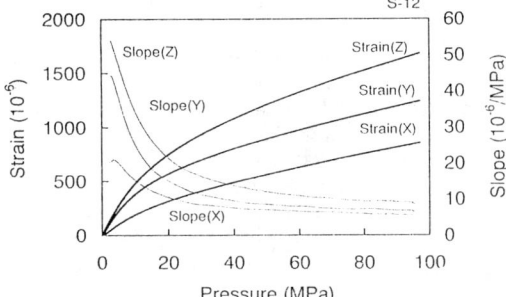

Figure 1. Example of pressure-strain curves and behaviors of their slope.

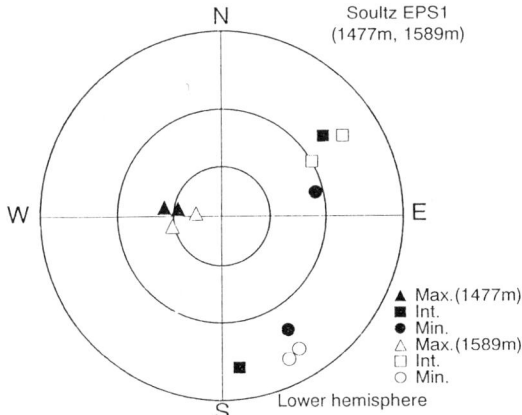

Figure 2(a). Estimated principal stress directions at 1477 m depth and 1589 m depth.

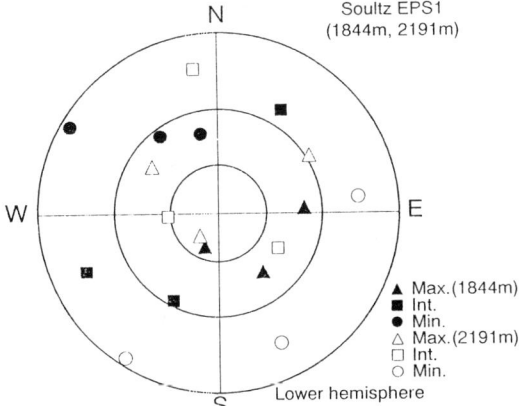

Figure 2(b). Estimated principal stress directions at 1844 m depth and 2191 m depth.

Table 2. Results of 3D analysis

Sample ID	Depth (m)	Ratio of principal stress magnitude			Principal stress magnitude*		
		Max.	Int.	Min.	Max. (MPa)	Int. (MPa)	Min. (MPa)
S-01	1477	1.00 :	0.98 :	0.83	38.4	37.8	32.0
S-02	1477	1.00 :	0.68 :	0.65	42.7	29.0	27.8
S-11	1589	1.00 :	0.93 :	0.63	41.1	38.1	25.7
S-12	1589	1.00 :	0.81 :	0.50	43.0	34.8	21.5
S-21	1844	1.00 :	0.81 :	0.74	54.5	44.3	40.2
S-22	1844	1.00 :	0.82 :	0.60	57.7	47.2	34.6
S-23	1844	1.00 :	0.84 :	0.72	48.2	40.6	34.7
S-31	2191	1.00 :	0.72 :	0.47	58.1	41.7	27.6
S-32	2191	1.00 :	0.66 :	0.61	76.3	50.3	46.6
S-33	2191	1.00 :	0.70 :	0.51	67.1	47.0	34.5

*: Magnitudes are estimated under an assumption that overburden pressure is equal to vertical stress magnitude. The overburden rock density is supposed to be 2.6g/cm^{-3}.

Table 3. Results of 2D analysis

Sample ID	Depth (m)	Ratio of principal stress magnitude Min./Max.	Principal stress magnitude*		Direction of max.principal stress
			Max. (MPa)	Min. (MPa)	
S-01	1477	0.90	37.7	33.8	N60E
S-02	1477	0.87	33.1	28.8	N102E
S-11	1589	0.76	38.2	29.1	N60E
S-12	1589	0.68	47.8	43.7	N67E
S-21	1844	0.85	49.6	42.4	N79E
S-22	1844	0.91	47.8	43.7	N109E
S-23	1844	0.87	41.6	36.2	N29E
S-31	2191	0.76	42.4	32.4	N178E
S-32	2191	0.68	70.4	47.7	N59E
S-33	2191	0.65	58.2	37.6	N124E

*: Magnitudes are estimated under an assumption that overburden pressure is equal to vertical stress magnitude. The overburden rock density is supposed to be 2.6g/cm-3.

overburden pressure, with an overburden density of 2.6g/cm^3, to calculate the principal stress values.

As for each direction of the principal stresses, specimens at 1477m and 1589 m show good agreement. The direction of the maximum principal stress (σ_1) is N-E and it deviates about 30° from vertical. The intermediate principal stress (σ_2) is NE-SW and it deviates 70° from vertical. The minimum principal stress (σ_3) is NNW-SSE and it deviates 75° from vertical. Specimens at 1844m depth show varied result and the direction of σ_1 is NW-SE and it deviates about 30° from vertical. The direction of σ_3 is NW-SE and it deviates about 60° from vertical. Specimens at 2191m depth show the most varied results and the directions of the principal stresses do not agreed from one specimen to another. As for all specimen, σ_1 is inferred to be deviated 30° from vertical and is ENE-WSW, and σ_3 is deviated 70°-80° from vertical and is NNW-SSE.

The principal stress ratio of σ_1, σ_2 and σ_3 of the specimen at 1477m and 1589m, which shows reasonably consistent results in the principal stress directions, are 1:0.90:0.65 respectively. According to each specimen, the highest ratio is 1:0.72:0.47 with specimen at 2191m depth and the lowest is 1:0.98:0.83 with specimen at 1477m depth.

The maximum horizontal stress (σ_H), the minimum horizontal stress (σ_h) and direction of σ_H were calculated from the three dimensional stress components estimated above, the results are shown in Table 3. In the horizontal plane, directions of σ_H are varied. Although N62E is a most frequent direction, N110E also occur.

5 DISCCUSION

At the Soultz experiment site the evaluations of stress state were conducted using various methods, including in-situ measurement. Two types of stress state estimated by those methods are considered to mainly reflect present stress state. One is N-S high type, and another is NW-SE high type. Moreover, a vertical stress (σ_v) is considered to be higher than σ_H at Soultz site ($\sigma_v > \sigma_H > \sigma_h$).

DSCA results of shallower specimens, at 1477m and 1589 m, show good agreement. σ_1 is N-E and it deviates about 30° from vertical. σ_3 is NNW-SSE and it deviates 75° from vertical. Only the direction of σ_1 is generally agreed with the stress state of high σ_v but σ_2 and σ_3 are not agree well with the stress state because results of DSCA in the horizontal plane are not agree well with the other investigations. The direction of N60E is strongly compressed from DSCA. Although deeper specimens show varied results, vertical stress tends to be high. As all cores, only the direction of σ_1 is generally agree with the stress state with high σ_v.

The shallower specimens show a good agreement but deeper specimens do not. This might be caused by a difference of degree of alteration. A varied grain size or fractures inside the specimen might cause the varied results of deeper specimens. For specimens at 2195m depth, a smaller diameter of the core might cause an additional influence because the coring could induce additional damages of crack in the specimen.

The principal stress ratio in the horizontal plane both at 1477m depth and at 1589 m depth is calculated to be 1:0.61 based on the result of the stress measurement by the hydraulic fracturing method in GPK1 conducted by Rummel and Baumgärtner. This ratio does not agree with the principal stress ratios determined by DSCA, which indicate a lower ratio of 1:0.78. This might be caused by an influence of cooling when obtaining the core and a local perturbation of the stress state between GPK1 and EPS1.

Two methods were conducted at 2200 m depth of EPS1. Klee and Rummel reported the principal stresses, σ_H and σ_h, were estimated as 50.2 MPa, 26.6 MPa respectively and the principal stress ratio in the horizontal plane became 1:0.53. Lienert et al. reported the stresses, σ_v, σ_H and σ_h, were estimated as 55MPa, 48MPa, 38MPa respectively. A principal stress ratio in the horizontal plane becomes 1:0.79 based on their results. The result of DSCA at 2191m depth is 1:0.70. This is lower than the hydraulic fracturing method and is higher than ASR method.

CONCLUSION

DSCA, an underground stress measurement method using oriented rock cores, was applied to estimate stress state at the Soultz hot dry rock test site.

Shallower specimens, at 1477m and 1589 m, show good agreement. The direction of the maximum principal stress, σ_1 is N-E and it deviates about 30° from vertical. The intermediate principal stress, σ_2 is NE-SW and it deviates 70° from vertical. The minimum principal stress, σ_3 is NNW-SSE and it deviates 75° from vertical. Only the direction of σ_1 generally agrees with the assumed stress state, i. e. high σ_v, but results of DSCA in the horizontal plane are not agreed well with the other investigations. The direction of N60E is high from DSCA. The principal stress ratio of σ_1, σ_2 and σ_3 using DSCA is 1:0.90:0.65 at 1477 m and 1589 m. Although deeper specimens show varied results, vertical stress tends to be high.

In the horizontal plane, directions of the maximum horizontal stress, σ_H and the minimum horizontal stress, σ_h are varied. Although N62E is a frequent direction of σ_H, N110E also occur.

The ratio of σ_H:σ_h of DSCA result at shallower depth is 1:0.78. This is lower than that of hydraulic fracturing method at the same depth in GPK1. The ratio of σ_H:σ_h at 2191m depth is 1:0.70. This is lower than that of hydraulic fracturing method but higher the ASR method.

The shallower specimens show a good agreement but deeper specimens do not. We will study further reasons that could cause varied results.

ACKNOWLEDGMENTS

The author would like to thank BRGM and Socomine for providing cores and their orientation.

REFERENCES

Dezayes, CH., et al. 1995. Analysis of fractures in boreholes of the Hot Dry Rock project at Soultz-sous-Forêts (Rhine graben,France). *Scientific Drilling.* 5: 31-41.

Genter, A., et al. 1995. Fracture analysis and reservoir characterization of the granitic basement in the HDR Soultz project (France). *Geotherm. Sci. & Tech.*,4(3): 189-214.

Klee, G. & F. Rummel 1992. Hydrofrac stress data for the European HDR research project test site Soultz-sous-Forêts as a part of the HDR feasibility study, *MeSy-Report*, 03.01.92.

Lienert, M., Wolter, K.E. & H. Berckhemer 1991. Berich über die Messung der zeitabhängigen Entspannungsdeformation und der akustischen Emission an Bohrkernen der Soultz-Bohrung EPS1 (HDR). *Ruhr-universität Bochum Report,* No.5.

Rummel, F. & J. Baumgärtner 1991. Hydraulic fracturing stress measurements in the GPK-1 borehole, Soultz-sous-Forets, *Geotherm. Sci. & Tech.*,3(1-4),119-148.

Strickland, F. G. & N. K. Ren 1980, Use of differential strain curve analysis in predicting in-situ stress state in deep wells, *Proc. 21st U. S. Sympo. on Rock Mech.*, 523-532.

Tenzer, H., et al. 1992. Fracture analysis in Hot Dry Rock drillholes at Soultz and Urach by borehole televiewer measurements. *Geothermal Resources Council Transactions.* 19: 317-321.

Laboratory investigation of controls of stress history on ASR response

D.F.Wang & P.J.Davies
Department of Geology and Geophysics, The University of Sydney, N.S.W., Australia

N.Yassir & J.Enever
Division of Petroleum Resources, CSIRO Australia, Australia

ABSTRACT: This paper presents a study of the anelastic strain relaxation (ASR) response of a synthetic sandstone to different applied stress histories. The experimental work presented herein is divided into two series: basic ASR response to a single applied stress field and ASR response to multiple stress fields. The first series includes ASR responses to isotropic and anisotropic stress fields with fixed stress magnitudes and loading times; this category demonstrates that the measured ASR responses reflect the applied stresses. The second test series includes the final ASR response to stress reversals, with varying stress magnitudes and loading times. It shows that although the final ASR measurement is controlled by many factors such as stress history and time of loading, it does reflect the last stress field that had acted on it. The results reveal some fundamental behaviour of ASR which could be born in mind when analysing real field data in core-based in situ stress measurement.

1. INTRODUCTION

Core-based stress measurement techniques, such as Anelastic Strain Recovery (ASR), are sometimes used by the petroleum industry to glean information on the stress field at depth (Voight, 1968; Blanton, 1983; Teufel & Warpinski, 1984). The attractiveness of these techniques lies in their simplicity: at their best, they can quickly and inexpensively provide a description of the stress ellipsoid and a continuous stress profile. However, in reality, they have generally proved more reliable in giving information on stress orientation rather than magnitude - even then, with mixed success. The assumption behind core-based techniques is that core will relax the most in the direction of the largest stress acting on it - the anisotropy in relaxation thus reflecting stress anisotropy. This assumption can break down, however, when dealing with factors such as a complex sample stress history, fabric, moisture conditions and temperature.

The experimental results described here are part of an on-going research programme which is systematically assessing the possible influences on core relaxation to aid us in better understanding core relaxation methods. To this end, a synthetic sandstone is used, with a known stress and cementation history.

2. DESCRIPTION OF EXPERIMENTS

The samples are created from a mixture of sand, silica flour and sodium silicate solution. The silicate reacts with CO_2 gas to form a cement, allowing "cementation" at any stage during testing. The detailed sample preparation procedure is described in Wang et al (1997). Two series of experiments are presented (Table 1): 1) ASR response to a single stress field, designed to understand the stress-strain behaviour of the synthetic sandstone and its ability to reflect stress anisotropy. 2) ASR response to multiple stress fields, designed to understand the ability of the material to "remember" a previous stress field after the stresses are changed. The details of the experiments in this paper are summarised in Table 1.

3. DISCUSSION OF RESULTS

3.1 ASR response to a single applied stress field

Fig. 1 shows typical results of the ASR response of the synthetic sandstone to different loading conditions for single stress field loading (Series I, Table 1). It can be seen that measured ASR magnitudes are approximately proportional to the

Table 1. Types of experiments presented in this paper

Test Series	I Single Stress Field	II Multiple Stress Fields	
Purpose ⇒ Type ⇓	Effect of stress anisotropy on stress-strain relationship and relative strain response ($\varepsilon_A/\varepsilon_R$)	Effect of multiple stress fields, final stress magnitude and duration of final applied stress field on anelastic strain recovery response	
Anisotropic	$\sigma_A=2\sigma_R=14$MPa 6, 12, 24 hr loading	Fixed loading time with reversed stress magnitude	Stress Field 1: $\sigma_R=2\sigma_A=14$MPa (or reverse) Stress Field 2: $\sigma_R=1/2\sigma_A=7$MPa (or reverse) 12 hours loading for each field.
Anisotropic	$\sigma_A=\frac{1}{2}\sigma_R=7$MPa 6, 12, 24 hr loading	Fixed stress magnitudes with varying loading times	Stress Field 1: $\sigma_A=10$MPa, $\sigma_R=20$MPa; Stress Field 2: $\sigma_A=20$MPa, $\sigma_R=10$MPa; 12 hr loading for the first loading stage; 12, 36 and 48 hr loading for the second loading stage
Anisotropic		Fixed loading times with varying stress magnitudes	Stress Field 1: $\sigma_A=10$MPa, $\sigma_R=14$MPa; Stress Field 2: $\sigma_A=14, 21, 28$ MPa; $\sigma_R=14$MPa; 12 hr loading for each loading stage.
Isotropic	$\sigma_A=\sigma_R=7,10,14,21,28$MPa 12 hr loading		

applied stress field with greater strain relaxation in the direction of the larger stress (Fig. 1 a and b), and similar radial and axial strain relaxation when isotropic stress was applied (Fig. 1c).

The ratio between the strains corresponds reasonably well to the ratio of the applied stresses for all the tests (Fig. 2). In Fig. 2a, $\varepsilon_A/\varepsilon_R$ tends towards 0.5 with elapsed time, as expected ($\sigma_A= 0.5\ \sigma_R$). Among them, the 12 hr loading case gave the most constant strain ratio of ASR . The variability of the initial ASR response will be further investigated. The duration of applied load clearly has an effect on ASR, which has led to the use of a minimum loading time of 12 hours in our subsequent tests.

Conversely, the ratio generally tends towards 2 in Fig. 2b ($\sigma_A=2\sigma_R$). It was found that the difference between the strain ratio curves for 12 and 24 hours loading in Fig. 2b was due to relatively increased axial strain and decreased radial strain in the 12 hr loading case. Repeated experiments gave the same result, suggesting that the material is affected by loading duration requiring further investigation. Finally, in Fig. 2c, the ratio tends towards 1, as expected from an isotropic test. Also it can be seen from the strain ratio curves that as stress magnitude increases, the sample's ASR response behaves more isotropically throughout the measurement time indicating an increased material isotropy.

It was noted in all the experiments that the relaxation strain/applied stress ratio (ε/σ) is generally the same in the axial and radial directions, indicating that the synthetic sandstone did not have an inherent material anisotropy. Fig. 3 demonstrates the relationship for the anisotropically loaded samples.

Note that samples loaded with a higher mean stress ($\sigma_R=2\sigma_A$), Fig. 3a, gave a lower ε/σ ratio than the samples loaded with the lower mean stress ($\sigma_A=2\sigma_R$), Fig. 3b. The same reduced relaxation strain with increased mean stress was observed for isotropically loaded samples (Fig. 4). This suggests increasing material stiffness with porosity reduction at the higher mean stresses.

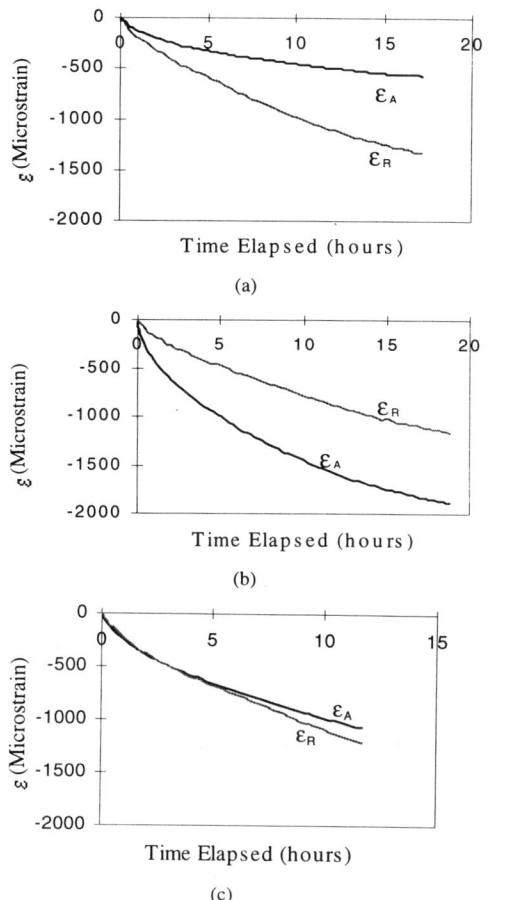
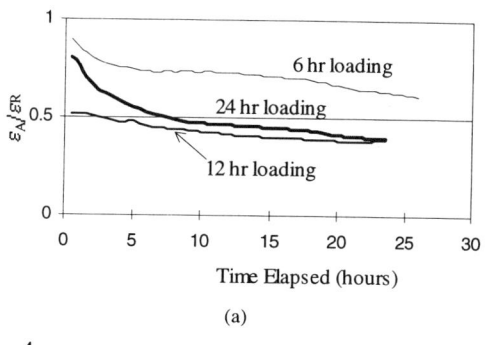
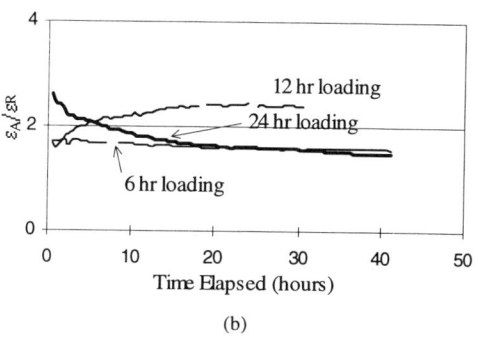
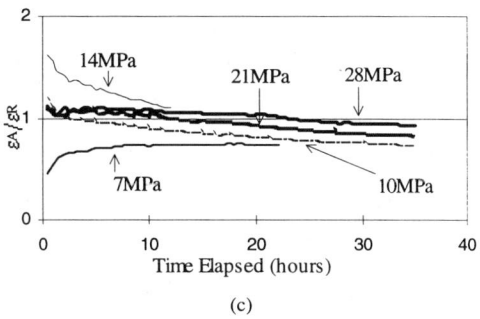

Fig. 1 ASR response to different loading conditions with a single stress field: (a) anisotropic stress field with $\sigma_R=2\sigma_A=14$MPa (24 hours loading); (b) anisotropic stress field with $\sigma_A=2\sigma_R=14$MPa (24 hours loading); (c) isotropic stress field with $\sigma_R=\sigma_A=10$MPa (12 hours loading)

Fig. 2 Ratio of axial to radial strains ($\varepsilon_A/\varepsilon_R$) with elapsed time for: (a) anisotropic stress field with $\sigma_R=2\sigma_A=14$MPa (loaded for 6, 12, 24 hours); (b) anisotropic stress field with $\sigma_A=2\sigma_R=14$MPa (loaded for 6, 12, 24 hours); (c) isotropic stress field with $\sigma_R=\sigma_A=7,10,14,21,28$MPa (12 hours loading)

3.2 ASR response to multiple stress fields

This test series was designed to assess the sample's ability to "remember" a previous stress state. The samples in these tests therefore experienced a stress reversal (series II, Table 1).

Typical ASR responses

When a sample was loaded with two stress fields (with equal loading time and reversed axial and radial stress magnitudes for each field), the measured ASR curves after unloading show a "memory" of both stress fields (Figs. 5 and 6).

In Fig. 5, the initial axial anelastic strain is greater than radial strain, which corresponds to the second applied stress. As measurement time elapses, the relative magnitude of ε_A and ε_R reverses, showing a strain relaxation condition corresponding to the previous stress field. The same phenomenon can be observed in Fig. 6 with the reversed stress fields.

Two types of test were further performed based on the above finding in order to investigate this

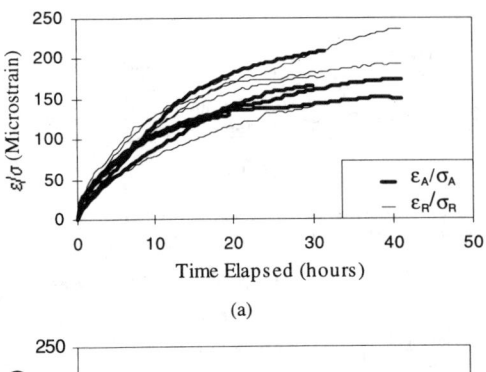

(a)

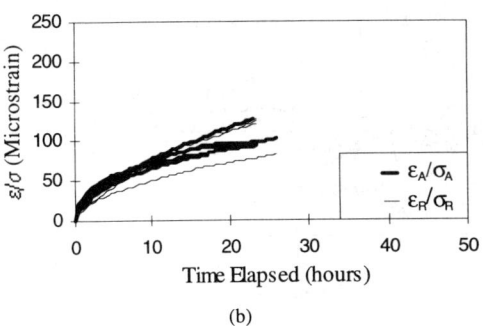

(b)

Fig. 3 Curves of relaxation strain-applied stress ratio (ε/σ) versus time for all anisotropically loaded samples: (a) $\sigma_R=2\sigma_A=14$MPa; (b) $\sigma_A=2\sigma_R=14$MPa.

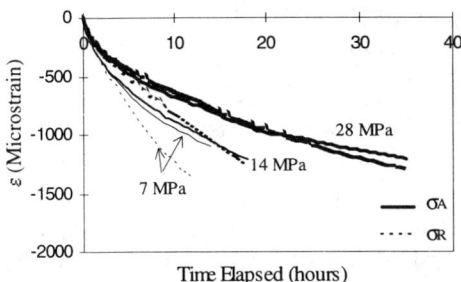

Fig. 4 Curves of relaxation strain (ε) versus time for samples isotropically loaded to 7 MPa, 14 MPa and 28 MPa.

stress memory phenomenon. Tests were conducted to examine the effects of loading duration and the stress magnitude in the second loading stage on the ASR response.

ASR response to loading time

Fig. 7 shows the effect of second cycle loading time on the ASR measurement.

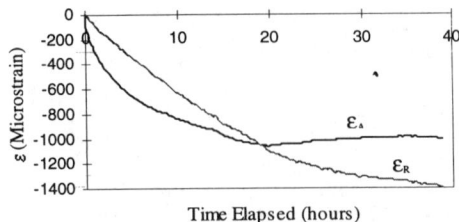

Fig. 5 Strain relaxation-time curves for a sample subjected to two anisotropic loads: $\sigma_R=2\sigma_A=14$MPa, followed by $\sigma_R=0.5\sigma_A=7$MPa. (12 hours loading each)

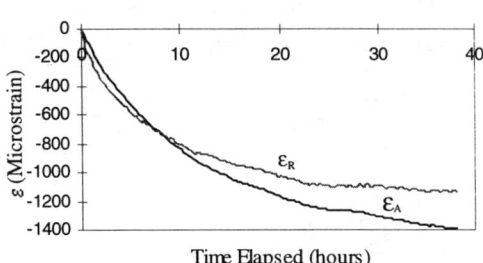

Fig. 6 Strain relaxation-time curves for a sample subjected to two anisotropic loads: $\sigma_A=2\sigma_R=14$MPa, followed by $\sigma_A=0.5\sigma_R=7$MPa. (12 hours loading each)

The strain ratio is clearly affected by both stress fields. The result for only one loading cycle is given in the $t_2=0$ curve, reflecting a ratio of ≤ 0.5. In the $t_2=t_1$ test, the $\varepsilon_A/\varepsilon_R$ ratio increases to around 2.25, the ratio then reverses in trend, reducing to approximates 1 with elapsed time, indicating that ε_R eventually exceeds ε_A. This reversal in strain ratio trend is not observed in the single stress loading cases (Figs. 1 and 2) and seems to reflect the effect of the first applied stress field on the final ASR response.

As the loading duration for the second stress field (t_2) increases, the reversal in strain ratio trend is less pronounced and the final strain ratio increases. This suggests that the "memory" of the first loading stage is reduced with increased t_2. It would be expected, therefore, that as $t_2 \gg t_1$, the ASR response in these tests would show no memory of the initial loading stage, giving a final $\varepsilon_A/\varepsilon_R$ ratio of 2. These results suggest that the earlier stress field influences the final strain ratio, the influence reducing with increased t_2.

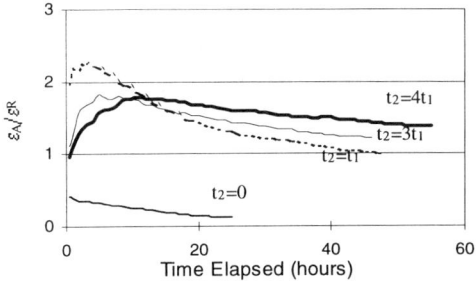

Fig. 7 Strain ratio ($\varepsilon_A/\varepsilon_R$) versus elapsed time for samples loaded with $\sigma_A=0.5\sigma_R=10$MPa, then with $\sigma_A=2\sigma_R=20$MPa, for increasing loading times in the second loading stage ($t_2 = t_1$, $3t_1$, $4t_1$; see series II, Table 1).

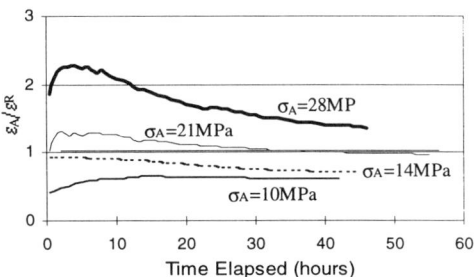

Fig. 8 Strain ratio ($\varepsilon_A/\varepsilon_R$) versus elapsed time for samples loaded with $\sigma_A=10$MPa, $\sigma_R=14$MPa then with $\sigma_A=14, 21, 28$ MPa, $\sigma_R=14$MPa ($t_2 = t_1= 12$ hr, see series II, Table 1).

ASR response to loading magnitude

Fig. 8 shows the effect of loading magnitude in the second loading stage on ASR response.

The strain ratio predicably increases for samples where the axial stress in the second loading cycle is higher. The initial strain ratios ($\varepsilon_A/\varepsilon_R$) can be related to applied stress ratio (σ_A/σ_R) at the second loading stage, with $\varepsilon_A/\varepsilon_R \approx 1$ for the case $\sigma_A=\sigma_R$, $\varepsilon_A/\varepsilon_R \approx 1.3$ for the case $\sigma_A=1.5\sigma_R$ and $\varepsilon_A/\varepsilon_R \approx 2.25$ for the case $\sigma_A=2\sigma_R$. The decrease of the ratios with elapsed time clearly shows that the original stress field (shown by the curve labelled "$\sigma_A=10$") affects the final strain response with elapsed time. This reversal in ratio is not reduced as the second stress magnitude is increased, which suggests that the "memory" of the earlier loading stage is not erased by higher stress magnitudes.

Fig. 9 shows the ASR curves for the case

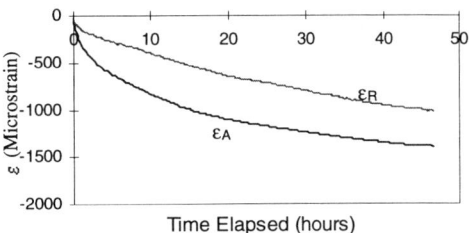

Fig. 9 Strain relaxation-time curves for a sample subjected to two stress field: (1) $\sigma_R=14$MPa; $\sigma_A=10$MPa; (2) $\sigma_R=14$MPa, $\sigma_A=28$MPa; 12 hours loading each.

$\sigma_A=28$MPa in Fig. 8. It was observed that, at the higher stress magnitude, the ASR curves no longer looked like those shown in Figs. 5 and 6, but more like those for the single stress magnitude cases (Figs. 1 and 2). This could be misleading, suggesting that only the last stress field affects the strain response. As seen from the $\varepsilon_A/\varepsilon_R$ curve in Fig. 8 (28 MPa), however, the ratio between strains does reflect the earlier stress field. The change in strain ratio should therefore be assessed in conjunction with the raw ASR data in analysing the stress field. This is a preliminary finding and will be the subject of further investigation.

4. CONCLUSIONS

Much of the information recovered with respect to the relative strain response (axial strain/radial strain) relates to the specific performance of the experimental material. In a very general sense, however, the logical radial and axial strain response to an applied single stress field suggest that anelastic strain measurements can in principle predict the shape of the corresponding stress ellipsoid. Based upon this conclusion, some useful information can be further concluded:

- With a single applied stress field, ASR always indicates the stress field by giving greater anelastic strain recovery in the direction where higher stress is applied, and the ratio of measured $\varepsilon_A/\varepsilon_R$ is close to the applied stress ratio.

- With multiple applied stress fields, the final ASR response is controlled by the whole past stress history. The ASR response shows reduced sensitivity to the earlier stress field with increased final loading duration. This sensitivity is not reduced with increased stress magnitude.

REFERENCES

Blanton, T.L.(1983). The relation between recovery deformation and in-situ stress magnitude, *SPE/DOE Symp. On Low Permeability Gas Reservoirs*, Denver, Colorado. **SPE/DOE 11624**, 213-218

Charlez, Ph., Hamamdjian, C. & Despax, D. (1986). Is the microcracking of a rock a memory of its initial state of stress? *Proc. Int. Symp. on Rock Stress and Rock Stress Measurements*, Stockholm, 341-368.

El Rabaa, A.W.M. & Meadows, D.L.(1986). Laboratory and field applications of the strain relaxation method, 56th California Regional Meeting of the SPE, Oakland, California, **SPE 15072**, 259-272.

Enever, J. & Mckay, L. (1976). Note of the relationship between anelastic strain recovery and virgin rock stresses - a possible method of stress measurement, *ISRM Symp. on Investigation of Stress in Rock - Advances in Stress Measurement*, Sydney, 37-40.

Holt, R.M., Unander, T.E. & Kenter, C.J.(1993). Constitutive mechanical behaviour of synthetic sandstone formed under stress, *Rock. Mech. Min. Sci. & Geomech. Abstr.* **Vol. 30, No.7**, 719-722.

Teufel, L.W. & Warpinski, N. R. (1984). Determination of in-situ stress from anelastic strain recovery measurements of oriented cores: comparison to hydraulic fracture stress measurements in the Rollins Sandstone, Piceance Basin, Colorado, *Proc. 25th U.S. Symposium on Rock Mechanics: Rock Mechanics in Productivity, Protection*, Northwestern University, Illinois, 176-185.

Voight, B. (1968). Determination of the virgin state of stress in the vicinity of the borehole from measurements of a partial anelastic strain tensor in drill cores, *Felsmechanik V. Ingenieureol*, **Vol. 6**, 201-215.

Wang, D.F., Yassir, N, Enever, J., and Davies, P.J., (1997) Laboratory Investigation of Core-based Stress Measurement Using Synthetic Sandstone, *Int. J. Rock Mech. & Min. Sci.* Vol. 34, No.3-4, ISSN 0148-9062 (in press)

Warpinski, N.R. & Teufel, L.W.(1986). A viscoelastic constitutive model for determining in-situ stress magnitudes from anelastic strain recovery of core, *61st SPE Annual Technical Conference and Exhibition*, New Orleans, **SPE 15368**, 1-12.

*Rock Stress, Sugawara & Obara (eds) © 1997 Balkema, Rotterdam, ISBN 90 5410 901 7*

Determination of in situ stress using DRA and AE techniques

M.Utagawa, M.Seto & K.Katsuyama
National Institute for Resources and Environment, Tsukuba, Japan

ABSTRACT: In this study, it is evaluated the possibility of AE and DRA techniques to measure in situ stress, in particular focusing on delay time effect on AE and DRA techniques in the range from one day to four hundreds days. Based on the technique established in the laboratory tests, in situ stress determinations were also conducted using rock cores obtained from a vertically drilled exploratory borehole. Not only axial pre-stress but also lateral one could be estimated from only one uniaxial cyclic loading test. And not only in-laboratory pre-stress specimen but also cored rock could be estimated by AE and DRA method, too. It can be concluded that the vertical geo-stress in this area has a strong effect of the weight of the overlying rock.

1 INTRODUCTION

Reliable evaluation of in situ stress is an important step in the analysis and design of underground excavations, particularly for evaluating the stability of underground structures to prevent failure or collapse of underground openings. Although a number of techniques have been proposed and developed to determine in situ stress, the determination of in situ stress is not an easy task and all suffer from deficiencies and limitations. The main deficiency of established techniques such as over coring method or hydraulic fracturing method is that they are usually expensive and time consuming. Other shortcomings of the techniques are that they are deficient for measuring the in situ stress at depth in remote regions which are hard to access from boreholes or mine workings.

An alternative method for determining the stress state at depth and in remote regions is to take advantage of the Kaiser effect of acoustic emission (AE) and deformation rate analysis by strain.

This "Kaiser effect", suggests that previously applied maximum stress might be detected by stressing a rock specimen to the point where there is a substantial increase in AE activity. Based on the Kaiser effect, the previous stress can be estimated from the curve of AE activity under monotonically increasing stress. A number of researchers have studied the Kaiser effect in geomaterials since the 1970's, and have discussed the factors that influence stress memory recollection of rocks under uniaxial and triaxial conditions (Kanagawa et al., 1976; Kurita and Fujii, 1979; Houghton and Crawford, 1987; Seto et al., 1989, 1992, 1995; Holocomb, 1993; Utagawa et al., 1995).

Deformation Rate Analysis (DRA) is one of the methods to estimate the initial-stress of rock mass using cored rock. In DRA, more than two cyclic compressive load are applied to a cored-rock specimen. The graph, stress vs difference of axial strain curve in cyclic loading test, have a bend point, as shown in Figure 1. This stress at the bend point expresses in-situ stress of rock mass. DRA is originally proposed by Yamamoto (Yamamoto et al, 1991).

The technique is functionally workable technology, and is anticipated that the rapid and economical determination of the in situ stress in the rock is possible.

These method, however, has some problems in its application to in situ stress measurement. One of the problems is that the Kaiser effect and DRA sign cannot always be clearly observed due to the disturbance by heat, water, and weathering (Yoshikawa and Mogi, 1981). Another problem is that the controversy still exists on that how long the stress memory can be retained. If the Kaiser effect recovered in a short time, it is impossible to apply the AE method to estimation of in situ stress.

In this paper, firstly, using the results of cyclic loading of previously stressed rock specimens, the AE method and DRA is proposed to accurately determine the previous stress using AE signatures in the repeated loading (Laboratory tests). In our method, the previous stress can be accurately estimated from AE take-off point and DRA in the second and third reloadings, even when the delay time from previous loading is long in the range up to 400 days. Secondly, the applicability of the AE and DRA method is discussed based on the estimation results of in situ stresses from cored rock specimens obtained in four different underground sites. The cored rock specimen was repeatedly loaded up to a certain stress level, and AE was measured in each loading to determine the in situ stress (In situ tests).

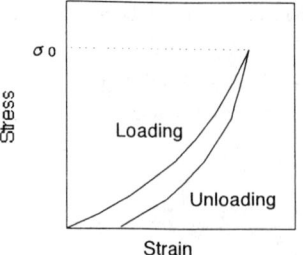

Figure 1 Stress Strain Curve

2 EXPERIMENTAL PROCEDURE

2.1 Rock specimen in laboratory tests

The rock specimens used in this study were Inada-Granite, Shirahama and Kimachi-Sandstones, Tage-Tuff, and in situ mudstone. The sandstones' uniaxial compressible strength is about 60 MPa. Granite's strength is about 185 MPa. And Tuff's strength is 40 MPa. The specimens are rectangular shape of which length of square was 30 mm, and height was 60 mm.

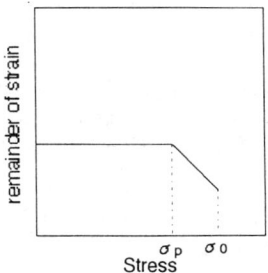

Figure 2 Stress-remainder of strain curve

2.2 Measuring system

In AE measurements, four sensors were put on the confronted sides of the specimen and these sensors formed a parallel oblong plane to the loading axis direction. The AE sensors used in this study were differential typed ones (5.0mm diameter, NF-AE-904DM model) and the resonance frequency was 500kHz. It had high gains between 200kHz and 550kHz. The response frequency band of this system was between 50kHz and 1MHz.

The signals from the AE sensors were amplified 40dB by the pre-amplifiers and sent to the AE measurement system (NF-9600 Local processor) and was amplified further by 40dB. When AE sensors detected AE, these sensors removed the noises which generated at the contact point between the rock specimen and the end piece, hydraulic pressure source etc from AE signals over threshold level (240mV) and detected AE generated only inside the rock specimen. The method to remove the noise was to get rid of the signals whose arrival time difference to these 4 sensors were longer than the prescribed figures. These prescribed figures were determined before the test by the way that we oscillated elastic waves through pressing propelling pencil leads (5mm diameter, 3mm length) on the surface of the specimen, endpiece etc not so as to measure signals from outside the rock specimen. The AE-strain-

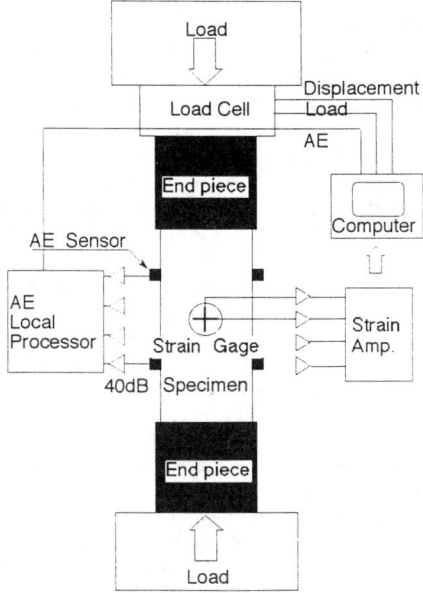

Figure 3 The AE-strain-load measuring system

load measuring system is shown in Figure 3. 4 strain gages were attached to each surface of a specimen to average the inclination of the value of each gage. Load, strain, and displacement data were converted to digital data, and recorded on a floppy disk.

2.3 Test Program

In the tests, at first, uniaxial cyclic loading experiments of rock specimen were conducted to know how accurately artificially applied previous stress can be estimated by AE and DRA. A rock specimen was previously stressed in two or three different directions. Then, after some times being elapsed, the pre-stressed rock specimen was again uniaxially loaded to estimate the previous stress. These rock are taken until 100 m from ground, so the effect of initial geostress is very little.

3. RESULT

3.1 AE method for estimating previous stress

Figure 4 shows a typical example that indicates the existence of Kaiser effect in a sandstone specimen. Data for a specimen tested 5 min. after the previous 50 repeated loading up to 10 MPa are shown. An arrow indicates the previous maximum stress. The take-off point of AE activity coincides with the maximum previous stress. In all experiments conducted within the short delay time, the existence of Kaiser effect in rock specimens could be clearly observed and the assigned stress from the take-off point of AE signature was within 5 %. Figure 2 represents the AE signature of sandstone which was previously stressed up to 10 MPa 7 days before the test. An arrow indicates the maximum previous stress, but lots of AEs were produced within the stress level of Kaiser effect. These AEs obscure the Kaiser effect. The longer the delay time is, the more the first reloading produces AEs within the stress level of Kaiser effect (delay time effect). The AEs produced before the maximum previous stress level are possibly due to the crack movements (closure, friction, or compaction) inside the specimen (Seto et al., 1995). Figure 3 represents the AE signatures from the second to fourth reloading of sandstone shown in Figure 5.

As shown in Figure 6, the AEs below the previous stress level were reduced by the repeated reloadings up to the same stress level, and the AE signature in the second and/or third reloadings gave clear indication of AE increase (AE take-off point). Consequently, based on the results of the laboratory test, even if Kaiser effect was obscured due to delay time effect, the AE signatures in the subsequent reloadings can allow us to determine the maximum previous stress.

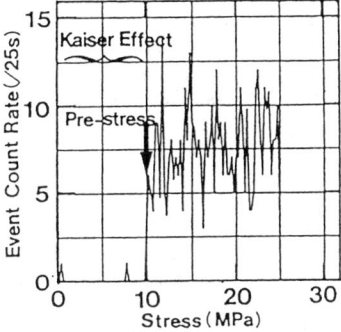

Figure 4 An example of Kaiser effect of sandstone

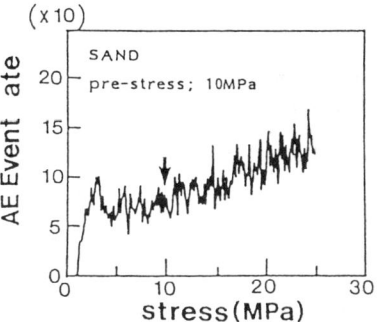

Figure 5 AE behavior of sandstone previously stressed up to 10 MPa 7days before.

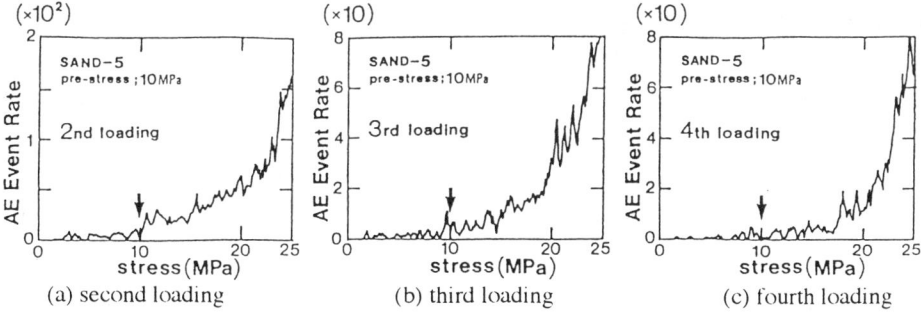

(a) second loading (b) third loading (c) fourth loading

Figure 6 AE events (elapsed time 7 days)

3.2 DRA for estimating previous stress

Figure 7 shows the relation between stress and differential strain of the Shirahama sandstone specimen previously uniaxial stressed 1 day ago. The differential strain was between the second loading and first loading. The previous stress value was 10 MPa. The DRA curve has a clear bend at near 10 MPa.

Figure 8 is a curve of stress and differential strain of the specimen previously stressed 7 days ago. This rock specimen is also Shirahama-sandstone, and the previous stress was 10 MPa. The DRA curve doesn't have a clear bend, while the DRA curve has a clearer bend when delay time is short. With the increase in delay time, the bend point of DRA curve became less clear. With the increase in elapsed time, error in the evaluated value became bigger.

Figure 9 is a curve of stress and differential strain of the rock specimen shown in Figure 8. This strain difference is between the third loading and second loading. The DRA curve has a clearer bend at near 10 MPa of pre-stress value than the one shown in Figure 7. The clear bend of the DRA curve appeared at the pre-stress point on and after the second loading.

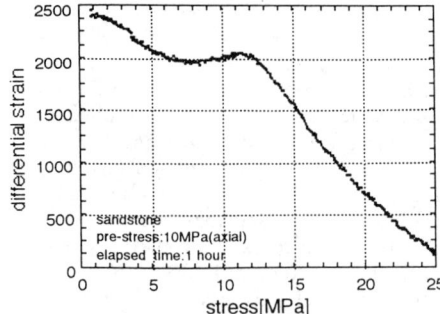

Figure 7 DRA Curve (elapsed time 1 hour)

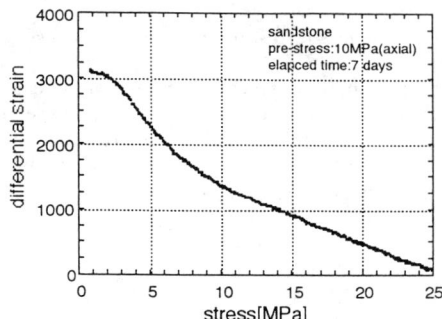

Figure 8 DRA Curve
(elapsed time 7days, First loading)

3.3 Conclusion in laboratory test

The laboratory test results indicate that the shorter the delay time is the more accurately the previous stress can be accurately estimated using Kaiser Effect and DRA principle, and that the estimation can be accuracy becomes worse with increase of delay time. But it was found out that AE increase point and inflection point in DRA curve could be clearly recognized at the previous stress level after the second reloading. It was possible to determine the previous stress level within the accuracy of 10%(AE) or 15%(DRA) even when the delay time is long and Kaiser Effect in the first reloading is not clear.

4 IN SITU STRESS MEASUREMENT RESULTS

There was significant correlation between the overburden pressure (estimated from depth and rock density) and estimated vertical stress from AE and DRA technique which are based on the laboratory tests. Figure 10 shows the relation between the depth(Z (m)) and the vertical stress estimated from AE. Figure 11 shows the relation between the depth(Z (m)) and the vertical stress estimated from DRA. The dotted line indicated the overburden pressure estimated from the depth and

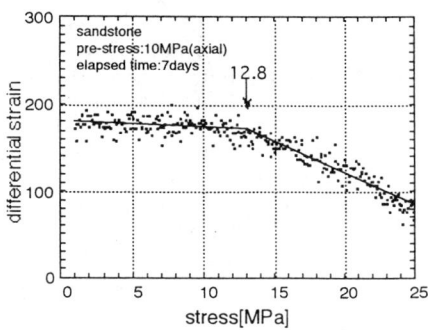

Figure 9 DRA Curve
(elapsed time 7days, Cyclic loading)

rock density. The estimated vertical stresses from acoustic emission behavior are consistent with the overburden pressure. The borehole was drilled up to the depth of 180 m from the surface five months before the tests, and rock type was sandy mudstone. And, as it can be seen from Figure 10 and 11, the results obtained from overcoring method and hydraulic fracturing method also agree with the stresses estimated from AE. The time lag of up to two years didn't deter to evaluate the critical in situ stress condition. Cored rock recollected the in situ stress condition reasonably well, when compared to the results from overcoring method and hydraulic fracturing method.

5 CONCLUSIONS

In situ rock stress measurements were performed by using AE and strain signatures in cyclic loading of rock core specimens. The cored rocks were uniaxially loaded to determine the in situ rock stresses in underground site, and the estimated stresses from AE method and DRA were compared with the results from other techniques such as over coring method or hydraulic fracturing method. The main conclusions obtained here are as follows:
(1) The time lag of up to eight months did not deter to evaluate the critical in situ stress condition. Rock core specimen recollected the in situ rock stress reasonably well (10%,AE 15%:DRA)
(2) Not only axial pre-stress but also lateral one could be estimated from only one uniaxial cyclic loading test.
(3) The determined stresses by AE were well consistent with the stresses from over coring method and hydraulic fracturing method. There was also significant correlation between the overburden pressure and estimated vertical stress from AE.
(4) The AE method suggested in the paper, in which AE activities after the second loading are utilized to determine the rock stresses, should be applicable to the in situ stress measurement with reasonable accuracy.
(5) It can be concluded that the vertical geo-stress in this area has a strong effect of the weight of the overlying rock.

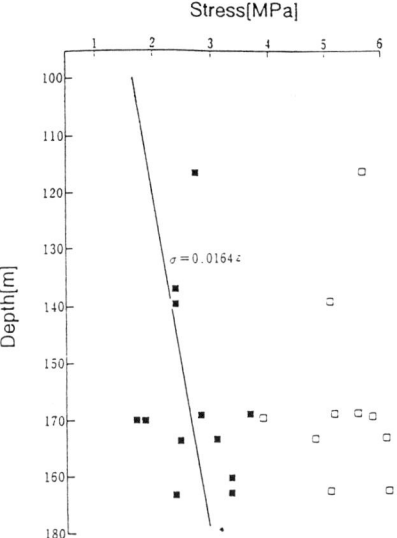

Figure 11 relation between the depth and the vertical stress estimated from DRA

REFERENCES

Houghton, D.R. and A.M. Crawford 1987. Kaiser effect gauging: The influence of confining stress on its response, Proc. 6th ISRM Congress, Montreal, Canada, Vol.2, pp.981-985

Holocomb, D.J. 1993. Observations of the Kaiser effect under multiaxial stress state: Implications for its use in determining in situ stress, Geophys. Res. Lett., 20, pp.2119-2122

Kanagawa, T., Hayashi, M. and H. Nakasa 1976. Estimation of spatial geostress components in rock samples using the Kaiser effect of acoustic emission, Rep. No. 375017, Central Res. Inst. of Electrical Power Industry, Abiko, Japan

Kurita, K. and N. Fujii 1979. Stress memory of crystalline rock in acoustic emission, Geophys. Res. Lett., 6, pp.9-12

Seto, M., Utagawa, M. and K. Katsuyama 1989. Estimation of geostress from AE characteristics in cyclic loading of rock (in Japanese), Proc. 8th Japan Symp. on Rock Mechanics, The Japan National Committee for ISRM, Tokyo, Japan, pp.321-326

Seto, M., Utagawa, M. and K. Katsuyama 1992. The estimation of pre-stress from AE in cyclic

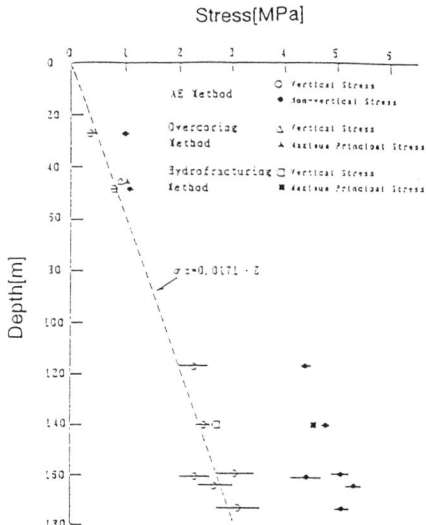

Figure 10 relation between the depth and the vertical stress estimated from AE

loading of pre-stressed rock, Proc. 11th Int. Symp. on Acoustic Emission, The Jap. Soc. for NDI, Fukuoka, Japan, pp.159-166

Seto, M., Utagawa, M. and K. Katsuyama 1995. The relation between the variation of AE hypocenters and the Kaiser effect of Shirahama sandstone, Proc. 8th Int. Cong. on Rock Mechanics, Vol.1, Tokyo, Japan, pp.201-205

Utagawa, M., Seto, M. and K. Katsuyama 1995. Application of acoustic emission technique to detrmination of in situ stresses in mines, Proc. 26th Int. Conf. Safety in Mines Research Institute Vol.4, Central Mining Institute, Katowice, Poland, pp.95-109

Yamamoto, K., Yamamoto, H., Kato, N.and Hirasawa, T. 1991) Deformation Rate Analysis for in situ Stress Estimation, Proc. of 5th AE/MS Activity in Creol. Struct. Mat., 1-13.

Yoshikawa, S. and K. Mogi 1981. A new method for estimation of the crustal stress from cored rock samples: Laboratory study in the case of uniaxial compression, Tectonophysics, 74, 323-339.

Numerical 2D-simulation of memory effects in rocks around a borehole

V.L.Chkouratnik & A.V.Lavrov
Moscow State Mining University, Russia

ABSTRACT: Two-dimensional computer simulation of emission memory effects in rocks around a borehole was carried out. Behaviour of an area of radius 0.5m containing 500 cracks was simulated in the course of three simulation stages: 1-loading with natural geostresses; 2-unloading through drilling a borehole; 3-loading of borehole walls with a pressuremeter creating uniform pressure in all directions. A theoretical model based on the concept of tensile cracks ("wing-cracks") was used. New quantitative features of emission memory effects in rock near a borehole have been established both for chaotic and preferential crack orientation. Memory effect while cyclically loading the borehole walls with a pressuremeter was also simulated. Simulation results are to be used for development of new rock state estimation techniques.

1 INTRODUCTION

Memory effects in rocks around a borehole take place when loading the borehole walls with a pressuremeter creating uniform pressure on the walls in all directions (Lord & Koerner 1985, Deutsch et al. 1989, Yamshchikov et al. 1991). The effects consist in an abrupt increase of acoustic and electromagnetic emission activities (pulse number/sec) when the pressure on the wall reaches a certain value P_*. The effects are similar to conventional Kaiser effect in rock samples and can be used to estimate rock stresses. The main problem here is interpretation of measurement data, namely, how the pressure value P_* ("memory effect pressure") is connected with in situ principal stresses. To solve the problem experimentally is difficult; this forces us to use computer simulation of the phenomenon.

The purpose of the study was to find out the quantitative correlations between principal stresses in the rock and the pressure on the hole walls at which memory effects take place.

2 THEORETICAL MODEL AND SIMULATION SETUP

Two-dimensional numerical simulation of memory effects in the area around a borehole was carried out. The simulation was based on a two-dimensional model of memory effects developed by the authors earlier using the concept of «wing-cracks» (Shkuratnik & Lavrov 1995, Yamshchikov et al. 1996).

A borehole was supposed to be drilled in the direction of one of the principal stresses σ_z in the rock mass. The borehole radius is 0.021m. A cylinder-shaped area of radius 0.5m surrounding the borehole was assumed to contain $N = 500$ randomly located initial cracks. Each initial crack is a thin 5mm long cut parallel to the borehole axis (Figure 1). There is no friction between crack faces.

Cases of both chaotically and preferentially oriented cracks were simulated. In the case of chaotic crack orientation, the angle between the initial crack plane and the X-axis is random. For preferential crack orientation, all initial cracks are inclined at the same angle φ to the X-axis (Figure 1).

Simulation was conducted in three stages: 1-loading the area with natural geostresses σ_x, σ_y perpendicular to the borehole axis; 2-unloading through drilling the borehole; 3-loading of the borehole walls with a pressuremeter creating equal pressure P in all directions. The stress state of the rock was assumed to be elastic. Inelastic deformation takes place in a narrow zone close to the borehole wall and does not have much influence on the memory.

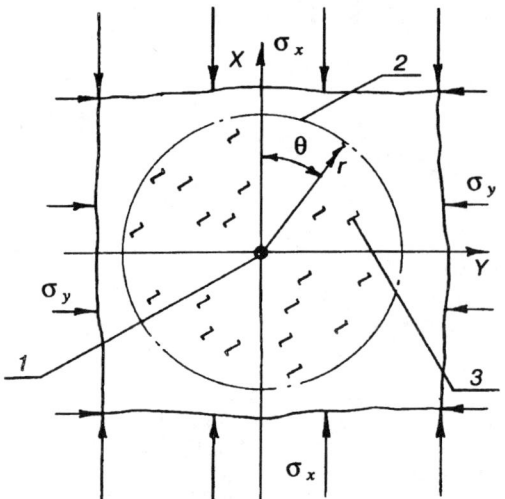

Figure 1. Area around a borehole: 1 − borehole; 2 − area boundary; 3 − crack; r, θ − crack coordinates

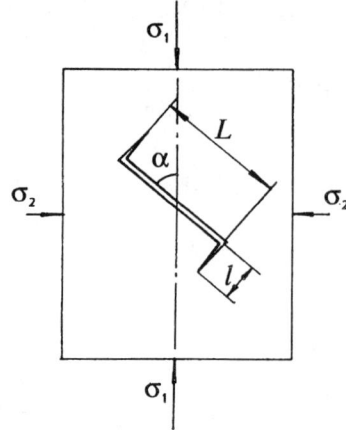

Figure 2. Initial crack with two tensile cracks

At each simulation stage, principal stresses σ_1, σ_2 were calculated for each crack location. The orientation of the principal axes was determined. Then, shear stress and displacement direction over each initial crack plane were determined.

At the first simulation stage, each initial crack generates two tensile cracks ("wings"). Their length is defined by the shear stress acting over the initial crack plane and is given by (Shkuratnik & Lavrov 1995):

$$l_i \approx \left(\frac{(\sigma_1 - \sigma_2) L \sin 2\alpha}{4 \zeta K_{Ic}} \right)^2 \qquad (1)$$

where i is the initial crack number; L is the initial crack length; α is the angle between the initial crack plane and the σ_1-axis (see Figure 2); K_{Ic} is the critical stress intensity factor; ζ is a coefficient.

Unloading at the second stage leads to redistribution in the stress field. Accordingly, lengths of the wing-cracks as well as directions of their growth (two directions are possible in all) were determined and memorized at the second stage. A tensile crack restarts growing when shear stress on the plane of the corresponding initial crack exceeds the maximum previously reached shear stress value, if the displacement direction is the same as earlier. If the displacement direction has changed, new tensile cracks begin to grow from the beginning of the loading.

Loading of the borehole walls at the third stage was carried out in steps: the pressure P was increased from zero to a maximum value P_{max} in equal steps. At each step, the total number W of initial cracks continuing or starting growth of wings was calculated. The value of W was assumed to be a measure for emission activity at a given pressure level. As a result, dependences «W versus P» were obtained.

3 SIMULATION RESULTS

The simulation has shown that in the case of uniform rock stress state ($\sigma_x = \sigma_y$) there is memory effect independent of the crack orientation type. This is the only case when complete restoration of the initial stress field with a pressuremeter is possible. Emission activity is zero at $P < P_*$. At $P = P_*$ there is an activity jump from $W = 0$ to $W = 500$, which remains constant at $P > P_*$ (Figure 3).

In the case of non-uniform stress state ($\sigma_x > \sigma_y$), memory effects take place if initial cracks are preferentially oriented with $10° < \varphi < 80°$. The dependences W versus P consist of two parts: At $P < P_*$ emission activity is low and fluctuates irregularly. When the pressure on the borehole wall reaches P_*, stable increase in emission activity starts (dotted line in Figure 4).

In most cases, the value of memory effect pressure P_* ranges between σ_x and σ_y, nearer the smaller stress σ_y. If one of the

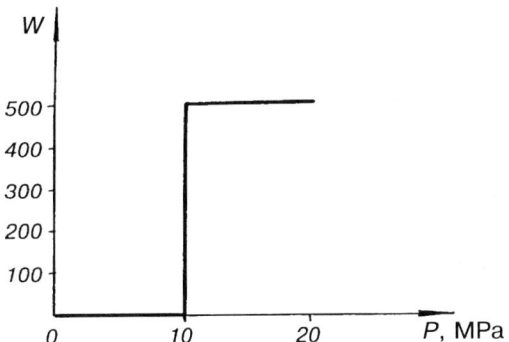

Figure 3. The dependence of emission activity measure on pressure for in situ stresses $\sigma_x = \sigma_y = 10$ MPa

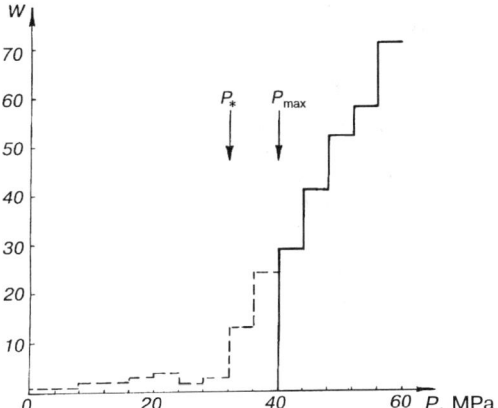

Figure 4. The dependence of emission activity measure on pressure in two loading cycles (1st cycle — dotted line; 2nd cycle — continuous line). Cracks are preferentially oriented at 15° to X-axis; $\sigma_x = 40$ MPa, $\sigma_y = 30$ MPa. Memory effect pressure in the first cycle ($P_* = 32$ MPa) and maximum pressure of the first cycle ($P_{max} = 40$ MPa) are marked

principal stresses is constant, P_* is linear dependent on the other principal stress:

$$P_* = A_1 \sigma_x + B_1 \qquad (2)$$

if $\sigma_y = $ const and

$$P_* = A_2 \sigma_y + B_2 \qquad (3)$$

if $\sigma_x = $ const. Coefficients A_1 and B_1 are functions of angle φ and stress σ_y. Coefficients A_2 and B_2 are functions of angle φ and stress σ_x.

In case the ratio σ_y/σ_x is constant, the value of P_* is proportional to one of the rock stresses (σ_y or σ_x). The coefficient of proportionality depends on crack orientation and the value of the ratio σ_y/σ_x:

$$P_*/\sigma_y = C\left[\frac{1}{1-(1-\sigma_y/\sigma_x)^2} - 1\right] + 1 \qquad (4)$$

where C depends on φ, e.g. for $\varphi = 25°$ $C = 0.58$, for $\varphi = 65°$ $C = 0.65$.

4 SIMULATION OF CYCLIC LOADING OF BOREHOLE WALLS

Experiments in situ show that cyclic loading of borehole walls with a pressuremeter is accompanied by memory effects. Emission activity increases abruptly when pressure reaches the maximum pressure value of the previous cycle (Lord & Koerner 1985).

To simulate this phenomenon, computer experiments were set up consisting of four stages. The first three simulation stages were the same as earlier. The fourth was similar to the third but the maximum pressure value was higher. Thus, two cycles of loading the borehole walls were simulated in all: the first one as the third simulation stage and the second one as the fourth.

The fourth stage was carried out in the same gradated way as the third, so that «emission activity versus pressure» dependences were obtained.

Simulation has shown that emission activity is zero while pressure is lower than the maximum pressure value of the previous cycle P_{max}. As soon as the value P_{max} is exceeded, stable increase in activity begins. Starting with that point, the emission curve looks like a continuation of the third cycle emission curve (Figure 4). This means that in this ideal case $P'_* = P_{max}$ in the second borehole wall loading cycle, i.e. the felicity ratio of the in situ rock is about 1.0. Here, P'_* is the pressure value of the memory effect in the second loading cycle.

The results obtained are independent of the crack orientation type. Both by random and preferential crack orientation, memory effects take place when cyclically loading borehole walls with a pressuremeter. The independence of the cracking features makes this result especially interesting for practical use.

5 STABILITY OF SIMULATION RESULTS

The results above were obtained for the following values of simulation parameters: initial crack length $L = 0.005$ m; critical stress intensity factor $K_{Ic} = 1.0$ MPa·m$^{1/2}$; $\zeta = 1.0$; crack number in the area of radius 0.5m $N = 500$. It is of interest to know to what extent the simulation results depend on the simulation parameters.

Computer experiments for different values of L, K_{Ic}, ζ, and N were set up to clear up this point. It has been found out that varying L, K_{Ic}, and ζ does not influence emission curves and the value of P_*. This is easy to explain because tensile crack length is defined by the shear stress value only. A tensile crack restarts propagating as soon as the maximum previous shear stress on the corresponding initial crack plane is exceeded. This condition is fulfilled (or not fulfilled) independently of parameter values.

Another case is the total initial crack number. Computer experiments for N ranging from 200 to 1000 have shown that the emission curve shape is influenced by varying N, but the pressure value P_*, at which stable activity growth begins, remains constant. Hence, the choosen value $N = 500$ is quite representative.

Stability of the simulation results allows us to consider them as a basis for developing new stress measurement techniques.

6 DISCUSSION

Based on the simulation results, two methods can be offered to estimate absolute values of geostresses using memory effects in rocks around a borehole.

It is possible to determine one of the principal stresses if another one is known. The former can be obtained using linear correlation with the memory effect pressure (see equations (2) and (3)).

Another approach can be used when the ratio of principal stresses is known. Their absolute values are directly proportional to the memory effect pressure (see equation (4)).

In both cases, supplementary geological information is needed to find out absolute values of principal stresses in situ. Another way is to use cyclic loading of borehole walls to estimate the rock condition on the whole. If the rock is little damaged, there will be a conventional memory effect (see Figure 4, continuous line) in each cycle at the pressure corresponding to the previous cycle's maximum pressure, as described earlier. In this case, the felicity ratio is about 1.0. The more fractured the rock, the worse its memory, and the lower the felicity ratio. Observing the Kaiser effect in two successive loading cycles with maximum pressure in the second cycle higher than in the first would allow to calculate the felicity ratio and to make conclusion about the overall rock state.

ACKNOWLEDGEMENTS

The authors would like to thank Dr.C.Li (Lulea University of Technology) for his useful discussion. The authors are sincerely grateful to Mt.Christopher Schmich for correcting the language and to Mrs.Olga Lavrova for her help in preparing the manuscript. The support of the International Soros Science Education Program (ISSEP), the Russian Foundation for Basic Research (RFBR project 95-05-14224) and the Acoustical Society of America is gratefully appreciated.

REFERENCES

Deutsch, W.L., R.M.Koerner & A.E.Lord 1989. Determination of prestress of in situ soils using acoustic emissions. *J.Geotech.Engrg.* 115(2): 228-245.

Lord, A.E., Jr. & R.M.Koerner 1985. Field determination of prestress (existing stress) in soil and rock masses using acoustic emission. *J.Acoustic Emission* 4(2/3):S11-S16.

Shkuratnik, V.L. & A.V.Lavrov 1995. Memory effects in rock. *J.Mining Science* 31(1):20-28.

Yamshchikov, V.S., V.L.Shkuratnik & A.V.Lavrov 1996. On the theoretical model of the Kaiser effect in rocks at different stages of loading. *Proc. Forum Acusticum 1996 - 1st Conv. of EAA. Acustica/Acta Acuctica* 82 (Suppl.1):S251.

Yamshchikov V.S., V.L.Shkuratnik, K.G.Lykov & V.M.Farafonov 1991. Rock stress state estimation on the basis of emission memory effects in rocks around a borehole. *Physico-Technical Problems of Mining* 27(2):26-29 (in Russian).

Three-dimensional simulation of memory effects in rock samples

A.V. Lavrov
Moscow State Mining University, Russia

ABSTRACT: Three-dimensional numerical simulation of emission memory effects in rocks was carried out using a theoretical model based on linear fracture mechanics. Two loading cycles were simulated. The first is axisymmetric compression, the second is uniaxial compression in the direction inclined at an angle to the axis of the maximum stress of the first cycle. New features of the memory effects under triaxial stress state were obtained. Dependence of the memory effects on the loading direction in the testing cycle was investigated. Conclusions are made on the preferable friction parameter values as well as on the effect features under triaxial stress state relevant for application of the memory effects to estimate geostresses.

1 INTRODUCTION

Memory effects take place when rock is loaded cyclically with the stress magnitude increasing from cycle to cycle. The effects consist in an abrupt increment of acoustic and electromagnetic emission activities when the stress reaches the maximum value of the previous cycle.

Although many experimental studies have been made on memory effects, especially memory effect in acoustic emission called the Kaiser effect (e.g. Yoshikawa & Mogi 1981, Rzhevskij et al. 1983, Holcomb 1983, Panasiyan et al. 1990, Li & Nordlund 1993), it is still very rare that these effects are used to measure rock stresses. The main difficulty here is that in situ rocks are usually under a triaxial stress state. In the laboratory test, they are reloaded uniaxially. Besides, the directions of principal stresses (principal axes) are often unknown, so that the laboratory test is carried out in a direction different from any of the original principal axes in the rock mass.

Some theoretical efforts have been made earlier to build a theoretical 2D-model based on the concept of wing-cracks (Kuwahara et al. 1990, Shkuratnik & Lavrov 1995, Yamshchikov et al. 1996a and 1996b, Li 1996). However, a two-dimensional model does not allow us to simulate memory effects under a triaxial stress state. The three-dimensional models offered before (Holcomb 1993, Li 1996) were qualitative and could not be used for numerical computer simulation of the effects.

The purpose of the study was to investigate theoretically features of memory effects under a triaxial axisymmetric stress state by means of computer simulation of the effects using a three-dimensional model based on linear crack mechanics.

2 THEORETICAL MODEL AND SIMULATION SETUP

Before original loading (1st cycle, "in situ", pre-loading), the rock is supposed to contain initial cracks. Each initial crack is a thin disk-like cut of radius a. The coefficient of friction between crack faces is μ. Distances between cracks are large enough so that cracks do not interact while loading.

Orientation of each crack is defined by three angles α, β, and γ between a normal to the crack plane and the directions of principal stresses (prestresses) in the 1st cycle σ_1^I, σ_2^I, and σ_3^I accordingly (I corresponds to the first loading cycle). Hereinafter, the three directions of the 1st cycle principal stresses are identified by three unit vectors $\vec{e}_1^I$, $\vec{e}_2^I$, $\vec{e}_3^I$.

Cracks were assumed to be oriented chaotically, α and β were random values ranging from 0 to 90°.

Two loading cycles were simulated. The first is "in situ" axisymmetric or uniaxial loading ("pre-loading"). The second is uniaxial laboratory loading ("testing loading" with measurement of acoustic and electromagnetic emissions). Uniaxial loading in the second cycle is conducted in the direction that makes angles α_1, β_1, and γ_1 with the unit vectors $\vec{e}_1^I$, $\vec{e}_2^I$, and $\vec{e}_3^I$. In the 1st cycle, the absolute value of normal stress on the plane of an initial crack is given by

$$|\vec{p}_n^I| = \sigma_1^I \cos^2\alpha + \sigma_2^I \cos^2\beta + \sigma_3^I \cos^2\gamma. \quad (1)$$

Shear stress on the same plane is expressed by

$$|\vec{p}_\tau^I| = [(\sigma_1^I)^2 \cos^2\alpha \sin^2\alpha + (\sigma_2^I)^2 \cos^2\beta \sin^2\beta +$$
$$+ (\sigma_3^I)^2 \cos^2\gamma \sin^2\gamma - 2\sigma_1^I \sigma_2^I \cos^2\alpha \cos^2\beta -$$
$$- 2\sigma_2^I \sigma_3^I \cos^2\beta \cos^2\gamma -$$
$$- 2\sigma_1^I \sigma_3^I \cos^2\alpha \cos^2\gamma]^{1/2}. \quad (2)$$

Shear direction over the initial crack plane is defined by the unit vector

$$\vec{e}_\tau^I = \vec{e}_1^I \cos\alpha \frac{\sigma_1^I \sin^2\alpha - \sigma_2^I \cos^2\beta - \sigma_3^I \cos^2\gamma}{|\vec{p}_\tau^I|} +$$
$$+ \vec{e}_2^I \cos\beta \frac{\sigma_2^I \sin^2\beta - \sigma_1^I \cos^2\alpha - \sigma_3^I \cos^2\gamma}{|\vec{p}_\tau^I|} +$$
$$+ \vec{e}_3^I \cos\gamma \frac{\sigma_3^I \sin^2\gamma - \sigma_1^I \cos^2\alpha - \sigma_2^I \cos^2\beta}{|\vec{p}_\tau^I|}. \quad (3)$$

The stress intensity factor on the contour of the initial crack is given by

$$K_{II} = 2|\vec{p}_{eff}^I|\sqrt{\frac{a}{\pi}}, \quad (4)$$

where

$$|\vec{p}_{eff}^I| = |\vec{p}_\tau^I| - \mu|\vec{p}_n^I| \quad (5)$$

is effective shear stress.

If for an initial crack condition $K_{II} \geq K_{IIc}$ is fulfilled in the 1st cycle, two tensile cracks (wing-cracks) appear on its contour (Figure 1)

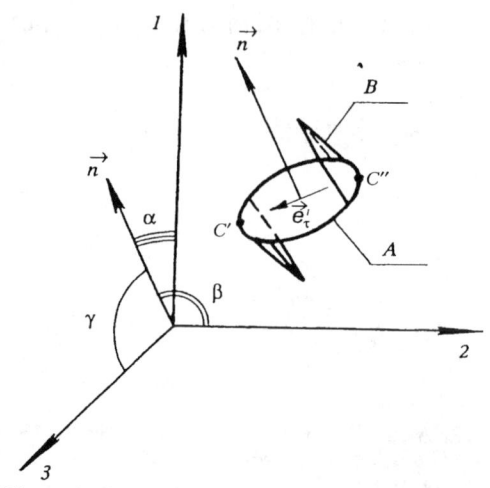

Figure 1. Initial disk-like crack (A) with two tensile cracks (B): 1, 2, 3 — axes of principal stresses of the first cycle σ_1^I, σ_2^I, σ_3^I

(Adams & Sines 1978, Dyskin et al. 1995). The wing-cracks arise from two diametrically opposite points C' and C''; diameter $C'C''$ is parallel to $\vec{e}_\tau^I$ (Figure 1). Length of the tensile cracks after completing the 1st loading cycle is determined by the value of $|\vec{p}_{eff}^I|$ reached in this cycle.

In the 2nd loading cycle, the stress tensor is given by

$$T_\sigma =$$

$$= \begin{Vmatrix} \sigma_1^{II}\cos^2\alpha_1 & \sigma_1^{II}\cos\alpha_1\cos\beta_1 & \sigma_1^{II}\cos\alpha_1\cos\gamma_1 \\ \sigma_1^{II}\cos\alpha_1\cos\beta_1 & \sigma_1^{II}\cos^2\beta_1 & \sigma_1^{II}\cos\beta_1\cos\gamma_1 \\ \sigma_1^{II}\cos\alpha_1\cos\gamma_1 & \sigma_1^{II}\cos\beta_1\cos\gamma_1 & \sigma_1^{II}\cos^2\gamma_1 \end{Vmatrix}. \quad (6)$$

where σ_1^{II} is the uniaxial compressive stress in the 2nd cycle, and II is the cycle number.

Normal stress acting on initial crack plane in the 2nd cycle is given by

$$|\vec{p}_n^{II}| = \sigma_1^{II} \cdot B^2 \quad (7)$$

where

$$B = \cos\alpha \cos\alpha_1 + \cos\beta \cos\beta_1 + \cos\gamma \cos\gamma_1. \quad (8)$$

Shear stress is

$$|\vec{p}_\tau^{II}| = \sigma_1^{II} B(1-B^2)^{1/2}. \quad (9)$$

The vector of full stress is given by

$$\vec{p}^{II} = \sigma_1^{II} B(\vec{e}_1^{I} \cos\alpha_1 + \vec{e}_2^{I} \cos\beta_1 + \vec{e}_3^{I} \cos\gamma_1). \quad (10)$$

The unit vector in the shear direction over the plane of an initial crack in the 2nd cycle is given by

$$\vec{e}_\tau^{II} = \vec{e}_1^{I} \frac{\cos\alpha_1 - B\cos\alpha}{(1-B^2)^{1/2}} + \vec{e}_2^{I} \frac{\cos\beta_1 - B\cos\beta}{(1-B^2)^{1/2}} +$$

$$+ \vec{e}_3^{I} \frac{\cos\gamma_1 - B\cos\gamma}{(1-B^2)^{1/2}} . \quad (11)$$

There are three cases possible for a crack in the 2nd cycle:
1. No wing-cracks appeared in the 1st cycle (condition $K_{II} \geq K_{IIc}$ was not fulfilled). Then in the 2nd cycle, wings do not arise while $K_{II} < K_{IIc}$. As soon as K_{II} exceeds K_{IIc}, two tensile cracks appear on the initial crack contour, and acoustic/electromagnetic emissions begin. K_{II} is here expressed through (4), where $|\vec{p}_{eff}^{I}|$ is to be replaced by $|\vec{p}_{eff}^{II}|$. The latter is defined in the same way as $|\vec{p}_{eff}^{I}|$ (see eq. (5)).
2. Tensile cracks appeared on the contour of the initial crack in the 1st cycle, and projection of the full stress in the 2nd cycle onto the shear direction of the 1st cycle is negative: $(\vec{p}^{II} \cdot \vec{e}_\tau^{I}) < 0$.

Tensile cracks, which appeared in the 1st cycle, close in the 2nd cycle because the 2nd cycle full stress does not have a positive component in the 1st cycle shear direction. The condition for new wing-cracks to arise in the 2nd cycle is $K_{II} \geq K_{IIc}$, where K_{II} is defined in the same way as earlier. This is also a condition for acoustic and electromagnetic emissions to begin from this crack.
3. Tensile cracks appeared from the initial crack in the 1st cycle, and the condition $(\vec{p}^{II} \cdot \vec{e}_\tau^{I}) > 0$ is fulfilled in the 2nd cycle.

In this case, effective shear stress has a positive component in the displacement direction of the 1st cycle given by

$$(\vec{p}_{eff}^{II} \cdot \vec{e}_\tau^{I}) = |\vec{p}_{eff}^{II}|(\vec{e}_\tau^{I} \cdot \vec{e}_\tau^{II}), \quad (12)$$

where $\vec{e}_\tau^{I}$ and $\vec{e}_\tau^{II}$ are defined by (3) and (11) respectively. This component causes mutual shear of the initial crack faces and reopening of the existing tensile cracks. The condition for the tensile cracks to restart propagating in the 2nd cycle is given by

$$(\vec{p}_{eff}^{II} \cdot \vec{e}_\tau^{I}) \geq |\vec{p}_{eff}^{I}|, \quad (13)$$

As soon as this condition is fulfilled, acoustic and electromagnetic emissions from the tensile cracks begin in the 2nd cycle.

Note that propagation of the tensile cracks is assumed to be the only reason for acoustic and electromagnetic emissions in our model. Friction processes between initial crack faces are not considered as a possible emission mechanism. It should be also noted that crack growth and emission restart are connected with the 1st cycle maximum stresses only for crack type 3. Tensile cracks of types 1 and 2 are new and start growing in the 2nd cycle as soon as the condition $K_{II} \geq K_{IIc}$ is fulfilled on the contour of the corresponding disk-like crack. This condition has no connexion with the 1st cycle stresses.

In the course of the computer simulation, a rock sample containing 1000 initial cracks was supposed to be loaded by stresses σ_1^{I} and $\sigma_2^{I} = \sigma_3^{I}$ in the 1st cycle. For each crack in the 1st cycle, it was determined whether the condition $K_{II} \geq K_{IIc}$ was fulfilled. Initial cracks giving wings in the 1st cycle were memorized.

The values of μ and K_{IIc} were assumed to be equal for all cracks (friction and strength homogenity).

The 2nd loading cycle was simulated by steps: testing uniaxial stress σ_1^{II} was increased from zero to its maximum value in equal steps (normally 1MPa). At each stress level for each crack, its type was determined (1, 2, or 3). Then growth conditions were checked for each crack according to its type. The total number of propagating cracks was calculated at each stress level. This number W was assumed to be a measure of emission activity at the given stress. As a result, dependences for emission activity versus testing stress in the 2nd cycle were obtained for various combinations of the principal prestresses and for different loading directions in the 2nd cycle.

3 SIMULATION RESULTS

In the case that the rock was loaded uniaxially in the 1st cycle, emission memory effects in the 2nd one appear at $\sigma_{1*}^{II} = \sigma_1^I$ (loading in the 2nd cycle in the direction of σ_1^I). Here σ_{1*}^{II} indicates the uniaxial stress value at which memory effect takes place in the 2nd cycle. Further in this paper, σ_{1*}^{II} is called the memory effect stress. If the rock was uniaxially loaded in the 1st cycle, emission activity is zero at $\sigma_1^{II} < \sigma_{1*}^{II} = \sigma_1^I$ in the second. At $\sigma_1^{II} = \sigma_{1*}^{II}$ there is an activity jump from $W = 0$ to $W = 672$ which remains constant during further increase of σ_1^{II}.

More interesting and more important from the practical point of view are simulation results for axisymmetric loading in the 1st cycle ($\sigma_1^I > \sigma_2^I = \sigma_3^I > 0$). In this case, memory effect takes place in the 2nd cycle only if σ_1^I in the 1st cycle exceeded a certain threshold value

$$\sigma_{1t}^I = (k+1)\sigma_2^I, \qquad (14)$$

where

$$k = \frac{2\mu}{(1+\mu)^{1/2} - \mu}. \qquad (15)$$

If the threshold was not exceeded in the 1st cycle, emission activity is high from the beginning of the uniaxial loading in the 2nd cycle, and there are no characteristic points on the emission curve $W = f(\sigma_1^{II})$. Of course, this does not mean that there is no memory in this case. It only means that the memory can not be displayed in a uniaxial test. If the 2nd cycle were carried out with non-zero confining stress equal to that in the 1st cycle ($\sigma_2^{II} = \sigma_2^I > 0$), there would be a memory effect at $\sigma_{1*}^{II} = \sigma_1^I$.

Hence, if a rock sample extracted out of a rock mass does not have the Kaiser effect in a uniaxial laboratory test, it does not mean that the rock stress state in situ was hydrostatic ($\sigma_1^I = \sigma_2^I = \sigma_3^I$). It only indicates that σ_1^I was below the threshold level σ_{1t}^I.

If the condition $\sigma_1^I > \sigma_{1t}^I$ was fulfilled in the 1st cycle, there is a memory effect when reloading the sample in the direction of σ_1^I in the 2nd cycle. Emission curve shape strongly depends on the value of K_{IIc} (Figure 2). The

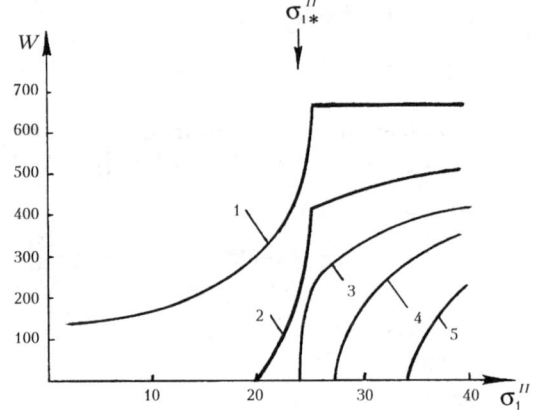

Figure 2. Dependences of emission activity measure on uniaxial compressive stress in the 2nd cycle for $K_{IIc} = 0$ (curve 1), $K_{IIc} = 0.2$ MPa·m$^{1/2}$ (curve 2), $K_{IIc} = 0.32$ MPa·m$^{1/2}$ (curve 3), $K_{IIc} = 0.4$ MPa·m$^{1/2}$ (curve 4), $K_{IIc} = 0.5$ MPa·m$^{1/2}$ (curve 5); $\sigma_1^I = 40$ MPa, $\sigma_2^I = \sigma_3^I = 5$ MPa, $\mu = 0.58$ for each curve

higher K_{IIc}, the lower the emission activity at lower stress values (at $\sigma_1^{II} < \sigma_{1*}^{II}$). But independent of the K_{IIc}-value, there is a characteristic point on each curve. The value of K_{IIc} may be chosen in such a way that emission activity is zero at $\sigma_1^{II} < \sigma_{1*}^{II}$, and there is an activity jump at $\sigma_1^{II} = \sigma_{1*}^{II}$ (curve 3 in Figure 2). This emission curve form is quite close to what is observed experimentally. Note that varying K_{IIc} does not influence the value of σ_{1*}^{II} (characteristic point). It allows us to choose the most convenient value of K_{IIc} for each combination of σ_1^I, σ_2^I.

The shape of the emission curve is also influenced by the coefficient of friction. Emission activity at $\sigma_1^{II} < \sigma_{1*}^{II}$ is lower in rocks with lower μ. If $\mu = 0$, there is zero activity at $\sigma_1^{II} < \sigma_{1*}^{II}$. In this case, memory effect takes place at $\sigma_{1*}^{II} = \sigma_1^I - \sigma_2^I$, which has been observed in some experiments (Hughson & Crawford 1987). Increasing μ is accompanied by increasing background emission activity at $\sigma_1^{II} < \sigma_{1*}^{II}$. The emission at lower stress hinders the display of memory effect at σ_{1*}^{II}.

Hence, rocks with lower friction are preferable to use the Kaiser effect.

Another influence of μ is that the memory effect stress is dependent on μ. The higher μ, the lower σ_{1*}^{II} for the same values of σ_1^I and σ_2^I. This is another reason why rocks with lower μ are more convenient to estimate prestresses on the basis of the Kaiser effect.

Computer experiments for various σ_1^I and σ_2^I have shown that if testing loading in the 2nd cycle is performed in the direction of σ_1^I, the memory effect stress is connected with the prestresses as follows:

$$\sigma_{1*}^{II} = (\sigma_1^I - \sigma_2^I) - k\sigma_2^I. \tag{16}$$

The equation is in complete agreement with experiment (Holcomb 1983, Holcomb & Martin 1985, Li & Nordlund 1993, Li 1996).

Uniaxial laboratory test with emission registration allows us to obtain only the right part of (16). Additional tests with non-zero confining stress σ_2^{II} do not give more information. The values σ_1^I and σ_2^I can be obtained only if the ratio $\lambda = \sigma_2^I/\sigma_1^I$ in situ is known. Then

$$\sigma_1^I = \frac{\sigma_{1*}^{II}}{1 - k(\lambda + 1)} \tag{17}$$

where σ_{1*}^{II} is the memory effect stress measured in the uniaxial test in the lab.

It was interesting to study how emission memory effects depend on the loading direction in the 2nd cycle. To determine this, two loading cycles were simulated. In the first one, rock was loaded with stress state $\sigma_1^I = 50$ MPa, $\sigma_2^I = \sigma_3^I = 10$ MPa (axisymmetric). Stress state in the 2nd cycle was uniaxial as earlier, but the loading was conducted at a non-zero angle α_1 to the σ_1^I-direction.

It was established that memory effects get worse when the angle between the axes of σ_1^{II} and σ_1^I is increased.

In rocks with lower friction ($\mu = 0.1 ... 0.2$), the effect exists for $0 \leq \alpha_1 \leq 5°$ and disappears at higher values of α_1.

In rocks with moderate friction ($\mu \approx 0.5$), the effect takes place for $0 \leq \alpha_1 \leq 7...8°$. Increasing α_1 leads to slightly rising σ_{1*}^{II}.

In rocks with $\mu \approx 0.7$, memory effects are to be observed up to $\alpha_1 = 10...12°$. But the memory effect stress σ_{1*}^{II} strongly depends on α_1: for $\alpha_1 = 0...5°$ $\sigma_{1*}^{II} = 13$ MPa, for $\alpha_1 = 10°$ $\sigma_{1*}^{II} = 16$ MPa, for $\alpha_1 = 13°$ $\sigma_{1*}^{II} = 23$ MPa.

Increasing μ leads to that background emission activity at $\sigma_1^{II} < \sigma_{1*}^{II}$ rises, and activity at $\sigma_1^{II} > \sigma_{1*}^{II}$ decreases.

Thus, in rocks with higher friction it is possible to observe the memory effects in a wider range of α_1. But the value of σ_{1*}^{II} obtained in this way is not representative because it may be up to twice as big as the real σ_{1*}^{II}-value measured in the direction of σ_1^I. This is one more reason why rocks with lower friction are better for estimating in situ stresses on the basis of the memory effects.

4 CONCLUSIONS

Simulation results allow us to make the following conclusions on the memory of the axisymmetric stress state:

1. For a given confining stress, there is a threshold value of axial stress to be revealed in a uniaxial test. The threshold axial stress is proportional to the confining pressure. If axial stress did not exceed the threshold level in the pre-loading cycle, there is no Kaiser effect in the uniaxial testing cycle.

2. Rocks with lower friction are more suitable for using memory effects to estimate prestresses in because of: a) lower threshold level; b) lower emission activity at the beginning of the testing loading; c) higher value of the memory effect stress for the same prestresses; d) lower error when testing the rock uniaxially in the direction different from the maximum stress axis in situ.

3. The critical stress intensity factor influences the shape of the emission curve in the testing cycle but not the stress value at which memory effect takes place.

4. Memory effect strongly depends on the direction of uniaxial loading in the testing cycle. Rocks with higher friction indicate memory effects for a wider range of the angle

between reloading direction and the principal axis of the maximum prestress, but memorized stress in this case may be strongly different from the real memory effect stress.

The next step in the theoretical research on the memory effects in rocks would be simulation with axisymmetric loading both in the 1st and in the 2nd cycles as well as investigation of memory under triaxial stress state with all different principal prestresses.

ACKNOWLEDGEMENTS

The work was supported through the International Soros Science Education Program (ISSEP) and the Acoustical Society of America (ASA). The author is grateful to Prof.Dr.Chkouratnik for his useful discussions. The author would like to thank Mr.Christopher Schmich for correcting the language and Mrs.Olga Lavrova for her help at preparing the manuscript.

REFERENCES

Adams, M. & G.Sines 1978. Crack extension from flaws in a brittle material subjected to compression. *Tectonophysics* 49(1/2):97-118.

Dyskin, A.V., L.N.Germanovich, R.J.Jewell, H.Joer, J.S.Krasinski, K.K.Lee, J.-C.Roegiers, E.Sahouryeh & K.Ustinov 1995. Some experimental results on three-dimensional crack propagation in compression. In H.-P.Rossmanith (Ed.), *Mech. Jointed & Faulted Rock*: 91-96. Rotterdam: A.A.Balkema.

Holcomb, D.J. 1983. Using acoustic emission to determine in-situ stresses: problems and promise. *Proc. Appl.Mech., Bioengng & Fluids Engng Conf.*:11-21.Houston.

Holcomb, D.J. 1993. Observation of the Kaiser effect under multiaxial stress states: implications for its use in determining in situ stress. *Geoph.Res.Letts.* 20(19): 2119-2122.

Holcomb, D.J. & R.J.Martin III 1985. Determining peak stress history using acoustic emissions. In E.Ashworth (Ed.), *Proc. 26th US Symp.Rock Mech. (Research and Engineering Applications in Rock Masses)*, v.2: 715-722.

Hughson, D.R. & A.M.Crawford 1987. Kaiser effect gauging: the influence of confining stress on its response. In G.Herget & S.Vongpaisal (Eds.), *Proc.6th Int.Congr.Rock Mech.*, v.2: 981-985. Rotterdam: A.A.Balkema.

Kuwahara, Y., K.Yamamoto & T.Hirasawa 1990. An experimental and theoretical study of inelastic deformation of brittle rocks under cyclic uniaxial loading. *Tohoku Geoph.J.* 33(1): 1-21.

Li, C. 1996. A theory for the Kaiser effect in rock and its potential applications. *Proc.6th Conf.Acoustic Emission/Microseismic Activity in Geological Structures & Materials:* 13 pp.

Li, C. & E.Nordlund 1993. Experimental verification of the Kaiser effect in rocks. *Rock Mech.Rock Engng* 26(4): 333-351.

Panasiyan, L.L., S.A.Kolegov & A.N.Morgunov 1990. Stress memory studies in rocks by means of acoustic emission. In H.-P.Rossmanith (Ed.), *Mech.Jointed & Faulted Rock:* 435-439. Rotterdam: A.A.Balkema.

Rzhevskij, V.V., V.S.Yamshchikov, V.L.Shkuratnik, V.M.Farafonov & K.G.Lykov 1983. Emission memory effects in rocks. *Doklady AN SSSR (DAN SSSR)* 273(5): 1094-1097 (in Russian).

Shkuratnik, V.L. & A.V.Lavrov 1995. Memory effects in rock. *J.Mining Science* 31(1):20-28.

Yamshchikov, V.S., V.L.Shkuratnik & A.V.Lavrov 1996a. On the theoretical model of the Kaiser effect in rocks at different stages of loading. *Proc. Forum Acusticum 1996 - 1st Conv. of EAA. Acustica/Acta Acustica* 82 (Suppl.1):S251.

Yamshchikov, V.S., V.L.Shkuratnik & A.V.Lavrov 1996b. Akustische Nachwirkung von Gesteinen bei geodynamischen Erscheinungen. *Gluckauf-Forschungshefte* 57(1): 18-19 (in German).

Yoshikawa, S. & K.Mogi 1981. A new method for estimation of the crustal stress from cored rock samples: laboratory study in the case of uniaxial compression. *Tectonophysics* 74(3/4): 323-339.

Interpretation of rock stresses

Interpretation of stress measurements in a Provence mine using a block modelling

F. Homand & M. Souley
LEGO, Ecole Nationale Supérieure de Géologie, Vandoeuvre-lès-Nancy, France

ABSTRACT : This study examines an interpretation of *in situ* stress measurements carried out in a *Provence* mine using a numerical modelling. Based on the geological setting and assumptions about historical tectonics, a large numerical model is developed. Calculations lead to a better explanation of stress distribution in the *Arc* syncline. Predicted magnitudes and orientations of natural stresses are in agreement with those measured.

1 INTRODUCTION

Natural stresses in rock masses are of considerable importance for determining the stability conditions of an underground excavation and depend on rock anisotropy, fracturing, tectonic history, topography, lithology, *etc*. All these factors are present in the region that we studied. It is a coal belt located in the *Arc* syncline in *Provence* (Southern France) where the HBCM company mines lignite at great depths. Numerous geological studies have been conducted in this region and detailed structural data are now available. *In situ* stress measurements using flat jack and hydraulic fracturing are available for this site. The stress measurements indicate that two different stress states can be distinguished: an isotropic state in the N-E and an anisotropic state in the southern.

The main objective of this paper is to explain the stress deviation towards the N-E currently observed using a numerical modelling based on the Distinct Element concept. A large scale numerical model including the major geological structures is developed and loaded on the basis of assumptions about the four recent tectonic events which have successively taken place in the Provencal area. The special feature of the study is that : in spite of the fact that the mechanical characteristics of faults are unavailable and magnitudes of tectonic stresses are prior unknown, it is possible to explain the natural stress distribution in this *Provence* mine. Numerical analyses described here were conducted using the two-dimensional UDEC code.

2 GEOLOGICAL SETTING

The *Arc* basin forms a 70-km-long syncline elongated from east to west ; from north to south it is 12 km wide. This asymmetric syncline is strongly affected by a dome-shaped anticline . The structure is overridden by a major thrust sheet overthrusting (Etoile unit, Fig. 1) due to the general N-S shortening which is the major tectonic event of the geological history of the region. In the eastern part of the *Arc* syncline, there are four major geological structures (1) The Etoile unit, which is an allochthonous unit, covers the meridional boundary of the basin and overthrusts the Regaignas dome.(2)The Diote fault, limiting the para-autochthonous wedge of *Gardanne*, brings the para-autochthonous unit and the autochthonous unit into contact.(3) The Meyreuil fault is a transverse fault crossing the basin from north to south and shaping a broken line formed of segments oriented N0° and N30-40°E.(4) The Regaignas dome, an autochthonous unit located on the meridional boundary of the *Arc* syncline, is a fold resulting from the *pyreneo-provencal* period and is the only visible part of the syncline bedrock.

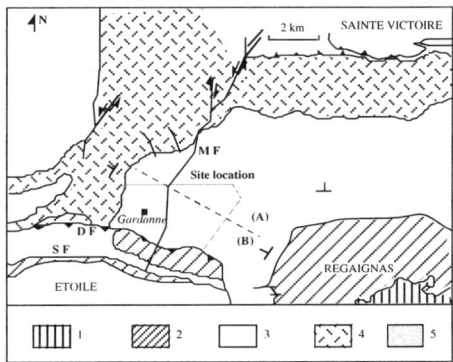

1 : Portlandian, 2 : Valdonian-Fuvelian, 3 : Begudian-Rognacian
4 : Eocene, 5 : Oligocene *MF* : Meyreuil fault, *DF* : Diote Fault *SF* : Safre fault

Fig.1-Geological map (Gaviglio *et al.* 1996).

The *Arc* syncline is essentially made up of superior Cretaceous and Eocene formations. Above the coal seam, the overburden is made up of Fuvelian, Begudian, Rognacian and Eocene, below the Fuvelian, lie Cretaceous and Jurassic. The investigated zone lies in the para-autochthonous wedge of *Gardanne,* just in front of the tectonic thrust wedge and bounded by Diote fault and Meyreuil fault.

Four major recent tectonic events took place successively in the Provencal area : (1) a N-S compression during the Eocene characterized by the positioning of the large overthrusts, (2) an extension dating from the Oligocene period, from which the effects are particularly marked in the Regaignas unit, (3) an ENE-WSW compression during the inferior Miocene period, and (4) a N-S compression starting from the superior Miocene period.

3 STRESS MEASUREMENTS

Several *in situ* measurements of the natural stresses were carried out in *Provence* colliery using first the flat jack method and later, the hydraulic fracturing. The synthetic results are shown in Table 1. The vertical stress is significantly smaller than the theoretical value calculated on the basis of the weight of overburden. No explanation for this difference has yet been found. Moreover, the ratio between the vertical stress and the weight of overburden ranges from 0.40 to 0.87.

The stress measurements show that the major principal stress is always horizontal and corresponds to the maximum horizontal stress, whereas the intermediate stress is almost vertical. The stress σ_1 is two to four times larger than σ_3. Except for sites ⑥ and ⑧, the stress σ_3 represents the minimum horizontal stress σ_h. It should be noticed that except for site ⑨, the orientation of the major principal stress (σ_1) varies between N40°E and N104°E.

Table 1 - Provence coalfield. Results of the natural stress measurements (*after* Gaviglio *et al.* 1996). F.J.: flat jack ; H.F.: hydraulic fracturing. $\gamma = 0.025$ MN/m^3.

Sector	Site n°	Method	Depth(m)	$\sigma_V/\gamma*z$	$\sigma_h/\gamma*z$	$\sigma_H/\gamma*z$
A	①	F.J.	390	0.82	0.72	0.82
A	②	F.J.	390	0.67	0.31	0.67
B	③	F.J.	700	0.40	0.14	0.91
B	④	F.J.	550	0.73	0.36	1.38
B	⑤	H.F.	700	0.63	0.91	1.71
B	⑥	H.F.	900	0.53	0.76	1.78
B	⑦	H.F.	1030	0.74	0.62	1.24
B	⑧	H.F.	1140	0.70	0.81	1.09
B	⑨	H.F.	1200	0.67	0.60	0.73
B	⑩	H.F.	1130	0.71	0.53	1.59
B	⑪	H.F.	1260	0.87	0.63	1.08

Moreover, there is a clear opposition in stress distribution between the sectors A and B (fig. 1). In sector B the stress state is strongly anisotropic with an E-W towards NE-SW direction. In sector A the stress is approximately isotropic.

The principal stress magnitudes and orientations vary from one site to another one. These stress heterogeneities are due to differences in mechanical properties from one bed to another.

4 - NUMERICAL MODELLING

Numerical modelling is of great importance in geology for understanding displacement, stress and strain phenomena, and even fault formation (Rosengren and Stephansson 1993, Homand *et al.* 1997, *etc.*). The modelling that we undertake must be viewed in this general framework. It consists of explaining the natural stress distribution in the *Arc* syncline which is characterized by the presence of major discontinuities (Meyreuil, Safre and Diote faults, layers limits) and affected by major tectonic events. This justifies the choice of UDEC.

4.1 Model and loading sequence

Only one numerical model is performed because of the major part of the stress measurements was 1030-1260 m depth (Table 1). This model is based on a horizontal cross section which is 1100 m deep. The geometrical model is about 27 km long, 22 km wide (Fig. 2) and involves all the major structures in the southern part of the *Arc* where the regional N-S compression prevails.

Based on geological assumptions, the geometrical model is loaded according to the four recent tectonic events. The involved tectonic events are successively : a N-S compression corresponding to the Eocene period and represented in Fig. 3(a), an E-W extension corresponding to the Oligocene (Fig. 3b), an ENE-WSW compression during the lower Miocene (Fig. 3c) and N-S compression during the upper Miocene period (Fig. 3d).

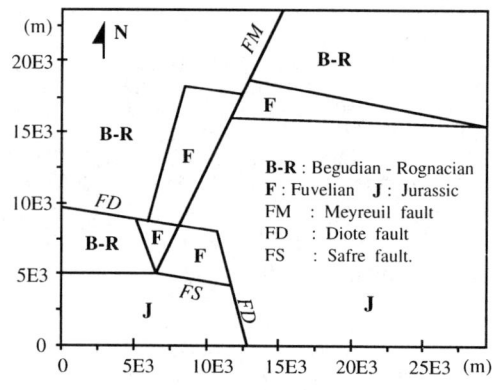

Fig.2 - Geometry of the model.

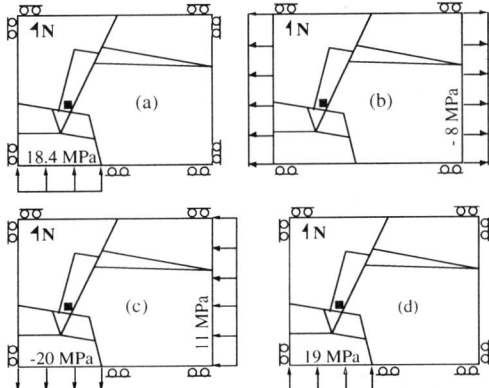

Fig. 3 - Loading involving tectonic history.
(a) - N-S compression during the Eocene period,
(b) - E-W extension dated from the Oligocene period,
(c) - ENE-WSW compression during the lower Miocene,
(d) - N-S compression starting from the upper Miocene.

The modelling sequences are : *firstly*, the model is consolidated under the initial and boundary stresses based on the gravity and the stresses due to the weight of overburden in order to produce the initial *in situ* stress field prior to any tectonic event, *secondly*, the four tectonic events are successively applied.

4.2 Choice of materials and joints characteristics

Table 2 and Table 3 summarize the elastic properties of rocks and the mechanical properties of joints. The choice of the parameters values presented here is based on some approaches encountered in the literature and detailed in Homand *et al.*(1997). Joint normal behaviour is assumed to be linear whereas, the joint shear is perfectly elasto-plastic and the shear stress is limited by Mohr-Coulomb's criterion.

Table 2 - Elastic properties of rock materials.

ROCK MATERIALS	ν	E (MPa)
Begudian (Rognacian or Eocene)	.25	3 000
Fuvelian	.25	24255
Jurassic	.25	37500

Table 3 - Mechanical properties of joints.

* GPa/m; ** MPa/m; φ is joint friction angle.
1- Begudian/Fuvelian, Begudian/Begudian, Begudian/Jurassic
2- Fuvelian/Fuvelian, Fuvelian/Jurassic
3- Coal/Fuvelian, Coal/Coal, Coal/Jurassic.

JOINT materials	Consolidation		DURING Tectonic loadings		
	k_n^*	k_s^*	k_n^{**}	k_s^{**}	φ (°)
1	188	75	3000	7.5	20
2	2625	1050	25000	100	22
3	200	80	2500	8	20

4.3 Results

Stress distribution around the tectonic wedge of *Gardanne* where all the stress measurements were carried out is examined. Calculations corresponding to the present state (*i.e.* the upper Miocene event) show a strong anisotropy in stress distribution. This anisotropy is highly increased in the more stiff formations (Jurassic and Fuvelian J1, J2, F4 and F2 showed in Fig. 4). A marked heterogeneity in stress distribution is also noted. The highest magnitudes of the major principal stress (σ_1) are observed in the Fuvelian blocks (F2 and F4), in the Jurassic (J1) located in the east of *Gardanne* and in the Jurassic (J2) situated to the south. The maximum value of σ_1 is observed close to the Meyreuil fault, in the block F4 and close to the Diote fault (at the west of *Gardanne*). More precisely, in the Fuvelian F4, the magnitudes of the principal stresses decrease from west to east. Also, close to the Diote fault, the value of σ_1 in the extreme west zone is around 53 MPa and decreases until 48 MPa in the east zone, whereas the value of σ_3 (minor principal stress) is almost constant. The magnitude of σ_3 is close to 28 MPa in the block F4. Generally speaking, the major stress deviates towards N-S. In particular, the orientation of σ_1 (θ : direction taken clockwise from north) increases from 34° close to the point of intersection between Diote and Meyreuil faults to 48° in the extreme SE zone of block F4.

In the Fuvelian F2, where all the stress measurements were carried out, σ_1 is oriented NE-SW and its magnitude decreases from south to north and from west to east. Particularly, in the vicinity of

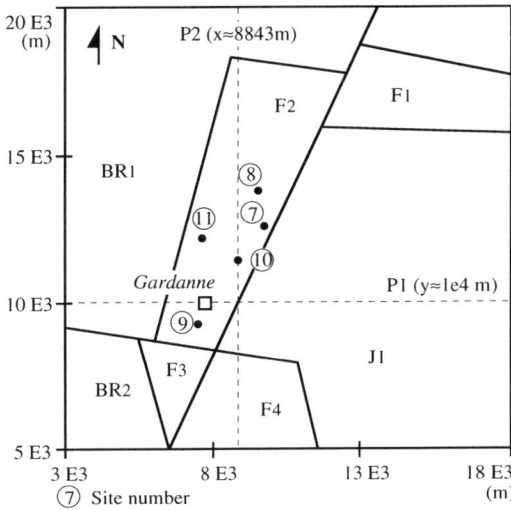

Fig. 4 - Part of horizontal section with the location of points of measurements.

the limit layer (BR1-F2), the value of σ_1 in the extreme S-W zone is around 50 MPa and decreases until 28 MPa in the N-E. Also, examination of the magnitude of σ_1 along an W-E profile crossing *Gardanne* and located in the block F2 showed that decreases progressively from west to east, reaching the value 36 MPa in the eastern. It is interesting to notice that on both sides of the Meyreuil fault, the magnitudes of σ_1 are less significant in the Fuvelian F2 (made up of fairly stiff materials), compared to those recorded in the Jurassic (Regaignas dome J1) which is quite stiff. The same phenomenon (decreasing of σ_1 in soft materials) is observed on both sides of the layer limit (BR1-F2) located in the west between the Begudian-Rognacian (BR1) and the Fuvelian (F2). Generally speaking, value of θ increases from west to east and decreases from south to north in the measurements area.

It is also interesting to notice that in the Fuvelian F3, no significant variation in magnitudes of the principal stresses is observed. The values of σ_1 and σ_3 in this block are close to 33 and 27 MPa, respectively. Consequently, no significant stresses anisotropy is noticed in comparison to the two others Fuvelian formations (F2 and F4). This stress distribution in the Fuvelian F3 is particularly related to the following factors : the proximity of the geological structures of the *Arc* (Meyreuil, Diote and Safre faults, the thrusted part J2, the Ragaignas dome J1), the orientations of faults delimiting the Fuvelian blocks, the N-S compression thrust but also, the presence of the Begudian BR2. In a recent study reported by Homand *et al.* 1997, the authors have clearly demonstrated the dependency of these geological structures on the natural stress in the *Arc* syncline, particularly in the south of the narrowest part of the Fuvelian where the measurements were carried out and the *Arc* presents some material heterogeneities.

Generally speaking, application of the different stress states during the four successive tectonic events can be summarized as follows :
(a) The N-S compression dated from the Eocene involves a deviation of the major principal stress towards N-E, except in the proximity of site ⑨. A decrease in the major stress magnitude is observed going from west to east and, from south towards the north, particularly in the Fuvelian F2 and F4 and the Jurassic J1.
(b) From the Eocene to the end of the Oligocene : numerical modelling results show that the principal stress magnitudes decrease. Also, the major principal stress is oriented according to NNE-SSW direction. Particularly, in the vicinity of *Gardanne*, the magnitudes of σ_1 and σ_3 are respectively reduced by 2 and 9 MPa, and the average orientation of σ_1 becomes N20°E.
(c) From the Oligocene to the end of the lower Miocene : the ENE-WSW compression is essentially characterized by a significant deviation of the principal stresses towards the east. In the south part of the *Arc*, the major principal stress deviates from NNE-SSE to ENE-WSE, independent to the materials. In the vicinity of *Gardanne*, θ varies from 70° to 90°.
(d) From the lower Miocene to the present state : this stage is characterized by an increase (from 3 to 10 MPa) of the principal stresses, and also by a new deviation of the major stress from ENE (lower Miocene) towards the North (upper Miocene).

Finally, we remarked that during the four periods which took place successively in the region, the global orientation of the major principal stress in the vicinity of *Gardanne* is N30°E, N20°E, N80°E and N40°E respectively during the Eocene, the Oligocene, the lower Miocene and the upper Miocene. Except for the Oligocene, where σ_1 is vertical by definition, these previous orientations of σ_1 are in agreement with those reported by Gaviglio et Gonzalès, 1987.

More precisely, Figs. 5-6 illustrate the evolution of σ_1 along two profiles P1 and P2 (see Fig. 4 for their locations) as a function of tectonic events. Fig. 5 indicates that for a given material, the magnitudes of σ_1 decrease going from west to east. To the east of *Gardanne*, σ_1 is practically uniform in the block F2 for a given event. It is interesting to note that the Begudian BR1 does not seem to be affected by the different tectonic events in comparison with the variations of s1 in the blocks F2 and J1. In fact the difference in σ_1 between two successive events does not exceed 2.5 MPa in the block BR1. The ENE-WSW compression (lower Miocene), representing the next stage of the Oligocene, shows that the major stress is almost uniform (near 28 MPa) along the profile P1. The other observation based on Fig. 5 is that crossing through discontinuities is clearly marked. A significant variation in σ_1 (reaching 15 MPa) can be noted between the left side of layer limit BR1-F2 and the right side for all events except the lower Miocene. Also, variations in magnitudes of σ_1 ranging between 5 and 9 MPa, can be noticed along the interface between F2 and J1 represented by the Meyreuil fault. In opposition to the reduction in σ_1 from west to east for a given material, the orientation of σ_1 (θ) increases from west to east for all tectonic events, except the lower Miocene. In this last case, θ is uniform at each side of Meyreuil fault : west to Meyreuil, σ_1 is oriented N80°E whereas east to Meyreuil, σ_1 is oriented N80°W. If the magnitude of σ_1 is characterized by an important variation crossing discontinuities, the orientation of σ_1 does not seem to be influenced by these discontinuities, except for the lower Miocene. Fig. 6 indicates that for a given material, the magnitudes of σ_1 decrease going from south to north. Also, Fig. 6 shows that the variations in magnitudes

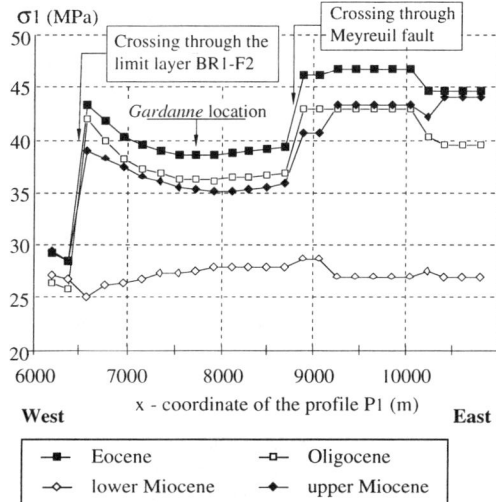

Fig. 5 - Major principal stress magnitude (σ_1) along P1 as a function of the tectonic history.

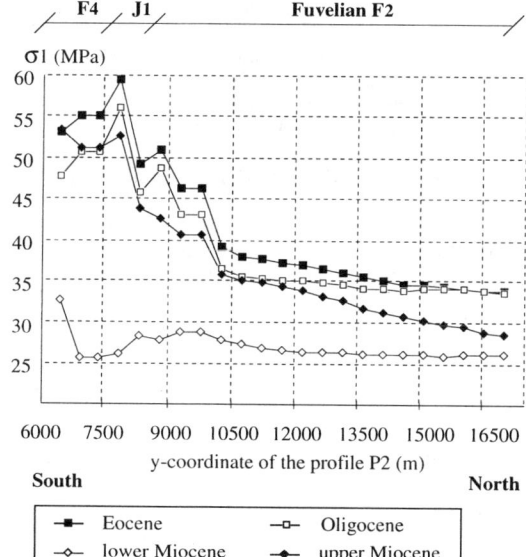

Fig. 6 - Major principal stress magnitude (σ_1) along P2 as a function of the tectonic history.

of σ_1 along the S-N profile (P2) are qualitatively similar for the three tectonic events : Eocene, Oligocene and upper Miocene. Except for the lower Miocene, magnitude of σ_1 is greater than 40 MPa in the southern part, whereas in the northern part of the Arc, σ_1 does not reach. It should be noted that in this northern part, the principal stresses are approximately isotropic at the end of the upper Miocene (σ_3 closed to 26 MPa). Examination of the orientation of σ_1 along the profile P2 showed that θ decreases from south to north for all tectonic events, except for the lower Miocene, where σ_1 is oriented N80°W in the southern part of the Meyreuil fault (i.e. in F4 and J1) or N80°E in the Fuvelian F2. Finally in the Fuvelian where most of the measurements were carried out, calculations corresponding to the present state indicate : (1) a decrease in the major stress magnitude going from west to east (profile P1) and, from south towards the north (profile P2) ; (2) the major stress deviates towards N-S. More precisely, θ increases from west to east in relation to the W-E direction, and decreases from south to north.

5 COMPARISON WITH MEASUREMENTS

In this section, we present a comparison between the calculations and measurements obtained from field investigations and corresponding to sites (⑦, ⑧, ⑨, ⑩ and ⑪ represented in Fig. 4) located on both sides of the modelled horizontal cross section.

Table 4 summarizes details of measured and computed principal horizontal stresses and orientations of the major principal stress. The predicted stress magnitudes and orientations involved the results of the tectonic loading stages. Based on this Table, comparison between measurements and calculations corresponding to the present state (i.e. upper Miocene) leads to the following comments.

• In the case of site ⑩ (1130 m depth) which is closest to the modelled cross section, the modelling provides a magnitude of σ_1 close to 35 MPa, whereas the measured value is equal 45 MPa. Recall that this measurement point is located 30 m below the modelled section. The predicted and measured orientations of σ_1 are identical. Concerning the site ⑨ (1200 m depth), examination of the stress state obtained by modelling shows that only the minor principal stress σ_3 remains in accordance with the measured value. It should be noted that this site is located in the narrowest part of the southern Fuvelian close to the Diote fault (Fig. 4). Obviously, site ⑨ is particularly influenced by numerous factors such as : location in the vicinity of the N-S regional compression, strong material heterogeneity, geological structures (Diote fault, Meyreuil fault, Safre fault and the westward layer limit between the Begudian-Rognacian and the Fuvelian) and also, orientations of these discontinuities (Homand *et al.* 1997). Natural stresses can be variable highly near geological structures, and stress orientations can rotate as much as 90° when geological structures cross.

This is effectively the case of site ⑨. *Site* ⑦ (1030 m depth) is located 70 m above the modelled cross section. The predicted value remains globally

Table 4 - Natural principal stresses : comparison between calculations and *in situ* measurements.

Site	EOCENE			OLIGOCENE			LOWER MIOCENE			UPPER MIOCENE			MEASUREMENTS		
	σ_1	σ_3	θ	σ_1	σ_3	θ	σ_1	σ_3	θ	σ_1	σ_3	θ	σ_1	σ_3	θ
⑨	39	22	N11E	38	10	N10E	29	20	N85E	34	24	N22E	22	18	N170E
⑩	38	26	N28E	35	19	N19E	27	22	N88E	35	25	N37E	45	15	N40E
⑪	38	26	N20E	37	18	N16E	27	21	N85E	33	26	N30E	34	20	N100E
⑦	36	26	N35E	33	19	N23E	26	23	N90E	34	25	N41E	32	16	N70E
⑧	35	27	N29E	32	19	N18E	26	23	N90E	32	25	N40E	31	23	N104E

σ_1 : major principal stress (MPa); σ_3 : minor principal stress and θ : orientation of major principal stress.

identical to the one determined based on the *in situ* measurements. The slight difference between the predicted and measured value of σ_1 must correspond to the lithostatic stresses due to 70 m overburden. Similarly to the site ⑩ analysis, calculations overestimate the magnitudes of the minor principal stress by about 10 MPa, compared to the measured value. Concerning the sites ⑧ and ⑪, it should be noticed that the predicted values of σ_1 and σ_3 are in agreement with those measured. However, predicted magnitude of σ_3 is 6 MPa greater than the measured value. The measured orientation of σ_1 is about N100°E. Predicted orientations of σ_1 are 60 - 70° lower than those measured. This is certainly connected to the geometry of the Meyreuil fault and/or the layer limit BR1-F2 geometry. Recall that in reality, the Meyreuil fault forms a broken line made of segments oriented N0° and N30-40°E (Fig. 1), whereas a N25°E average orientation was assumed. The layer limit BR1-F2 between is really oriented N0° in depth, whereas in our modelling, an average orientation of about N15°E has been considered. It should be noted that the effect of Meyreuil fault and the layer limit orientations on the stress distribution has been widely developed in Homand *et al.* 1997.

• Also, Table 4 shows the evolutions of stress distribution at the measurement points with respect to the geological history of the *Arc* syncline. In particular, results indicate : *(a)* a reduction of σ_3 from Eocene to Oligocene and from Oligocene to the lower Miocene, *(b)* a reduction of σ_3 from Eocene to Oligocene and an increase of σ_3 from Oligocene to the lower Miocene, *(c)* an increase of σ_3 and a decrease of σ_1 from the end of lower Miocene to the present state.

6 CONCLUSION

Large scale numerical modelling using UDEC code for a horizontal cross section at 1100 m depth allows the geological hypothesis of the N-S compression prevailing in the *Arc* basin to be reconciled with the currently observed stress deviations towards the N-E. Calculations lead to a better explanation of the orientations of the principal stresses which are in accordance with the observation of a NE-SW stress deviation. Finally, results show that natural stresses magnitudes and orientations in the *Arc* syncline can generally be explained based on geological information. *In situ* stress measurements carried out in the *Arc* syncline, using flat jack and hydraulic fracturing methods, enabled the numerical modelling to be validated. Calculations were compared with *in situ* measurements concerning five sites located on both sides of the modelled horizontal cross section. Results indicate that the predicted magnitudes and orientations of natural stresses are globally in agreement with those measured. Finally, we remarked that during the four tectonic periods which took place successively in the region, the global orientation of the major principal stress in the vicinity of *Gardanne* is N30°E, N20°E, N80°E and N40°E respectively during the Eocene, the Oligocene, the lower Miocene and the upper Miocene.

ACKNOWLEDGEMENTS - The authors wish to thank the HBCM-Unité d'Exploitation de *Provence* for the permission to use their *in situ* stress measurement data. Also, authors wish to aknowledge Professor P. Gaviglio for the geological comments.

REFERENCES

Gaviglio P., Bigarré P., Baroudi H., Piguet J-P and Monteau R. 1996. Measurements of natural stresses in a Provence Mine (Southern France). *Engng Geology* **44**, pp 77-92.

Gaviglio P. and Gonzalès J-F. 1987. Fracturation et histoiretectonique du bassin de Gardanne. *Bull.Soc.Géol.France* , **8-III**,pp675-682.

Homand F., Souley M., Gaviglio P. and Mamane I. 1997. Modelling of natural stresses in the Arc syncline and comparison with *in situ* measurements. *Int. J. Rock Mech. Min. Sci & Geomech. Abstr.* in press.

Rosengren L. and Stephansson O. 1993. Modelling of rock mass response to glaciation at Finsjön, Sweden. *Tunnelling and Underground Space Technology,* **8,** No 1, pp. 75-82.

Recent advances in the interpretation of the overcoring test

K. Fouial, M. Alheib & P. Bigarre
Laboratoire Environnement Géomécanique et Ouvrages, INERIS, Ecole des Mines de Nancy, France

ABSTRACT : The overcoring method is one of the methods the most frequently used in geotechnics for stress measurements. It has been shown to be highly suitable for measuring the stresses in "hard and sound" rocks. But applied to some rock formations and under some local conditions, many overcoring stress measurement campaigns have ended to failure. Interpretation of the measurements by the conventional method produces erroneous results. These failures are due mainly to the worst assumption that the behaviour of the rock is elastic and that a sound core is obtained. So it is impossible to use the interpretative conventional method.

To overcome these problems and in order to determine the stress tensor from deformations recorded under such conditions we have been developed a new method which is based on an analysis of the start of the deformation curves ; this method is the subject of our paper.

1 SURVEY OF THE CONVENTIONAL METHOD OF INTERPRETATION

The determination of the in-situ state of stress in a rock mass is one of the most challenging problems in geotechnics. A common method of stress determination is the overcoring method (cf. Fig. 1) : a small diameter borehole is drilled in rock mass ; an instrument for measuring strain or deformation in several directions is placed in the borehole ; and a larger hole is then drilled around the instrument. Because the specimen is now released from the in-situ stress field, the resulting deformations give a measure of the amount of stress released.

The conventional method of processing the data from an overcoring test includes the following steps (cf. Fig. 2) :
- determination of the deformations arising from the total release of the core, corresponding to the final deformations recorded at the end of the test, from 12 gauges of the CSIRO measurement cell mounted in the central extension hole.
- inversion of the equation system linking the recorded deformations to the investigated stresses by the relationship :

$$[\varepsilon] = [A][\sigma] \qquad (1)$$

where $[\varepsilon]$ is the single-column vector of the 12 measured plateau values, $[\varepsilon] = [\varepsilon_1, \varepsilon_2, ..., \varepsilon_{12}]^T$

$[\sigma]$ is the single-column vector of the investigated stresses, $[\sigma] = [\sigma_{xx}, \sigma_{yy}, ..., \sigma_{zx}]^T$
and [A] is the 12 x 6 influence matrix determined by :

$$a_{ij} = \frac{\varepsilon i}{\sigma j} \qquad (2)$$

where a_{ij} are the influencing coefficients whose value corresponds to the deformation recorded by gauge i as a function of a unitary load σ_j.

Each coefficient a_{ij} depends on the geomechanical properties as well as the technical and geometrical parameters of the overcoring tests (diameters of boreholes, cell position, etc.). An analytical solution making it possible to calculate these influencing coefficients is available only for the phase of total release of the core.

Nevertheless, the application of this method is based mainly on the validity of the assumption that the behaviour of the rock is elastic and linear during the overcoring operation.

Figure 3 shows the various phases recorded during the overcoring operation, a distinction is made between :
- **phase a** : where the overcoring has not yet reached the measurement region.
- **phase b** : where the overstressing caused by the undercutting of the overcoring reaches the measurement

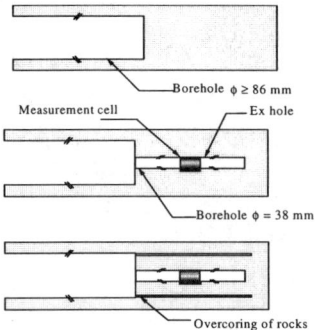

Figure 1 : The various stages in an overcoring test

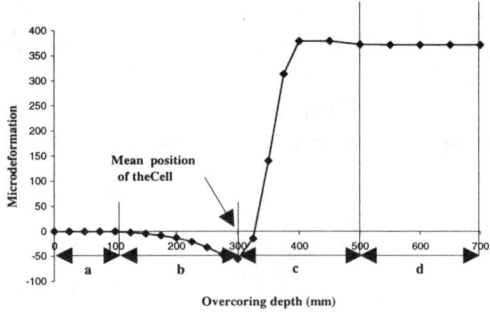

Figure 3 : The various phases recorded during the overcoring operation

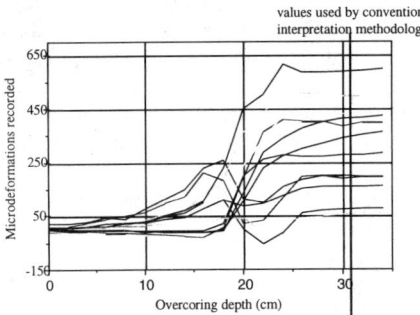

Figure 2 : Deformations used by conventional interpretation methodology

region, **the transient deformation** is due to loading phase.
- **phase c** : where the release of the core takes place progressively and the **transient deformation** recorded is the result at one and the same time of a total loading and a partial unloading phases.
- **phase d** : where the release of the core is complete ; **the final deformation** recorded on this occasion is the resultant of total loading and unloading.
In the unloading phases (phases c and d) the non-elastic behaviour of the rock may occur after the core-drill has passed through at measurement cell level. This is the case with certain argillaceous or marly rocks.

2 FACTORS RESTRICTING THE APPLICATION OF THE CONVENTIONAL INTERPRETATION METHOD

As we have just seen, the conventional method of interpreting the overcoring tests is based on :
- the obtaining of a sound core (no fractures) from the overcoring operation.
- the validity of the assumption that the behaviour of the rock is elastic,

Unfortunately, the following factors restrict the application of this method and compel the operator to abandon these measurements :
- **Presence of natural fractures** : An overcoring test carried out in a highly fractured rock formation cannot produce correct and interpretable results [Worotnicki, 1993], particularly if the measurement cell is surrounded by one or more fracture planes.
- **Disking phenomenon** : This is a phenomenon frequently encountered in measurement campaigns. The rupture mechanism of the core depends not only on the state of the initial stresses but also on the drilling method [Kutter, 1991]. According to Cornet [1981] the disking is the result of the appearance of tensile stressing parallel to the drilling axis. If these tensile stresses are sufficiently intense, they can lead to the disking phenomenon. If they are small, they may simply re-open pre-existing or badly cemented micro-cracks.
The presence of fractures, be they of natural origin or induced by the drilling operations, makes it impossible for the stabilisation stage to correspond to the release of the core [Cai et al, 1995] which means that the conventional interpretation method cannot be used. However, during the overcoring operation, the disking phenomenon is observed only from a certain overcoring depth, thus making it possible to obtain the correct transient deformations at the start of this operation.
- **Behaviour of the rock :** the hypothesis of the linear elasticity of the rocks is not always valid. In fact, because of their mineralogical composition, their heterogeneity and the presence of microfractures, the majority of rocks do not always have linear elastic behaviour. Furthermore, with certain types of rock, other factors such as the viscosity and the plasticity determine the behaviour of the rock, reducing the reliability of the results and can even give rise to erroneous results.
- **Technical factors** : The use of the conventional method of interpretation assumes that the overcoring test has taken

place under good conditions right to the end. Unfortunately, several technical factors (skewing of the boring rods, sudden breakage of the conducting wires, poor adaptation of the drilling method, etc.) result in automatic failure of the test. In this case, determination of the stress state requires that other tests be carried out and therefore that additional investments are made.

However, in the majority of cases, despite the existence of the above factors, it is still possible to record partial deformations down to a certain overcoring depth. So as not to abandon these tests, we propose to utilise these partial deformations.

3 DETERMINATION OF THE STRESS TENSOR FROM THE TRANSIENT DEFORMATIONS

In fact, it is a matter of improving the method of interpreting the stresses by including not just the data relating to the total release of the core, but also all the information not used so far and contained in the recorded curves, from the moment the cell is put under pressure by the overcoring.

The use of the part of the curves representing the initial phases of the measured deformations, or transient deformations, is of considerable value for the following reasons :

1 - the rock, at gauge level, undergoes a compression phase (loading) whereas the final deformations correspond to a behaviour of the rock resulting from a loading-unloading of much greater amplitude ; often this phase is accompanied by a permanent deformation (i.e. plastic deformation).

2 - the significant deformations measured before the passage of the core-drill through the cell are small compared with those obtained at the end of the test. In this case, they may represent a reversible behavioural phase of the rock, i.e. the rock remains in the elastic range.

3 - similarly, as for the disking of the core head at the start of the overcoring operation, it may be considered that the deformations are recorded before the start of the disking phenomenon or at this side of the existing fractures.

4 DESCRIPTION OF THE RECOMMENDED METHOD

For a given stage of **advancement j** of the core-drill it is possible to estimate initial stresses from the **measured deformations** $[\varepsilon]_j$ provided that the **influence matrix** $[A]_j$ for this particular stage is determined. The latter can be estimated using the numerical methods which enable the overcoring operation to be simulated with parameter conditions (geometry, mechanical properties) similar to those in situ (cf. Fig.4).

In fact, at each overcoring step C_j, the deformation

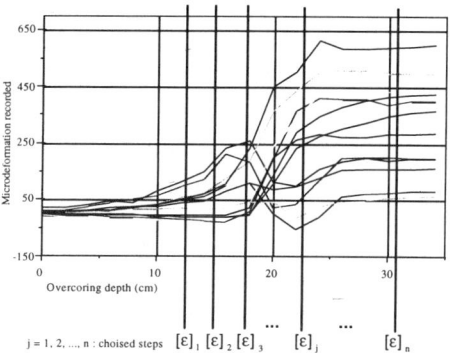

Figure 4 : Deformations used in the new interpretation methodology

recorded by **gauge i** is a **linear combination** linking this deformation with the tensor of the initial stresses. This relationship can be formulated simply as :

$$\varepsilon_{ij} = a_{ij1}\sigma_{xx} + a_{ij2}\sigma_{yy} + a_{ij3}\sigma_{zz} + a_{ij4}\sigma_{xy} + a_{ij5}\sigma_{yz} + a_{ij6}\sigma_{zx} \quad (3)$$

or $\varepsilon_{ij} = \sum_{k=1}^{k=6} a_{ijk} \cdot \sigma_k$

where ε_{ij} is the deformation measured by **gauge i** at overcoring step C_j ;

$\sigma = [\sigma_1, \sigma_2, ..., \sigma_k, ..., \sigma_6]^T = [\sigma_{xx}, \sigma_{yy}, \sigma_{zz}, \sigma_{xy}, \sigma_{yz}, \sigma_{zx}]^T$ is the stress tensor ;

$a_{ij1}, a_{ij2}, ..., a_{ij6}$ are the influencing coefficients dependent on the geometrical characteristics of the test notably the advancement of the core drill, and the geomechanical characteristics of the rock.

Since we are working with the assumption of linear elasticity, it is possible to apply the superposition principle of the deformations. Thus, each coefficient a_{ijk} can be determined by numerical simulation of the overcoring test provided that the model is loaded with a tensor having a single component σ_k from among the six components of the tensor. This component has a unitary value making it possible to determine the coefficient relating to the loading of this component. For example, if we wish to determine the coefficients of the twelve gauges corresponding to the unitary stress σ_{xx} and to the overcoring step C_j, our model will be loaded with the following tensor : $[1, 0, 0, 0, 0, 0]^T$. We repeat the same operation for the six component of the stress tensor.

Then we determine, for an advancement stage j, and for each gauge i the influencing coefficients a_{ijk}, we can denote these by a vector $[a]_{ij} = [a_{ij1}, a_{ij2}, a_{ij3}, a_{ij4}, a_{ij5}, a_{ij6}]^T$ where the terms are equal to the particular values of ε_{ij}, successively computed for each one of these loadings.

Let $[A]_{ij}$ be the matrix of the influencing coefficients corresponding to the 12 gauges i, the tensor of initial stress [σ] may be obtained by solving the following matrix system :

$$[\varepsilon]_{ij} = [A]_{ij} [\sigma] \qquad (4)$$

where $[\varepsilon]_{ij}$ is the single-column vector of the measured deformations for an advancement stage j, by all gauge i of the cell, $1 \leq i \leq 12$;

[σ] is the single-column vector of the investigated stresses $[\sigma_{xx}, \sigma_{yy}, \sigma_{zz}, \sigma_{xy}, \sigma_{yz}, \sigma_{zx}]^T$;

$[A]_{ij}$ is the matrix of the influencing coefficients with (12x6) terms.

In the case where the advancement travel of core drill, which equal to the sum of the preceding advancement stages C_j, is largely greater than the position spacing of the measurement cell, $[\varepsilon]_{ij}$ is the single-column vector of the total deformations corresponding to the conventionally used plateau values. The numerically determined matrix $[A]_{ij}$ is then equal to the analytically resolved matrix [A].

This approach can be generalised by quantising all the 12 deformation curves recorded by the 12 gauges of the cell during an overcoring test for a number **N of advancement stages**.

The procedure then becomes :
1 - after fixing N advancement stages judiciously positioned on the 12 measured deformation curves, the influencing matrices $[A]_{ij}$ ($1 \leq j \leq N$) are determined numerically by three-dimensional modelling. The method used is the finite elements method. Six numerical simulations are required for each advancement stage, in total 6 x N calculations ;
2 - plotting of the deformation measurements for each advancement stage j ;
3 - inversion of the equation system (4) linking the measured deformations with the investigated stresses.
Thus for each selected advancement j we have a matrix of influencing coefficients $[A]_{ij}$, and deformation measurements at the same overcoring depth $[\varepsilon]_{ij}$.

This system can be solved by the method of least squares or by the combination method. Thus, we obtain the average tensor of initial stress with these standard deviations (caused by the variation of the recorded measurements).

In practice, it is necessary to remove the measurements which appear to be unreliable. For this we need to be able to :
- eliminate one or more advancement stages, where the measured deformations are not representative because of the pressure effect of the core drill during the overcoring operation and the influence of the measurement cell position ;
- eliminate one or more measurements carried out at the same overcoring depth.

5 APPLICATION ON A REAL SITUATION

The different stages of this approach : numerical calculation, deformation calculation method and inversion method were checked against known analytical solutions before a validation was made based on real data.

After the method has been set up and the necessary checks made on the tools used, it is necessary to perform a validation for a real situation. To do this, the test to be chosen requires that :
1 - the rock must have a linear elastic behaviour during the first phases of the test ;
2 - the overcoring test must be carried out successfully at least to a certain overcoring depth ;
3 - the deformations must be plotted carefully over the entire overcoring depth. Continuous recording of these deformations is recommended.

Our choice went to a test performed by the Australian company MINDATA PTY. LTD which is well known in the field of stress measurements. The test was carried out in a granitic rock for the purpose of measuring the stresses induced in a mine pillar.

The data of the selected test is complete (cf. Fig.5) and makes it possible therefore to carry out validation of the new method of interpreting the overcoring test.

A model has been done with CESAR-LCPC software in 3D to take account of the specific geometry of the test. A total 15 advancement steps has been simulated.

For each step of overcoring, six calculations has been carried out for each of the six terms of the stress tensor, in order to determine each matrix of influencing coefficients $[A]_{ij}$. Each calculate give 12 terms from this matrix, which contain 6x12 terms in total.

Fig.6 illustrates the dimensions and the boundary conditions of the model. The mesh is also shown in Fig.7.

The numerical calculations have made it possible to construct the influence matrix for the 15 advancement stages of the core drill.

Similarly, a simulation was performed with the stress tensor obtained from the final deformations of the test by the conventional method of interpretation.

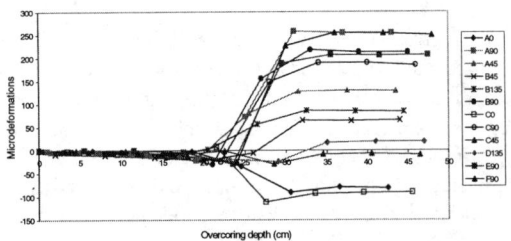

Figure 5 : Deformations curves obtained by in situ measurements

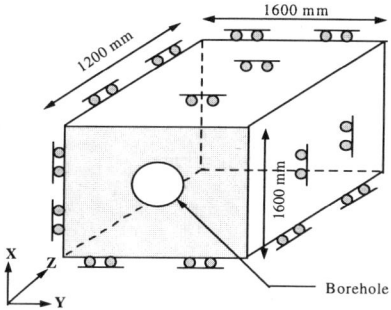

Figure 6 : Dimensions of the model and the displacements imposed U = V = W = 0

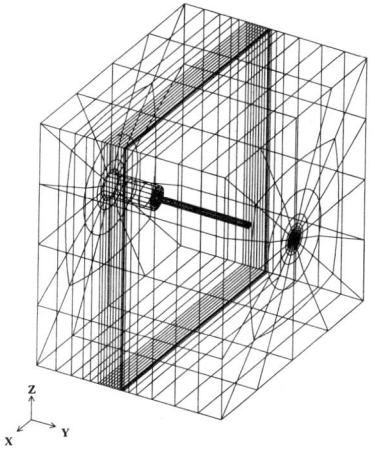

Figure 7 : Mesh created with the CESAR finite elements code

From now on, the tensor determined by the conventional method will be called the reference tensor. Fig.8 shows the deformation curves obtained by using the reference tensor as initial loading tensor.

We find that the shapes of the curves obtained by the three-dimensional modelling with the CESAR-LCPC code are similar to those recorded in situ. Figure 9 compares the final deformations of the 12 gauges obtained by numerical modelling, by analytical solution due to the reference tensor and by the values measured in situ. Major differences can be noted for gauges A45, B135, C45 and D135. The latter are supposed to measure the axial deformation ε_Z, the tangential deformation ε_θ and the shear deformation $\gamma_{\theta z}$ at the same time.

From the deformations obtained in situ we have calculated the tensor of the stresses for two advancement stages of the core drill :
- a stage located at 185 mm before the position of the measurement cell,
- the second stage corresponds to the final parts of the curves at 425 mm.

For the two stages we have used calculated the mean value m and standard deviation Δ of each component of the stress tensor.

Table 1 and Table 2 summarise the results of two advancement steps as well as the stress reference tensor determined by a conventional method based on the final deformations.

We find that the two calculated stress tensors are comparable for the two intermediate and final stages. The stresses (σxx and σzz) are correctly estimated relative to the reference tensor. The maximum standard deviation for these two components relative to those determined by conventional method is equal to 19 %.

The stress σyy and the shear stresses were estimated with larger standard deviations The stress orientations are very much dependent of those deviations. This is due partly to a

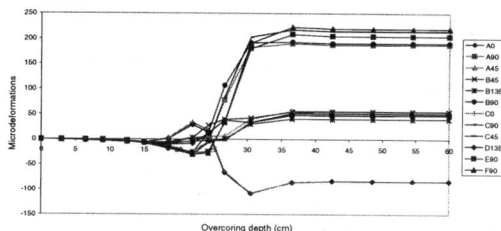

Figure 8 : Deformations curves obtained by the numerical modelling

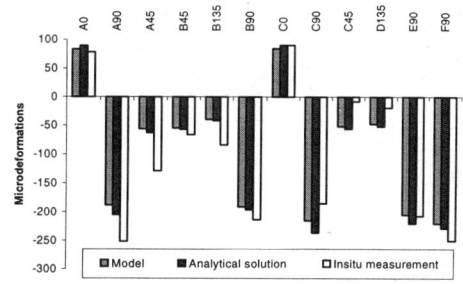

Figure 9 : Comparison between the deformations obtained by numerical modelling, analytical solution and those measured in situ

stress tensor with tensile stresses and very low, almost zero, shear stresses.

These results show that the new method for interpretation of overcoring tests makes it possible to determine the tensor of the stresses in situ for intermediate

Table 1 : Stresses calculated for two advancement steps 185 mm and 425 mm
m : mean value of the stress component (MPa)
Δ : standard deviation of the stress component (MPa)

tensor component	Obtained tensor (in MPa) by :					
	New method				Conventional method	
	at 185 mm		at 425 mm		Final phase	
	m	Δ	m	Δ	m	Δ
σ_{xx}	6.20	0.57	5.96	0.18	5.56	0.15
σ_{yy}	-2.07	0.37	-1.36	0.39	-1.33	0.37
σ_{zz}	6.10	0.66	6.62	0.19	5.12	0.15
σ_{xy}	2.12	1.02	-0.09	0.17	-0.11	0.15
σ_{yz}	-1.15	1.45	0.82	0.21	-0.53	0.17
σ_{zx}	0.77	0.41	0.45	0.12	-0.28	0.09

Table 2 : Principal stresses calculated for two advancement steps 185 mm and 425 mm

Value of the principal stresses (MPa)	Obtained tensor by :		
	New method		Conventional method
	at 185 mm	at 425 mm	Final phase
σ_1	7	6.9	5.72
σ_2	6	5.76	5
σ_3	-2.81	-1.44	-1.4

Dip of the principal stresses (°)	Obtained tensor by :		
	New method		Conventional method
	at 185 mm	at 425 mm	Final phase
σ_1	31.82	64.63	65
σ_2	56.78	24.58	32
σ_3	8.56	5.87	4

Azimuth of the principal stresses (°)	Obtained tensor by :		
	New method		Conventional method
	at 185 mm	at 425 mm	Final phase
σ_1	261	258.5	262
σ_2	62	93.7	93
σ_3	19	1	1

stages before the total release and complete culmination of the overcoring test.

The validation of the methodology was performed on data from tests carried out by MINDATA in a mine pillar. The tensor obtained is close to that measured by the conventional method. The biggest deviations relate to the shear stresses. It can be estimated that in the case of an homogeneous isotropic elastic rock we can determine the stress tensor by using the intermediate deformations provided that we have available a sufficient number of measurements between 100 and 200 mm of travel for a cell positioned at 250 mm.

6 GENERAL CONCLUSION AND FUTURE PROSPECTS

A new methodology has been developed to improve the processing of data from overcoring stress measurements. This methodology makes it possible to utilise virtually all the measurements recorded during testing whereas the conventional method can only handle the final recordings corresponding to the complete release.

The implementation of this methodology is based on the determination of the influencing coefficients linking the investigated stresses with the measured deformations for each advancement step of the core drill. For this purpose a three-dimensional numerical modelling approach has been adopted.

The methodology was validated for a rock having relatively controlled mechanical behaviour. We have shown that it is possible to determine the stress tensor in situ for intermediate stages before total release and before completion of the overcoring test. A data base is being developed which will enable rapid interpretation of measurements made in situ without the need to resort to extremely cumbersome numerical calculations.

ACKNOWLEDGMENTS

The authors thank Walton R. J. of Mindata Australia Pty Ltd for his technical contribution to the development of this method. This work was sponsored by ANDRA which we thank for its support.

REFERENCES

Cai M., Qiao L.and Yu J. 1995. Study and tests of techniques for increasing overcoring stress measurement accuracy. Int. J. Rock. Mech. Min. Sci. & Geomech. Abstr., 32 : 375-384.

Cornet F. H. 1981. La mesure in situ des contraintes dans un massif rocheux. Tunnels et ouvrages souterrains - Novembre - Décembre Revue bimestrielle 48 : 262 - 273.

Kutter H. K. 1991. Influence of drilling method on borehole breakouts and core disking. International Society for Rock Mechanics Aachen. Belkama, Rotterdam, 3 : 1659-1664.

Worotnicki G. 1993. CSIRO Triaxial Stress Measurement Cell. Comprensive Rock Engeinnering : Priciples, Practiceand Projects. Rock Testing and Site Characterization. Pergamon Press, Oxford, England. Volume 3, pp. 329-394.

Data processing in rock stress measurement

Shixiong Zhang, Mingliang Yang & Jian Zhang
Department of Resources and Environment Engineering, Wuhan University of Technology, People's Republic of China

Jianmin Jia
Henan Gold Administration Bureau, Zhengzhou, People's Republic of China

ABSTRACT: Using the stress relief method to measure the *in-situ* stresses, while a triaxial strain cell has twelve strain gauges, at most twelve observations can be obtained, so the least square method is usually used to obtain the best possible values of the measured stresses. According to some directive rules for the engineering rock tests, a calculating method, which gives up the observation with the greatest residual error one by one, is suggested. The authors of this paper indicate that the random abandonment of the observations with an equal precision violates the basis of the statistics, and leads to the way of the subjective indeterminacy. The authors also give the correct consummation of errors and recommend the method of compounding the principal stresses according to the average of the stress components of all the measured points in a hole.

1 INTRODUCTION

Since the crust rock masses are in the complex stress states, the rock stresses *in-situ* have a great effect on the stability of an underground rock project before setting out. Nowadays there are probably some larger differences among the measured rock stresses *in-situ*. Besides the rock masses themselves are in some quite complex stress states, it's also because the measuring methods and some improper data processing bring errors. This paper focuses on how to correct the latter problem.

2 THE LEAST SQUARE METHOD IN STRESS MEASUREMENT

2.1 Principle of measuring the rock stress by holewall strain method

The holewall strain method is the most popular way used in the world now to get 3-D stresses of several points of the rock mass in one hole.

Firstly, drill a hole of 36 mm diameter and 400 mm depth at a measured point in the rock mass. Secondly, paste 3 rosettes which has 4 or 3 resistance wires at the middle of the holewall. Then, operate the stress-relief with a bit of 110 mm diameter, and get less than 12 or 9 strain values. Finally, calculate the rock stress values based on the elastic theory and the consummation of errors.

Suppose, before drilling, the rock stress components are σ_x, σ_y, σ_z, τ_{xy}, τ_{yz}, and τ_{zx}, in a Cartesian system respectively, and after drilling, the rock stress components are σ_r, σ_θ, $\sigma_{z'}$, $\tau_{r\theta}$, $\tau_{\theta z'}$ and $\tau_{z'r}$ in a cylindrical coordinate system. According to the elastic theory, the stress components in these two systems are defined by:

$$\sigma_r = ((\sigma_x + \sigma_y)/2)(1 - a^2/r^2) + ((\sigma_x - \sigma_y)/2)$$
$$(1 + 3a^4/r^4 - 4a^2/r^2)\cos 2\theta + \tau_{xy}$$
$$(1 + 3a^4/r^4 - 4a^2/r^2)\sin 2\theta \quad (1)$$

$$\sigma_\theta = ((\sigma_x + \sigma_y)/2)(1 + a^2/r^2) - ((\sigma_x - \sigma_y)/2)$$
$$(1 + 3a^4/r^4)\cos 2\theta - \tau_{xy}(1 + 3a^4/r^4)\sin 2\theta \quad (2)$$

$$\sigma_{z'} = -\mu[2(\sigma_x - \sigma_y)a^2/r^2 \cos 2\theta + 4\tau_{xy} a^2/r^2 \sin 2\theta] + \sigma_z \quad (3)$$

$$\tau_{r\theta} = -((\sigma_x - \sigma_y)/2)(1 - 3a^4/r^4 + 2a^2/r^2)\sin 2\theta$$

$$+\tau_{xy}(1-3a^4/r^4+2a^2/r^2)\cos 2\theta \quad (4)$$

$$\tau_{\theta z'} = (\tau_{yz}\cos\theta - \tau_{zx}\sin\theta)(1+a^2/r^2) \quad (5)$$

$$\tau_{z'r} = (\tau_{zx}\cos\theta - \tau_{yz}\sin\theta)(1-a^2/r^2) \quad (6)$$

where r is radius vector, θ is polar angle, a is the drilled hole's radius, and μ is rock Poisson's ratio.

When $r=a$

$$\sigma_r = \tau_{r\theta} = \tau_{z'r} = 0 \quad (7)$$

$$\sigma_\theta = (\sigma_x+\sigma_y)-2(\sigma_x-\sigma_y)\cos 2\theta - 4\tau_{xy}\sin 2\theta \quad (8)$$

$$\sigma_{z'} = -\mu[2(\sigma_x-\sigma_y)\cos 2\theta + 4\tau_{xy}\sin 2\theta]+\sigma_z \quad (9)$$

$$\tau_{\theta z'} = 2\tau_{yz}\cos\theta - 2\tau_{zx}\sin\theta \quad (10)$$

Suppose arrange S rosettes at a measured point, the sequence number is i, the respective angle is θ_i, every rosette is made up by T resistance wires, the sequence number is j, and the respective angle is φ_j. The relation between the measured strain values and holewall stresses may be written:

$$E\varepsilon_{ij} = (\sigma_{z'i}-\mu\sigma_{\theta i})\cos^2\varphi_j + (\sigma_{\theta i}-\mu\sigma_{z'i})\sin^2\varphi_j$$
$$+(1+\mu)\tau_{\theta z'i}\sin 2\varphi_j \quad (11)$$

where $i=1,2,...,S$; $j=1,2,\cdots,T$; E is the elastic modulus.

Take Equations 8 — 10 into Equation 11, and suppose $k=(i-1)T+j$, Then get the relation of the holewall strain values and the rock stresses:

$$E\varepsilon_k = A_{k1}\sigma_x + A_{k2}\sigma_y + A_{k3}\sigma_z + A_{k4}\tau_{xy} + A_{k5}\tau_{yz} + A_{k6}\tau_{zx}$$
$$(12)$$

where
$$A_{k1} = [1-2(1-\mu^2)\cos 2\theta_i]\sin^2\varphi_j - \mu\cos^2\varphi_j$$
$$A_{k2} = [1+2(1-\mu^2)\cos 2\theta_i]\sin^2\varphi_j - \mu\cos^2\varphi_j$$
$$A_{k3} = \cos^2\varphi_j - \mu\sin^2\varphi_j$$
$$A_{k4} = -4(1-\mu^2)\sin 2\theta_i \sin^2\varphi_j$$
$$A_{k5} = 2(1+\mu)\cos\theta_i \sin 2\varphi_j$$
$$A_{k6} = -2(1+\mu)\sin\theta_i \sin 2\varphi_j$$

Determine the elastic modulus E, Poisson's ratio μ and the strain observations, reference them to Equation 12, probably get 6 stress components at this point, further, work out 3 principal stresses and their directions depended on the relative formula.

2.2 The consummation of errors

In common, every point may get 12 or 9 observations and list out 12 or 9 linear equations, only 6 unknowns require solution. Selecting 6 equations from them in random the stress values could be shown differently in terms of measurement errors. But there are the true stress values in the point. To acquire the best possible values of the measured stresses from the observations, the least square method is adopted.

2.2.1 List error equations

If ε_k are the strain true values, ε'_k are the measured strain values with the same measurement accuracy, the accidental error υ_k of the measured values and the true values is illustrated as follow:

$$\upsilon_k = \varepsilon'_k - \varepsilon_k \quad (13)$$

where $k=1,2,\cdots,n$. The number of the measured strain values is n.

Nevertheless, for the existence of measurement errors, the true values can't be acquired. In calculation use the best possible values ε''_k instead of true values, the error equation can be demonstrated as follow:

$$\upsilon_k = \varepsilon'_k - \varepsilon''_k = \varepsilon'_k - (A_{k1}\sigma''_x + A_{k2}\sigma''_y + A_{k3}\sigma''_z + A_{k4}\tau''_{xy}$$
$$+A_{k5}\tau''_{yz} + A_{k6}\tau''_{zx})/E \quad (14)$$

where $\{\sigma''\}$ — the best possible values of the measured stresses.

2.2.2 Make up and solve the system of equations

The least square method means making the sum of square of the accidental errors smallest, i.e.

$$\sum_{k=1}^{n}\upsilon_k^2 = \sum_{k=1}^{n}(\varepsilon'_k - \varepsilon''_k)^2 = Min \quad (15)$$

Hereafter, write without "'" and "''" for convenience.

Calculation of the measured stress components requires that:

$$\frac{\partial}{\partial \sigma_x}\left(\sum_{k=1}^{n} v_k^2\right) = \frac{\partial}{\partial \sigma_y}\left(\sum_{k=1}^{n} v_k^2\right) = \cdots\cdots = \frac{\partial}{\partial \tau_{zx}}\left(\sum_{k=1}^{n} v_k^2\right) = 0 \quad (16)$$

Take Equation 14 into Equation 16, then get the equation to solve the measured stress components:

$$\begin{bmatrix} \sum_{k=1}^{n} A_{k1}^2 & \sum_{k=1}^{n} A_{k1}A_{k2} & \cdots & \sum_{k=1}^{n} A_{k1}A_{k6} \\ \sum_{k=1}^{n} A_{k2}A_{k1} & \sum_{k=1}^{n} A_{k2}^2 & \cdots & \sum_{k=1}^{n} A_{k2}A_{k6} \\ \vdots & \vdots & \ddots & \vdots \\ \sum_{k=1}^{n} A_{k6}A_{k1} & \sum_{k=1}^{n} A_{k6}A_{k2} & \cdots & \sum_{k=1}^{n} A_{k6}^2 \end{bmatrix} \begin{bmatrix} \sigma_x \\ \sigma_y \\ \vdots \\ \tau_{zx} \end{bmatrix} = E \begin{bmatrix} \sum_{k=1}^{n} A_{k1}\varepsilon_k \\ \sum_{k=1}^{n} A_{k2}\varepsilon_k \\ \vdots \\ \sum_{k=1}^{n} A_{k6}\varepsilon_k \end{bmatrix} \quad (17)$$

2.2.3 Pick out the observations which are out of the error limit

Solve Equation 17, and take the probably best possible stress values into equation 14, then get the residual errors v_k of the observed strain values, now their mean square error's assessment m can be expressed as follow:

$$m = \left(\left(\sum_{k=1}^{n} v_k^2\right)/r\right)^{1/2} \quad (18)$$

where r is the surplus observations' number, $r = n-t$, n is the observation' number, t is the unknowns' number in the equations.

In common, three times of the mean square error's assessment is considered as the limiting error Δ_L of accidental errors, i.e.

$$\Delta_L = 3m \quad (19)$$

Because a measurement accidental error Δ is a random variable which is subordinate to the normal distribution, where $\Delta_L = 3m$, the probability of beyond the limiting error is only 0.3%, similar to a little probability near zero, i.e. an improbable incident. It should be considered as a mistake and the respective measured values should be pick out.

Without the measured values which are beyond the limiting error, the calculated best possible value is the most suitable value.

2.2.4 Accuracy evaluation

The mean square error's assessment of the measured stress components' best possible value are defined by

$$m_i = mQ_{ii}^{1/2} \quad (20)$$

where $i = 1,2,\cdots,6$; Q_{ii} is the weight reciprocal of stress components, it contents the following equation:

$$\begin{bmatrix} \sum_{k=1}^{n} A_{k1}^2 & \sum_{k=1}^{n} A_{k1}A_{k2} & \cdots & \sum_{k=1}^{n} A_{k1}A_{k6} \\ \sum_{k=1}^{n} A_{k2}A_{k1} & \sum_{k=1}^{n} A_{k2}^2 & \cdots & \sum_{k=1}^{n} A_{k2}A_{k6} \\ \vdots & \vdots & \ddots & \vdots \\ \sum_{k=1}^{n} A_{k6}A_{k1} & \sum_{k=1}^{n} A_{k6}A_{k2} & \cdots & \sum_{k=1}^{n} A_{k6}^2 \end{bmatrix} \begin{bmatrix} Q_{11} & Q_{12} & \cdots & Q_{16} \\ Q_{21} & Q_{22} & \cdots & Q_{26} \\ \vdots & \vdots & \ddots & \vdots \\ Q_{61} & Q_{62} & \cdots & Q_{66} \end{bmatrix}$$

$$= E^2 \begin{bmatrix} 1 & 0 & \cdots & 0 \\ 0 & 1 & \cdots & 0 \\ \vdots & \vdots & \ddots & \vdots \\ 0 & 0 & \cdots & 1 \end{bmatrix} \quad (21)$$

In terms of the specimens which is subordinate to the normal distribution, T-distribution is used to assess the sample error. The assessment of the best possible value's error of rock stress components is:

$$\Delta_i = \pm T(n-t)m_i \quad (22)$$

2.3 The indefiniteness of data processing in some rules

A rock test rules regulate : " Using 12 measured strain values with a triaxial strain cell to solve 6 unknowns, there may be 324 composite samples. To the measured values of a survey point, data analysis must be carried on, i.e. firstly get the best values of the measured stress components from 12 survey values ,secondly abandon the one of the survey values that has the biggest residual error, then continue calculating with the remainders , repeat above process, finally 6 survey values are remained .Only after all the measured data and the calculated data have been analyzed can the rock triaxial stresses *in-site* being estimated at a point be affirmed."

It's demonstrated in a paper with above method

Table 1. The principal stresses in two holes

Hole	Point	Depth (m)	σ_1 (MPa)	Pitch (degree)	Bearing (degree)	σ_2 (MPa)	Pitch (degree)	Bearing (degree)	σ_3 (MPa)	Pitch (degree)	Bearing (degree)
1	1	4.1	24.3	-4	245	13.1	-17	156	6.5	72	143
1	2	5.1	12.0	-17	255	7.3	52	142	5.5	-33	177
1	3	5.8	17.7	-39	167	12.8	-44	129	12.2	-20	240
2	1	4.2	56.8	-2	71	36.6	-39	-17	26.4	51	-21
2	2	4.7	14.7	-26	53	6.5	36	-15	0.7	-42	117
2	3	5.3	14.6	11	230	5.3	4	140	4.1	-78	72
2	4	5.8	13.3	2	223	6.7	36	135	0.4	-54	130

Table 2. The compounded principal stresses according to the value's sizes of the pricipal stresses

Hole	Point		Value (MPa)		Bearing (degree)		Pitch (degree)	
			Average	Range	Average	Range	Average	Range
1	2,3	σ_1	14.9	12.0~17.7	211	167~255	-28	-17~-39
1	2,3	σ_2	10.1	7.3~12.8	136	129~142	-86	-44~52
1	2,3	σ_3	8.8	5.5~12.2	209	177~240	-27	-20~-33
2	2,3,4	σ_1	14.2	13.3~14.7	229	223~233	13	2~26
2	2,3,4	σ_2	6.2	5.3~6.7	147	135~165	1	-36~36
2	2,3,4	σ_3	1.8	0.4~4.1	106	72~130	-58	-42~-78

that abandoning different observations, the difference between the calculated normal stress and its best possible value may be 35%, and shear stress may be times larger. The rules don't make it clear that the observations with how much residual error should be abandoned. This makes the calculation of stress value random.

The authors consider, the observations, if they are not beyond the limiting error, have same survey accuracy, the best possible value of stress calculated from all the qualified samples according to the statistic method is the best value. It must be pointed out that, the observations are few, abandoning them in random could lead to the decrease of confidence.

3 CALCULATION OF COMPOSITE PRINCIPAL STRESSES ACCORDING TO STRESS DIRECTIONS

While using the holewall strain method to measure the rock stress *in-situ*, several points can be measured systematically in a hole, and the distance among these points is only a few meters. All of them are only a part, even to say, a point relative to the rock mass area which is probable several hundred or several thousand meters long. Then, the question that how to compound the principal stresses belonging to the series of points to a position's principal stresses come out.

The authors have measured the rock stresses *in-situ* in two holes at Tongkuangyu Mine in China, and the measured principal stresses are shown as Table 1.

Table 1 demonstrates that when the point depth is deeper than 4.5 meters, the rock stresses tend to be stable, i.e. the induced stress field is less than 4.5 meters, when calculating the original rock stresses, the readings of these points which are in the field should be picked out.

3.1 Compounding the principal stresses according to stress values' sizes

Table 2 illustrates the result of compounding the principal stresses according to the values' sizes of the principal stresses at the points. It is not satisfactory. As shown in Table 2, the composite σ_1 of Hole 1 is the average based on that the difference of the two respective bearing angles in Table 1 is 88°, almost perpendicular.

3.2 Compounding the principal stresses according to their directions

Using this method, the result of Hole 1 changes greatly as shown in Table 3, the fluctuating range

Table 3. The composite principal stresses according to principal stresses directions

Hole	Point		Value (MPa)		Bearing (degree)		Pitch (degree)	
			Average	Range	Average	Range	Average	Range
1	2,3	σ_1	12.1	12.0~12.2	248	240~255	-19	-17~-20
1	2,3	σ_2	11.7	5.5~17.7	172	167~177	-36	-33~-39
1	2,3	σ_3	10.1	7.3~12.8	136	129~142	-86	-44~52

Table 4. The average stress components (MPa)

Hole	σ_x	σ_y	σ_z	τ_{xy}	τ_{yz}	τ_{zx}
1	11.3	10.9	11.5	-1.1	0.1	-0.5
2	5.2	4.2	12.7	1.4	-2.7	2.4

Table 5. The composite principal stresses according to the average of stress components (MPa)

Hole	σ_1			σ_2			σ_3		
	Value (MPa)	Pitch (degree)	Bearing (degree)	Value (MPa)	Pitch (degree)	Bearing (degree)	Value (MPa)	Pitch (degree)	Bearing (degree)
1	12.4	-32	282	11.3	-26	209	10.0	47	150
2	13.9	-14	49	6.2	37	138	2.0	-49	119

of the directions of the principal stresses which are compounded can be reduced greatly. The principal stresses of Hole 2 do not change.

3.3 *Compounding the principal stresses according to the average of stress components*

At first, calculate the average of the stress components of all the measured points in a hole according to their coordinate directions (see Table 4), then calculate the composite principal stresses from them (see Table 5). It conforms to the mechanic principal.

4 CONCLUSIONS

1. The consummation of errors of the measured stresses should use the least square method. Abandoning the observations with same survey accuracy in random would bring the indefiniteness to stress measurement.
2. Compounding the principal stresses according to the average of the stresses components of all the measured points in a hole conforms to the mechanic principle, the authors recommend this method.

A geostatistical approach to evaluate differences in results between hydraulic fracturing and overcoring

J. Andersson
Golder Associates AB, Sweden

C. Ljunggren
Vattenfall Hydropower AB, Luleå, Sweden

ABSTRACT: Three-dimensional overcoring and two-dimensional hydraulic fracturing are the two most commonly used methods to measure rock stresses in-situ. A linear regression analysis on overcoring measurements of vertical stress has been performed and shows that some of the variance in the measurements can be explained by the depth dependence, but the remaining variance is large and apparently random. A second set of statistical analyses were performed in order to substantiate to what extent this variability could be attributed to the small measurement scale of overcoring data. The analysis shows that the variance of overcoring data is significantly larger than the variance of the hydraulic fracturing data, and that it is in the same order of magnitude as the large scale variability. Consequently, care is required when extrapolating results of a limited number of stress measurements.

1 INTRODUCTION

Three-dimensional overcoring and two-dimensional hydraulic fracturing are the two most commonly used methods to measure rock stresses in-situ. In Sweden, overcoring was first introduced in the beginning of the 1950:s (Hast, 1958) whereas the first hydraulic fracturing attempts were made in the beginning of the 1980:s (Doe et al., 1983). Today, the methods are commonly used in Scandinavia and the choice of method normally depends on the data required and on economical and practical limitations in each project.

Overcoring is based on the principle of strain relaxation when the rock volume containing the strain gauges is cut off from the outer stress field. The stresses are then calculated from the strains resulting from the overcoring process. Most overcoring equipments uses strain gauges with a length at the order of 10 - 20 mm. Hence, the measurement is affected of the small heterogeneities that exists in the rock. It also follows that the rock volume involved in a measurement is relatively small. Hydraulic fracturing on the other hand is based on the principle of counteracting forces. By application of a controlled force an equilibrium is disturbed, and the counteracting force that is balanced at the point when equilibrium is disturbed, is thus determined. In an hydraulic fracturing test the volume incorporated is in the order of m^3, which is substantially larger than that of the overcoring.

In Sweden and Finland a relatively large amount of overcoring and hydraulic fracturing tests have been conducted at the same sites, and in a few cases also in the same boreholes (Ljunggren and Klasson, 1996, Bjarnason et al., 1989, Lee et al., 1993, Litterbach et al., 1994, Ljunggren and Wikman 1996). When comparing results between the methods at these sites it is seen that there is a larger variability in the overcoring results between neighbouring points. Furthermore an overall larger variability is often seen in the overcoring results.

The discrepancies in results between the methods rise some questions when applying rock stress measurement results. To what extent are they representative in the application scale? What is the cause of the variability seen in the results? Is the observed variability due to natural variations of the rock stresses or are they due to measuring errors?

Although stress per definition is scale independent, there does exist a scale dependency from an engineer point of view. Since the rock mass is heterogeneous the result from a measurement will depend on the nature of the rock at the measurement location. In the case of overcoring, with a small measuring scale, the placement of the strain gauges across grain boundaries or within larger grains may affect the result. Hydraulic fracturing on the other hand, though based on an entierly different measuring technique, involves a much larger volume and is therefore not sensitive to the small scale variation in the rock.

2 STATISTICAL ANALYSIS OF ROCK STRESS MEASUREMENTS

In exploring variability in stress it needs to be realised that stress is a dependent parameter of rock structure and external loadings. It is thus necessary to consider both small scale variations due to the variability in small scale structures and to consider larger scale trends due to loadings and major structures. In order to substantiate these general observations a set of statistical analyses have been performed on actual rock stress measurements.

2.1 Depth dependence

Evidently depth is one reason for large scale variations in rock stress. Theoretically the vertical stress should depend on ρgz, where ρ is the rock density, g the gravitational acceleration and z is the depth. In order to evaluate how much of a measured variability in rock stress that could be associated with this depth dependence a linear regression analysis was performed on measurements of vertical stress, measured by overcoring in deep boreholes and in short boreholes from the tunnel at the Äspö Hard Rock Laboratory constructed and operated by the Swedish Nuclear Fuel and Waste Management Company (see e.g. SKB, 1995). In general the geology of Äspö is crystalline granitic rock. The rock stress data are assembled in a special database (Ljunggren and Persson 1995).

Figure 1 displays the measured vertical stresses. Already from this Figure it is evident that there is significant variability apart from the depth dependence. These observations were also confirmed by a stepwise multiple regression analysis of the data. Independent parameters tried included measurement depth, the modulus of Elasticity, the Poisson ratio and the horizontal co-ordinates. The following results were obtained:

- Some of the variance in vertical stress can be explained by the depth dependence - the R^2, see e.g. Dewore (1987), is in the order of 30%.
- The slope of the regression line is close to the slope of the theoretical line given by the weight of the overburden
- The remaining variance is large and apparently random. No other suggested parameter contributes to the regression.

2.2 Difference between overcoring and hydraulic fracturing.

A possible explanation for the large remaining variance in the analysed data could be that the measurements are performed with overcoring and has not been locally averaged. From a theoretical standpoint, large variability in overcoring data would be expected since measurements are performed at a scale of just o few centimeters. In

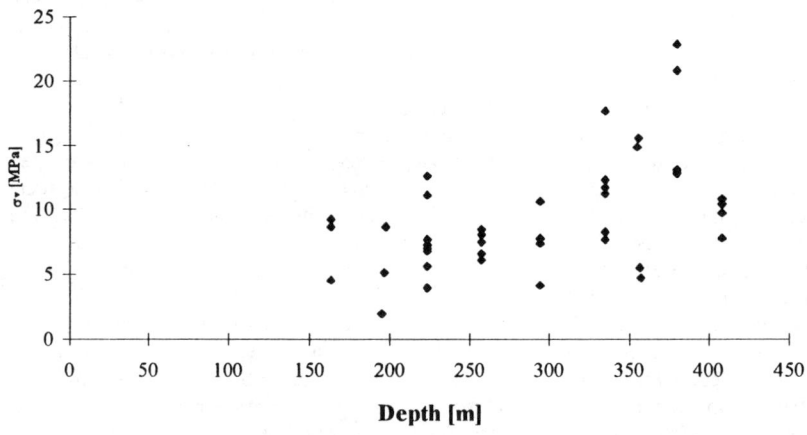

Figure 1. Vertical stress σ_v, as function of depth below ground surface. Data from overcoring rock stress measurements at the Äspö Hard Rock Laboratory.

contrast, hydraulic fracturing concerns stresses over a larger scale and could thus be expected to be less variable. A second set of statistical analyses of field data were performed in order to substantiate these differences.

As hydraulic fracturing primarily measures the minimum horizontal principal stress it seams appropriate to primarily compare estimates of the magnitude of this quantity with both methods. Data were obtained from two sites were measurements have been conducted with both methods. These sites were the Äspö HRL already used in the previous example, and Kivetty which is one of four sites presently being investigated in the nuclear waste programme in Finland. Kivetty is also a crystalline granitic site.

At the Äspö HRL hydraulic fracturing was applied in two deep boreholes, whereas overcoring was used in another, closely situated deep borehole and in some holes drilled from the tunnel. Clearly, one would not expect a perfect comparison of these data due to the large scale variability, but Figure 2 clearly displays that the overcoring data are much more variable than the hydraulic fracturing data. This observation is further supported by the data from Kivetty, displayed in Figure 3, where in fact the stresses were first measured using overcoring and then later with hydraulic fracturing in the same borehole.

Statistical analysis including descriptive statistics and analysis of variance provide further support to Figures 2 and 3. Figure 4 displays normal cumulative histograms of the hydraulic fracturing and overcoring stress data from Kivetty, subtracted by the general depth dependence (i.e. ρgz). The Figure shows that both the medians and the variance differ between the methods. For the Kivetty case the

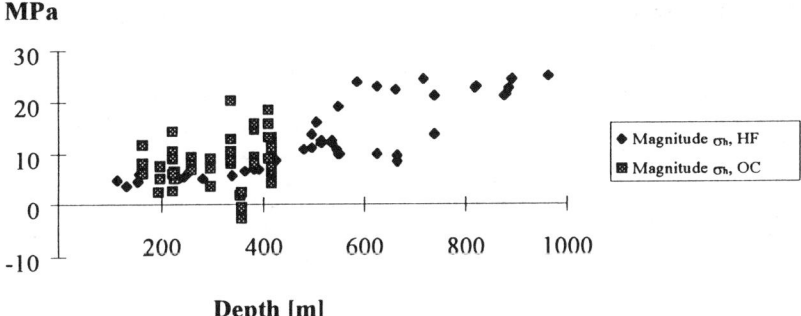

Figure 2. The minimum horizontal principal stress as a function if depth measured at Äspö using overcoring (squares) and hydraulic fracturing (diamonds).

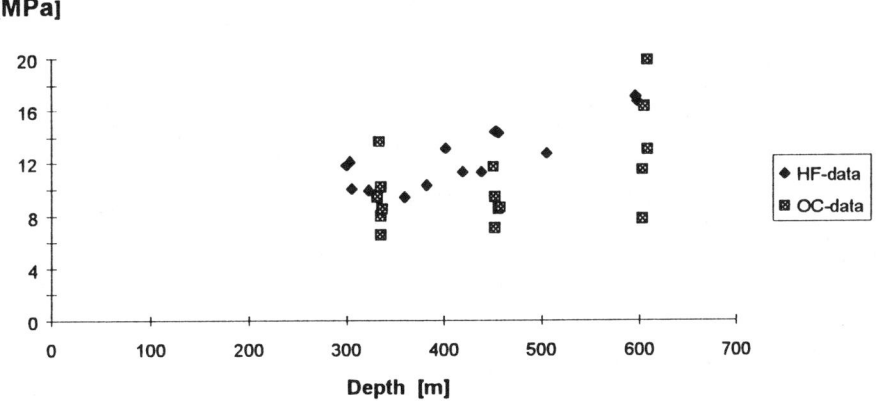

Figure 3. Minimum horizontal principal stress as a function of depth in one borehole at Kivetty using overcoring (squares) and hydraulic fracturing (diamonds).

median for the hydraulic fracturing data is about 2 MPa above the median of the overcoring data. For the Äspö data the medians are approximately the same. The standard deviation of the hydraulic fracturing data measured at Kivetty is in the order of 1.5 MPa, whereas the standard deviation of the overcoring data is in the order of 3.5 MPa. This means that an hypothesis that the two standard deviations are equal could be rejected at a significance level above 95%.

The following conclusions may be drawn from the analyses:

- The variance of overcoring data is significantly larger than the variance of the hydrofracturing data.
- The standard deviation of overcoring data appears to be in the order of 4-5MPa and are thus in the same order of magnitude as the large scale variation of stress data down to the 500 m level.
- In the mean the difference between the methods is less pronounced even if the Kivetty example suggest a significant difference. However, the difference is small in relation to the variance and it is furthermore not self-evident how to properly average the stress data.
- There is a large scale variability in data apart from the small scale variability.

The comparison between overcoring data and hydraulic fracturing data supports the suggestion that a significant part of the remaining variance in the earlier regression analysis could be explained by the fact that stresses were measured with overcoring, and without subsequent averaging. It should also be noted that the variance difference is reasonable considering the large scale difference between the methods. Clearly, the micro-structure of the crystalline rock could account for quite a significant stress variability also in the centimeter scale.

3 CONCLUSIONS

The analysis shows that rock stress varies over both small and larger scales. This implies that estimates of rock stress needs to be coupled to the scale of the engineering problem. In particular, data obtained from overcoring show a strong variability also over a very short scale, which suggests that just one or two overcoring stress measurements seems to be insufficient. More measurement would be needed and properly averaged.

Stresses show spatial variability apart from depth dependence and small scale variability. The reason for this variability could intuitively be explained by the distribution of larger structures and blocks. In order to study such stress variation comparison between measured stresses and results of numerical modelling would be of high interest.

Categorized Normal Plot for Variable: RESID

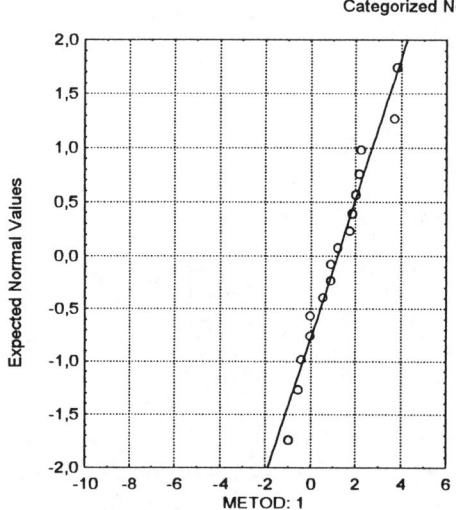
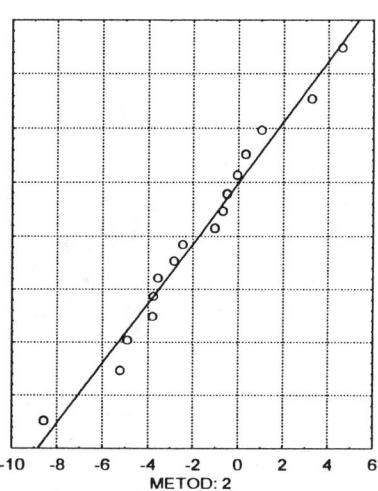

Figure 4. Normal histogram of minimum horizontal principal stress, subtracted for depth dependence, measured at Kivetty using hydraulic fracturing (method 1) and overcoring (method 2).

ACKNOWLEDGEMENTS

This work has been sponsored by the Swedish Rock Engineering Research (SveBeFo) and the Swedish Nuclear Fuel and Waste Management Co. (SKB).

REFERENCES

Devore J.L., 1987. Probability and Statistics for Engineering and the Sciences, Brooks/Cole Publishing Co, California, USA.

Doe, T.W., Ingevald, K., Strindell, L., Leijon, B., Hustrulid, W., Majer, E. and H. Carlsson, 1983. In-situ stress measurements at the Stripa Mine, Sweden. Report LBL-15009, SAC44. Swedish-American Cooperative Program on Radioactive Waste Storage in Mined Caverns in Crystalline Rock. 251 p.

Bjarnason, B., Klasson, H., Leijon, B., Strindell, L. and T. Öhman, 1989. Rock stress measurements in boreholes KAS02, KAS03 and KAS05 on Äspö. Progress Report 25-89-17. Swedish Nuclear Fuel and Waste Management Co.

Hast, N., 1958. The measurement of rock pressure in mines. Swedish Geological Survey, Ser. C, No. 560, 183 p.

Lee, M., Bridges, M. and B. Stillborg, 1993. Äspö virgin stress measurement results in sections 1050, 1190 and 1620 m of the access ramp. Progress report 25-93-02. Swedish Nuclear Fuel and Waste Management Co.

Litterbach, N., Lee, M., Struthers, M. and B. Stillborg, 1994. Virgin stress measurement results, boreholes KA2870A and KA3068A. Progress Report 25-94-32. Swedish Nuclear Fuel and Waste Management Co.

Ljunggren, C. and H. Klasson, 1996. Rock stress measurements at the Zedex test area, Äspö HRL. Äspö Hard Rock Laboratory Technical Nore TN-96-08z. Swedish Nuclear Fuel and Waste Management Co., 34 p.

Ljunggren, C. and H. Klasson, 1996. Rock stress measurements at the three investigation sites, Kivetty, Romuvaara and Olkiluoto, Finland, volume 1. Work Report PATU-96-26e. Posiva OY, Finland. 99 p.

Ljunggren, C. and M. Persson, 1995. Beskrivning av databas - bergspänningsmätningar i Sverige, SKB Djupförvar Projekt Rapport, PR D-95-017, Swedish Nuclear Fuel and Waste Management Co., (in Swedish), 21 p.

SKB, RD&D Programme 95. Treatment and final disposal of nuclear waste. Programme for encapsulation, deep geological disposal, research, development and demonstration. The Swedish Nuclear Fuel and Waste Management Co., 1995.

Validation of far field overcore stress measurement data using an integrated geomechanical analysis

W. F. Bawden
Queens University, Kingston, Ont., Canada

J. D. Tod
ESG Canada Inc., Kingston, Ont., Canada

ABSTRACT: An approach is presented whereby data from multiple in situ stress campaigns at a given site are combined using tensor statistics to derive a local in situ stress tensor for input into numerical models. The validity of the resulting mean stress tensor is then evaluated using an integrated technique incorporating conventional geomechanics, numerical stress analysis and microseismic monitoring. A recent case study of the extraction of the 2151-6W sill pillar at Campbell Mine, Balmertown, Ontario, was analyzed using this approach; the resulting mean stress tensor was found to be representative of the stress conditions at the site.

1. INTRODUCTION

Far field in situ stress measurements are commonly performed at Canadian hard rock mining operations. This data is generally used to provide input for numerical stress analyses which, at most modern operations, are run as a routine part of the geomechanical mine design and ground control studies. Overcore stress measurements represent the technique used most commonly, although other techniques, such as hydraulic fracturing and the bore hole slotter technique, are occasionally used. Under reasonable conditions overcore and borehole slotter measurements give similar results and are subject to the same types of limitations. These include:

- high cost [instrument cost, drilling cost, etc.],
- considerable data scatter, both within individual test locations and between test locations at a given mine site, and
- limited data.

In fact, all geomechanical data is statistical in nature and, as such, should be sampled in a manner which permits treatment of the data using conventional statistical techniques. With in situ stress measurements, cost limitations always result in data limited samples and a high degree of uncertainty in the data interpretation. Therefore, the fundamental questions that result are:

- how reliable is the in situ stress data for use in underground mine design studies;
- how can the engineer relate data from different locations in the mine, different measurement campaigns, etc.; and
- how can confidence in the data set be evaluated?

An approach has been applied to several case studies whereby data from multiple in situ stress campaigns at a given mine site are combined using appropriate tensor statistics to derive a local mine site in situ stress tensor for input into numerical models. This technique has the advantage of helping to smooth some of the initially more erratic field data. While clearly such an approach depends on both the (i) quality and (ii) quantity of available in situ stress data, techniques for filtering out poor quality data from individual tests at least are well known. At that point, however, the validity of the resulting far field stress tensor must still be determined

An approach for the validation of the mean far-field stress tensor, which has been used at several mining test sites, is described below. Input stresses for numerical modelling of the test sites are derived using the statistical approach discussed in section 2. The mean far field stresses are then used as input into the numerical models. The results of the models are then evaluated using an integrated technique incorporating conventional geomechanics, numerical stress analysis and microseismic monitoring. The degree of similarity between the observations and the model results gives an indication of the validity of the calculated far field stress tensor. This technique is briefly discussed in section 3 of this paper. Most recently, a case study of extraction of the 2151-6W sill pillar in the P-Zone at Placer Dome's Campbell mine in Balmertown, Ontario, Canada was done. The results from this case history are discussed in section 4.

2. THEORY

Because stress is a tensor, the average of several stress measurements cannot be calculated using the same statistical methods as would be applied to a series of scalar values (Dyke *et al.*, 1987; Walker *et al.*, 1990). To determine the average of several stress measurements, the average of the six individual components of the measured tensor must be determined. These average values will then represent the mean stress tensor (Walker *et al.*, 1990).

2.1. Determination of mean stress tensor

Prior to calculation of the average stress tensor, it is first necessary to transform the individual stress measurements to the same coordinate axes. The stress transformation is accomplished by the matrix operation

$$[\sigma^*] = [R][\sigma][R]^T$$

where $[\sigma^*]$ is the stress matrix in the new coordinate system, $[\sigma]$ is the stress tensor in the original coordinate system, and $[R]$ is the rotation matrix. The rows of the rotation matrix are formed by the row vectors of direction cosines of the new axes relative to the old axes (Brady & Brown, 1985).

The mean stress tensor of the transformed stress tensors is calculated using the relation (after Walker *et al*, 1990)

$$\bar{\sigma}_{xyz} = \begin{bmatrix} \frac{1}{n}\sum_{i=1}^{n}\sigma_{xi} & \frac{1}{n}\sum_{i=1}^{n}\tau_{xyi} & \frac{1}{n}\sum_{i=1}^{n}\tau_{yzi} \\ \frac{1}{n}\sum_{i=1}^{n}\tau_{xyi} & \frac{1}{n}\sum_{i=1}^{n}\sigma_{yi} & \frac{1}{n}\sum_{i=1}^{n}\tau_{yzi} \\ \frac{1}{n}\sum_{i=1}^{n}\tau_{xzi} & \frac{1}{n}\sum_{i=1}^{n}\tau_{yzi} & \frac{1}{n}\sum_{i=1}^{n}\sigma_{zi} \end{bmatrix}$$

The principal stresses are represented by the eigenvalues of the mean stress tensor, whereas the principal stress directions are represented by the eigenvectors of the respective eigenvalues (Brady & Brown, 1985). The standard deviation for the mean stress tensor is calculated first by rotating the raw stress measurement data to the coordinate axes represented by the principal stress axes, as determined using the technique described above. The standard deviations for each component of the mean stress tensor can then be calculated using the relation

$$S_\sigma = \begin{bmatrix} \sqrt{\frac{1}{n-1}\sum_{i=1}^{n}(\sigma_{xi}-\bar{\sigma}_x)^2} & \sqrt{\frac{1}{n-1}\sum_{i=1}^{n}(\tau_{xyi}-\bar{\tau}_{xy})^2} & \sqrt{\frac{1}{n-1}\sum_{i=1}^{n}(\tau_{xzi}-\bar{\tau}_{xz})^2} \\ \sqrt{\frac{1}{n-1}\sum_{i=1}^{n}(\tau_{xyi}-\bar{\tau}_{xy})^2} & \sqrt{\frac{1}{n-1}\sum_{i=1}^{n}(\sigma_{yi}-\bar{\sigma}_y)^2} & \sqrt{\frac{1}{n-1}\sum_{i=1}^{n}(\tau_{yzi}-\bar{\tau}_{yz})^2} \\ \sqrt{\frac{1}{n-1}\sum_{i=1}^{n}(\tau_{xzi}-\bar{\tau}_{xz})^2} & \sqrt{\frac{1}{n-1}\sum_{i=1}^{n}(\tau_{yzi}-\bar{\tau}_{yz})^2} & \sqrt{\frac{1}{n-1}\sum_{i=1}^{n}(\sigma_{zi}-\bar{\sigma}_z)^2} \end{bmatrix}$$

3. VALIDATION OF STRESS MEASUREMENT DATA

In situ rock masses are, generally, in a state of natural compression. Creating underground excavations disturbs the pre-existing force equilibrium, leading to rock mass movements as the ground attempts to find a new equilibrium that accommodates the newly created excavation's free surface. The rock mass movements, which are generally most pronounced adjacent to the excavation, may include slip along existing discontinuities, creation of new fractures, or continuous deformation of intact rock. These processes can occur at any depth, although they generally become more significant with increasing depth.

Slip along existing discontinuities and/or creation and propagation of new fractures results in the release of seismic energy. The magnitude of the resulting events can vary over a wide range, with larger energy releases (i.e. M > 1) possibly resulting in damage to surrounding mine openings. In such instances the event is called a rockburst.

It has been postulated that, for any rock mass, a relationship exists between the induced stresses, the stiffness (which may reflect ongoing failure), the seismic wave propagation characteristics, and the seismic energy released as a result of failure. This connection can be called the rock mass *stress-stiffness-velocity-seismicity* (σ-E-v-s) *relation* [Bawden, 1993]. The basic premise of this relation is the observation that, at increasing stress levels there is an increase in crack closure, resulting in a stiffer rock mass and, generally, a higher seismic velocity in the rock mass. The reverse is also true. Additionally, observations of seismicity generated in triaxial testing of laboratory samples indicate that low rates of seismicity can begin at stresses less than half the peak strength, with seismicity rates and magnitudes increasing to a maximum around peak strength. In the post-peak regime, seismicity rates and magnitudes tend to fall off rapidly.

This simple model of the stress-stiffness-velocity-seismicity (σ-E-v-s) relationship can be used to validate in-situ stress data by evaluating the results of 3D numerical model predictions compared to mine induced seismic data, visual observations underground, and conventional geomechanical instrumentation data. Results are evaluated based on failure zone locations, areas of de-stressing, and areas of stress concentration. In this way the 3D in-situ stress tensor used for the model input is evaluated. This approach is particularly useful where linear elastic modelling is applicable since, in this case, the material properties do not affect the predicted stresses.

It is also possible to directly compare the stress changes predicted by the model with those measured using conventional geomechanical instrumentation. However, direct comparison, while theoretically correct, can be fraught with practical problems due to the 'point source' nature of conventional instrumentation, combined with perturbations in the stress field 'local' to the instruments due to nearby geological structures. The use of mine induced seismicity for model validation is less affected by the local stress field perturbations, and provides a more 'global' validation of the in-situ stress data. Both of the above techniques were followed in the present study.

4. CASE STUDY – CAMPBELL MINE 2151-6W SILL PILLAR EXTRACTION

4.1. Background

Placer Dome Canada's Campbell Mine is a primary gold producer located in Balmertown in Northwestern Ontario. The 2151-6W Sill Pillar is located in the P-Zone orebody, a subvertically oriented pod- or pipe-like orebody. The P-Zone stopes were originally mined using cut and fill methods, which were converted to longhole sill recovery mining when the thickness of the remaining sill pillar reached 14 m. The 2151-6W sill pillar, located between 900 and 914 m depth, was extracted via a series of 7 blasts during the spring and summer of 1993.

A linked geomechanical – microseismicity – numerical stress analysis study was conducted on this sill pillar between 1992 and 1996 (Tod, 1996). During this time, a 64 channel full waveform microseismic system was installed in a closely spaced array around the sill pillar, and microseismicity associated with the sill pillar extraction was recorded. The stress change in the orebody footwall due to the sill pillar extraction was also monitored through the use of 4 IRAD gauges, oriented parallel and perpendicular to the orebody. IRAD gauge locations are shown in Figure 1a.

Detailed geomechanical mapping of the study area was conducted during this study. Data collected included in-situ stress measurement data, discontinuity orientations and properties, large scale structural features, and rock strength characteristics. The sill pillar extraction was simulated using the three dimensional linear elastic continuum boundary element model, *examine*^{3d}.

4.2. Mean Stress Tensor and Stress Gradient Calculations

Two series of in-situ stress measurements have been carried out at Campbell Mine. Both measurement campaigns used triaxial strain cells and overcoring techniques to collect the data. During the first campaign, a total of 3 measurements were taken at depths of 625 m, 990 m, and 1220 m (Arjang, 1986). The second series of measurements were taken in two perpendicular boreholes located at 1220 m depth, from which 5 measurements were considered repeatable, and were used to determine the stress magnitudes and orientations at the test locations (AECL Research, 1994).

Table 1. Magnitudes and orientations of Mean Principal Stresses.

Depth (m)	Data Set	Field Stresses in MPa		
		Sigma 1 (trend/plunge)	Sigma 2 (trend/plunge)	Sigma 3 (trend/plunge)
625	CANMET	20 ± 1 (041/04)	15 ± 4 (313/30)	10 ± 4 (123/59)
990	CANMET	52 ± 11 (075/16)	24 ± 6 (335/31)	12 ± 16 (189/54)
1220	CANMET	71 ± 15 (249/17)	41 ± 9 (346/21)	29 ± 15 (124/63)
1220	AECL	56 ± 17 (091/03)	43 ± 14 (000/11)	27 ± 10 (194/79)
1220	AECL & CANMET	60 ± 9 (259/06)	42 ± 8 (350/11)	29 ± 6 (189/54)
945	CANMET	45 ± 16 (070/01)	26 ± 6 (340/25)	20 ± 8 (161/65)
945	AECL & CANMET (using means from each level)	42 ± 32 (073/07)	27 ± 21 (341/17)	19 ± 17 (187/72)
1013	AECL & CANMET (using raw values)	48 ± 10 (285/01)	33 ± 9 (015/15)	23 ± 6 (190/74)

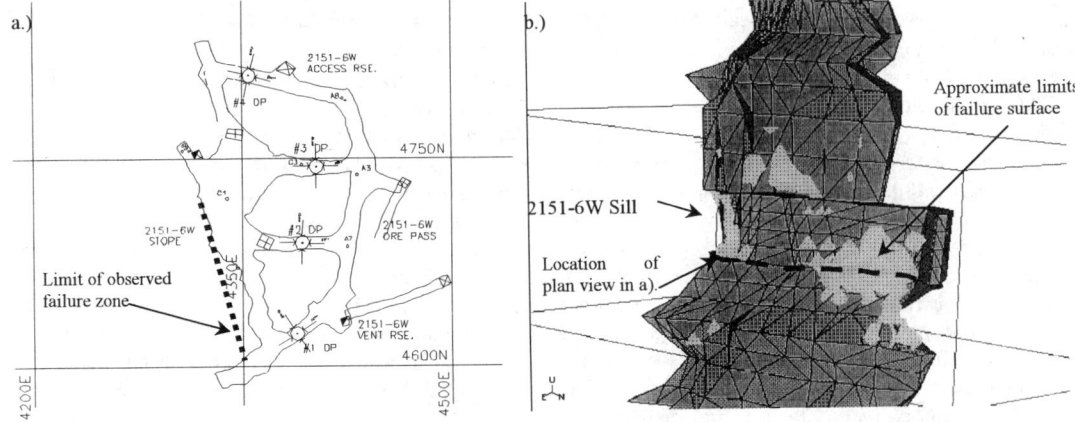

Figure 1. Approximate limits of hanging wall failure zone: a.) observed failure zone, and b.) failure zone predicted by numerical model.

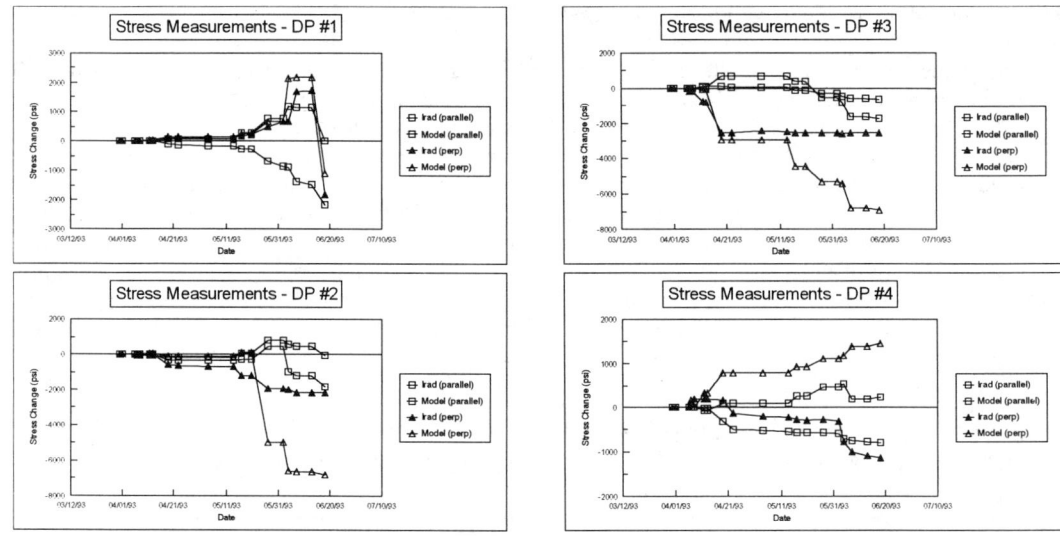

Figure 2. Comparison of IRAD gauge monitoring data and numerical model stress change values. Note limit of IRAD gauges is approximately 2500 psi.

Tensor statistics, as described earlier, were applied to the in-situ stress measurements to determine an average far-field stress tensor. Due to the limited number of tests performed at the site, all of the in-situ stresses were used in the determination of the average principal stresses. Mean tensors, and the corresponding principal stress magnitudes and directions, were calculated at each depth for which measurements were taken, as well as for an overall stress tensor. The overall stress tensor corresponds to the mean stresses at a depth of 945 m. Because the area of interest is between 900 m and 914 m depth, this value was considered representative of the study area, and was used as an input parameter into the numerical modelling portion of this study. The results of all tensor calculations are shown in Table 1.

4.3. *Model Calibration*

Model calibration was accomplished based on the back analysis of a failure, which occurred from the hanging wall of the stope excavation following the extraction of the final blast cut. The outline of this failure zone, caused by relaxation of the lower portion of the hanging wall, is shown in plan view in Figure 1a. Using the in-situ stresses determined above, the numerical modelling predicted the failure surface shown in Figure 1b, which occurs due to de-stressing of the hanging wall area. The model uses the Hoek Brown failure criteria (UCS=175 MPa, m=5.45, s=0.0319). As can be seen from these figures, the model predicted failure surface is very similar to that which was observed.

Figure 2 shows the stress change measurements from the IRAD gauge data compared to the changes predicted by the numerical modelling at the gauge locations over the extraction sequence. As can be seen from this figure, there is reasonable calibration between the stress changes predicted by the model, and those measured by the IRAD gauges, particularly at Drawpoints 1, 2 and 3. The results from Drawpoint 4 do not compare as favourably, and it is suspected that the gauges at this location are influenced by near-field stress perturbations due to local structure.

4.4. Evaluation of Microseismic Data

A total of 1605 microseismic events were recorded in the study area during the extraction of the 2151-6W Sill Pillar. These events were manually processed, and corrected for first arrivals of the compressional (i.e. P-) wave energies, and the corresponding polarities of first motions. Spatially, microseismic events tended to occur close to the excavations, and more specifically, to cluster around the blast locations, as shown for Blast 3 in Figure 3. Temporally, most of the events occurred immediately following the blasts, with the frequency of events dropping off to the background level of near zero within a few hours following each blast (Fig. 4).

The results from the numerical modelling are consistent with the observed microseismicity. First, the modelling predicted no zones of failure due to redistribution around the excavations, and ongoing microseismicity long after the blasts. Second, the microseismicity occurs close to the excavation surfaces. Based on the numerical modelling, these are the areas where deviatoric stresses in excess of 0.4 to 0.5 of the UCS occur. As mentioned above, this is the range in which low rates of seismicity can begin to occur. The microseismic observations also confirm the correct selection of an elastic model for the rock mass in this case.

4.5. Geomechanical / Microseismic Calibration

Focal mechanism analyses of microseismic data

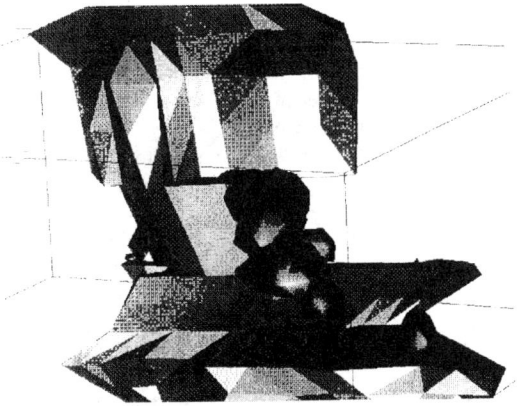

Figure 3. Clusters of microseismic events for Blast 3.

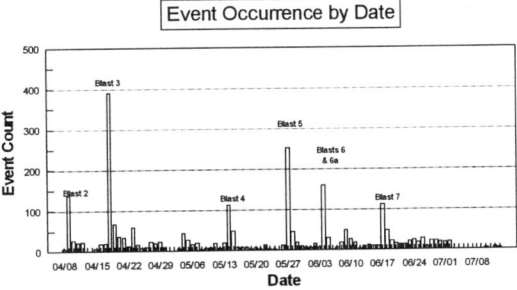

Figure 4. Temporal distribution of events over study interval.

attempt to determine the orientation of the feature along which a microseismic event occurred by examining the emitted seismic waves. A total of 889 focal mechanism solutions were obtained from the microseismic data, and following spatial and temporal analysis of the events, eight clusters with populations greater than 20 events were selected for further analysis. Most of these events were found to occur by a reverse faulting mechanism, with failure planes similar to the mapped regional foliation (117°/71°) and flat-lying joint sets (343°/20°). A ubiquitous joint analysis was performed using the numerical model to evaluate the slip potential of the various discontinuity orientations at the locations of microseismic data clusters (Kazakidis & Diederichs, 1993). Based on this analysis, it was found that slip was possible on the planes suggested by the focal mechanisms, giving more confidence in the in-situ stress orientations used in the numerical modelling.

5. CONCLUSIONS

1. Tensor statistics provide a reliable technique to assimilate diverse in situ stress measurements obtained over a broad area.
2. The use of an integrated stress – geomechanics – seismicity analysis has provided confidence in the statistically derived in situ stress tensor used as input in the 3D elastic model.
3. The comparison of measured mine induced stress change to 3D elastic model predicted stress change has, in this case, provided additional confidence to the statistically generated stress tensor.

6. ACKNOWLEDGEMENTS

The authors graciously acknowledge the support and assistance of Placer Dome Canada's Campbell Mine and CAMIRO (formerly the Mining Research Directorate) throughout this project.

7. REFERENCES

AECL Research, 1994. Overcore in situ stress determinations in drillholes 487 and 488 at the Campbell Mine. Report prepared for Placer Dome Inc., February.

Arjang, B. 1986. *Field and pillar stress determination at Campbell Red Lake Mine.* CANMET Division Report M&ET/MRL 86-57, April.

Bawden, W. F., 1993, Some ideas on the use of mine induced seismic monitoring to characterize a fractured rockmass based on a conceptual stress-velocity-seismicity-geomechanical model, in Proceedings of Geotechnical Instrumentation and Monitoring in Open Pit and Underground Mining, Szwedzicki (ed.), Balkema.

Brady, B.H.G and E.T. Brown, 1985. Rock Mechanics for Underground Mining. George, Allen and Unwin, London.

Dyke, C.G., A.J. Hyett and J.A. Hudson, 1987. *A preliminary assessment of correct reduction of field measurement data: scalars, vectors and tensors.* Proceedings of 2nd Int. Symp. On Field Measurements in Geomechanics, Kobe, Japan, Vol. 2, pp. 837-848.

Herget, G. 1988. Stresses in Rock. A.A. Balkema, Rotterdam.

Kazakidis, V.N and M.S. Diederichs, 1993. *Technical note: understanding jointed rock mass behaviour using a ubiquitous joint approach.* Int. J. Rock. Mech. Min. Sci. & Geomech. Abstr., Vol. 30, No. 2, pp. 163 – 172.

Tod, J.D. 1996. A Linked Microseismic – Geomechanical – Mine Induced Stress Analysis of the 2151-6W Sill Pillar Extraction at Placer Dome Canada's Campbell Mine. M.Sc. Thesis, Queen's University at Kingston, July.

Walker, J.R., C.D. Martin and E.J. Dzik, 1990. *Technical Note: Confidence intervals for in situ stress measurements.* Int. J. Rock Mech. Min. Sci. & Geomech. Abstr., Vol. 27, No. 2, pp. 139-141.

On determination of large scale stresses and moduli

A.N.Galybin, A.V.Dyskin & R.J.Jewell
The University of Western Australia, Nedlands, W.A., Australia

ABSTRACT: Results of *in-situ* stress measurements obtained by the conventional overcoring technique are related to a small scale (centimetres). To extrapolate them to the scales of interest to Rock Mechanics (from meters to kilometres) requires a large number of individual stress measurements followed, by statistical analysis if one is to avoid a considerable scatter of the measured values. In this paper, a measuring scheme for near surface measurements of stress using the cylindrical jack technique is proposed that allows the simultaneous reconstruction of the stress components and of the elastic moduli of the rock mass at a scale considerably larger than for the conventional methods such as overcoring. The scheme allows interpretation of the measurements near the surface of excavation in both isotropic and orthotropic rocks with a plane of symmetry parallel to the plane of measurements.

1. INTRODUCTION

With an increasing emphasis on the exploitation of large low-grade and of deeper ore bodies by underground mining techniques, concern arises for the safety of mining operations. Knowledge of the stress fields acting in the rock mass corresponding to both the original (pre-mined) regional stress state and the local stress concentrations caused by mining is necessary for the control the fracture processes in existing excavations and for the design of new ones.

This paper outlines the shortcomings associated with traditional small scale measurements (eg, overcoring) and methods of direct large-scale stress reconstruction: the under-excavation method as well as a proposed modification to the cylindrical jack method from which a measurement scheme has been devised to enable large-scale surface measurements.

Mathematical aspects of the problem for isotropic rocks have been developed earlier (Galybin at al, 1997). In this paper the scheme will be extended to the case of a 2-D orthotropic elastic medium such as exists in foliated rocks.

2. LARGE- AND SMALL-SCALE STRESS MEASUREMENTS

The major drawback to the use of the overcoring technique for the determination of *in-situ* stress is the irrelevance of extrapolating the results obtained by a small measuring device (tens of centimetres) to the scales of mining operations (from meters to kilometres). As a result, any one particular stress measurement can become non-representative as is illustrated by Figure 1 which shows a fragment of the photoelastic representation of the heterogeneous stress field created in a blocky rock mass under uniform external loading (Ergun 1970). If one attempts to reconstruct the external load by conducting a single small-scale measurement (the circle at A in Figure 1 which represents a borehole used in overcoring relative to the block size) the resulting data may have any value depending on the point of the measurement (cf. points A and B).

Obviously, the correct reconstruction of the external (large-scale) stresses requires a number of measurements scattered over the area in question from which to determine the mean value. If Δ is the range of the stress variation within the area and N measurements are conducted in random and at independently chosen points, then the standard error of the stress reconstruction will be $ERR=\Delta N^{-1/2}$. In particular, if the local stresses vary by 100% (which is not unusual given that at a contour of a circular hole under uniaxial compression p, the stress concentration varies from $-p$ to $3p$, 400%), measurements at $N=100$ points are required to reach an accuracy of 10%. Thus reaching the proper scale requires a large number of point measurements and becomes a very expensive exercise.

A potentially attractive method of obtaining a representative value for stresses at a larger scale is the under-excavation technique (Wiles & Kaiser 1994) in which the driven excavation itself is used as a measuring device. In this situation the scale of stress determination corresponds to the dimensions of the excavation. The method is based on displacement and stress measurements made within

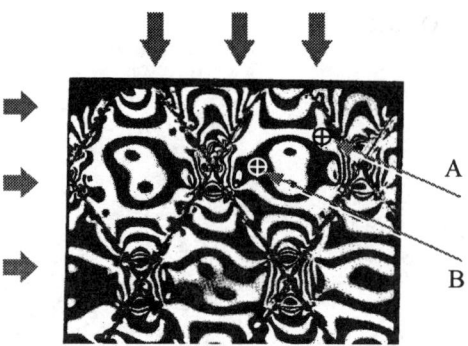

Figure 1. A fragment of photoelastic representation of the heterogeneous stress field created in a blocky rock mass under uniform external loading (after Ergun 1970).

the excavation as it advances and then the recalculation of the actual *in situ* stresses by back analysis based on a 3-D elastic solution. However, in this method the stress measurements around the excavation are still obtained by the overcoring technique and hence are of a scale much less than the one involved in the elastic solution.

The stress measurements at the larger scale required for the under-excavation technique can, in principle, be obtained by the flat-jack (slot) method in which the scale of the measurements is determined by the slot dimensions (the volume of rock involved in the measurement is of the order of 1-2 m^3, eg. Cuisiat & Haimson (1992)). However the method is laborious and expensive since in the conventional form of the method each slot allows the determination of only one stress component.

A simpler option is to use the cylindrical jack method (eg, Dean & Beatty (1968)) which allows a number of displacement measurements in different directions around a borehole after the drilling and subsequent pressurising phases and hence, potentially, recovery of the full 2-D stress tensor and the elastic moduli. The importance of determining the *in-situ* moduli simultaneously with the stresses should be emphasised, for these are required for the calculation of the stress concentrations at the excavation and hence for the evaluation of its stability.

3. SURFACE STRESS MEASUREMENTS AT LARGER SCALES

Three characteristics of an *in-situ* stress field can be determined by measurements near a free excavation surface. They are the two non-zero principal stresses, σ_1, σ_2 ($\sigma_3=0$ on the free surface) and their orientation θ_p at the surface. There are also deformation characteristics of the rock, generally unknown, which should be determined. For the case of isotropic elastic rock there are only two: Young's modulus, E, and Poison's ratio, ν. Therefore, in this case, five parameters of the stress-strain state have to be determined. Three of them, σ_1, σ_2, E, have the units of stress, the other two, θ_p and ν, are dimensionless. This means, that in an ideal situation five independent measurements should be performed and at least one of them must have the units of stress.

The cylindrical jack method indeed provides an independent measurement of stress: the jack pressure. However, the variant employed in the 1960's by Dean & Beatty (1968) has some shortcomings. These shortcomings mainly come from the measuring scheme adopted which is (1) based on monitoring only radial displacements, which is not sufficient to recover Poisson's ratio (since it requires an extra measurement in a perpendicular direction); and (2) the measuring pins are located close to the borehole contour, hence the scale of measurement is only of the order of the borehole diameter.

A new measurement system proposed by Galybin et al. (1997) described below has been developed to overcome these shortcomings and thus enables *in-situ* stress and full moduli determination over a larger scale. The key innovations are the proposed arrangement of measuring points and the adoption of modern displacement measurement transducers with the level of resolution necessary to enable the system to work.

The measurement system is based on a number of extensometers (eg vibrating wire extensometers) placed as shown in Figure 2 to monitor the displacement (elongation/contraction) in both radial and circumferential directions. Since the measuring pins in this arrangement are spread over a large area, the scale of the stress and moduli reconstruction is determined by the size of this area rather than the borehole diameter. In addition, the extensometers do not obstruct the drilling and pressurising operations and do not have to be removed during drilling.

In this arrangement N measurements are obtained in radial directions (lines 1-1', 2-2', ..., N-N' denote the radially placed extensometers of base length d) and N measurements in the circumferential directions (lines 1-2, 2-3, ..., $(N-1)$-N denote the circumferentially placed extensometers of base length $2r_0\sin(\pi/N)$). The number of measuring pairs, N, is to be chosen to satisfy the redundancy requirement (4 minimum) and to be sufficient for the desired accuracy of the stress determination, while the choice of the extensometer base lengths, d and $2r_0\sin(\pi/N)$ will be a compromise between the necessity to ensure appreciable scale of measurements and the sensitivity of the extensometers.

The mathematics of the stress and moduli reconstruction in elastic isotropic situation is described by Galybin et al. (1997). It has however been found that the accuracy of the reconstruction is not uniform: the most accurate are the reconstruction of the hydrostatic component of the stress state ($\sigma_1+\sigma_2$) and the shear modulus $G=E/2(1+\nu)$. There are cases in which the reconstruction of Poisson's ratio is not accurate, eg when the stress state is close

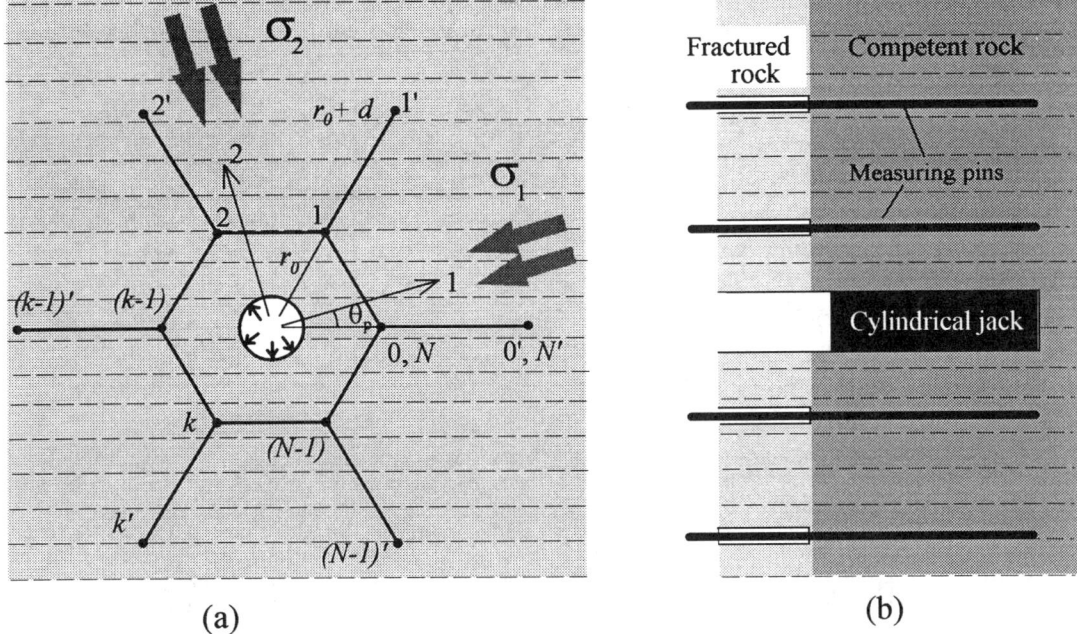

Figure 2. The measuring scheme for the cylindrical jack method in isotropic or foliated (dash lines) rocks.

to the hydrostatic one. In this case the influence of Poisson's ratio is minor anyway. For the stress states close to the hydrostatic, the deviatoric parts ($\sigma_1-\sigma_2$) being small reconstructed with high relative errors. Nevertheless, the orientation of the principal stresses can still be reconstructed accurately.

To demonstrate how well the original stress state and the Poison's ratio can be reconstructed using the proposed method three artificial examples of moduli and stress reconstruction are presented in Table 1. In these examples the moduli and the stress states have been specified, the ideal readings of the extensometers computed and then distorted by introducing random errors uniformly distributed within the range of (-10%, 10%). The reconstruction was undertaken with N=3, 4, .., 8 measuring pairs.

Analysis of the variation coefficients for the reconstructed parameters for different number of measuring pairs has shown that N=6 measuring pairs are sufficient for reasonable accuracy. The accuracy of the determination of the shear modulus is not considered here, for it will obviously be the best one since it uses all $2N$ measurements for determination of this single parameter. It should be noted that by monitoring the displacements during the process of pressurising, the non-linear behaviour of the rock mass and the dependence of the shear modulus on the pressure can also be examine.

The technique described above permits surface stress determination only. Section 5 discusses the ways of extending this to the full 3-D stress reconstruction. It is however worth noting that information on the surface stresses is important per se, for it reflects stress concentration developed at the surface and hence the risk of failure.

4. ORTHOTROPIC ROCKS

The discussion to date has related to isotropic conditions. Orthotropic conditions such as exist in foliated rocks or rocks with two orthogonal sets of fractures are more complicated and will now be considered. In this, 2-D consideration it is assumed that the surface of measurement is parallel to a symmetry plane (ie the fractures or foliation are perpendicular to the surface as shown in Fig. 2 by dash lines).

Displacements in an orthotropic plane with a circular hole can be expressed through complex potentials Φ_1, Φ_2 as follows (Lekhnitskii, 1968)

$$u(x,y) = 2\operatorname{Re}[p_1\Phi_1(x,y) + p_2\Phi_2(x,y)] \qquad (1)$$
$$v(x,y) = 2\operatorname{Re}[q_1\Phi_1(x,y) + q_2\Phi_2(x,y)]$$

where

$$p_k = (\mu_k^2 - \nu_1)E_1^{-1}, \quad q_k = -\mu_k \nu_1 E_1^{-1} + \mu_k^{-1} E_2^{-1} \qquad (2)$$

$$\mu_k = \sqrt{\nu_1 - \frac{E_1}{2G} - (-1)^k \sqrt{\left(\nu_1 - \frac{E_1}{2G}\right)^2 - \frac{E_1}{E_2}}} \qquad (3)$$

Table 1. Comparison of the average values of the reconstructed principal stresses σ_{1rec}, σ_{2rec}, the principal direction θ_{prec} and the elastic modulus $\kappa_{rec}=3-4\nu$ with the original ones (shown in the table head, in all cases $\kappa=1.5$) for isotropic rocks. The stresses are in MPa.

	$\sigma_1 = 32$, $\sigma_2 = 18$, $\theta_p = -20°$				$\sigma_1 = 22$, $\sigma_2 = 18$, $\theta_p = -20°$				$\sigma_1 = 22$, $\sigma_2 = 18$, $\theta_p = -50°$			
N	σ_{1rec}	σ_{2rec}	θ_{prec}	κ_{rec}	σ_{1rec}	σ_{2rec}	θ_{prec}	κ_{rec}	σ_{1rec}	σ_{2rec}	θ_{prec}	κ_{rec}
3	31.8	18.2	-20.2	1.72	21.8	18.2	-19.7	2.00	21.8	18.2	-51.3	1.98
4	30.0	20.0	-13.7	2.00	21.5	18.6	-14.5	2.00	21.0	18.9	-52.3	2.00
5	32.1	18.0	-20.0	1.50	22.0	18.1	-20.5	1.55	21.6	18.5	-49.4	1.01
6	32.0	17.9	-20.3	1.50	22.0	18.0	-19.9	1.54	22.0	18.0	-50.0	1.51
7	32.0	17.9	-20.0	1.49	22.0	18.0	-20.3	1.56	21.8	18.2	-50.3	1.29
8	31.9	18.0	-20.2	1.51	22.0	18.0	-20.0	1.51	22.0	18.0	-50.1	1.51

Here E_1, E_2 are Young's moduli along the principal directions of elasticity, ν_1 is the Poisson's ratio in x-direction, G is the shear modulus which characterises changes of angles between principal directions.

If the plane is subjected to biaxial compression at infinity (σ_1, σ_2) and internal pressure Q inside the hole, the potentials have the following form

$$\Phi_k(x,y) = A_k \zeta_k(x,y)^{-1}, \quad k=1,2 \qquad (4)$$

where

$$A_1 = -\frac{R}{2}\frac{(P+Q)(i-\mu_2)-(\sigma+i\tau)(i+\mu_2)}{\mu_1-\mu_2}$$

$$A_2 = \frac{R}{2}\frac{(P+Q)(i-\mu_1)-(\sigma+i\tau)(i+\mu_1)}{\mu_1-\mu_2}$$

$$\zeta_k(x,y) = \frac{x+\mu_k y + \sqrt{(x+\mu_k y)^2 - R^2(1+\mu_k)^2}}{R(1-i\mu_k)} \qquad (5)$$

Here the new parameters characterising the applied stresses in the plane: P, σ, τ are

$$P = \frac{\sigma_2+\sigma_1}{2}, \quad \sigma = \frac{\sigma_2-\sigma_1}{2}\cos\varphi, \quad \tau = \frac{\sigma_2-\sigma_1}{2}\sin\varphi \qquad (6)$$

These parameters and any of the four independent deformation moduli in Hook's law (or their combinations), form the full set of unknown parameters in the orthotropic case; μ_1, μ_2, $a_{11}=E_1^{-1}$, $a_{12}=-\nu_1 E_1^{-1}$ will be used as independent parameters.

If the displacement field $\mathbf{V}(x,y)=\{u(x,y),v(x,y)\}$ is known, the change of the length, $\rho_{i,j}$, of the segment connecting any two points (x_i, y_i) and (x_j, y_j) can be expressed in the form

$$\rho_{i,j} = \Delta \mathbf{V}_{i,j}\{\cos\theta_{i,j},\sin\theta_{i,j}\}, \quad \Delta \mathbf{V}_{i,j} = \mathbf{V}(x_i,y_i)-\mathbf{V}(x_j,y_j) \qquad (7)$$

where $\theta_{i,j}$ is the angle between the segment and the positive direction of x-axis. For the arrangement shown in Fig. 2, the relative elongation between pins can be expressed though a single index. Let the index j be equal to $j=2k+1$ for the internal pins and $j=2k$ for the external pins denoted in Fig. 2 as 1'...N', ($k=1...N$). Then coordinates of the pins are

$$x_{2k+1} = r_0 \cos\frac{2\pi k}{N}, \quad y_{2k+1} = r_0 \sin\frac{2\pi k}{N} \qquad (8)$$

for the internal pins and

$$x_{2k} = (r_0+d)\cos\frac{2\pi k}{N}, \quad y_{2k} = (r_0+d)\sin\frac{2\pi k}{N} \qquad (9)$$

for the external pins.

The elongations/contractions between the pins can now be expressed as

$$\delta_{2k-1} = \rho_{2k-1,2k+1}, \quad \delta_{2k} = \rho_{2k-1,2k}, \quad k=1...N \qquad (10)$$

The current angles between the line connecting the adjacent pins and the x-axis can be easily calculated from formulae (8), (9).

The number of readings available is proportional to $2N$ times the number of steps in the cylindrical jack loading. When readings δ_j are known with sufficient redundancy, the problem of simultaneous determination of the moduli and stresses can be reduced to the problem of minimisation of a proper functional in the space of seven variables

$$F(\mu_1,\mu_2,a_{11},a_{12},P,\sigma,\tau) \to \min \qquad (11)$$

In particular, one can use the following functional

$$F(\mu_1,\mu_2,a_{11},a_{12},P,\sigma,\tau) = \\ = \left\| \delta_j - 2\operatorname{Re}\sum_{k=1}^{2}(p_k\cos\theta+q_k\sin\theta)A_k\eta_{k,j} \right\| \qquad (12)$$

where $\|.\|$ stands for a norm, and

$$\eta_{k,j} = \zeta_k(x_{j+1}, y_{j+1})^{-1} - \zeta_k(x_j, y_j)^{-1} \quad (13)$$

Similar to what was done in the isotropic case (Galybin et al. 1997), a numerical experiment has been undertaken to estimate the accuracy of the stress and modulus reconstruction. In the model the geometrical parameters are $R=0.025$m, $r_0=2R$, $d=2r_0\sin(\pi/N)$. The moduli are: $E_1=11.8$GPa, $E_2=5.88$GPa, $G=0.686$GPa; the Poisson's ratio is $\nu_1=0.071$. The principal compressive stresses at infinity, $\sigma_1=-32$MPa, $\sigma_2=-18$MPa, are inclined to the x-axis at an angle $\varphi=20°$.

The readings are modelled as the ideal ones computed for the above stress state using the formulae (1)-(10) and then distorted by adding to each of them an independently generated random error which is uniformly distributed within the range of (-10%, 10%). That is, if the ideal readings form the vector δ with the components δ_j, then the readings used for the reconstruction will have the components $Y_j(1+0.1\xi_j)$ where ξ_j, $j=1,..,2N$ are independent random variables uniformly distributed over (-1, 1).

The reconstruction was performed with the number of measuring pairs $N=5, 6, 7, 8$. Only two values of the cylindrical jack pressure were used: $Q=0$ and 10 MPa.

The functional (12) written for the Euclidean norm was minimised using a procedure built into MATHCAD 6 PLUS with the initial value obtained from the exact values of the parameters randomly disturbed within ±30%. It should be emphasised that the minimisation procedure used is very sensitive to the initial value, which suggests that a search for a more robust minimisation method is necessary.

For each stress state, and for each number of measuring pairs, 50 sets of readings were independently generated, the values of P, σ, τ and μ_1, μ_2, $a_{11}=E_1^{-1}$, $a_{12}=-\nu_1 E_1^{-1}$ were reconstructed for every set of readings. The averages over 50 sets of readings and the variation coefficients (the standard deviation over the average) were then computed.

The principal stresses and the principal direction computed from the average values of the reconstructed parameters may be compared with the original ones from the results presented in Table 2 for different numbers of measuring pairs N.

Table 3 shows the variation coefficients representing the relative errors of the reconstruction.

It can be seen that the errors do not vary much when N changes from 5 to 8, which suggests that the minimum number of 2*2*5=20 already gives sufficient redundancy to determine the 7 unknown parameters.

Table 2. The parameters estimated for the case of orthotropic rock.

N	5	6	7	8	16	Exact
$-i\mu_1$	4.11	4.11	4.11	4.11	4.11	4.11
$-10i\mu_2$	3.44	3.44	3.45	3.44	3.44	3.44
E_1^{-1} 10^3MPa	8.50	8.50	8.49	8.51	8.50	8.50
$\nu_1 E_1^{-1}$ 10^4MPa	5.88	6.05	5.69	6.24	5.92	6.03
P/MPa	-25	-25	-25	-25	-25	-25
σ/MPa	5.34	5.35	5.32	5.36	5.37	5.36
τ/MPa	4.50	4.52	4.49	4.49	4.49	4.50

Table 3. The variation coefficients.

N	5	6	7	8	16
μ_1	0.002	0.001	0.002	0.002	0.007
μ_2	0.008	0.004	0.008	0.005	0.012
E_1^{-1}	0.011	0.005	0.003	0.006	0.011
$-\nu_1 E_1^{-1}$	-0.202	-0.164	-0.216	-0.257	-0.21
P	-0.002	-0.004	-0.004	-0.004	-0.01
σ	0.028	0.025	0.023	0.021	0.029
τ	0.025	0.027	0.025	0.017	0.025

5. FULL *IN-SITU* STRESS RECONSTRUCTION

The technique proposed for measurements of surface stress and moduli values can form the basis for complete, large scale *in-situ* stress reconstruction. Since a single installation can recover only a 2-D stress tensor related to the surface of measurements, measurements from at least two installations on differently oriented surfaces are required to compute all stress components. In order to extend these data and recover the original stress state in the rock mass itself further computations are required.

This can be achieved by combining the results of the stress measurements at different locations on the excavation walls by means of back analysis of the solution for the excavation (Goodman 1989). In order to do this the deformation characteristics of the rock mass are required. In the case of an elastic isotropic rock mass, only the Poisson's ratio is required and this may be obtained simultaneously with the stress measurements. In the case of a non-elastic and/or anisotropic rock mass a number of additional moduli measurements might be necessary.

Another method of large scale *in-situ* stress reconstruction is the under-excavation technique (Wiles & Kaiser 1994) in which the stress measurements are combined with excavation surface displacement monitoring during advance of the excavation face. This provides the necessary redundancy for accurate stress determination and, in principal, takes into account the time effects.

The above discussion relates to the situation when the rock near the excavation surface is representative of the rock mass as a whole ie; the damage at the excavation walls is insignificant. In the case of heavily fractured surface layers, the measuring pins and the cylindrical jack must be installed at a depth sufficient to penetrate competent rock, Figure 2b.

A more complicated situation arises when the fractured zone is so extensive that it is not possible to install the measuring device in the representative part of the rock mass. Despite that, the proposed method can still be used if an enhanced mathematical model of the excavation is available which takes the fractured zone into account.

It should be emphasised that whatever sophisticated method is used to obtain the physical stress and moduli measurements, the true large scale stress reconstruction can only be achieved by employing an adequate model (or a system of models) of the rock mass containing the excavation (or excavations) in question.

6. CONCLUSIONS

The measuring scheme proposed allows the simultaneous reconstruction of the stress components and the elastic moduli of an isotropic rock mass at a scale considerably larger than the conventional methods such as overcoring, albeit only near the surface of the excavation. The method also allows interpretation of the measurements (near the surface of the excavation) in orthotropic rocks with a plane of symmetry parallel to the plane of measurements.

The transition to full large-scale stress and moduli reconstruction can then be achieved by employing mathematical models of the excavation.

An advantage of the proposed measurement scheme is that the extensometers do not interfere with the drilling operations and therefore do not have to be dismantled, which will increase the accuracy of the measurements. A sufficiently robust measuring system could be left in place after the test and for example monitored during and after blasting to estimate the effect of such operations on the rock structure and the local stress distribution.

The next step in the investigating the value of this technique will be to conduct appropriate laboratory and field experiments.

REFERENCES

Cuisiat F.D. & Haimson B.C. 1992. Scale effects in rock mass stress measurements. *Int. J. Rock Mech. Min. Sci. & Geomech. Abstr.*, **29**: 99-117.

Dean A.H. & Beatty R.A. 1968. Rock stress measurements using cylindrical jacks and flat jacks at North Broken Hill Limited. *Broken Hill Mines Monograph No 3*: 1-8, Melbourne: Australian Inst. Min. Metal.

Ergun I. 1970. Stress distribution in jointed media. *Proceedings of the 2nd Congress of the Int. Soc. Rock Mechanics*, V.1, Paper No. 2-31, Belgrade.

Galybin, A.N., A.V. Dyskin & R. J. Jewell 1997. A measuring scheme for determining in situ stresses and moduli at large scale. *Int. J. Rock Mech. Min. Sci. & Geomech. Abstr.* **34**: 157-162.

Goodman R.E. 1989. *Introduction to Rock Mechanics*. New York: John Wiley & Sons.

Lekhnitskii, S.G. 1968. *Anisotropic plates*. NY: Gordon and Breach, Science Publishers, Inc.

Wiles T.D. & Kaiser P.K. 1994. In situ stress determination using the Under-excavation Technique. Parts I, II. *Int. J. Rock Mech. Min. Sci. & Geomech. Abstr.*, **31**: 439-446, 447-456.

Sound velocity as a measure of small stress change

O. Sano & Y. Mizuta
Department of Civil Engineering, Yamaguchi University, Ube, Japan

T. Murakami & Y. Tanaka
Nishimatsu Construction Co., Ltd, Japan

ABSTRACT: A travel-time of a dilatational wave in a granitic rock in situ has been measured every one hour interval for the past three years. The testing site was 450m deep in the Kamaishi Mine, northeastern Japan. A measurement path was 15 m long, and the best resolution of the travel-time was an order of ppm. Sudden changes in the travel-time were often observed in relation to earthquakes. Possible stress changes were discussed in terms of the stress sensitivity of Vp for dry rocks in laboratories. For the stress change associated with the Far East Off Sanriku earthquake, the stress change was estimated as 15 kPa, which agrees with the strain estimated by using source parameters of the earthquake. This result suggests a possibility to use sound velocities as a measure of very small stress changes in rocks in situ.

1 INTRODUCTION

A sound velocity is one of the useful parameters for monitoring long-term stability of underground structures in rocks, because the sound velocity is significantly influenced by the opening and closure of dry cracks. When the differential stress is high enough to create new cracks, a sudden decrease in the sound velocity can be observed with a formation of the crack. When the differential stress is not high enough to form new surfaces, the sound velocity may still decrease due to opening of preexisting cracks in response to decreasing compressive stresses. The sound velocity may contrarily increase due to closure of these cracks with increasing compressive stresses. The monitoring of the sound velocity can, therefore, be a tool for estimating small stress variations [Reasenberg and Aki, 1974; Gladwin, 1982], when the differential stress is sufficiently low.

Many laboratory data showed that the sound velocity increased with confining pressure due to closure of preexisting cracks [Birch, 1960; Birch, 1961]. The increment of the sound velocity with pressure decreased with increasing pressure. These results suggest that the stress sensitivity of the sound velocity should decrease with depth in situ. At a depth of 500 meters, for example, the stress sensitivity of the sound velocity, V_p, of Oshima granite [Sano et al., 1992] should be down to the order of 10 ppm/kPa. A very high accuracy and/or resolution is, therefore, needed to estimate small stress changes at depth.

A pulse transmission method was usually employed in a measurement of V_p in situ. In this method, a travel-time of the wave propagation was measured between the pulse application time and the time of the first arrival of the incident wave at a given distance. In order to create wave propagations in rock, explosives have been used by many authors. One of the reasons can be attributable to a fact that the explosives could easily produce strong motion within rocks. However, this property can not be suitable for a long-term monitoring and/or a highly precise monitoring of V_p, because of possible damages around striking points. An air-gun was used by Reasenberg and Aki [1974]. A magnetostrictive transducer and a piezo-electric transducer were used by Gladwin [1982] and Yukutake et al. [1988], respectively. Damage-free transmitters were particularly important when a stacking method was employed to get such a high resolution of 10 ppm as shown above.

When multiple samplings are needed for stacking data, each waveform should be recorded in a digital form. A simple calculation shows that memories more than 1 Mbytes are necessary for a full record of the waveform with a time-base required for getting a resolution of ppm in the sound velocity. In the early 1980s, it was very difficult to get a high-speed transient event recorder with such a large amount of memories. Gladwin [1982] employed a counter method where the base clock was counted during transit time between a transmitter and a detector. This method did not require a full record of the waveform but the travel-time. Although the counting method had a big advantage, the results might have lost any information that the waveform could show.

In either way, an accuracy and reproducibility depend on the accuracy and stability of the base clock. A timing error in transmitting wave propagation may occur for both ways. An error in the identification of the arrival of the first motion may also occur when the first break of the received wave is not sufficiently sharp.

When cracks are filled with water, Vp increases [Nur and Simmons, 1969; Thill et al., 1969]. Any change in the water saturation ratio of the cracks can be an environmental disturbance in the estimation of the stress change.

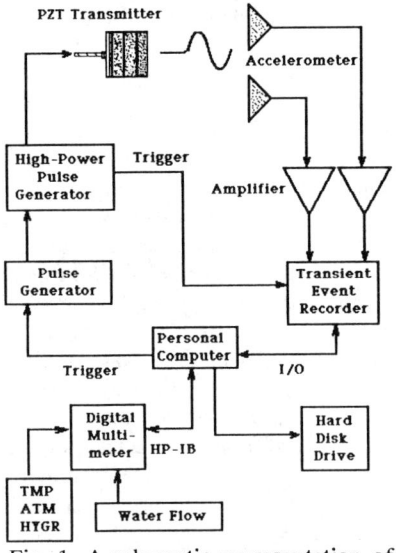

Fig. 1. A schematic representation of the system for soud velocity measurement.

2 EXPERIMENTAL CONDITIONS

A test site was an underground 450 m deep in a drift of the 550 m level of the Kamaishi Mine Co. Ltd, Iwate Prefecture, north-eastern Japan. The measurement site was more than 2 km inside from the entrance of the 550 m level. The rock was very hard granodiorite. Any mining-induced stress change could not be expected, because no excavation was carried out within several hundred meters from the test site. Any artificial air-ventilation was not used, because the testing site was in one of the branch drifts, and nobody works in this branch.

The experimental system was very similar to the one which Yukutake et al. [1988] was used. A schematic representation of the system is shown in Fig. 1. A laminated piezo-electric transducer was used as a transmitter on which a box car pulse of 1 kV with a duration of 20 microseconds was applied. Two accelerometers were set at a distance of about 15 m from the source. Two waveforms received by the detectors were recorded on a transient-event-recorder with a resolution of 10 bit and a sampling rate of 50 nanoseconds. The recorded seismograms were transferred on to a memory of a personal computer. In an each sampling, 4000 waveforms were accumulated in the memory of the computer. In order to check timing errors in transmitting wave, 1000 waveforms of the pulse applied on the source were also recorded. A rock temperature, an air temperature, humidity and atmospheric pressure in a drift were simultaneously monitored. The seismograms and other environmental parameters were recorded every one hour interval from 29th August 1994 to 12th December 1996 except for several periods of the power line down. The measurement still continues now, June 1997, at an interval of 30 minutes.

The accuracy and the stability of the base clock of the transient-event-recorder were better than 200 ppm and 10 ppm/K, respectively. A very precise and stable clock having an accuracy of 0.8 ppm and a stability of 0.01 ppm/K was used as a reference clock.

3 TRAVEL-TIME CALCULATION

The first quarter of the first motion was fitted by arbitrary cubic function by means of the least-squares-method. The arrival time was then estimated by an intersection of two lines, namely, a line defined by the maximum tangent of the cubic function and a zero level line defined by the observed signals just before the arrival. The travel-time was calculated between the time of transmitting pulse and the arrival of the first motion of the received wave, and could be determined with a fluctuation less than 50 ppm. A time at the first peak of the received wave was not easily affected by possible errors in the estimation of the zero level which might have affected the estimated travel-time. The time at the apex could be another measure of the travel-time which was denoted the travel-time of the second kind in this study. Fluctuations of this kind of the travel-time were smaller, by one order of magnitude, than the travel-time of the first kind.

4 RESULTS AND DISCUSSIONS

Neither daily nor seasonal variation of the rock temperature was observed within the accuracy of 0.1 K. Observed travel-time variations more than ppm should, therefore, be free from thermal effects on the length of the measurement path. The air temperature was almost constant within the resolution of 0.5 K. This environment is favorable for a highly precise measurement of the sound velocity.

Eighty-six sudden jumps in the travel-time were observed between 3rd November 1994 and 31st December 1995. The largest jump was found between 21:00 JST and 22:00 JST on 28th December 1994. This jump can be associated with the M 7.5 earthquake, Far East Off Sanriku, occurred at 21:19 JST on the same day. The epicenter was about 270 km apart from the observation site. The variation of the travel-time of the second kind is shown in Fig. 2 for twenty days including 28th December. The second largest jump shown in Fig. 2 was related to the largest aftershock occurred at 7:37 JST on 7th January 1995. In Fig. 2, several small jumps can also be found. In relation to all the small jumps shown in Fig. 2 as asterisk symbols, we could easily find aftershocks which might have affected these jumps, partly because many small aftershocks occurred after the main shock.

Coseismic changes in elastic strains for the main shock and the largest aftershock were calculated by Heki [1996] in the work of Heki et al. [1997]. The equation and the program used in the calculation were developed by Okada [1992]. His results are shown in Fig. 3 by letters (A) and (B) for the main shock and the largest aftershock, respectively.

For other small earthquakes, we could not easily obtain source parameters in detail, needed in the Okada's equation, but the magnitudes and location of the epicenters. The data of

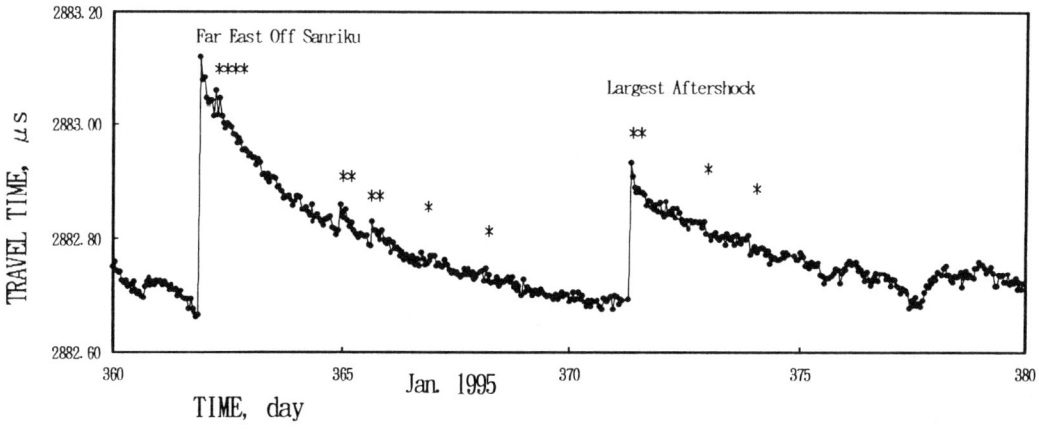

Fig. 2. Temporal variation of the travel time of the second kind defined by the peak of the first motion. Two large coseismic jumps were related to the M7.5 Far East Off Sanriku earthquake and its largest aftershock. Asterisk symbols indicate small coseismic jumps.

earthquakes, which occurred in an area enclosed by the lines, 138th degree and 146th degree of east longitude, 35th degree and 44th degree of north latitude, were then collected among the database of the Meteorological Agency Japan. The threshold magnitude was 3.0. As a first approximation for obtaining coseismic elastic strain change, we used the equation developed by Chinnery [1961], namely

$$u(x) = D/\pi \; \arctan(W/x) \quad (1)$$

where $u(x)$ is a displacement at a distance, x. D and W are a discontinuity and a width of source parameters, respectively. In addition to this, we used empirical scaling laws [Kanamori and Anderson, 1975], namely

$$\begin{array}{l} D/L = 2.0 \times 10^{-5} \\ W/L = 0.5 \\ Ms = \log(L^2) \end{array} \quad (2)$$

where L and Ms are a length and a surface wave magnitude of earthquakes. The calculated elastic strains and relating coseismic changes in the travel-time are shown in Fig. 3. The induced strains for two major earthquakes were also calculated and compared with the results by Heki [1996]. When we consider that neither radiation pattern nor gap between the epicenter and the moment center was involved in the approximate calculations, we can conclude that the coseismic travel-time jumps have a good correlation with the estimated elastic strains, inspite of the wide scattering of the results. We can also conclude that the coseismic change in length of the measurement path should be too small to explain the coseismic Vp change.

Reasenberg and Aki [1974] measured the Vp in situ with a resolution of about 100 ppm, and found a good correlation between the temporal variation of Vp and the earth tide. They suggested that the small stress change associated with the earth tide should have brought in the opening and closing of preexisting cracks, and could be responsible for observed variations of the travel-time. Yukutake et al. [1988] also found a good correlation between the travel-time variation and the earth tide. Based on the pressure dependence of Vp, they suggested that the observed variation was not directly affected by the stress change itself, but was mainly affected by water migration into or out of the rock in response to the stress change.

When the opening and closing of cracks due to stress changes were assumed to be responsible for the travel-time jumps, we can estimate the magnitude of the coseismic stress change. When we use the stress sensitivity of Oshima granite [Sano et al., 1992], we can obtain about 15 kPa for the travel-time jump of 120 ppm corresponding to the main shock of the Far East Off Sanriku earthquake. Employing elastic moduli of Oshima granite, we assume Young's modulus and Poisson's ratio as 80 GPa and 0.28, respectively.

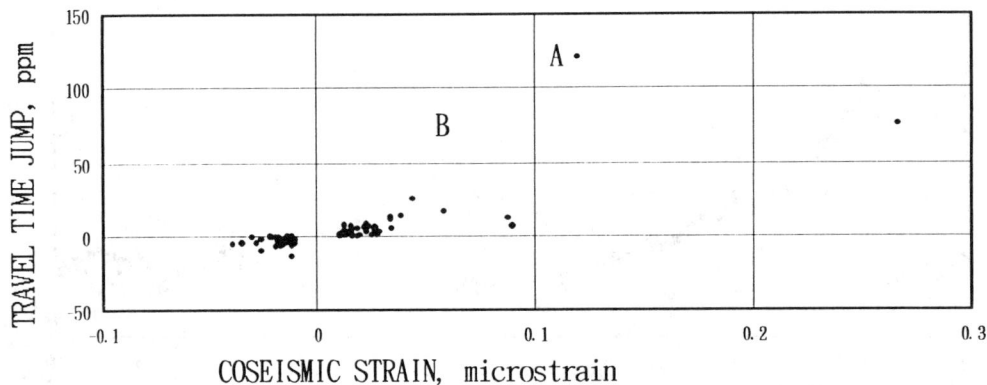

Fig. 3. Observed coseismic jumps in the travel-time are plotted against calculated induced strains. Eqautions by Okada [1992] and Chinnery [1961] were used in the calculation for two major earthquakes and other small earthquakes, respectively. The results by the former formula are shown in the letters (A) and (B), and others are shown in solid circles. In spite of wide scattering, a clear correlation can be seen.

The stress change of 15 kPa may correspond to the change in the elastic strain of 0.20 and 0.15 microstrains for plane stress and plane strain conditons, respectively. These estimated strains agree well with the calculated elastic strain shown in Fig. 3. Because the smallest coseismic change detected in this study was a couple of ppm, stress changes of several hectopascals could be detected in this system.

As suggested by Yukutake et al. [1988], we can also explain these coseismic changes in terms of the change in water content within cracks. Using the data shown in Sano et al. [1991], and assuming the water saturation ratio as 85 %, we can estimate possible change in the water content as 0.02%. The time domain of the coseismic change is, however, much smaller than the time domain of the earth tide which Reasenberg and Aki [1974] and Yukutake et al. [1988] discussed. Among the eighty-six coseismic events, we found a sudden jump within a couple of minutes just after the earthquake. It seems too short for sufficient water to diffuse out of the area of the wave propagation in hard rocks.

5 CONCLUSION

A laminated piezo-electric transducer was used as a transmitter to obtain sufficiently precise and non-damaging source for a measurement of the sound velocity. The measurement has been carried out for the past three years and still continues in June 1997. More than eighty coseismic jumps in the travel-time were observed in the period between November 1994 and December 1995. The coseismic velocity change was discussed in terms of the very small stress change due to earthquakes. The maximum coseismic change associated with the Far East Off Sanriku earthquake (28th December 1994) was 120 ppm, which corresponds to the stress change of 15 kPa. Although the discussions in this study were almost limited within the order estimation, the present study suggests the possibility to use sound velocities as a measure of very small stress change of several hectopascals.

ACKNOWLEDGMENT

Authors express sincere gratitude to Dr Yukutake who told us details of his system used in his work in 1988 and passed away in 1994. Authors express many thanks to Mr Takahara, Mr Saburi and other miners in Kamaishi Mine Co. Ltd. Discussions with Drs Fujii, Yanagidani and Hirata were particularly important for me to continue this long-term experiment in a distant site. Dr. Heki showed me his result. Drs Yamashita and Yoshii helped me to obtain earthquakes data through the network of the Earthquake Research Institute of the University of Tokyo.

REFERENCES

Birch, F., 1960. The velocity of compressional waves in rocks to 10 kilobars, part 1. J. Geophys. Res. 65; 1083-1102.

Birch, F., 1961. The velocity of compressional waves in rocks to 10 kilobars, part 2. J. Geophys. Res. 66; 2199-2224.

Chinnery, M.A., 1961. Deformation of the ground around surface faults. Bull. Seismol. Soc. Amer. 51; 355-372.

Gladwin, M.T., 1982. Ultrasonic stress monitoring in underground mining, Int. J. Rock Mech. Min. Sci. & Geomech. Abstr. 19; 221-228.

Heki, K., 1996. personal communications.

Heki., K., S. Miyazaki and H. Tsuji., 1997. Silent fault slip following an interplate thrust earthquake at the Japan trench. Nature. 386; 595-598.

Kanamori, H. and D.L. Anderson, 1975. Theoretical basis of some empirical relations in seismology. Bull. Seismol. Soc. Amer. 65; 1073-1095.

Nur, A. and G. Simmons, 1969. The effect of saturation on velocity in low porosity rocks. Earth Planet. Sci. Lett. 7; 183-193.

Okada, Y., 1992. Internal deformation due to shear and tensile faults in a half-space. Bull. Seismol. Soc. Amer. 82; 1018-1040.

Reasenberg P., and K. Aki, 1974. A precise, continuous measurement of seismic velocity for monitoring in situ stress. J. Geophys. Res. 79; 399-406.

Sano, O, Y. Kudo, T. Mizota and Y. Mizuta,1991. Influence of capillary water on the brittle fracture of granite. Suiyokwai-shi. 21; 390-396.

Sano,O., Y. Kudo, Y. Mizuta, 1992. Experimental determination of elastic constants of Oshima granite, Barre granite and Chelmsford granite. J. Geophys. Res. 97; 3367–3379.

Thill, R.E., T.R. Bur, and R.C. Steskey, 1973. Velocity anisotropy in dry and saturated rock spheres and its relation to rock fabric. Int. J. Rock Mech. Min. Sci. 10;535–557.

Yukutake, H., T. Nakajima, and K. Doi, 1988. In situ measurements of elastic wave velocity in a mine, and the effects of water and stress on their variation. Tectonophysics. 149; 165–175.

Estimation of regional in-situ stress field controlling subsurface fracture system by using microseismic multiplets

H. Moriya & H. Niitsuma
Faculty of Engineering, Graduate School of Tohoku University, Sendai, Japan

J.T. Rutledge
Nambe Geophysical Inc., USA

M. Fehler
New Mexico Institute of Mining and Technology, N.Mex., USA

ABSTRACT: We examine a method for determination of regional (field scale) in-situ stress field which controls fracture systems such as in geothermal reservoirs, oil and gas reservoirs, by using microseismic multiplets observed in downhole three-component microseismic measurement. A group of microseismic events with similar waveforms, which is called multiplet, are introduced to the stress field estimation method. In this paper, the structural planes which would behave as seismic sources are estimated from the source distribution of multiplets. The slip motion of the structures are estimated by the grid test on a moment tensor analysis using P-wave polarities and S/P amplitude ratios. The principal stress directions and stress ratios are calculated by the inversion using the orientations and the slip directions of the structural planes which are independently evaluated from the source location of multiplets and the grid test, respectively. This method is examined using the microseismicity at an oil field, and the feasibility of the proposed method for evaluating in-situ stress field is discussed.

1. INTRODUCTION

Microseismic events with very similar waveforms and high correlation to each other, in spite of different origin times, are observed in downhole microseismic measurement during hydraulic fracturing experiments, oil productions and in natural seismicity. A group and a pair of such the similar events are called a multiplet or a doublet. It is postulated that these events are the expression of stress release on the same part of fault. It is reported that precise relative location of multiplets can delineate subsurface structure such as hydraulically induced fracture in geothermal fields (Frechet et al. 1989: Moriya et al. 1994). Under a basis of an consideration that the multiplet source locations would represent the structures such as a fracture plane or adjacent subparallel fractures, we would be able to estimate principal stress directions and stress ratio by using the orientations and the dynamic behaviors of delineated structures. The authors are examining a method for determining stress field, which controls the dynamic behavior of reservoirs, from the precise relative locations of multiplets and the expected slip directions of the delineated structural planes. The aim of this study is to develop a method which allows us to understand three dimensional principal stress directions and principal stress ratios on reservoir scale by the deployment of a few three-component seismic detectors.

In this paper, the microseismicities observed during oil production at Clinton County oil field are analyzed. The result of stress field estimation and the feasibility of the method is discussed.

2. MONITORING OF MICROSEISMICITY

Microseismic events analyzed in this paper were observed during oil production in Clinton County, Kentucky, USA. The monitoring of microseismicity was carried out using three 3C geophones installed in two wells. Although, no injection activity was conducted before and during monitoring, a lot of microseismic events were induced. The both temporal and spatial relationships between the microseismicity and production was also indicated (Rutledge et al. 1996). The composite fault plane solutions are also estimated using P-wave first motions, and the set of low angle thrust faults have been revealed. These faults strike about N65° E and dip to both the NW and SE at angles ranging from approximately 15 to 35 degrees. The nodal planes of the composite fault plane solutions are well agree with the orientation of structures derived from the extensive hypocenter distributions. The principal stress directions and the relative stress magnitude ratio has been also estimated using Gephart's focal mechanism stress inversion method, where the high compressive horizontal stress condition is suggested (Gephart & Forsyth 1984: Rutledge et al. 1996).

From the original 29 spatial/temporal clusters which consist of the original 1720 located events, 91 multiplet/doublet groups were identified, where the ratio of multiplet/doublet in the data set is 57%.

3. ESTIMATION OF STRUCTURAL PLANES USING MULTIPLETS

We have applied the multiplet/doublet analysis to estimate the precise relative location of multiplets.
This relocation method is based on re-readings of arrival times, and the relative difference of arrival times among similar events are detected using the cross spectral moving window technique. The phase of the cross spectrum between two windowed waveforms is computed in frequency domain, and then the relative time delay is detected (Moriya et al. 1994). It is not necessary to pick P- and S-wave onsets in this cross spectrum analysis, the accuracy of the locations are remarkably improved.

Figures 2 and 3 show the source location of a multiplet group, where the absolute location and the relative location are shown, respectively. A structure is delineated clearer in relative location.

Because the events in each multiplet have very similar waveforms each other, and it is considered that they are the expression of stress release on the same fault planes, we have calculated the planes determined from the eigenvectors fitting the distribution of microseismic locations within each multiplet (Flynn 1965). Figure 4 shows the stereographic projection of the planes for eight multiplets, where the open circles denote the direction of vectors that represent the relative directions among the source locations. It is suggested that the multiplet locations are distributed in general along the planes which is striking WSW-ENE and have gentle dip.

4. EVALUATION OF SLIP DIRECTION OF STRUCTURAL PLANES

We have introduced the grid test on a moment tensor analysis to estimate the dynamic behavior of structural planes by using the waveforms of events detected using downhole 3C microseismic detectors. Although the unique solution of shear dislocation direction can not be determined, we can obtain the estimates of all the possible slip directions along the structural planes (Moriya et al. 1995). In this paper, we have used the P-wave polarities and the S/P ratios to calculate the possible fault orientations and their slip directions. The possible slip directions corresponding to each plane structure are summarized in table 1. It is suggested that most of the structural planes are suggested to have possibility of behaving as thrust or lateral strike slip faults.

5. ESTIMATION OF STRESS FIELD

Through the relocation analysis and focal mechanism analysis, we have obtained the estimates of eight structural planes and their expected slip direction of structural planes. Then, we have calculated the principal stress directions and stress ratios, where an inversion method using the orientation of structural planes and the slip directions are introduced (Hayashi & Masoka 1995).

Figure 5 shows the lower hemisphere equal-area projection showing the principal stress directions which are estimated using eight planes. Figure 6

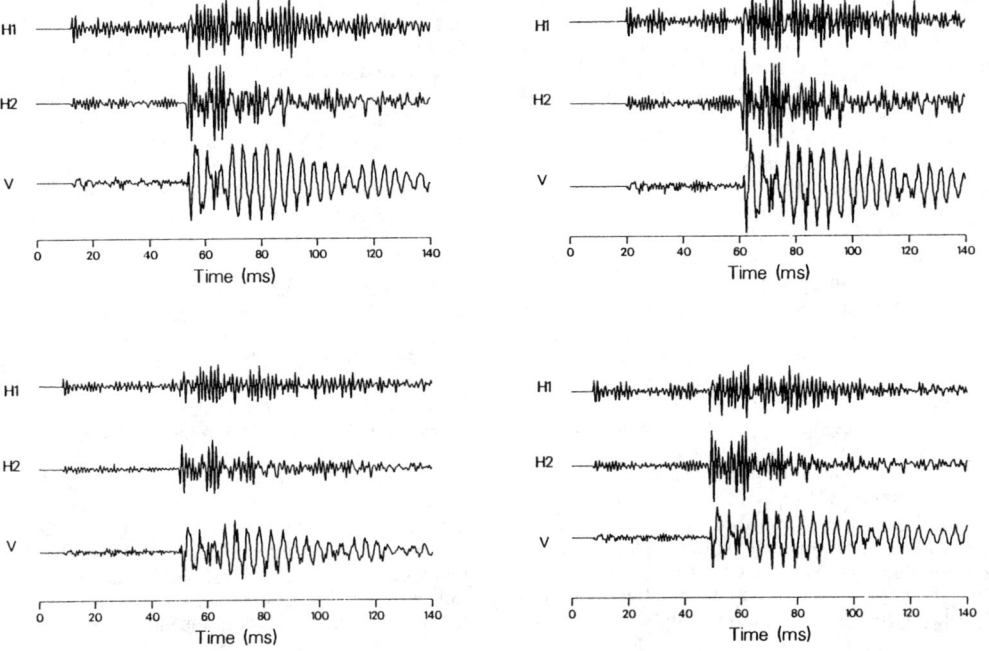

Figure 1. 3 component waveforms of a multiplet.

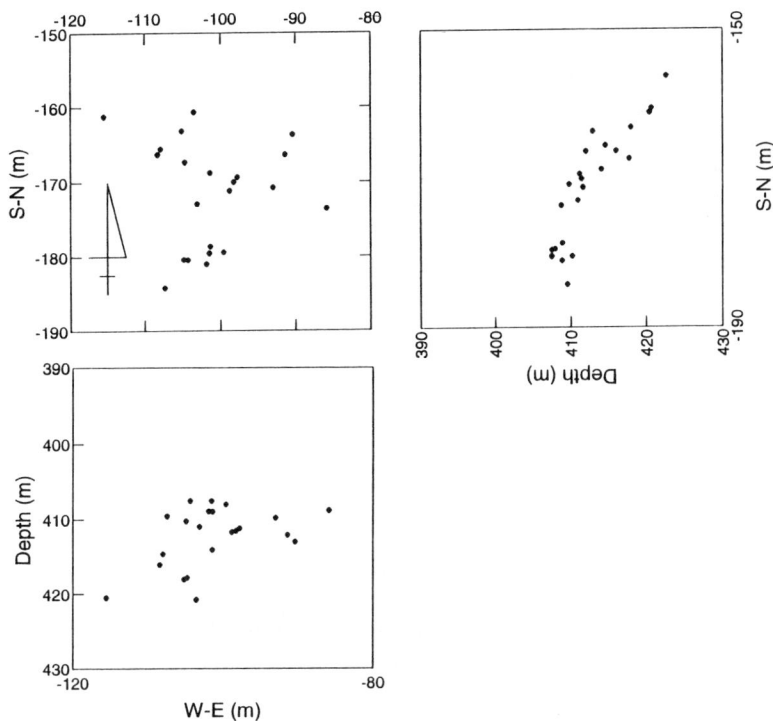

Figure 2. Source location of a multiplet (Absolute location).

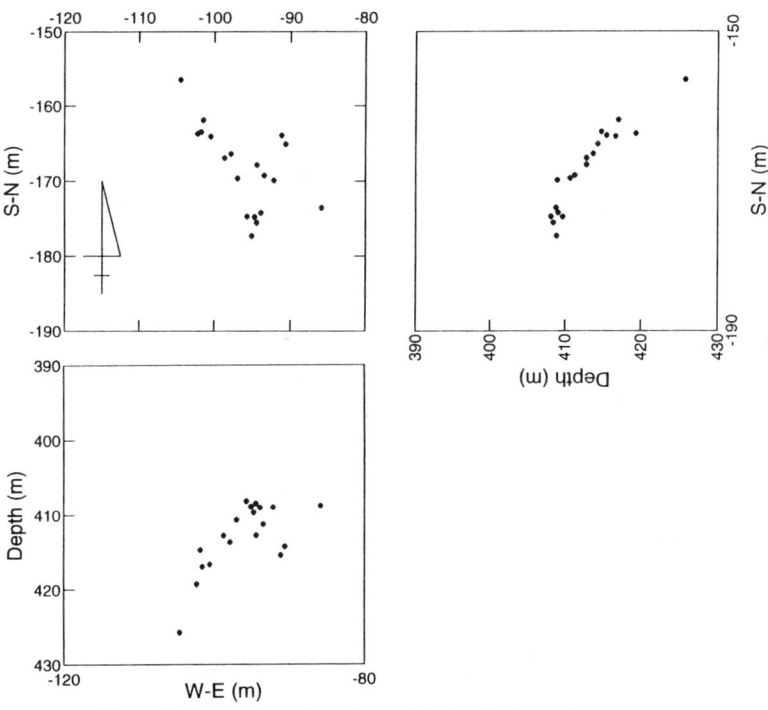

Figure 3. Source location of a multiplet (Relative location).

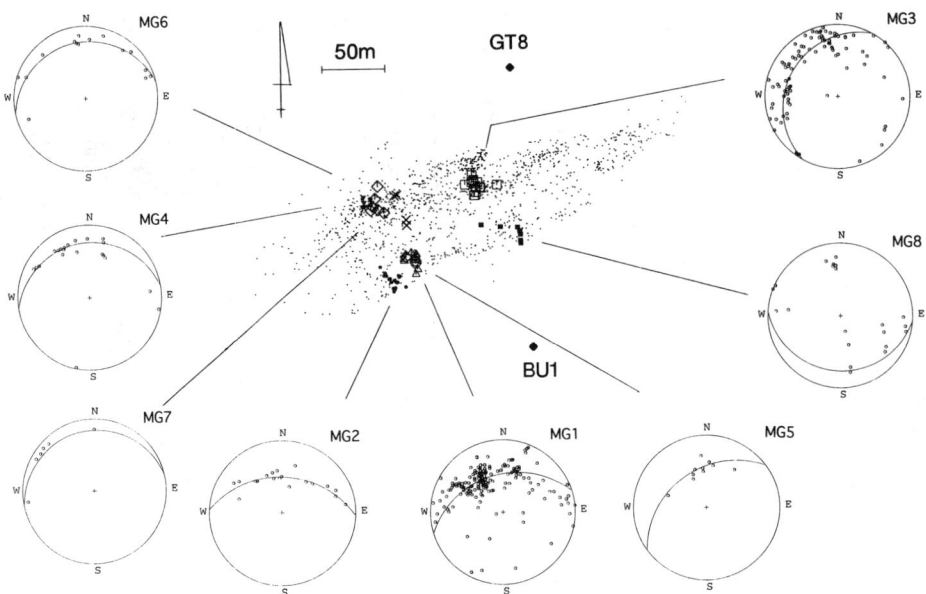

Figure 4. Structural planes derived from source distribution of multiplets.

Table 1. Orientation and slip direction of each structural plane derived from multiplet relative locations.

Multiplet (Number of Events)	Strike (deg.)	Dip (deg.)	Cr_2 (Cr_1)	Slip (deg.)
MG1 (19)	N254E (± 2.8)	35N (±0.8)	96.7 (84.1)	80
MG2 (7)	N273E (± 3.3)	38N (±1.0)	99.5 (78.3)	70-100
MG3 (14)	N209E (± 1.2)	19N (±0.2)	98.7 (64.7)	310-50
MG4 (7)	N262E (± 0.8)	16N (±0.2)	99.8 (95.4)	50-110
MG5 (5)	N235E (± 1.4)	35N (±2.3)	99.9 (95.5)	30-70
MG6 (6)	N258E (± 1.5)	14N (±1.4)	98.4 (85.5)	50-90
MG7 (4)	N251E (±39.8)	9N (±4.7)	99.9 (97.7)	40-90
MG8 (7)	N 94E (± 3.7)	15S (±5.0)	96.1 (87.6)	350

from the composite focal mechanisms (Rutledge et al. 1996). All the possible directions are calculated, where the errors in the estimates of plane orientations are taken into consideration. A total of 46200 sets of solutions has been obtained, and 80% of the solutions are included within the area encircled with the counter lines. The stress ratios are the function of normalized pore-pressure. In practical analysis, the coefficient of friction is given as 0.8. The stress ratio is also calculated using eight planes, and the relative stress magnitude R ($R=(\sigma_2 - \sigma_1)/(\sigma_3 - \sigma_1)$) is ranging from 0.71 to 0.76, where the normalized pore-pressure is changed from 0 to 1.

6. DISCUSSION

As mentioned, the estimate of stress field by Gephart's method in figure 6 agrees with the stress directions in figure 5. Since the stress change due to

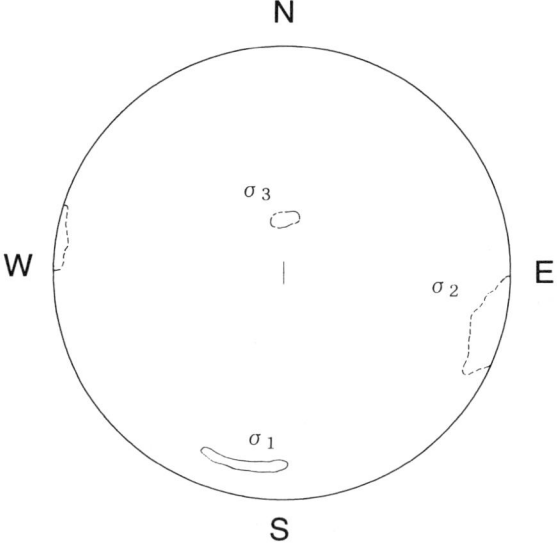

Figure 5. Calculated principal stress directions. Lower hemisphere equal-area projection showing the principal stress directions which are estimated using eight planes.

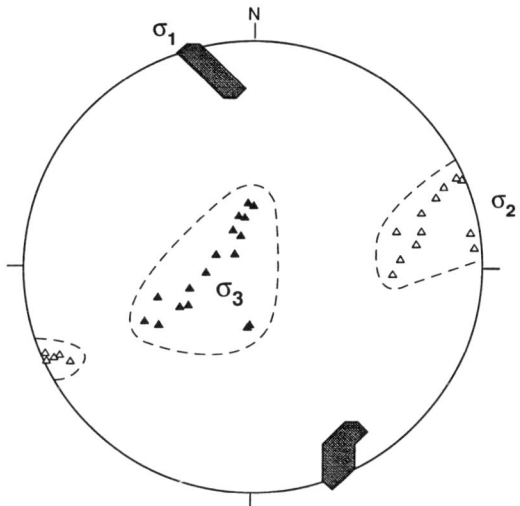

Figure 6. Principal stress orientations determined from the composite focal mechanisms. Equal-area, lower-hemisphere projection (Rutledge et al., 1996).

the drain of oil is evaluated to be small and the sense of slip motion at structural planes are similar, we could consider that the dynamic behavior of the structures is much depending on the background state of stress. Therefore, the estimated principal stress directions would represent the global and originally existing stress state which is controlling the dynamic behavior of fractures and faults in and around the reservoir.

On the other hand, it is reported that the borehole breakouts in western Kentucky indicates an orientation of the maximum horizontal stress of N81° E (Plumb & Cox, 1987). The maximum horizontal stress orientation suggested by earthquake was N71° E (Herrman et al. 1982). These stress directions are not consistent with our result. One of the reason would be that the rotation of principal stress directions due to the local structural controls at shallow depth, and this phenomenon is also appeared in the stress field estimated using Gephart's method.

Our method is a variation of focal mechanism techniques. However, the difference is that the orientation of structural planes estimated from the precise relative locations of multiplets and the expected slip directions of the structural planes are introduced in the inversion analysis for stress field calculation. In this method, the dynamic behavior is evaluated as to the structural planes and not as to a single microseismic event. Therefore, although we need more examinations and discussions, it would be able to consider that the effect of local stress heterogeneity is smaller in the estimate of stress field, and that a global stress field which controls the dynamic behavior of fractures in and around the reservoir can be evaluated.

7. CONCLUSION

It has been revealed that the estimate of stress field can be obtained through our method. As a result, the stress field similar to the result of stress inversion using the composite fault plane solutions has been estimated. A merit of presented method is that we can estimate stress field by using more than two multiplets and a few 3C seismic detectors, and which is the advantage of engineering applications such as Hot Dry Rock (HDR) and oil and gas field development.

ACKNOWLEDGEMENT

This research was made as a part of the MTC (More Than Cloud) international collaborative project. We are grateful for the support of NEDO (International Joint Research Grant).

REFERENCES

Flynn, E. A. 1965. Signal analysis using rectlineality and direction of particle motion. *Proc. IEEE* : **53**, 1725-1743.

Frechet, J., L. Martel, L. Nikolla & G. Poupinet 1989. Application of the cross-spectral moving window technique (CSMWT) to the seismic monitoring of forced fluid migration in a rock mass. *Int. J. Rock Mech. Min. Sci. & Geomech. Abstr.*: 26, 221-233.

Gephart, J. W. & D. W. Forsyth 1984. An improved method for determining the regional stress tensor using earthquake focal mechanism data: Application to the San Fernando earthquake sequence. *J. Geophys. Res.* : **89**, 9305-9320.

Hayashi, K. & M. Masoka, 1995. Estimation of tectonic stress from slip data obtained from fracture in core samples. *Proc. Int. Workshop on Rock Stress Measurement at Great Depth, 8th Int. Cong. on Rock Mech.* : 35-39.

Herrmann, R. B. & C. A. Langston & J. E. Zollweg 1982. The sharpsburg, Kentucky, earthquake of 27 July 1980. *Bull.Seismol. Soc. Am* : 72,1219-1239.

Moriya, H. & N. Niitsuma 1994. Precise source location of AE doublets by spectral matrix analysis of triaxial hodogram. *Geophysics*: **59**, 36-45.

Moriya, H. & H. Niitsuma 1995. Characterization of subsurface crack systems by combining triaxial doublet analysis and focal mechanism analysis. *Geotherm. Sci. & Tech.*: **5**, 123-146.

Poupinet, G., W. L. Ellsworth, & J. Frechet 1984. Monitoring velocity variations in the crust using earthquake doublets: An applications to Calaveras Fault, California: *J. Geophys. Res.*, **89**, 5719-5713.

Plumb, R.A. & J. W. Cox 1987. Stress directions in eastern North America determined to 4.5km from borehole elongation measurement. *J. Geophys. Res.*: 92, B6, 4805-4816.

Rutledege, J. T., W. S. Phillips & B. K. Schuessler 1996. Reservoir characterization using oil-production induced microseismicity, Clinton County, Kentucky, *Techtonophysics* (submitted).

Development of high sensitivity borehore strainmeters and application for rock mechanics and earthquake prediction study

Hiroshi Ishii
Earthquake Research Institute, The University of Tokyo, Japan

Tuneo Yamauchi
School of Science, Nagoya University, Japan

Futosi Kusumoto
Shimizu Corporation, Japan

Abstract

We have developed multi-component borehole strainmeters with a sensitivity more than 10^{-8} strain for earthquake prediction study. The instruments have sizes with 4 to 10 cm of diameter and 50 cm of length. Mechanical enlargement system invented are equipped inside of it and amplify about forty times diameter change of a vessel due to applied stress. Displacement sensors can transfer change of a vessel diameter into output voltage change. Based on these instrument, we have also developed a multi-component borehole instrument (diameter: 10 cm, length: 200 – 500 cm) which can observe three components of strain, two components of tilt, three components of seismic waves and temperature equipped with a gyro system.

For earthquake prediction study the multi-component borehole instruments were installed into boreholes at depths from 150m to 800m in seismically active areas. They are recording well data relating to earthquake activities and crustal deformations.

We also applied the strainmeters for rock mechanics and civil engineering purposes. We employed them for investigating rock behavior and 3 dimensional deformation of the rock at a tunnel diverging point during tunnel excavation. The measuring system was useful to clarify rock behavior in the diverging tunnel

1. INTRODUCTION

Crustal movement observation (especially strain) is important for earthquake prediction research. Up to now Japan Meteorological Agency distributed volume strainmeters (Sacks and Evertoson,1971) in 31 places in the Kanto Tokai area. Sakata (1981) developed 3 components strainmeter applying Sacks type principle. The principle of these instruments is to transfer strain change into movement of silicon oil sealed up in a cylindrical vessel. Sensitivity of instruments is high but instruments are very large as usually 8 to 10 m long and heavy. On the other hand Gladwin (1984) developed 3 component strainmeter whose measuring principle is to measure diameter change of vessel by using capacity sensor.

Multi-component observation by small instruments with high sensitivity must be performed in deep borehole in order to progress earthquake prediction observation, by looking at the present situation.

2. DEVELOPMENT OF HIGH SENSITIVITY BOREHOLE STRAINMETER

We have developed multi-component borehole strainmeters with a sensitivity more than 10^{-8} strain for earthquake prediction study. The instruments have sizes with 4 to 10 cm of diameter and 50 cm of length and are observable for long period as more than ten years. Mechanical enlargement system invented is equipped inside of it and amplify about forty times diameter change of a vessel due to applied stress. Displacement sensor is magnetic sensor and can transfer change of a vessel diameter into output voltage change. The mechanical enlargement system is schematically shown in Fig.1. Principle of lever is employed to amplify a displacement applied to the system and amplification reach to about 40 times. Strain meters usually equip with three enlargement system for recording 3 components strain. Strain meters are fixed with rocks by expansion cement grout with expansion coefficient of 0.15 %.

For earthquake prediction study the strain meters were installed into bore holes at

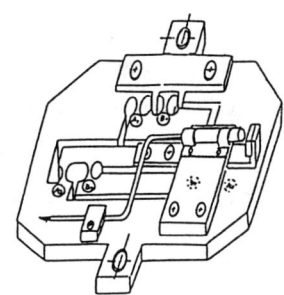

Fig.1: Enlargement part of strainmeter

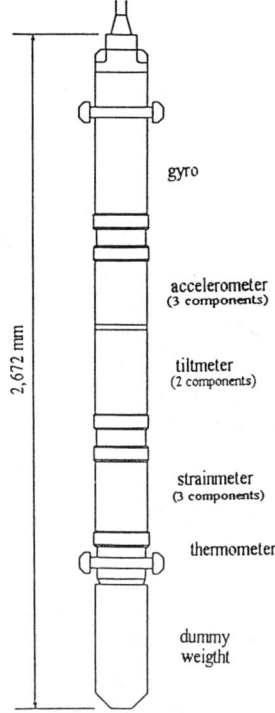

Fig.2: Multi-component borehole instrument

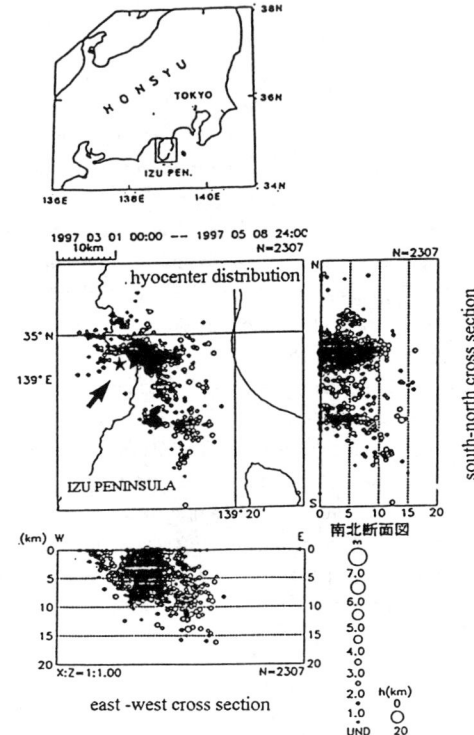

Fig.3: Hypocenter distribution of earthquake swarms (after J.M.A.) and location of borehole observation station (star mark)

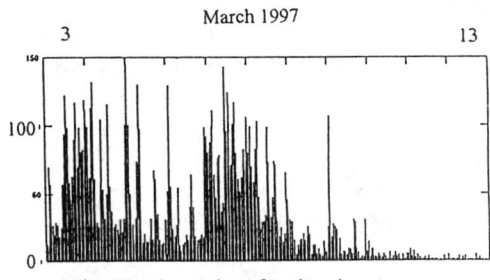

Fig.4: Hourly number of earthquake swarms at Kamata station (after J.M.A.)

depths from 150m to 800m in seismically active areas. They are recording well data relating to earthquake activities and crustal deformations.

3. MULTI-COMPONENT BOREHOLE INSTRUMENTS

We have also developed a multi-component borehole instruments which can observe three components of strain, two components of tilt, three components of seismic waves and temperature (Fig.2).

The tiltmeter was also newly developed for this instrument. Two parallel leaf springs support a weight and movement of the weight is recorded for measuring tilt by using a displacement to voltage transfer sensor.. A special metal whose elastic constant is stable for temperature changes is utilized as leaf springs.

The length of the spring is 5 cm and width of that is 5 mm. In this tiltmeter a damping oil is not used. There is no mechanical damper but natural period of pendulum is removed by filtering of electrical circuit. Therefore, this tiltmeter can well record co-seismic tilt steps as well as Earth tide. The multi-component borehole instrument has a size with 10 cm of diameter and 200 cm to 500 cm of length depending on how many observation sensors are installed. The instrument is equipped with a small gyro system developed by us so that we can set up a multi-component instrument in deep boreholes up to 1 km as can continuously record the direction of the instrument from surface to the last stage of borehole bottom during installation.

The instruments were set up at depths from 150m to 800m for earthquake prediction observation up to now and have recorded well data. Some examples of observed data are reported in the next section.

4. AN EXAMPLE OF OBSERVED DATA

We will present an example of observation results by multi-component borehole instruments. Earthquake swarms often occurs

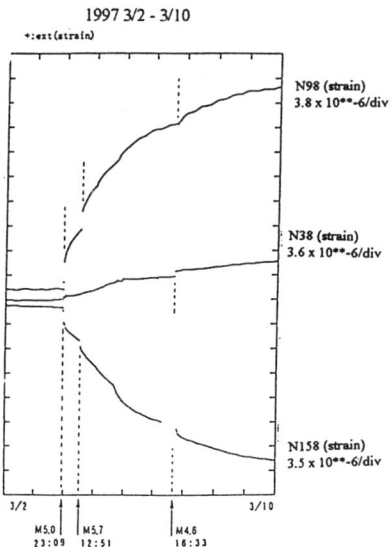

Fig.5: Anomalous strain changes (3 components) observed by multi-component borehole instrument during earthquake swarms

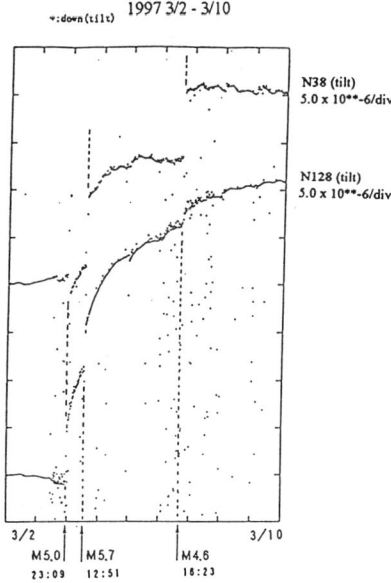

Fig.6: Anomalous tilt changes (2 components) observed by multi-component borehole instrument during earthquake swarms

in the off east coast of Izu peninsula located about 120 km southeast of Tokyo in Japan. In 1989 undersea volcanic eruption occurred off

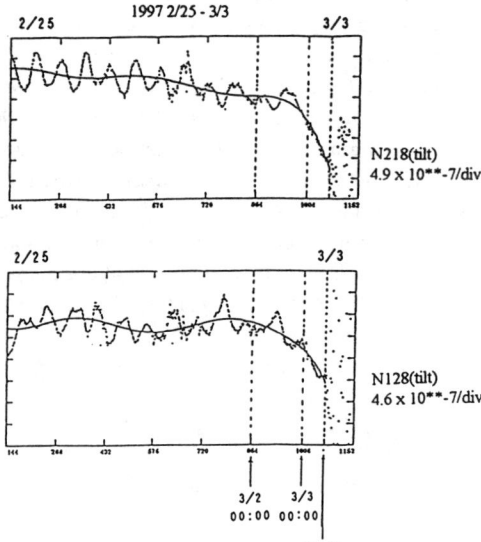

Fig.7: Anomalous tilt variation preceding the earthquake swarms. Solid lines are approximated curves by Chebyshev function

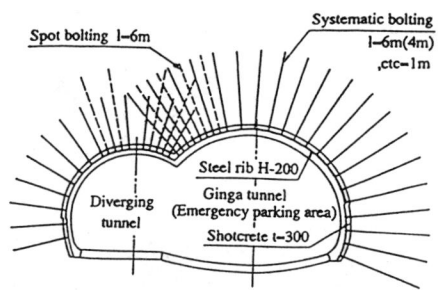

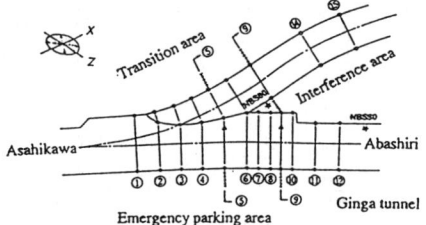

Fig.8: Cross section (upper) and plane figure (lower) for transition area of the Ginga tunnel. Borehole strainmeters NBS60 and NBS90 are installed at star marks.

east coast of Izu peninsula. Earthquake swarms occurred from 3rd of March in 1997. Our borehole observation station is located very close to the earthquake swarm area. Hypocenter distribution of the earthquakes are shown in Fig.3. The location of our observation station is also indicated in Fig.3 and the depth of the borehole is 150 m. Hourly number of earthquakes observed at Kamata station of J.M.A. is plotted in Fig.4 and total number of earthquakes reached to more than 9,000. Three strain components observed by the multi-component borehole instrument are illustrated in Fig.5 from 2nd of March to 10th of March in 1997. It is found that from 3rd of March anomalous strain variation started and became stable after about 10th of March. We can also realize strain steps as co-seismic behavior. The anomalous variations were also recorded by tiltmeter as in Fig.6. We can see a similar variation as the case of strains. That is considered to be related to movement of material like magma or hot water near the surface in the upper part of the crust. The variation at a time of beginning of the swarms are presented in Fig.7. It is realized that the anomalous change started from at noon of 2nd of March before the start of the earthquake swarms (0:20 o'clock of 3rd of March). Therefore, these variation may be precursory phenomena preceding the earthquake swarms. By these data mechanism of earthquake swarms can be discussed and the detailed analysis will be reported elsewhere.

5. ROCK BEHAVIOR OF DIVERGING TUNNELS

We also applied the instruments for rock mechanics and civil engineering purposes. The Ginga tunnel is beiing constructed as a by-pass tunnnel of National Highway 39 at a location in Daisetuzan National Park in the So-unkyo region of Kamikawa-cho, Hokkaido where columnar joints stand in a row. Cross section and plane figure of the transition area are shown in Figs.8 . In Fig.8 two star marks indicate 3 component strainmeters NBS60 and NBS90 installed.

The NBS60 was placed about two meters away from a boring hole in the orthogonal direction to the axis of the diverging tunnel almost horizontally from the surface of the wall of the Ginga Tunnel. The NBS90 was placed downward from the bottom of the Ginga Tunnel and was distant about 30 m from the diverging tunnel. The instruments monitored strain changes by redistribution of equivalent excavation stress during tunnel excavation work. Upper in Fig.9 illustrates strain change of NBS60 caused by the excavation of diverging tunnel. The vertical strain ε_y extended about 10^{-4} by the excavation of the diverging tunnel. The horizontal strain ε_x of tunnel axis direction and the shear strain γ_{xy} became minus about 2.5×10^{-4} with pass of the heading face by the strain meter.

Lower in Fig.9 indicated strain change of NBS90 caused by the excavation of diverging tunnel. ε_x and ε_z are extended about 10^{-5} but γ_{xz} became minus about 10^{-4}. During the head excavation the tunnel axial strain ε_x was larger, but after the bench excavation the horizontal strain ε_z became larger than ε_x.

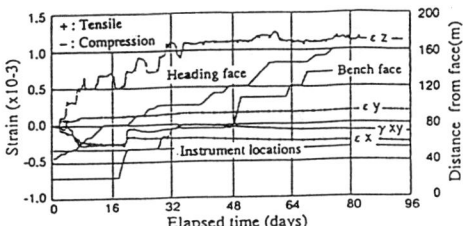
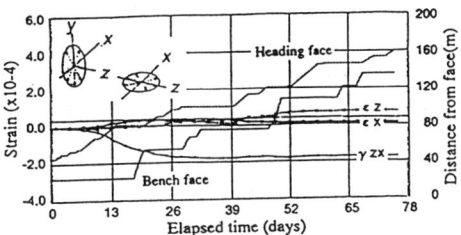

Fig.9: (Upper) Rock strain in the wall obtained from NBS60 for tunnel excavation.
(Lower) Rock strain in the bottom obtained from NBS90 for tunnel excavation.

6. CONCLUSIONS

We have developed multi-component borehole strainmeters with a sensitivity more than 10^{-8} strain for earthquake prediction study and engineering purposes . The instruments are small with sizes of 4 to 10 cm of diameter and 50 cm of length and long period observation is possible as not using gage sensor. Mechanical amplification systems invented are equipped inside of it and amplify about forty times diameter change of a vessel due to applied stress. We have also developed a multi-component instrument (diameter: 10 cm, length: 200 – 500 m) that can record three components of strain, two components of tilt, three components of seismic waves and temperature. The instrument can also attach a gyro system developed by us so that we can set up it in deep boreholes upto 1 km. The instruments are fixed with base rock by utilizing expansion cement of 0.15 % expansion rate.

For earthquake prediction study the instruments were installed into boreholes at depths from 150m to 800m in seismically active areas. The instrument set up at Izu recorded anomalous precursory and coseismic variation of strains and tilts for earthquake swarms occurring in March 1997. By this example it became sure that these instruments well contribute to earthquake prediction study.

We also applied the strainmeters for rock mechanics and civil engineering purposes. We employed the instruments for investigating rock behavior of diverging tunnels and 3-dimensional deformation of the rock at a tunnel diverging point during excavation. The measuring system was useful to clarify rock behavior in the diverging tunnel.

REFERENCES

Sacks,I.S., and D.W.Evertoson ,1971a、A sensitive borehole strain-rate meter, CarnegieInst.Washington Yearb.,68,448-453.

Sakata,S.,1981. On the concept os some newly-invented borehole three-component strainmeters (in Japanese with English abstract). Rep. Nat. Res. Center Disaster Prev.,25,95-126.

M.T.Gladwin,1984.High-precision multicomponent borehole deformation monitoring, Rev.Sci.Instrum,55,2011-2016.

Ishii,H.,S.Matsumoto,Y.Hirata,T.Yamauchi,T. Takahashi,K.Suzuki,S.Watanabe,T.Wakasugi, T.Kato,S.Nakao,1992.Development of new multi-component small bore hole strain meter and observation. Prodeedings of the 86th SEGJ Conference, 32 (in Japanese with English abstract).

Ishii,H.,T.Yamauchi,S.Matsumoto,Y.Hirata,K. Suzuki,T.Takahashi,T.Wakasugi,S.Watanabe, S.Nakao,G.Chen,1993.Development of a new portable tilt meter(ERI-93 type).1993 Japan Earth And Planetary Science Joint Meeting Abstracts(in Japanese).

Ishii,H., 1994. Development of wide range and multi-component bore hole strain meter and application of stress measurement. 1994 Japan Earth And Planetary Science Joint Meeting Abstracts (Japanese with English abstract).

Kusumoto,F., H.Ishii and K.Soma, 1997. A study on rock behavior of diverging tunnels using the new measuring system. Proceedings of ISRM 8th Congress.

Estimation of far-field stresses from borehole strainmeter observations

Hiroshi Ishii
Earthquake Research Institute, The University of Tokyo, Japan

Guangqi Chen & Yuzo Ohnishi
Kyoto University, Japan

ABSTRACT: A numerical method have been presented to estimate the far-field stresses from the observations of borehole strainometers by using Stimulation Response Method (SRM) combined with Boundary Element Method (BEM). A 3-ring model based on $ERI-92$ borehole strainometer has been investigated in detail, and the coupling effects between the instrument wall, the grout and the rock are considered in the model for the first time. The hydrostatic and shear response factors of the borehole strainometer can also be evaluated simultaneously, which is very useful to the instrument design and implant. Finally, the tidal stress field around the Nokogiriyama Geophysical Observatory have been obtained by using the method based on the borehole strainometer observations.

1 INTRODUCTION

Borehole strain observation is an efficient way to reliably monitor the small strains and to avoid extensive near-surface disturbances. Since the first borehole hydrostatic-strain instrument was installed in the Japan islands in 1971 (Sacks et al., 1971), a variety of borehole strainometers have been developed (Gladwin, 1984). More and more of them have been put into operation in recent decade. The observations have played an important role in earthquake predication and geophysics research.

One of the most important and interesting targets of such observation is to estimate the corresponding far-field strains or stresses. However, this is not direct and easy because the instruments merely record the disturbed near-field deformations due to the so-called cavity effect and the effects from the presence of instrument and grout within a borehole.

The problem of how to estimate the corresponding far-field stresses from the observations made in a disturbed near-field has been discussed by several authors. For example, Jaeger and Cook (1976) have given an analytical solution for an empty borehole model. Savin (1961) has made analytical solutions for more general n-ring models, and later, some errors in the solutions were found and corrected by Gladwin and Hart (1985).

In this paper, we present a numerical method for calculating the far-field stresses from borehole strainometer observations by using Stimulation Response Method (SRM) combined with Boundary Element Method (BEM) (Chen, 1993). Since the method is derived under much less assumptions than the analytical methods, it may be adaptable for more complicated models in practice. The coupling effects between the instrument wall, the grout and the rock have been considered in the method for the first time, and the hydrostatic and shear response factors of the instrument can also be calculated for the instrument design and implant. The efficiency of the method has been shown by practical evaluations of the tidal stress field in Nokogiriyama area based on the borehole strainometer observations at Nokogiriyama Geophysical Observatory Tunnel.

2 THE NUMERICAL METHODS

We take $ERI-92$ three-component borehole strainometer as an example to introduce the presented method, but, it is easy to extend the discussions to the other types of the borehole strainometers. The instrument was developed in Earthquake Research Institute, the University of Tokyo (Ishii et al., 1992). The three radial deformations of the instrument rosette cylinder holder are recorded with a resolution up to 10^{-9}. For a installed borehole strainometer, the instrument, grout, and rock consist of a 3-ring model in numerical calculations.

Suppose that the three components of radial displacements are observed as U_1, U_2 and U_3 and the corresponding far-field stress components are σ_{xx}, σ_{yy}

and τ_{xy}. The Stimulation Response Method (SRM) (Chen, 1993) for this case can be stated as follows.

The relationship between the observations and the far-field stresses can be expressed as:

$$\begin{pmatrix} U_1 \\ U_2 \\ U_3 \end{pmatrix} = \begin{pmatrix} \frac{\partial U_1}{\partial \sigma_{xx}} & \frac{\partial U_1}{\partial \sigma_{yy}} & \frac{\partial U_1}{\partial \tau_{xy}} \\ \frac{\partial U_2}{\partial \sigma_{xx}} & \frac{\partial U_2}{\partial \sigma_{yy}} & \frac{\partial U_2}{\partial \tau_{xy}} \\ \frac{\partial U_3}{\partial \sigma_{xx}} & \frac{\partial U_3}{\partial \sigma_{yy}} & \frac{\partial U_3}{\partial \tau_{xy}} \end{pmatrix} \begin{pmatrix} \sigma_{xx} \\ \sigma_{yy} \\ \tau_{xy} \end{pmatrix}. \quad (1)$$

Take the far-field stresses as the following three sets of values $(1\ 0\ 0)^\top$, $(0\ 1\ 0)^\top$ and $(0\ 0\ 1)^\top$, called stimulation stresses, in turn, and use BEM modeling technique to calculate the three radial displacements responding to each set of the stimulation stresses. The corresponding models are shown in Fig. 1. Then, we can get the relationship matrix in Eq. (1) as follows:

$$\begin{pmatrix} U_1 \\ U_2 \\ U_3 \end{pmatrix} = \begin{pmatrix} U_1^1 & U_1^2 & U_1^3 \\ U_2^1 & U_2^2 & U_2^3 \\ U_3^1 & U_3^2 & U_3^3 \end{pmatrix} \begin{pmatrix} \sigma_{xx} \\ \sigma_{yy} \\ \tau_{xy} \end{pmatrix}, \quad (2)$$

where U_j^i is the component j of the radial deformations corresponding to the stimulation stress of set i, The matrix in the right side of Eq. (2) is also called the response matrix, denoting as $\mathbf{A}$ here.

Therefore, the far-field stresses can be obtained as follows:

$$\begin{pmatrix} \sigma_{xx} \\ \sigma_{yy} \\ \tau_{xy} \end{pmatrix} = \begin{pmatrix} U_1^1 & U_1^2 & U_1^3 \\ U_2^1 & U_2^2 & U_2^3 \\ U_3^1 & U_3^2 & U_3^3 \end{pmatrix}^{-1} \begin{pmatrix} U_1 \\ U_2 \\ U_3 \end{pmatrix}. \quad (3)$$

Now, as we can see, the inverse problem is converted into the numerical modeling problem. Therefore, the method is adaptable for any complicated model providing the numerical modeling is possible.

There is another way to use SRM for the same estimation, which is based on the relationship between radial displacement observations and the corresponding far-field areal and maximum shear stresses.

For a n-ring model, SAVIN (1961, Chap. 5) has derived the radial displacement of the instrument inner wall at angle θ clockwise from a uniaxial stress P applied at a large distance as follows:

$$U_r = \frac{R_1 P}{8G_1}(a + b\cos 2\theta), \quad (4)$$

where a and b are dimensionless constants, functions of the elastic constants and the radii of the instrument, the grout and the borehole system. R_1 and G_1 are the inner radius and the rigidity of the instrument.

According to linear elastic superposition, the displacement arising from principal stresses σ_1, i.e. the maximum compression (most negative), and σ_2 can be then expressed as

$$U_r = \frac{R_1}{4G_1}(aV - bS\cos 2\theta), \quad (5)$$

where V is the areal stress and S is the maximum shear stress, and they are related to the principal stresses σ_1 and σ_2 as follows:

$$\begin{cases} V = (\sigma_1 + \sigma_2)/2 \\ S = -(\sigma_1 - \sigma_2)/2 \end{cases} \quad (6)$$

If the three components of the radial displacement with 60° apart each other have been measured, we can get from Eq. (5):

$$\begin{cases} U_1 = \frac{R_1}{4G_1}(aV - bS\cos 2\theta) \\ U_2 = \frac{R_1}{4G_1}(aV - bS\cos 2(\theta + 60°)) \\ U_3 = \frac{R_1}{4G_1}(aV - bS\cos 2(\theta + 120°)) \end{cases} \quad (7)$$

where the component U_1 is measured at angle θ clockwise from the axis of maximum compression.

Then, we can express V, S and θ in terms of U_1, U_2 and U_3 by inverting above equations:

$$\begin{cases} V = 4G_1(U_1 + U_2 + U_3)/(3aR_1) \\ S = 4G_1\sqrt{2((U_1 - U_2)^2 + (U_2 - U_3)^2 + (U_3 - U_1)^2)}/(3bR_1) \\ \theta = 0.5\tan^{-1}(\sqrt{3}(U_3 - U_2)/((U_1 - U_2) + (U_1 - U_3))) \end{cases} \quad (8)$$

It can be seen that if constants a and b are known, the far-field V, S and θ can be calculated from the three-component borehole strainometer observations.

Now, we also apply SRM combined with BEM to determine the constants a and b by the following procedures.

First, let $V = -1\ bar$ and $S = 0$, and calculate the responded radial displacement U_r^1 by using BEM modeling technique (Fig. 2). In this condition, the Eq. (5) becomes

$$U_r^1 = -\frac{R_1}{4G_1}a . \quad (9)$$

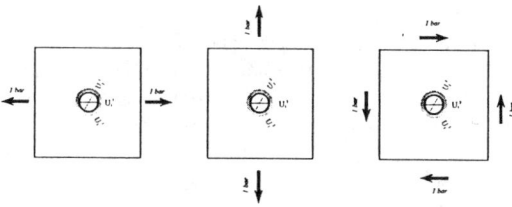

Fig. 1 BEM models correspond to the three sets of stimulation stresses.

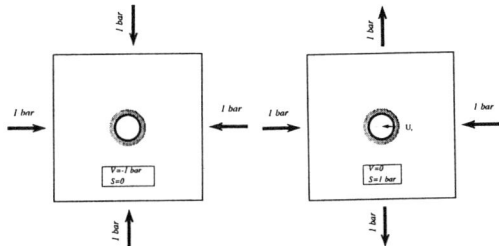

Fig. 2 BEM models correspond to the conditions $V = -1\ bar$, $S = 0$ and $V = 0$, $S = -1\ bar$.

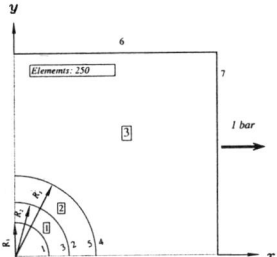

Fig. 3 BEM model for practical calculation.

Then, constant a can be obtained as follows:

$$a = -\frac{4G_1 U_r^1}{R_1}\ . \quad (10)$$

In the second step, let $V = 0$ and $S = -1\ bar$, and calculate the responded radial displacement U_r^2 by using BEM modeling technique (Fig. 2). In this condition, the Eq. (5) becomes

$$U_r^2 = -\frac{R_1}{4G_1} b \cos 2\theta\ . \quad (11)$$

Using the calculated response radial displacement at the point in the σ_1 axis $U_r(\theta = 0°)$, we have

$$U_r(\theta = 0°) = -\frac{R_1}{4G_1} b\ . \quad (12)$$

Then, we can obtain the constant b as follows:

$$b = -\frac{4G_1 U_r(\theta = 0°)}{R_1}\ . \quad (13)$$

3 BEM MODELING

In order to determine the response matrix **A** or the constants a and b, numeric modeling technique is necessary. In this paper, BEM technique is used for this purpose.

It is unnecessary to calculate the three models in Fig. 1 and two models in Fig. 2 one by one. We only need to calculate the model shown in Fig. 3, since the other models can be obtained from it based on linear elastic superposition principle and/or by axis rotation.

In the model, the axial symmetry of the problem has been considered, and there are three regions: region 1, instrument wall with inner radius R_1, has two boundaries (1 and 2); region 2, grout with inner radius R_2, has two boundaries too (3 and 4); region 3, rock with a hole of radius R_3, has three boundaries (5, 6, and 7).

The boundaries 6 and 7, 50 meters long for each,

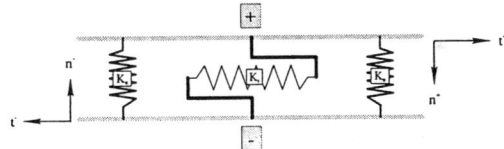

Fig. 4 Boundary conditions for common boundaries.

are divided into 50 elements respectively while the others are divided into 30 elements for each.

Boundary 7 has 1 bar prescribed traction acted in x direction and is traction free in y direction; Boundaries 1 and 6 are traction free for both directions; Boundaries 2 and 3, 4 and 5 are common boundaries.

In order to investigate the coupling effects between the instrument wall, the grout and the rock, so-called coupling friction elements, as shown in Fig. 4, have been used in these common boundaries. The corresponding boundary conditions for a coupling friction element are treated as

$$\begin{cases} u_n^+ = -u_n^-,\ \ t_n^+ = t_n^- \\ t_t^+ = t_t^-,\ \ t_t^+ = k_t(u_t^+ + u_t^-)\ , \end{cases} \quad (14)$$

where local coordinate systems are used and the rigidity k_n of the spring is taken infinity. The rigidity k_t of the spring can be viewed as friction factor because we know that from the Eq. (14):

$$u_t^+ = -u_t^- \quad if\ \ k_t = \infty\ , \quad (15)$$

which represents the case of complete coupling between the two regions; and

$$t_t^+ = t_t^- = 0 \quad if\ \ k_t = 0\ , \quad (16)$$

represents the case of free contact between two regions. Therefore, we can model any coupling state between the instrument, the grout and the rock by changing friction factor k_t, which is impossible for analytical methods presented up to now.

In order to verify the method and computer program, the model with the parameters $R_1 =$

Table 1: Numerical and analytical results

method	numerical modeling	analytical solution
θ	$U_r(\theta)$	$U'_r(\theta)$
0°	0.1729	0.1729
30°	0.1153	0.1153
60°	0.0000	0.0000
90°	-0.0577	-0.0576
a	3.2251	3.2258
b	6.4520	6.4516

$37mm$, $R_2 = 45mm$, $R_3 = 60mm$ and $E_1 = E_2 = E_3 = 6.42 \times 10^5 bar$, $\nu_1 = \nu_2 = \nu_3 = 0.24$, $k_t = \infty$ has been calculated. In this case, the 3-ring model is equivalent to the empty borehole model with radius $R = 37mm$, for which the analytical solutions are known.

The calculated results together with the analytical solutions are presented in Table 1. The unit of radial displacements $U_r(\theta)$ and $U'_r(\theta)$ is μm. It can be seen that the results from both methods are quite good in agreement. Therefore, the numerical method presented in this paper has been proved correct and precise enough.

4 RESPONSE FACTORS

According to Hooke's low, we can also easily get the relationship between the radial displacement and the areal strain v, the maximum shear strain s from Eq. (5) as follows:

$$U_r = R_1(cv - ds\cos 2\theta), \quad (17)$$

where constants c and d can be derived from the constants a and b as follows:

$$c = \frac{a(1+\nu_3)G_3}{2(1-\nu_3)G_1}, \quad (18)$$

$$d = \frac{bG_3}{2G_1}, \quad (19)$$

where ν_3 and G_3 are the Poisson's ratio and rigidity of rock.

On the other hand, the radial displacement of the instrument inner wall would be as follows if the rock is undisturbed by the instrument installation:

$$U_r = R_1(v - s\cos 2\theta). \quad (20)$$

Comparing Eq. (20) with Eq. (17), we can see that the areal strain is amplified by c times, and the shear

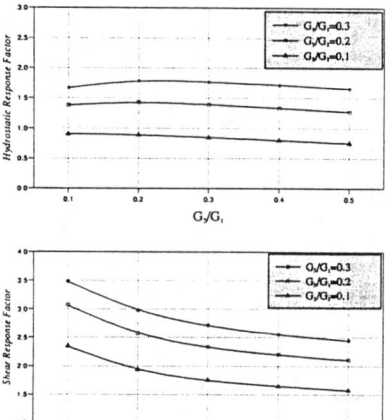

Fig. 5 Variation of response factors with the rigidity of grout.

strain is amplified by d times because of the presence of the instrument and the grout within the borehole. Therefore, c and d may be viewed as the hydrostatic and shear response factors for the in-situ instrument. In general, there are $c \geq 1$ and $d \geq 1$.

The knowledge of the hydrostatic and shear response factors is very important for the instrument design and implant. For $ERI - 92$ borehole strainmeters, both factors have been investigated by a lot of numeric calculations. It has been found that the response factors are affected by the following things:

1. The inner radius of instrument The shear response factor will decrease and the hydrostatic factor will increase if the inner radius of instrument increases; the effect on the hydrostatic factor is larger than that on the shear response factor.

2. The thickness of instrument wall Both the hydrostatic and the shear factors will decrease if the thickness of instrument wall increases.

3. The thickness of grout The shear response factor increases very largely but the hydrostatic factor remains unchanged when the thickness of grout wall increases.

4. The rigidity of grout When the grout rigidity increases, the shear response factor decreases, and the hydrostatic factor will increase if the grout rigidity is less than the rock rigidity, otherwise, it will decrease. (Fig. 5).

5. The coupling state between instrument and grout People pay much attention to the coupling state between instrument, grout and rock when they install

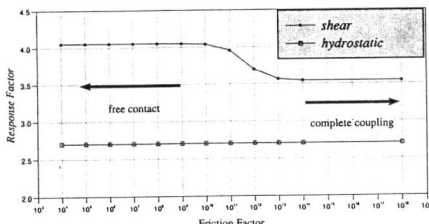

Fig. 6 Coupling effects on the response factors.

borehole instruments, since it affect the response factors (Fig. 6). It is found that the shear response factor could change 30% from free contact to complete coupling, but, the hydrostatic response factor is not affected by the coupling state. When the rigidity of the friction spring is less than 10^{10}, the shear response factor is the same as the free contact case, and when the rigidity is larger than 10^{14}, the shear response factor is the same as complete coupling case.

5 EXAMPLE OF PRATICAL ESTIMATION

We have applied the method to the estimation of the tidal stress field in Nokogiriyama area from the borehole strainmeter observations. The instrument is installed in a vertical borehole located at the Nokogiriyama Geophysical Observatory Tunnel. One component of the instrument is oriented in north south direction (N-S), which is taken as U_1 of the BEM model shown in Fig. 3; the other two components are 60° apart from north to west noted as WN-ES and WS-EN corresponding to U_2 and U_3 of the BEM model respectively.

The parameters needed in the modeling are taken as follows: $E_1 = 2.16 \times 10^6$ bar, $E_2 = 2.62 \times 10^5$ bar, $E_3 = 6.42 \times 10^5$ bar, $\nu_1 = 0.30$, $\nu_2 = 0.25$, $\nu_3 = 0.24$, $R_1 = 37mm$, $R_2 = 45mm$, $R_3 = 60mm$ and $k_t = 10^{18}$, where the subscript 2 and 3 represent grout and rock respectively.

The response matrix is determined as follows:

$$\mathbf{A} = \begin{pmatrix} 0.316478 & -0.162833 & 0.000000 \\ -0.043005 & 0.196650 & -0.415103 \\ -0.043005 & 0.196650 & 0.415103 \end{pmatrix} \quad (21)$$

and the constants are obtained as $a = 6.900$, $b = 21.52$, $c = 1.754$, and $d = 3.354$ by BEM modeling calculation.

The observations from Feb. 1 to Feb. 28 in 1993 have been used. The time series of each component observations has been separated into two parts: linear

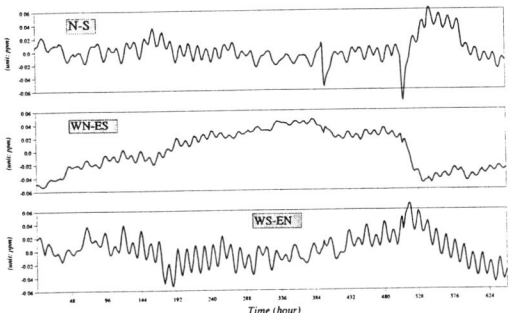

Fig. 7 The observed apparent tidal strains.

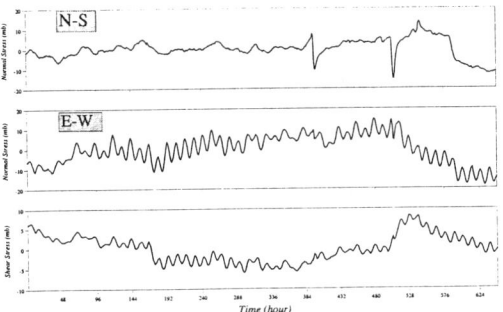

Fig. 8 The calculated far-field tidal stresses.

long-term trend variation and earth tide. Here, only tidal field is processed.

Fig. 7 shows the apparent strains calculated from the observations by simply dividing the instrument diameter. The maximum amplitudes are 6×10^{-8} for WS-EN, 4×10^{-8} for N-S and 2×10^{-8} for WN-ES.

The calculated tidal stresses from the practical observations are shown in Fig. 8. The tide amplitude of the E-W component is larger than the other two components. The maximum amplitude is about $15mb$ for E-W component of normal stresses, $5mb$ for shear

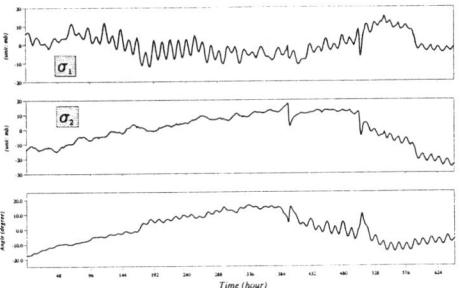

Fig. 9 The corresponding principal stresses.

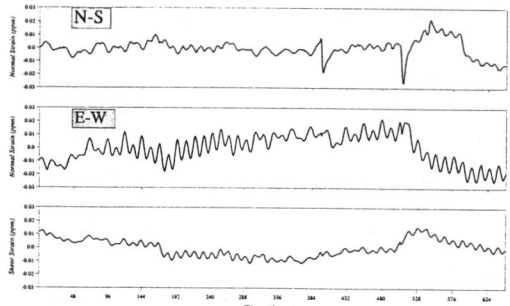

Fig. 10 The corresponding far-field tidal strains.

component and $2mb$ for N-S component of normal stresses. Fig. 9 shows the corresponding principal stresses.

The corresponding tidal strains are shown in Fig. 10. The maximum tide amplitudes of the E-W component is about 2×10^{-8}. Therefore, it is obvious that the observed strains are amplified by about three times because of instrument installation.

6 CONCLUSIONS

A practical numerical method has been presented by using SRM combined with BEM in this paper for estimating far-field stresses from three-component borehole strain meter observations. The correctness and precision of the method have been verified by a lot of calculations.

It has been shown that the deference between the observed local-field and the corresponding far-field stresses depends on the hydrostatic and shear response factors, which are the functions of the materials, the radii and the coupling states of the instrument, the grout and the borehole.

The coupling effects between the instrument, the grout and the rock have been investigated for the first time. It has been found that the hydrostatic response factor is not affected by the coupling state of common boundaries, but, the shear response factor corresponding to free contact state is about 30% larger than complete coupling state.

The practical calculation have been made based on the observations of a $ERI - 92$ borehole strainometer installed at Nokogiriyama Geophysical Observatory. The hydrostatic response factor for the instrument has been estimated as 1.754 and the shear response factor as 3.354. The maximum tidal stress amplitudes have been estimated as $15mb$ for E-W component of normal stresses, $5mb$ for shear component and $2mb$ for N-S component of normal stresses; the maximum tidal strain amplitude of the E-W strain component has been estimated as about 2×10^{-8}, which is about 3 times smaller than the observed maximum tidal strain amplitude. That is, the observed strains have been amplified by about 3 times because of instrument installation. Therefore, it is necessary to do this work when one hopes to study on tide analysis using borehole strain meter observations.

REFERENCES

Chen, G. (1993): Study on Crustal Deformation and Stress Fields – Modeling by Using SRM Combined with BEM, Ph.D. Thesis, The University of Tokyo, 223p.

Gladwin, M. T. (1984): High precision multi-component borehole deformation monitoring, Rev. Sci. Instr. 55, No.12, 2011-2016.

Gladwin, M. T. , and R. Hart (1985): Design parameters for borehole strain instrumentation, PAGEOPH, vol.123, 59-80.

Ishii, H. , Matsumoto, S., Hirata, Y., Yamauchi, T., Takahashi, T., Suzuki, K., Watanabe, S., Wakasugi, T., Kato, T., and S. Nakao (1992): Development of new multi-component small borehole strainmeter and observation, Presentation to 1992 Japan Earth and Planetary Science Joint Meeting.

Jaeger, J. C. , and N. G. W, Cook (1976): *Fundamentals of Rock Mechanics,* 2nd ed., Chapman and Hall.

Sacks, I. S. , Suyehiro, S., Evertson, D. W., and Y. Yamagishi (1971): Sacks-Evertson strainmeter, its installation in Japan and some preliminary results concerning strain steps, Papers Meterol. Geophys. 22, Nos. 3-4, 195-208.

Savin, G. N. (1961): *Stress Concentration around Holes,* Pergamon Press.

Determination of the in-situ stresses at Sellafield, UK: A case study

A.S. Batchelor & K.A. Kwakwa
GeoScience Limited, Falmouth, UK

A.J. Proughten
GIBB Ltd, UK

N. Davies
United Kingdom Nirex Limited, UK

ABSTRACT: This paper presents a comprehensive case study in the assessment of in-situ stress using four independent methods. The determinations were made at the Sellafield site on behalf of Nirex. The paper presents an overview of the techniques used and a description of the data from ten boreholes which provided seventy-seven discrete spatial locations at which stress assessments were made. The paper is presented in three parts:

Part A, in which the various techniques employed are discussed and the data is considered.
Part B, in which the orientation of the maximum principal stress and spatial variation in orientation are considered.
Part C, in which the magnitudes of the three principal stresses and variations in magnitudes are discussed.

PART A: INTRODUCTION TO TECHNIQUES AND DATA

The model

The state of stress at a point in a rock mass may be specified by means of a six-component tensor whose magnitudes are related to arbitrarily selected orientations of reference axes. In the case of an isotropic rock mass, the complete state of stress at a point can be defined by determining the magnitudes and attitudes (azimuths and inclinations) of the principal stresses. Also, as the principal stresses are orthogonal, only the three magnitudes and the attitudes of two of the principal stresses are required to characterise the state of stress at the point.

Conventionally, principal stresses are ordered in descending magnitude and referred to as the maximum (σ_1), intermediate (σ_2) and minimum (σ_3) principal stresses. Where the principal stresses are (or have been assumed to be) oriented in the vertical and horizontal directions, they are referred to as the vertical (σ_V), minimum horizontal (σ_{Hmin}) and maximum horizontal (σ_{Hmax}) principal stresses. In the latter case, only the three magnitudes and the azimuth of one of the horizontal principal stresses are required to define the state of stress completely.

The techniques and simplifying assumptions

In assessing stress orientations and magnitudes from field data, all the methods described in this paper assume that the rocks at the locations of measurement in the borehole are homogeneous and isotropic with linearly-elastic deformational responses in the region of the measurement. Four techniques have been used to assess the stress field. These are:
- Hydrofracture Stress Measurement (HFSM)
- Breakout analysis
- Density log analysis
- Overcoring Stress Measurement (OCSM)

Implicit in HFSM and breakout analysis is the assumption that the principal stresses are oriented vertically and horizontally. Thus the derived parameters from these methods relate to σ_{Hmin}, σ_{Hmax} and σ_V. In contrast, OCSM theory does not make such an assumption and enables the magnitudes and orientations of σ_1, σ_2 and σ_3 to be computed. An additional assumption in HFSM analysis is that the overburden stress magnitudes are equivalent to those of σ_V, allowing the magnitudes of σ_V to be calculated by integrating the corrected density logs obtained from the borehole.

The in-situ stress parameters which may be obtained from these four methods are summarised in Table 1. It is important to note that results derived from any one individual method will be independent of any results obtained from any (or all) of the other three.

Table 1. Summary of in-situ stress parameters determined from the various methods

In-situ stress measurement method	In-situ stress parameters determined		Comments
	Directly	By computation	
HFSM	σ_{Hmin} magnitude σ_{Hmax} azimuth	σ_{Hmax} magnitude σ_{Hmin} azimuth	May require P_p magnitude and mechanical properties of rock
Breakout Analysis	σ_{Hmin} azimuth	σ_{Hmax} azimuth	Also good indicator of nature/orientation of principal stresses
Density Log Analysis	Trend of σ_v magnitudes with depth	----	Requires lithology versus depth data
OCSM	Induced strains	σ_1, σ_2 and σ_3 magnitudes and orientations	Requires the elastic properties of the recovered overcore

Table 2. Summary of boreholes in which methods were deployed

In-situ stress measurement method	Boreholes in which method deployed	Comments
HFSM	2, 3, 5, 8A, 10A	29 tests in all
Breakout Analysis	3, 5, 10A, 11A, 12A, 13A, 14A	
Density Log Analysis	2, 3, 5, 8A, 10A	
OCSM	10B	Over depth interval 150 - 250 mbGL

Table 3. Summary of results of in-situ stress field data at Sellafield

BH 2 Ground Level elevation (maOD)				60.18										
BH ID	Mid MD	X	Y	Z	mbGL$_{TVD}$	Type	Lith	$\theta\sigma_{Hmax}$	$\theta\sigma_{Hmax}$ SD*1.96	σ_v (MPa)	σ_{Hmin} (MPa)	σ_{Hmax} (MPa)	P_p (MPa)	Top MD	Base MD
BH 2	675.25	305553.85	503429.50	-609.67	669.85	HF	Fleming	325.2	13.89	16.67	9.8	17.3	6.82	671.10	679.40
BH 2	750.25	305555.58	503433.01	-684.56	744.74	HF	Fleming	7.0	NA	18.66	10.1	19.1	7.58	746.10	754.40
BH 2	1186.25	305561.20	503462.40	-1119.48	1179.66	HF	Bleawath	320.0	19.89	30.18	18.8	35.3	12.16	1182.10	1190.40
BH 2	1205.25	305561.12	503464.10	-1138.41	1198.59	HF	Bleawath	344.9	32.15	30.69	17.8	31.8	12.33	1201.10	1209.40
BH 2	1314.25	305560.42	503474.16	-1246.94	1307.12	HF	Bleawath	346.0	NA	33.56	22.1	38.7	13.30	1310.10	1318.40
BH 2	1447.25	305559.44	503487.23	-1379.29	1439.47	HF	Bleawath	343.5	1.39	37.07	23.5	-	14.49	1443.10	1451.40

BH 3 Ground Level elevation (maOD)				9.07										
BH ID	Mid MD	X	Y	Z	mbGL$_{TVD}$	Type	Lith	$\theta\sigma_{Hmax}$	$\theta\sigma_{Hmax}$ SD*1.96	σ_v (MPa)	σ_{Hmin} (MPa)	σ_{Hmax} (MPa)	P_p (MPa)	Top MD	Base MD
BH 3	1444.01	302624.91	502670.64	-1427.42	1436.49	HF	Brockram	335.1	19.46	35.26	32.8	41.8	15.14	1442.00	1446.02
BH 3	1477.39	302626.45	502672.22	-1460.72	1469.79	IF	Urswick	350.9	4.11	36.13				1477.26	1477.51
BH 3	1490.46	302627.06	502672.85	-1473.76	1482.83	WD	Urswick	358.9	11.20	36.48				1488.89	1492.03
BH 3	1499.01	302627.46	502673.27	-1482.29	1491.36	HF	Urswick	325.0	NA	36.71	33.0	48.0	15.75	1497.00	1501.02
BH 3	1514.02	302628.18	502674.02	-1497.27	1506.34	AD	Urswick	331.3	8.95	37.11				1513.85	1514.18
BH 3	1522.20	302628.59	502674.43	-1505.43	1514.50	WD	Frizington	342.0	10.74	37.32				1519.16	1525.25
BH 3	1527.60	302628.85	502674.71	-1510.81	1519.88	WD	Frizington	342.0	14.87	37.47				1526.24	1528.98
BH 3	1533.01	302629.12	502674.99	-1516.21	1525.28	HF	Frizington	344.0	24.95	37.61	32.8	48.4	16.12	1531.00	1535.02
BH 3	1564.35	302630.66	502676.71	-1547.46	1556.53	WD	Frizington	359.8	47.79	38.44				1564.28	1564.42
BH 3	1575.55	302631.21	502677.33	-1558.63	1567.70	WD	Frizington	343.2	10.05	38.74				1575.50	1575.59
BH 3	1578.01	302631.33	502677.47	-1561.09	1570.16	HF	Frizington	3.0	NA	38.81	31.6	39.4	16.61	1576.00	1580.02
BH 3	1583.30	302631.59	502677.77	-1566.36	1575.43	WD	Frizington	347.3	31.34	38.95				1581.72	1584.88
BH 3	1585.01	302631.68	502677.87	-1568.07	1577.14	HF	Frizington	349.8	16.90	38.99	33.4	46.7	16.69	1583.00	1587.02
BH 3	1612.94	302633.09	502679.52	-1595.91	1604.98	WD	Frizington	326.7	11.51	39.73				1612.72	1613.16
BH 3	1684.56	302636.66	502684.16	-1667.29	1676.36	WD	Ignimbrite	346.5	14.62	41.62				1684.30	1684.81
BH 3	1711.52	302638.03	502686.04	-1694.15	1703.22	WD	Volc Sst	321.9	12.01	42.33				1711.10	1711.95
BH 3	1725.23	302638.74	502687.05	-1707.81	1716.88	WD	Ignimbrite	338.8	28.58	42.69				1713.45	1737.00
BH 3	1833.42	302644.10	502695.59	-1815.52	1824.59	WD	Volc unit B2	333.2	11.88	45.54				1833.37	1833.46
BH 3	1845.01	302644.66	502696.55	-1827.06	1836.13	HF	Ignimbrite	332.1	12.82	45.85	33.4	63.3	19.64	1843.00	1847.02
BH 3	1874.70	302646.12	502699.02	-1856.61	1865.68	WD	Ignimbrite	320.5	13.72	46.63				1864.77	1884.63

The data

In this case study, data from 77 zones in ten boreholes (Nos. 2, 3, 5, 8A, 10A, 10B, 11A, 12A, 13A and 14A) were processed to estimate the in-situ principal stress magnitudes and orientations at Sellafield. All the boreholes are nominally vertical. Figure 1 shows a map of the Sellafield area with the borehole locations identified. The relationship between test method and borehole number is summarised in Table 2.

Data processing for stress orientation

In a vertical borehole subject to anisotropic horizontal stresses, the tangential stresses around the borehole wall are unequal, with the maximum and minimum magnitudes occurring along the azimuths of σ_{Hmin} and σ_{Hmax} respectively. The high tangential or hoop stress magnitudes along the azimuth of σ_{Hmin} can cause the borehole wall to fail in compression, the 'breakout' phenomena. Breakout processing is widely accepted as a method of defining the σ_{Hmax} azimuth and excellent agreement with other techniques has been reported in a variety of geological environments (e.g. Zoback, 1992; Barr, 1993; Batchelor et al, 1995). Alternatively, the borehole can fail in tension along the σ_{Hmax} azimuth when the magnitude is reduced below the tensile strength of the rock.

Figure 2 illustrates the relationship between the failure features and the horizontal stresses. As the failure zones are at right angles to each other, determination of the azimuths of one of the two features enables assessment of the mean azimuths of both σ_{Hmax} and σ_{Hmin}.

Figure 3 shows a typical example of a breakout zone, at 1872-1874m MD in Borehole No. 3, on the travel time image of the Borehole Televiewer (BHTV). The breakout zones can be seen on the log. The processed view of the hole shape is clearly visible in Figure 4. It shows the relatively narrow zone of failure corresponding to the high stress magnitudes along the σ_{Hmin} direction. A cross-section through the image showing the inferred direction of σ_{Hmin} is presented in Figure 5. The small dots (labelled 'HOSANA flag') in Figure 3 show where the automatic processing method, HOSANA, picked the azimuths of the breakouts in this section. Each represents an individual data point (also referred to as a 'breakout level') that was subsequently processed to provide a mean and an estimate of uncertainty over the individual breakout zones.

According to the theory of HFSM, induced hydraulic fracturing initiates at two diametrically opposite locations on the vertical borehole wall, parallel to the direction of σ_{Hmax}. A typical illustration of induced fracturing is presented in Figure 6 which compares the unwrapped images of a borehole section 'before' and 'after' an HFSM test at 1045m MD in Borehole No. 5. Determination of the mean orientation of the fracture traces provides the estimated azimuth of σ_{Hmax}.

Data processing for in-situ stress magnitudes

Hydrofracture tests were undertaken in Borehole Nos. 2, 3, 5, 8A and 10A. Magnitudes of σ_{Hmin} were estimated mainly from analysis of pressure versus flowrate data obtained from the slow refracture operations. Where the slow refracture results were not readily amenable to unambiguous interpretation because of operational difficulties during testing (e.g. leakage of surface flowlines and inaccurate flow metering), the shut-in pressure versus time data were used to estimate the σ_{Hmin} magnitudes. In the latter, it was found that the shut-in pressure versus logarithm of Horner time plot provided consistent results. The application of these alternative techniques ensured that suspect data were not used in the analysis.

29 HFSM tests were carried out. 28 of these provided useful data from which σ_{Hmin} and σ_{Hmax} were obtained. σ_V magnitudes were assumed to be equivalent to the overburden pressures and were calculated by integrating the density logs of all five HFSM boreholes.

Data processing for overcore stress method

In the OCSM method, a cell containing three strain rosettes (all mounted on external pads) was glued onto the surface of a pilot hole in the rock. The cell was subsequently overcored whilst the recovered strains due to stress relief are monitored and recorded by a downhole datalogger. The in-situ state of stress was computed from the strain readings after determining the deformation properties of the rock in a laboratory biaxial test on the recovered overcore.

The OCSM tests were carried out in Borehole No. 10B. Unlike the HFSM test which assumes vertical and horizontal principal stresses, the OCSM test determines the complete state of stress (magnitudes and orientations of the principal stresses) in 3-dimensions.

Summary of results for Sellafield: Orientation and magnitude

Table 3 presents the interpretation results for the in-situ stress field for all the 77 zones studied in the Sellafield area. The results are from Borehole Nos. 2, 3, 5, 8A,

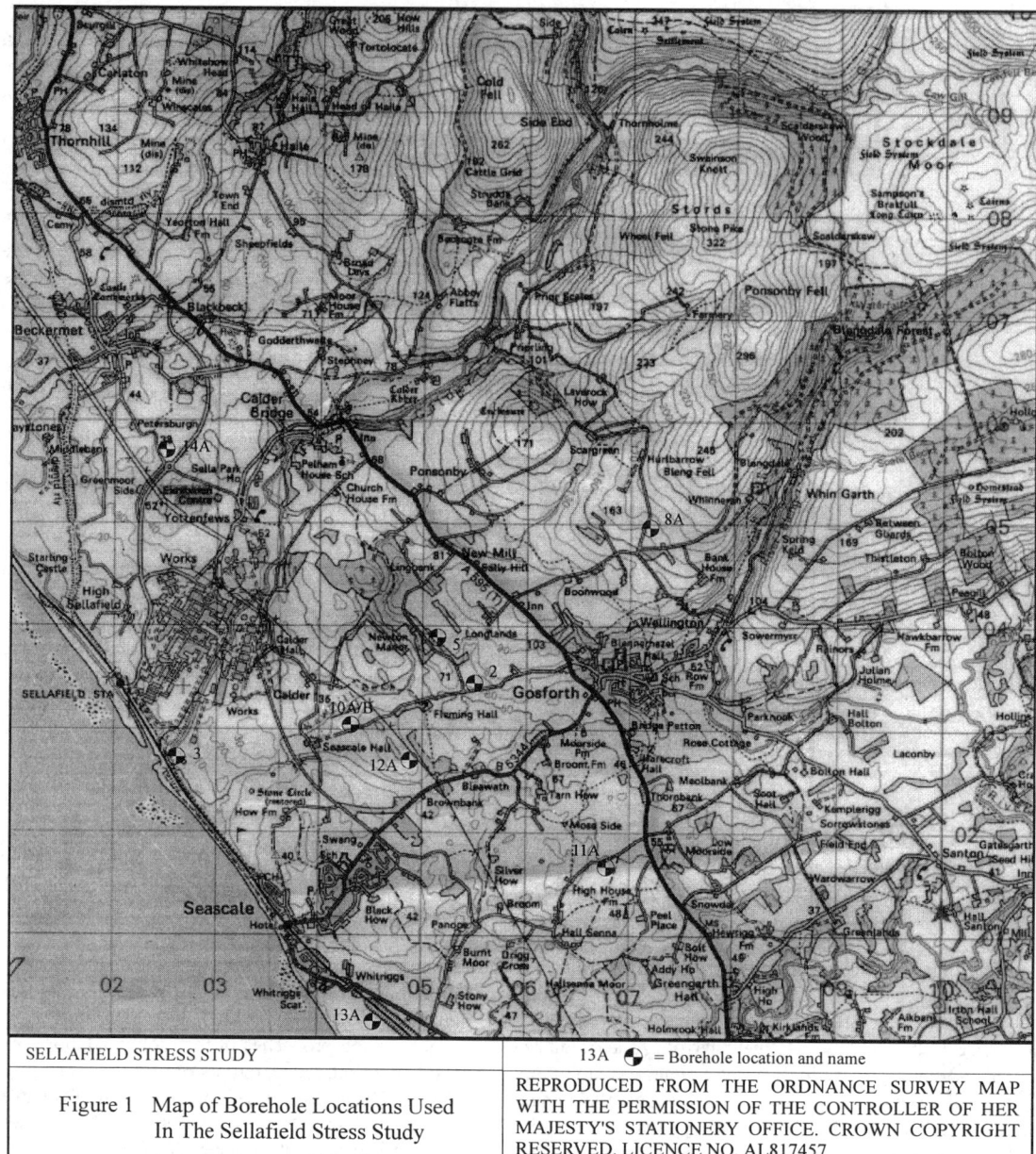

Figure 1 Map of Borehole Locations Used In The Sellafield Stress Study

13A ⊕ = Borehole location and name

REPRODUCED FROM THE ORDNANCE SURVEY MAP WITH THE PERMISSION OF THE CONTROLLER OF HER MAJESTY'S STATIONERY OFFICE. CROWN COPYRIGHT RESERVED. LICENCE NO. AL817457

10A, 10B, 11A, 12A, 13A and 14A. Orientation results were derived for all 77 zones (44 breakouts, 28 HFSM and 5 OCSM) and full magnitude results were estimated for 33 (28 HFSM and 5 OCSM) locations.

Table 3 contains eight types of data that have been derived (or collated) from different sources and processed to give the final results. They are:

a) Borehole name and test interval
b) National Grid coordinates
c) Depth below ground level
d) Type of result
e) Formation name
f) σ_{Hmax} azimuth data
g) Stress magnitude data (where appropriate)

Table 3. Summary of results of in-situ stress field data at Sellafield (continued)

BH 5 Ground Level elevation (maOD)			80.61										
BH ID	Mid MD	X	Y	Z	mbGL$_{TVD}$	Type	Lith	$\theta\sigma_{Hmax}$	$\theta\sigma_{Hmax}$ SD*1.96	σ_v (MPa)	σ_{Hmin} (MPa)	σ_{Hmax} (MPa)	P$_P$ (MPa)	Top MD	Base MD
BH 5	847.99	305171.72	503878.78	-762.30	842.91	HF	Intrusion	337.0	NA	21.42	13.0	24.3	8.44	845.91	850.06
BH 5	960.99	305170.53	503881.53	-875.26	955.87	HF	Bleawath	328.0	NA	24.41	17.3	29.8	9.87	958.91	963.06
BH 5	1043.99	305169.18	503884.03	-958.22	1038.83	HF	Bleawath	321.0	8.32	26.61	25.4	49.2	10.80	1041.91	1046.06
BH 5	1072.99	305168.63	503885.01	-987.19	1067.80	HF	Bleawath	350.5	22.37	27.37	22.0	41.7	11.08	1070.91	1075.06
BH 5	1088.99	305168.31	503885.56	-1003.18	1083.79	HF	Bleawath	341.0	NA	27.80	27.3	52.9	11.28	1086.91	1091.06
BH 5	1145.56	305167.10	503887.51	-1059.70	1140.31	WD	Bleawath	338.1	26.30	29.29				1144.63	1146.50
BH 5	1225.99	305164.92	503890.34	-1140.06	1220.67	HF	Bleawath	342.0	NA	31.42	27.0	50.5	13.37	1223.91	1228.06
BH 5	1234.99	305164.66	503890.66	-1149.05	1229.66	HF	Bleawath	345.0	13.86	31.66	24.3	46.3	13.51	1232.91	1237.06

BH 8A Ground Level elevation (maOD)			162.99										
BH ID	Mid MD	X	Y	Z	mbGL$_{TVD}$	Type	Lith	$\theta\sigma_{Hmax}$	$\theta\sigma_{Hmax}$ SD*1.96	σ_v (MPa)	σ_{Hmin} (MPa)	σ_{Hmax} (MPa)	P$_P$ (MPa)	Top MD	Base MD
BH 8A	263.06	307209.00	504981.46	-96.26	259.25	HF	Fleming	335.0	NA	6.58	7.2	11.8	2.27	262.00	264.12
BH 8A	770.06	307211.04	504980.78	-603.26	766.25	HF	Fleming	339.0	NA	19.82	14.9	27.1	7.60	769.00	771.12
BH 8A	978.06	307211.61	504979.74	-811.25	974.24	HF	Fleming	303.0	NA	25.25	17.7	31.9	10.04	977.00	979.12

BH 10A Ground Level elevation (maOD)			35.46										
BH ID	Mid MD	X	Y	Z	mbGL$_{TVD}$	Type	Lith	$\theta\sigma_{Hmax}$	$\theta\sigma_{Hmax}$ SD*1.96	σ_v (MPa)	σ_{Hmin} (MPa)	σ_{Hmax} (MPa)	P$_P$ (MPa)	Top MD	Base MD
BH 10A	251.15	304312.94	503063.36	-210.66	246.12	HF	St Bees Sst	325.0	22.17	5.76	7.0	10.0	2.39	249.00	253.29
BH 10A	344.15	304313.81	503064.35	-303.65	339.11	HF	St Bees Sst	326.0	NA	8.03	6.8	8.8	3.34	342.00	346.29
BH 10A	377.25	304314.16	503064.76	-336.74	372.20	WD	St Bees Sst	310.3	5.50	8.83				377.21	377.29
BH 10A	386.15	304314.26	503064.87	-345.64	381.10	HF	St Bees Sst	335.0	NA	9.05	9.8	15.0	3.75	384.00	388.29
BH 10A	509.15	304315.78	503066.66	-468.62	504.08	HF	St Bees Sst	327.0	8.54	12.04	10.7	15.0	4.98	507.00	511.29
BH 10A	582.56	304316.87	503068.01	-542.01	577.47	WD	St Bees Sst	345.8	3.86	13.83				582.37	582.76
BH 10A	701.76	304318.85	503070.56	-661.16	696.62	WD	NHM	325.4	15.51	16.73				697.46	706.07
BH 10A	717.00	304319.11	503070.92	-676.40	711.86	IF	NHM	336.6	3.82	17.10				716.60	717.40
BH 10A	729.18	304319.33	503071.21	-688.57	724.03	WD	NHM	330.2	16.62	17.39				724.62	733.73
BH 10A	743.82	304319.58	503071.57	-703.21	738.67	IF	St Bees Shl	333.1	1.98	17.76				743.82	743.82
BH 10A	744.94	304319.60	503071.60	-704.32	739.78	IF	St Bees Shl	339.5	21.52	17.79				744.03	745.85
BH 10A	779.15	304320.22	503072.47	-738.52	773.98	HF	St Bees Shl	359.0	24.20	18.67	12.9	17.4	7.72	777.00	781.29
BH 10A	796.85	304320.54	503072.92	-756.21	791.67	AD	St Bees Shl	359.6	9.04	19.13				796.63	797.07
BH 10A	936.07	304323.24	503076.63	-895.35	930.81	WD	Frizington	5.5	6.11	22.76				936.00	936.14
BH 10A	952.15	304323.57	503077.09	-911.42	946.88	HF	Frizington	341.0	NA	23.19	22.8	33.4	9.52	950.00	954.29
BH 10A	1123.32	304327.36	503082.35	-1082.47	1117.93	BD	Brown Bank	298.6	10.38	27.71				1122.78	1123.86

BH 10B Ground Level elevation (maOD)			35.72										
BH ID	Mid MD	X	Y	Z	mbGL$_{TVD}$	Type	Lith	$\theta\sigma_1$	$\theta\sigma_1$ SD*1.96	σ_2 (MPa)	σ_3 (MPa)	σ_1 (MPa)	P$_P$ (MPa)	Top MD	Base MD
BH10B	144.49	304268.30	503080.30	-108.77	144.49	OC	Calder	338.8	NA	4.7	4.0	7.1		-	-
BH10B	149.00	304268.30	503080.30	-113.28	149.00	OC	Calder	323.8	NA	2.8	1.4	7.3		-	-
BH10B	201.47	304268.30	503080.30	-165.75	201.47	OC	St Bees Sst	332.8	NA	5.0	2.9	7.8		-	-
BH10B	205.99	304268.30	503080.30	-170.27	205.99	OC	St Bees Sst	324.8	NA	4.6	2.2	5.3		-	-
BH10B	251.74	304268.30	503080.30	-216.02	251.74	OC	St Bees Sst	335.8	NA	6.1	1.7	8.3		-	-

BH 11A Ground Level elevation (maOD)			44.59										
BH ID	Mid MD	X	Y	Z	mbGL$_{TVD}$	Type	Lith	$\theta\sigma_{Hmax}$	$\theta\sigma_{Hmax}$ SD*1.96	σ_v (MPa)	σ_{Hmin} (MPa)	σ_{Hmax} (MPa)	P$_P$ (MPa)	Top MD	Base MD
BH 11A	844.39	306801.21	501672.64	-793.50	838.09	WD	NHM	356.4	8.63					844.34	844.44
BH 11A	847.40	306801.26	501672.79	-796.51	841.10	WD	St Bees Shl	10.5	6.25					847.17	847.63
BH 11A	851.19	306801.32	501672.99	-800.29	844.88	WD	St Bees Shl	345.8	9.93					851.10	851.28
BH 11A	888.77	306801.90	501674.91	-837.82	882.41	IF	Brockram	354.1	17.15					887.16	890.38

BH 12A Ground Level elevation (maOD)			38.45										
BH ID	Mid MD	X	Y	Z	mbGL$_{TVD}$	Type	Lith	$\theta\sigma_{Hmax}$	$\theta\sigma_{Hmax}$ SD*1.96	σ_v (MPa)	σ_{Hmin} (MPa)	σ_{Hmax} (MPa)	P$_P$ (MPa)	Top MD	Base MD
BH 12A	648.61	304941.78	502650.65	-603.84	642.29	WD	NHM	337.4	2.19					648.59	648.63
BH 12A	670.38	304942.34	502651.52	-625.58	664.03	IF	NHM	343.2	13.07					655.43	685.34
BH 12A	699.07	304943.05	502652.68	-654.24	692.69	WD	NHM	349.1	7.71					699.01	699.14
BH 12A	702.67	304943.14	502652.83	-657.83	696.28	WD	NHM	325.5	12.10					702.54	702.79
BH 12A	730.92	304943.86	502654.03	-686.05	724.50	AD	St Bees Shl	337.5	9.44					730.63	731.20
BH 12A	757.60	304944.52	502655.20	-712.70	751.15	IF	Brockram	342.7	2.81					757.55	757.65
BH 12A	790.42	304945.36	502656.68	-745.47	783.92	IF	St Bees Shl	332.0	13.22					758.09	822.75
BH 12A	834.34	304946.47	502658.73	-789.33	827.78	BD	St Bees Shl	339.2	6.21					834.10	834.58

BH 13A Ground Level elevation (maOD)			18.50										
BH ID	Mid MD	X	Y	Z	mbGL$_{TVD}$	Type	Lith	$\theta\sigma_{Hmax}$	$\theta\sigma_{Hmax}$ SD*1.96	σ_v (MPa)	σ_{Hmin} (MPa)	σ_{Hmax} (MPa)	P$_P$ (MPa)	Top MD	Base MD
BH 13A	1376.06	304539.51	500176.76	-1351.58	1370.08	WD	St Bees Shl	300.6	12.12					1375.59	1376.53
BH 13A	1620.40	304550.07	500194.46	-1595.03	1613.53	WD	Frizington	351.9	16.58					1620.10	1620.70
BH 13A	1622.23	304550.15	500194.81	-1596.85	1615.35	IF	Frizington	348.6	8.10					1621.80	1622.67
BH 13A	1628.84	304550.45	500195.35	-1603.43	1621.93	WD	Frizington	341.4	11.49					1623.27	1634.42
BH 13A	1634.54	304550.70	500195.82	-1609.11	1627.61	WD	Basal Beds	344.4	1.08					1634.54	1634.55
BH 13A	1636.32	304550.78	500195.97	-1610.88	1629.38	WD	Ignimbrite	350.0	18.56					1636.15	1636.50

BH 14A Ground Level elevation (maOD)			41.20										
BH ID	Mid MD	X	Y	Z	mbGL$_{TVD}$	Type	Lith	$\theta\sigma_{Hmax}$	$\theta\sigma_{Hmax}$ SD*1.96	σ_v (MPa)	σ_{Hmin} (MPa)	σ_{Hmax} (MPa)	P$_P$ (MPa)	Top MD	Base MD
BH 14A	337.04	302488.62	505697.06	-290.75	331.95	WD	St Bees Sst	349.1	3.84					336.93	337.15

h) Pore pressure data (determined separately, by Environmental Pressure Measurements)

Under column d (type of result) the tests are categorised as follows:
- HF : obtained from HFSM
- OC : obtained from OCSM
- IF : mean breakout azimuth determined from intact borehole sections (i.e. test zone is free from discontinuities)
- WD : mean breakout azimuth determined from borehole sections containing discontinuities

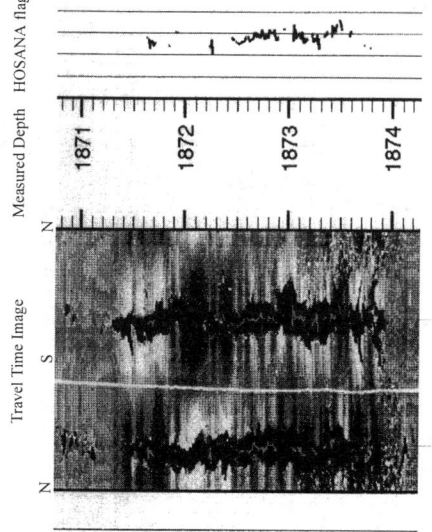

Figure 3 An Example Of The HOSANA Processing to Identify Breakout In The BVG In Sellafield Borehole No. 3

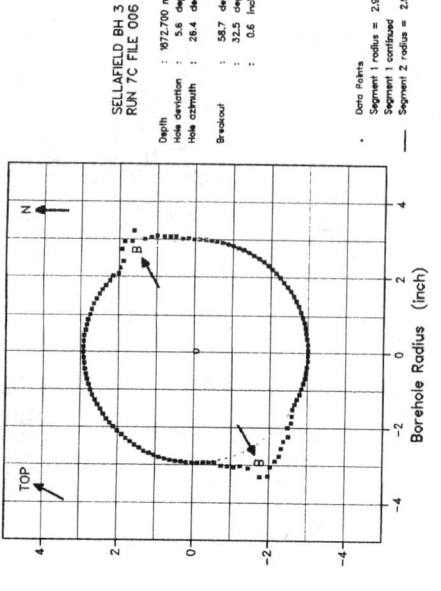

Figure 5 An example cross-section through the section shown in Figure 3 showing a breakout azimuth of 58.7 degrees

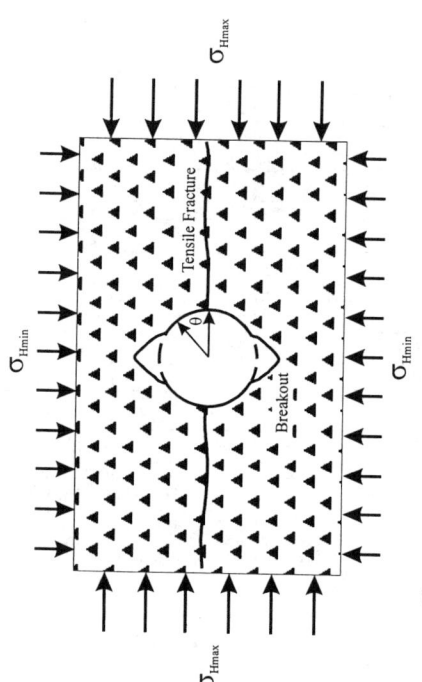

Figure 2 Schematic Cross-Section Through A Vertical Borehole Showing Location Of Tensile Fracture And Breakout

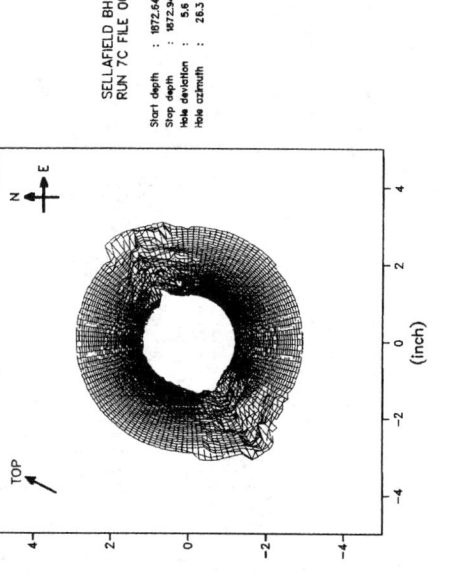

Figure 4 A view down the borehole at the section shown in Figure 3

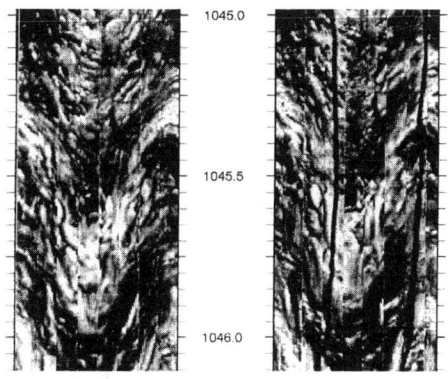

Figure 6 σ_{HMAX} Azimuth Variations With Stress Measurement Type Versus Depth

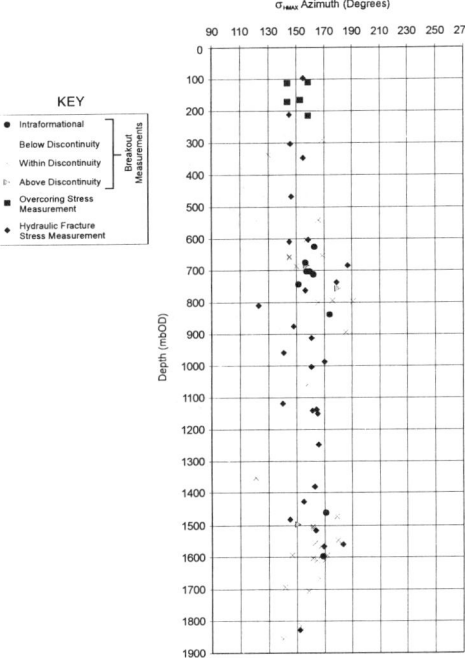

Figure 7 σ_{HMAX} Azimuth Variations With Stress Measurement Type Versus Depth

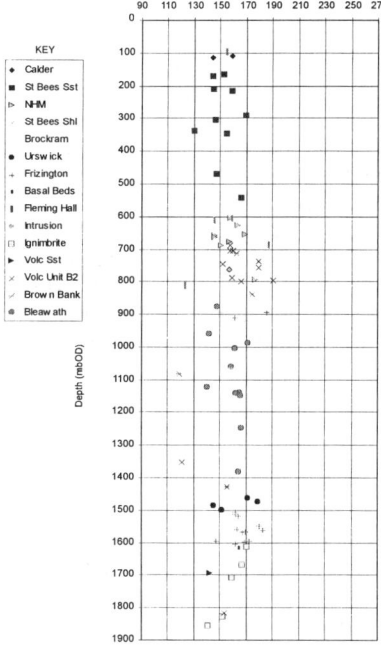

Figure 8 σ_{HMAX} Azimuth Variations With Lithology Versus Depth

AD : mean breakout azimuth determined from intact borehole sections above a discontinuity

BD : mean breakout azimuth determined from intact borehole sections below a discontinuity

PART B: THE ORIENTATION OF THE MAXIMUM PRINCIPAL STRESS AND ITS SPATIAL VARIATIONS

The orientation data which are summarised in Table 3 were analysed statistically to seek reliable and valid correlations. An overall mean azimuth of all the data was derived. Mean values were also derived by borehole, by depth range and by lithology. They were then tested against fault plane data, local structural data and the overcoring results. Also, the mean values and the variances were compared statistically.

Overall trend

Figures 7 and 8 show depth plots of orientation data by measurement type and lithology. The orientation data appear to be a single population of azimuths normally distributed about a mean value. Figure 9 shows the distribution of the azimuth data; giving a mean azimuth of 159.2-339.2°N with a standard deviation of 14.6° and a confidence level of the mean value of ± 3.5° (95%).

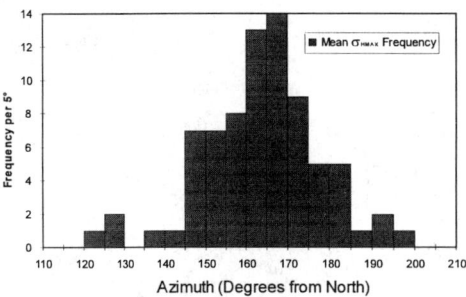

Figure 9 Histogram Of Data For The Azimuth Of The Maximum Horizontal Stress

Trend by borehole and trend by lithology

The mean azimuths from the individual boreholes were found to be generally in excellent agreement with the overall average orientation, with the apparent exception of the results for Borehole No. 11. Statistical testing indicated that the very limited number of data points from Borehole No. 11 could be part of the overall population and the results may not be significantly different from those of the other holes. This observation could only be confirmed by further measurements in the Borehole No. 11 area.

The data for each borehole and each formation were tested for normality (i.e. a Gaussian distribution) using the Shapiro-Wilks' test (Shapiro et al, 1983). Data from Borehole No. 13A and the Bleawath Formation just failed the test, suggesting that it is possible that the data from these samples are not distributed normally.

No significant differences were found between boreholes but a small difference was identified between the stress direction measured in the St Bees Sandstone and the Frizington formations.

Check for correlation of azimuth with depth

The dataset has been checked for correlations between azimuth and depth by borehole and, considering the dataset as a whole, no significant correlation has been found. It may therefore be concluded that there is no correlation with depth, confirming the lack of visual correlation apparent from Figures 7 and 8.

Comparison of data type

The HFSM, OCSM and breakout processing were all independent operations, 29 HFSM tests were carried out in five boreholes over a depth range of approximately 660 to 1840 mbGL (true vertical depth).

Of these 29 HFSM tests, 28 provided useful results. 15 OCSM tests were attempted in a single borehole at 102 to 252 mbGL; five provided useful results. 44 groups of breakout data from various lithologies in seven boreholes were used to estimate the inferred σ_{Hmax} azimuth.

As the HFSM and breakout tests sample larger volumes of rock compared with an OCSM test, and there were 28 successful HFSM orientation tests and 44 sets of breakout data compared with five from the OCSM tests, it can be concluded that the combined HFSM and breakout results form the primary data for the Sellafield stress field with the OCSM data providing confirmatory results.

Overcoring results

The overcoring results were found to be not significantly different from the overall results and showed excellent agreement with the breakout and hydraulic fracturing data. The data also showed maximum principal stress azimuths trending approximately NNW to SSE, indicating consistency with the mean maximum horizontal stress direction derived from HFSM and breakout data. Furthermore, the stress tensors calculated from overcoring data showed a steeply-dipping principal stress (generally σ_3 at shallow depth and σ_2 with increasing depth). Therefore, the assumption that one principal stress is vertical (used in the analysis of HFSM and breakout data) would appear to be generally valid. In broad terms, it was concluded that the overcoring data may be compared with the breakout and HFSM data without the need to resolve stresses in the horizontal plane.

Seismological data

The orientation data related to fault plane solutions of selected seismic events has shown that the stress direction generally is NW-SE (Nirex, 1996). As fault plane solutions have a relatively large error and the spread of results is in excess of 30°, it can therefore be concluded that the fault plane solution from seismic data are broadly in agreement with the results of the direct measurements reported here.

Overall geological structure

Figure 10 shows the Level Plan at 650 mbOD (Nirex, 1996) with the mean stress directions and the local stresses superimposed on the fault data. It can be seen that none of the measurements is very far from a fault or the associated damage zone. The overall strike of

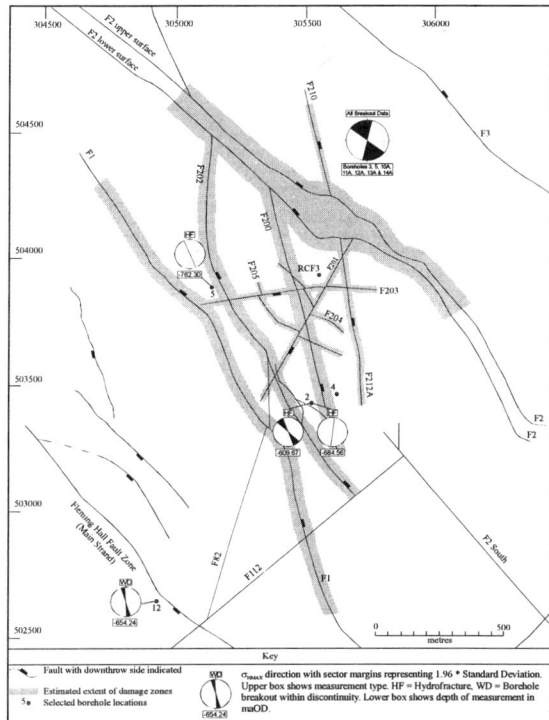

Figure 10 Fault Map At -650 maOD Showing Damage Zones Estimated From Borehole Data With Stress Data Superimposed

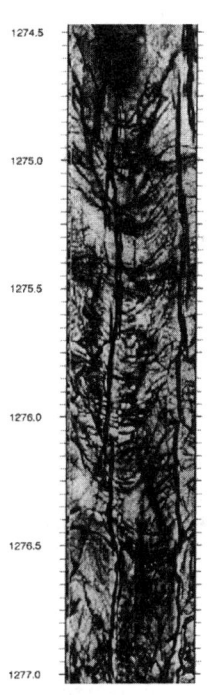

Figure 11 Borehole No. 10A: An Example of Drilling Induced Fracturing On The FMI Image

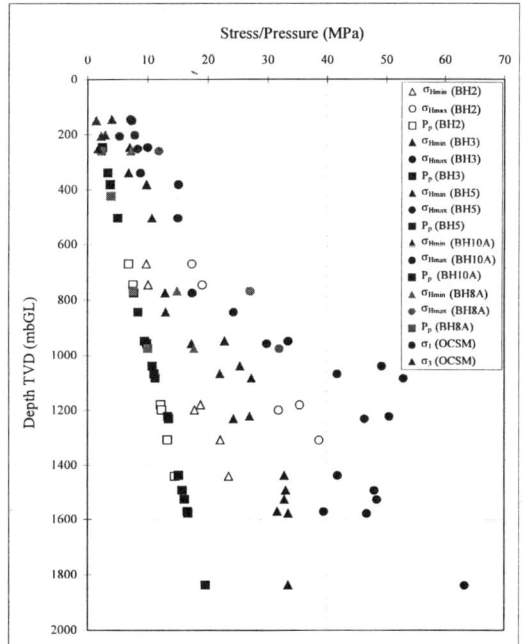

Figure 12 Graphical Representation of HFSM, OCSM and P_p Data

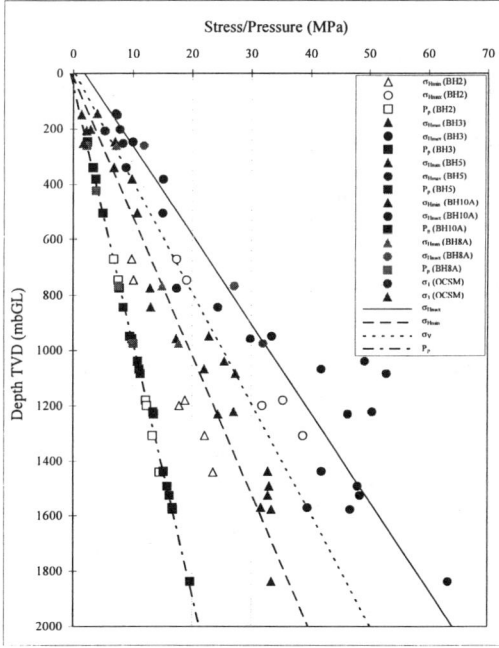

Figure 13 Mean In-situ Stresses and P_p Trends At Sellafield

the features in the Level Plan is approximately 315°. This means that the mean azimuth of the maximum stress is aligned at approximately 25° to the dominant strike direction of the faults. This alignment produces the optimum condition for strike-slip motion. As strike-slip motion has been identified as the predominant earthquake mechanism in the Sellafield area, this alignment provides further support for the estimated value for the direction of maximum principal stress.

Local perturbations to the direction of maximum stress

Statistically, the data presented in Table 3 combine to give an estimate of the overall stress direction, but some of the individual readings do show local perturbations that are real. For example, orientations in Borehole No. 10A display a tendency for the azimuth of the maximum principal stress to rotate slightly to the north with depth and then, suddenly, rotate to the west by nearly 60°. These rotations are not intrinsic uncertainties in the readings, they are real observations.

Similarly, the azimuth of the maximum stress inferred from the breakout data at 1123.32 mbRT is 298.55° in the Brown Bank formation. By chance, there is a drilling induced hydraulic fracture at 1250 mbRT to 1282 mbRT in Borehole No. 10A. The average orientation of this fracture is 300° with standard error (95%) of ± 4.5° and is directly comparable to the breakout data at 1123.32 mbRT. Figure 11 shows part of the drilling induced fracture which can be seen in full on the FMI log of the borehole. It is concluded that local perturbations of the stress field do occur on a scale of a few tens of metres, although such variations only become apparent in closely spaced data such as that available for Borehole No. 10A.

Conclusions regarding orientation of maximum principal stress

The work to define the azimuth of the in-situ maximum principal stress at Sellafield involved processing and orientating data from many different sources. In particular, the various ultrasonic imaging (pre-UBI) measurements had to be checked and aligned to the orientation of the Formation Micro Imager/Micro Scanner logs. The close agreement and consistency of the results shows that this process was successful and did not introduce any systematic errors.

Agreement has been obtained between the datasets and it has been concluded that the mean azimuth of σ_{Hmax} is 339° (± 3.5°). It is possible that the in-situ stress direction in the vicinity of Borehole No. 11 is rotated 15° towards the north, but insufficient data are available to confirm this difference.

Local perturbations in direction of maximum stress have been observed that may be related to both formation and fault positions.

PART C: THE MAGNITUDE OF THE PRINCIPAL STRESSES

Graphical presentations of the magnitudes of HFSM principal stresses, OCSM horizontal principal stresses and pore pressure are shown in Figure 12. Consistency of the derived stress magnitudes have been checked by comparing stress estimates for hydraulic fracturing and borehole breakout at specific locations where these features were found close to each other. The checks also confirmed the need for further evaluation of the rock strength parameters obtained from laboratory testing on cores during these investigations (Nirex, 1996).

The depth trends of the principal stress magnitudes were determined using linear regression analyses. The derived trends were then used to predict the stresses in the RCF region.

Pore pressure (P_p) trend with depth

An excellent linear correlation (coefficient of 0.999) for the trend of the pore pressure magnitudes was obtained. The equation of the trend is given by:

$$P_p \text{ (MPa)} = (0.01088 \pm 0.000113)D - (0.53189 \pm 0.12265) \quad (1)$$

where, D = true vertical depth in metres below ground level.

σ_V trend

Regression analysis on the computed σ_V data indicated that the mean depth trend of the σ_V magnitudes for the HFSM boreholes at Sellafield can be described with the composite equation:

$$\sigma_v \text{ (MPa)} = (0.02494 \pm 0.00025)D + (0.26622 \pm 0.25326) \quad (2)$$

where, D is true vertical depth in metres, measured from ground level. An excellent coefficient of correlation (0.9985) was obtained.

Trend of σ_{Hmin} magnitudes with depth

Magnitudes of σ_{Hmin} were obtained during overcoring and by equating fracture opening pressure to σ_{Hmin}. The equation for the computation of the least stress with depth was derived as:

$$\sigma_{Hmin} (MPa) = (0.01996 \pm 0.00113)D - (0.31619 \pm 1.15545) \quad (3)$$

where, D = true vertical depth in metres below ground level.

The 95% confidence limits approximate to ± 2 MPa over the depth range 100 to 1000 mbGL$_{TVD}$. The coefficient of correlation for this equation using the σ_{Hmin} data presented in Table 3 is 0.954.

The scatter in the data increases with depth and the higher than expected values at 1000 - 1200 mbGL$_{TVD}$ are predominantly in the Bleawath in Borehole No. 5. The majority of the induced fractures in this interval show a tendency to be inclined so these data points (in the Bleawath) may either reflect the fact that the stress field is slightly inclined or that a component of the vertical stress is included in the measurements.

Trend of σ_{Hmax} magnitudes with depth

Magnitudes of σ_{Hmax} were computed either directly from the induced strains during overcoring or calculated from HFSM results and pore pressure data.

Two major sources of uncertainty influence the values of σ_{Hmax}; firstly, the value of σ_{Hmin} is scaled by a factor of 3 and therefore it contributes three times the intrinsic variability of the σ_{Hmin} value. In this case, for example, the σ_{Hmax} value may be expected to have a ± 6 MPa confidence limit because the σ_{Hmin} value has a ± 2 MPa limit. Secondly, the value of effective tensile strength of the formation is always uncertain.

The derived equation for σ_{Hmax} is:

$$\sigma_{Hmax} (MPa) = (0.03113 \pm 0.00227)D + (1.88747 \pm 2.28402) \quad (4)$$

where, D = true vertical depth in metres below ground level and the coefficient of correlation, r, is 0.93.

The trends of the in-situ principal stresses and pore pressure are presented in Figure 13.

Conclusions regarding magnitudes of principal stresses

The magnitudes of the principal stresses have been calculated from:

a) Hydraulic fracturing stress measurements
b) In-situ density measurements
c) Overcore stress measurements

The consistency of the results has been tested by predicting the occurrence of breakout at certain depths and comparing the image logs where breakout was located.

The variation of the principal stresses with depth

The principal stresses are oriented generally in the vertical and horizontal planes. The trends have been estimated as:

σ_V = (0.02494 ± 0.00025)D + (0.26622 ± 0.25326)MPa
σ_{Hmin} = (0.01996 ± 0.00113)D - (0.31619 ± 1.15545)MPa
σ_{Hmax} = (0.03113 ± 0.00227)D + (1.88747 ± 2.28402)MPa

where, D = true vertical depth in metres below ground level.

These predictions are valid over the depth range of the dataset only (140 to 1830 metres below ground level) and must not be extrapolated.

The averaging process for the horizontal stresses masks some real variations in the magnitudes of the stresses. The most notable perturbation is the group of higher than expected values for the maximum stresses in Borehole No. 5. These are all associated with the Bleawath Formation but similar values were not found in this formation in Borehole No. 2. It is possible that the results were all obtained on slightly inclined features or that the stresses themselves are inclined thus increasing the pressure on near vertical fractures. This type of perturbation is not seen at depths shallower than 1000m in the existing boreholes.

ACKNOWLEDGEMENTS

The work described in this paper was carried out under contract to United Kingdom Nirex Limited and their permission to publish the paper is gratefully acknowledged.

Schlumberger GeoQuest undertook the HOSANA processing and Jury van Doorn's assistance was particularly helpful.

Many groups participated in different aspects of the work and the input from Golder Associates (UK) Ltd, Soil Mechanics Ltd, Schlumberger, Vattenfall, Baker Oil Tools, Nowsco and Kenting Drilling Services is acknowledged.

REFERENCES

Barr, S. 1993. *The Kaiser effect of acoustic emissions*

for the determination of in-situ stress in the Carnmenellis granite, PhD Thesis, Camborne School of Mines, University of Exeter, UK.

Batchelor, A.S., Kwakwa, K.A., Pearson, R.A., Lanyon, G.W. & Thin, I.G.T. 1995. *Stresses in the North Sea (with an example from Northern Scotland)*, Proceedings of the Workshop on 'Rock Stresses in the North Sea', Fejerskov, M. & Myrvang, A.M. (Eds), University of Trondheim, February, 127-146.

Nirex. 1996. Assessment of the in-situ stress field at Sellafield - Main Report, 2 Vols., Nirex Report No. SA/96/010. United Kingdom Nirex Limited, Curie Avenue, Harwell, Didcot, Oxfordshire OX11 0RH.

Shapiro, S.S., Wilk, M.B. & Chen, H.J. 1983. *A comparative study of various tests of normality*, J. Am. Stats. Assoc. 63, 1343-1372.

Zoback, M.L. 1992. *First and second-order patterns of stress in the lithosphere: the world stress map project*, J. Geophys. Res. Vol. 97, No. 8, 30 July, 11703-11728.

SYMBOLS

English

BHTV	-	Borehole Televiewer
RCF	-	Rock Characterisation Facility
mbOD	-	metres below Ordnance Datum
FMI	-	Formation Micro Imager*
HOSANA	-	hole size analysis*
UBI	-	Ultrasonic Borehole Imager*
TVD	-	true vertical depth
mbGL	-	metres below Ground Level
m	-	metre
MPa	-	Mega Pascals
MD	-	measured depth
HFSM	-	hydrofracture stress measurement
OCSM	-	overcoring stress measurement
P	-	Pressure

* Schlumberger Trade Marks

Greek

ν	-	Poisson's Ratio
σ_1	-	maximum principal stress
σ_2	-	intermediate principal stress
σ_3	-	minimum principal stress
σ_V	-	vertical stress
σ_{Hmax}	-	maximum horizontal principal stress
σ_{Hmin}	-	minimum horizontal principal stress

Subscripts

p	-	pore pressure
TVD	-	true vertical depth

Interpretation of rock fracture phenomena

On rock stress in rockburst risk assessment of deep gold mines

Xia-Ting Feng – *Dept. of Mining Engineering, Northeastern University, Shenyang, People's Republic of China*
M. Seto & K. Katsuyama – *National Institute for Resources and Environment, Tsukuba, Japan*
M. Özbay – *Department of Mining Engineering, The University of Witwatersrand, South Africa*
S. Webber – *Mining Technology Division, CSIR, South Africa*

ABSTRACT: Rock stress has nonlinear effect on rockburst risks in deep gold mines. Neural network techniques can be used to find nonlinear representation of features and retrieve missing features. It is proposed that the data collected from rockburst events can be structured to form a database that can be used to train neural networks to assess effect of rock stress in a given mining situation. The results from the test cases for mining of various reefs, for both stopes and gullies, are presented. The control level of rock stress on risks of rockburst was recognized. The results show that, for different geological conditions and energy release rates, effect of rock stress on risks of rockburst is different. Sometimes high rock stress condition did not result in occurrence of rockburst. For other 5 rockburst cases, the field rock stress decreases were successfully recognized by using the trained neural network model if rockburst would not occur. It is shown that the proposed artificial intelligent approach has the potential to assess effect of rock stress on risks of rockburst, this is highly dependent on the accuracy of the data collected.

1 INTRODUCTION

Rockbursts and rockfalls exact a heavy toll in South African gold mines in terms of injuries and fatalities and in lost production. It is shown from statistical data (Webber 1996) that rate of rock related fatality per 1000 workers was running up 0.5 to 0.75 and 5 for rate of rock related injury per 1000 workers. Ratio of rock related fatalities and injuries with totals were 50 to 70% and 30% respectively. With some mines intending to extract ore at depths of 4500 m and deeper within the next years, clearly serious steps are required to minimize the risks related rockbursts and rockfalls implicit in mining at great depth. In essence, the safety of underground workers is paramount. Therefore, it is imperative to look for reasonable measurement to decrease rockburst catastrophes in South African gold mines at great depth.

Some researchers have obtained information on influence of the field stress to the rockburst. Gay (1974) encountered discing when using strain-relief techniques to measured the *in situ* state of stress in a large dyke at ERPM. From the stress measurement, deviatoric stresses of the order of 100 to 160 MPa were calculated-sufficient to induce the observed discing in the very strong dyke rock (with a uniaxial comprehension strength of 360 MPa). Gay and Van der Heever (1982) found that large horizontal stresses (48 to 56 MPa) act at high angles to fault planes, enhancing the strain energy stored in the quartzite adjacent to the faults. Moreover, modelling by Brummer and Rorke (1990) showed that these structures have the potential to generate large (magnitude 4+) seismic events. The values of k ratios determined from the *in situ* stress measurement cited vary from 0.6 at the ERPM dyke site to 1.0 in the Klerksdorp district. The lower the value of the k ratio, the greater the potential for sudden seismic slip on the structure. Significantly, the minimum k ratios (i.e. $\sigma h_{min}/\sigma v$) encountered in deep South African mines range between 0.3 and 0.4; k ratios of this order probably indicate that normal fault slip could readily occur during mining, supporting Brummer and Rorke's (1990) conclusions.

Many factors have influence on occurrence of rockburst. The field stress is one of important factors. These factors also interact each other, which results in rockburst modelling problem is in data-limited range and little or some understanding. It is hard or impossible to bring these factors to the model by using traditional mathematical methodologies. This paper concentrates on influence of the field stress on

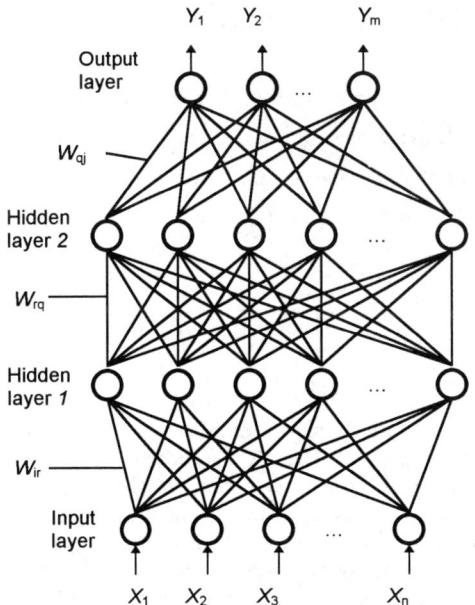

Fig 1. A feedforward neural network

rockburst risk in deep gold mines and its estimation at rockburst case. The methodology involved is application of artificial neural network.

2 NEURAL NETWORK METHODOLOGY

Unlike the conventional modeling methods, which use mathematical expressions to approximate the relationship between the field stress and other factors and rockburst, neural networks offer a fundamentally different approach to model an intrinsic connection of factors and rockburst and have the capability to avoid some basic shortcomings in the mathematical modeling techniques. Neural networks use the learning capabilities, and are massively parallel computational models for knowledge representation and information processing. They have unique learning capabilities that can be used in learning complex nonlinear relationships (Rumelhart, Hinston, and Williams, 1986; Kohonen, 1988; Grossberg, 1988). The learning capabilities encourage us to investigate applicability of neural networks to describe the influence of the field stress on rockburst.

Grossber (1991) testified that the neural network with one (at most two) hidden layer(s) is suitable for any complicated problem. Accordingly, the rockburst problem with influence of field stress can be expressed by the feedforward neural network with at most two hidden layers shown in Fig.1. The parallel distribution model can be written as follows

Table 1 Data for test samples

Parameters	45*	46*	47*	48*	49*
x_1	1980	3150	3565	1372	1595
x_2					
Fault				×	
Dyke	×	×	×		×
Joint					
None					
x_3					
Longwall		×	×		
Scattered	×			×	×
x_4	25	20	19	17	25
x_5	200	270	240	120	230
x_6	no	no	no	no	no
x_7					
Carbon leader		×			
VCR	×				×
Composite reef			×		
Others				×	
x_8					
Pack		×	×	×	×
Backfill					
Hydraulic props					
x_9					
None	×				×
Backfill				×	
Stabilizing pillar			×		
Backfill + Stabilizing pillar		×			
x_{10}					
None		×			
Mechanical props	×				×
Mine pole				×	
Hydraulic props			×		
x_{11}	1.19	0.9	0.9	1.3	1.2
x_{12}	50	24	200	180	200
x_{13}	Yes	Yes	Yes	Yes	Yes
Height of fall	1.5	0.8	0.7	0.9	0.7
Width of fall	4	2.4	2.0	2.7	2

• Sample no.

Table 2 Comparison of neural network estimation with the measurement of stress

No.	Measured (MPa)	Predicted (MPa)	Absolute Error	Relative Error
45	53	51.8	1.2	0.02
46	72	71.6	0.4	0.01
47	141	149.3	8.3	0.06
48	85	8.72	2.2	0.03
49	42	4.85	6.5	0.15

$$(y_1, y_2, \Lambda, y_m) = NN(in, h_1, h_2, o)(x_1, x_2, \cdots, x_n) \quad (1)$$

Where, y_j $(j = 1, 2, \cdots, m)$ is the jth output variable, x_i $(i = 1, 2, \cdots, n)$ is the ith input variable, in is number of the input nodes, h_i is the number of nodes the ith hidden layer, o is the number of the output nodes.

2.1 Estimation of the field stress

The neural network model for estimating the field stress can be expressed by

$$y = NN(n, h_1, h_2, o)(x_1, x_2, x_3, x_4, x_5, x_6, x_7, x_8, x_9, x_{10}, x_{11}, x_{12}, x_{13}) \quad (2)$$

where, y: the field stress; x_1: depth below surface; x_2: geological structure (fault, dyke, joint, none); x_3: mining method (longwall, scattered); x_4: dip; x_5: dip span (m); x_6: pillar; x_7: reef description (Carbon Leader, VCR, composite reef, others); x_8: permanent support (pack, backfill, hydraulic props); x_9: regional support (none, backfill, stabilizing pillar); x_{10}: temporary support (none, mechanical props, mine pole, hydraulic props); x_{11}: stope width (m); x_{12}: strike span (m); x_{13}: rockburst.

$NN(n, h_1, h_2, o)$ in Eq.(2) can be learned by training the network using case data set. The 49 rockburst cases have been selected from the database developed by Mining Technology Division at CISR, South Africa. They were divided to two parts. The 44 cases have been selected random to train the network to obtain the model. The rest 5 cases have been used to test the model, which data is shown in Table 1. Many network architectures have been evaluated to get the best output. The best network was found to be NN(13, 21, 1).

Table 2 shows those estimations of the model NN(13, 21, 1). It is seen that average relative errors on the field stress are 5.4%. Fig.2 shows the acquisition of parameters.

2.2 The influence of the field stress on rockburst

The model describing the influence of the field stress on rockburst can be expressed by

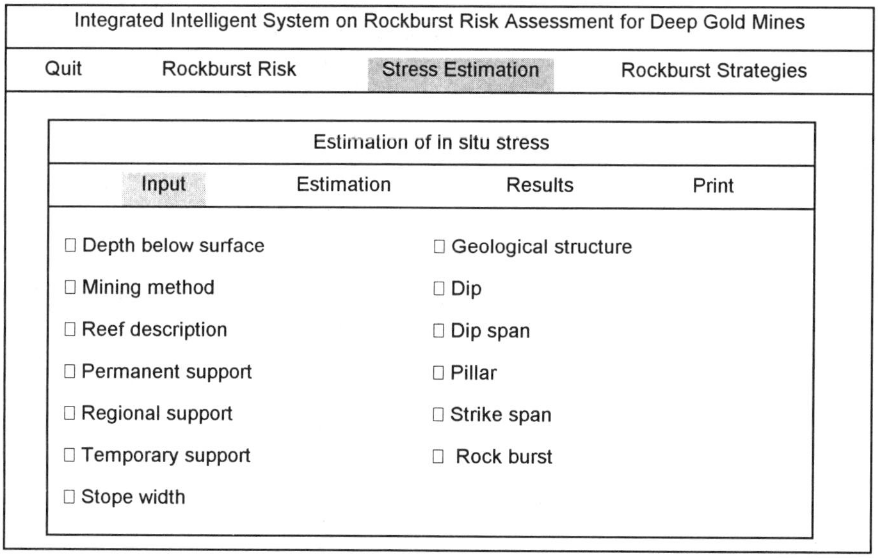

Table 3 The field stress decrease estimated by the model NN(14,14,14) without rockburst occurrence

No.	Measured field stress at rockburst occurrence (MPa)	Field stress estimated by the model without rockburst occurrence (MPa)
40	67	56.7
41	212	189
42	67	46.1
43	95	92.3
44	115	105.5

Fig 2. Acquisition of geological information for stress estimation

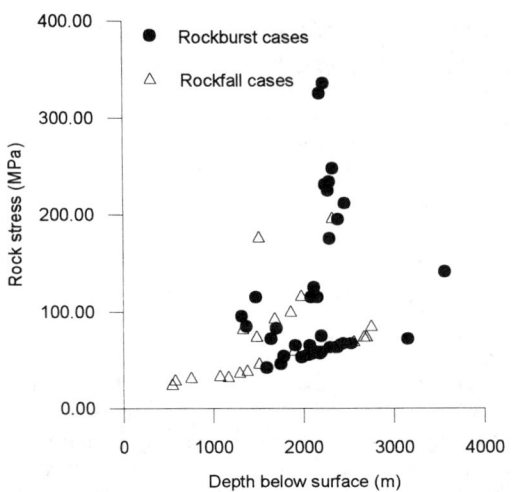

Fig 3. Field rock stress in rockburst and rockgall cases

$(x_1, x_2, x_3, x_4, x_5, x_6, x_7, x_8, x_9, x_{10}, x_{11}, x_{12}, x_{13}, y)$
$= NN(n, h_1, h_2, o) (x_1, x_2, x_3, x_4, x_5, x_6, x_7, x_8, x_9, x_{10}, x_{11}, x_{12}, x_{13}, y)$ (3)

The 44 cases used in above have been used to construct the model. The parameter "rockburst" in 5 cases was replaced by "without rockburst" to become new cases. Decreases of the field stresses were estimated by the model for these new cases.

Many network architectures have also been evaluated to get the best outputs. The best network was found to be NN(14, 14, 14). Table 3 shows the results of the model. They indicate that in these 5 cases if rockburst does not occur the field stress might decrease to 56.7 MPa from 67 MPa, 189 MPa from 212 MPa, 46.1 MPa from 67 MPa. 92.3 MPa from 95 MPa, 105.5 MPa from 115 MPa, respectively. This is useful guide to design more reasonable mining and support strategies to ameliorate the hazards of rockburst.

3 DISCUSSION

The influence of the field stress on rockburst occurrence is not unitary and controlled by other factors (see Fig.3). It is very difficult to describe it by traditional mathematical model. Learning with neural network is possible for highly nonlinear associations in the presence of noise and uncertainty. The learning capabilities allow neural networks to be directly trained with the results of measurements. They learn the intrinsic relationship between factors and rockburst and then "memorize" as knowledge in their connection weights. If the training data contains the relevant information of rockburst, then the trained neural network can generalize from its training data to novel cases. The investigations show higher accuracy has been obtained from the novel method.

ACKNOWLEDGEMENT

Mining Technology at CSIR, South Africa, and Japanese Governmental ITIT Program for Xia-Ting Feng, and China Natural Science Foundation financially supported this research and are gratefully appreciated. Rockburst data base was provided by Mining Technology at CSIR, South Africa are gratefully acknowledged.

REFERENCES

Brummer, R. K. and Rorke, A. J. 1990. Case studies on large roxkbursts in South African gold mines, Rockbursts and Seismicity in Mines. Fairhurst (ed.) Rotterdam, Balkema, 323-329.

Gay, N. C. 1974. State of stress in a large dyke on ERPM, Boksburg, South Africa. *Int. J. Rock Mech. Min. Sci. & Geomech. Abstr.*, 16.

Gay, N. C. and Van Der Heever, P. K. 1982. *In situ* stresses in the Klerksdrop gold mine district, South Africa - a correlation between geological strucures and seismicity, *Issues in Rock Mechanics*, Proc. 23rd Symposium on Rock Mechanics. Berkeley, Goodman and Heuze(eds.) Now Year, AIME. 176-182.

Ghaboussi, J., Sidarta, D. E., and Lade, P. V. 1994. Neural network based modelling in geomechanics, in *Computer methods and Advances in Geomechanics*, Siriwardane & Zaman (eds.) 153-164.

Grossberg, S. 1988. Nonlinear neural networks: principles, mechanisms, and architectures, *Neural Networks*, 1, 17-61.

Kohonen T. 1988. An introduction to neural computing, *Neural Networks*, 1, 3-16.

Rumelhart, D. E., Hinton G. E., and Williams, R. J. 1988. Learning internal representations by error propagation, in *Parallel Distribution Processing*, Rumelhart, D. E. and McClelland, J. L. (eds), MIT Press, Cambridge , MA.

S. Webber 1996. Rockburst risk assessment on South African gold mines: an expert system approach, *Proc. of Eurock'96*, Italy.

Crack kinematics and stress intensity factors by acoustic emission

Munwam C. Muzo
Graduate School of Science and Technology, Kumamoto University, Japan

Masayasu Ohtsu
Department of Civil Engineering and Architecture, Kumamoto University, Japan

Hans P. Rossmanith
Institute of Mechanics, Technical University of Vienna, Austria

ABSTRACT: The moment tensor analysis of acoustic emission (AE) can provide quantitative information on cracking mechanisms. Relations between moment tensor components and parameters in fracture mechanics are examined. In bending tests of notched beams, direction of crack propagation are determined from the moment tensor analysis of AE. In the mixed-mode cracking, based on the linear elastic fracture mechanics (LEFM), crack nucleation can be analyzed by the criterion of the maximum circumferential stress. The relation between the direction of crack propagation and the stress intensity factors (K_I and K_{II}) is applied to estimate the relative values of K_I / K_{IC} and K_{II} / K_{IC}.

1 INTRODUCTION

Fracture toughness is a material property which can be defined as the critical stress intensity factor (K_{IC}), the critical energy release rate (G_{IC}), the strain energy density factor (S_C) and so forth. Fracture mechanics was first introduced for brittle materials, such as glass by Griffith. The application of fracture mechanics to concrete structures appear to have been made by Kaplan (1961). Griffith model has been applied by numerous researchers with a goal to understand the modes of mechanical failure in concrete.

Previously, a moment tensor analysis of acoustic emission (AE) was attempted to identify cracking mechanisms of glass due to indentation, assuming the components (Kim & Sachse 1984). A simplified and stable procedure has been developed (Ohtsu 1987) with aim to determine the moment tensor components in the general cases. Based on the eigenvalue analysis of the moment tensor, the procedure for the classification of crack type and the determination of crack orientation is developed. The procedure is known as SiGMA code (Ohtsu 1995).

In the present paper, the directions of crack motion and crack normal determined by AE analysis are applied to the maximum circumferential stress concept, based on the linear elastic fracture mechanics (LEFM). The relative stress intensity factors K_I / K_{IC} and K_{II} / K_{IC} are estimated.

2 DETERMINATION OF STRESS INTENSITY FACTORS.

2.1 Moment tensor

Mathematically, crack kinematics is modeled by crack motion vector (Burgers vector) b and unit normal vector n to crack surface F as shown in Fig 1. Crack motion vector $b(y, t)$ at point y, is set to be equal to $b(y)$ l $S(t)$, where $b(y)$ represents the magnitude of crack displacement, l is the direction vector of crack motion, and $S(t)$ is the source-time

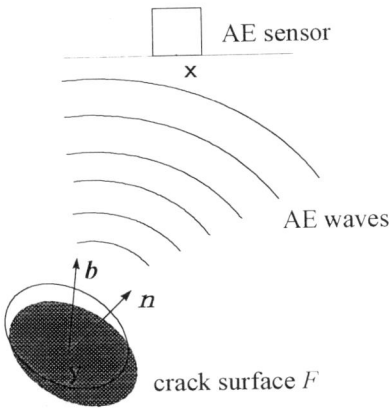

Figure 1 Generation of AE waves due to cracking

function of crack motion. The following integration over crack surface F leads to a product of moment tensor m_{pq}, source-time function $S(t)$, and crack volume ΔV.

$$\int_F C_{pqkl}[b(y)l_k S(t)]n_l ds$$
$$= [C_{pqkl}l_k n_l]S(t)\left[\int_F b(y)ds\right] = m_{pq}S(t)\Delta V, \quad (1)$$

where C_{pqkl} are elastic constants. From the theory of elastodynamics, elastic displacement $u(x, t)$ at location x due to the crack motion $b(y, t)$ is represented, assuming a point source,

$$u_i(x,t) = \int_F C_{pqkl}G_{ip,q}(x,y,t)*[b(y)l_k S(t)]n_l ds$$
$$= G_{ip,q}(x,y,t)*m_{pq}S(t)\Delta V, \quad (2)$$

where $G_{ip,q}(x,y,t)$ represent the spatial derivatives of Green's function and the asterisk * represents the convolution integral. The moment tensor m_{pq} can be represented in an isotropic material, as follow:

$$m_{pq} = [C_{pqkl}l_k n_l]$$
$$= \begin{pmatrix} \lambda l_k n_k + 2\mu l_1 n_1 & \mu l_1 n_2 + \mu l_2 n_1 & \mu l_1 n_3 + \mu l_3 n_1 \\ \mu l_2 n_1 + \mu l_1 n_2 & \lambda l_k n_k + 2\mu l_2 n_2 & \mu l_2 n_3 + \mu l_3 n_2 \\ \mu l_3 n_1 + \mu l_1 n_3 & \mu l_3 n_2 + \mu l_2 n_3 & \lambda l_k n_k + 2\mu l_3 n_3 \end{pmatrix}.$$
(3)

where λ and μ are Lame constants. $l_k n_k$ follows the summation convention.

2.2 Mixed-mode fracture

Erdogan and Sih (1963) has proposed the maximum circumferential stress concept in mixed-mode fracture, based on the LEFM theory. The direction θ of crack propagation is determined from Eq.5 (Carpinteri 1986),

$$\cos\frac{\theta}{2}\left[K_I\cos^2\frac{\theta}{2} - \frac{3}{2}K_{II}\sin\theta\right] = K_{IC}, \quad (4)$$

$$K_I\sin\theta + K_{II}(3\cos\theta - 1) = 0. \quad (5)$$

In the case that direction θ is given, two vectors l

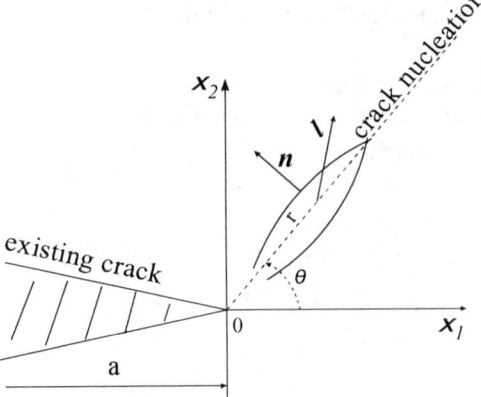

Figure 2 Direction of crack propagation and crack normal.

and n are shown in Fig. 2. Then the direction n corresponds to $(\cos(\theta + \pi/2), \sin(\theta + \pi/2))$.
Directions l and n are theoretically obtained from eigenvectors of the moment tensor. Three eigenvectors are determined from Eq.3 (Ohtsu 1995):

$$\begin{aligned} &l + n, \\ &l \times n, \\ &l - n. \end{aligned} \quad (6)$$

where $\times$ means the vector product. In the SiGMA code, unit vectors $\vec{e_1}, \vec{e_2}, \vec{e_3}$ of direction $l + n$, $l \times n$ and $l - n$ are determined, respectively. Thus, vectors l and n can be recovered from the following relations,

$$\begin{aligned} l &= \sqrt{(2 + 2l_k n_k)}\vec{e_1} + \sqrt{(2 - 2l_k n_k)}\vec{e_3}, \\ n &= \sqrt{(2 + 2l_k n_k)}\vec{e_1} - \sqrt{(2 - 2l_k n_k)}\vec{e_3}. \end{aligned} \quad (7)$$

2.3 Estimation of the stress intensity factors.

To combine crack normal n and Eqs.4 and 5, the three-dimensional (3-D) coordinate system is transformed, as the direction of vector $\vec{e_2}$ corresponds to the x_3-axis in the new (2-D) coordinate system (Fig. 3). Then, the directions of two vectors are determined as,

$$\begin{aligned} l &= \frac{\sqrt{2 + 2l_k n_k}\,\vec{e_1}^* + \sqrt{2 - 2l_k n_k}\,\vec{e_3}^*}{2}, \\ n &= \frac{\sqrt{2 + 2l_k n_k}\,\vec{e_1}^* - \sqrt{2 - 2l_k n_k}\,\vec{e_3}^*}{2}. \end{aligned} \quad (8)$$

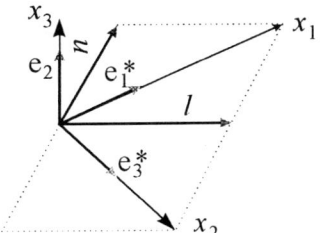

Figure 3 Eigenvectors and crack vectors in new 2-D coordinates system.

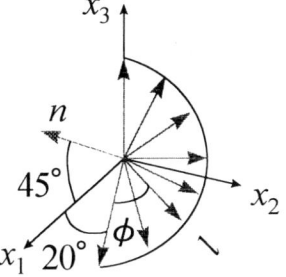

Figure 4(a) Normal vector **n** is fixed, and crack vector **l** is varied.

Here, $\vec{e}_1^*$ and $\vec{e}_3^*$ are transformed vectors of $\vec{e}_1$ and $\vec{e}_3$, respectively. Taking into account $n = (-\sin\theta, \cos\theta)$ in Eq.5 (Ohtsu 1996), relative stress intensity factors K_I/K_{IC} and K_{II}/K_{IC} can be estimate from Eq.4.

2.4 Numerical experiment

An applicability of Eq.8 to the determination of relative stress intensity factors K_I/K_{IC} and K_{II}/K_{IC} was investigated by numerical experiments. As given in Eq.7, two vectors **l** and **n** were assumed. Then, new vectors **l** and **n** in Eq.8 were determined in the new coordinates system. By substituting the vector **n** into Eqs.4 and 5, relative stress intensity factors K_I^* and K_{II}^* were obtained. Two cases considered are shown in Fig.4. In the case of Fig.4 (a), the angles between two vectors **l** and **n** are slightly changed, while those vary from 0 to 70° in the case of Fig.4 (b). Corresponding to these cases, relative stress intensity factors are determined as shown in Fig.5. In Fig.5 (a), even though crack motion vectors are varied, dominant mode is mode I as K_I^* is always greater than K_{II}^* and values of K_I^* are almost equal to 1.0. In contrast, K_I^* decreases and K_{II}^* increases with the increase of the angle of crack normal. Around 55°, the dominant mode shifts from the mode I to mode II. Thus, it is confirmed that relative stress intensity can be determined from the direction of crack motion, which could be obtained from the eigenvectors of moment tensor components in AE analysis.

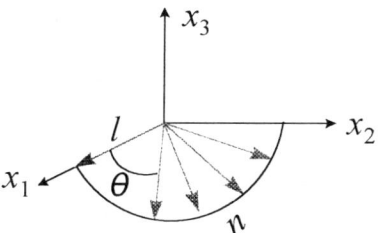

Figure 4(b) Crack vector **l** is fixed, and normal vector **n** is varied.

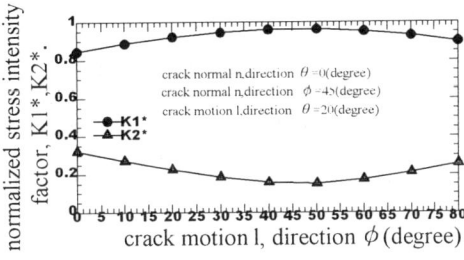

Figure 5(a) Numerical stress intensity factor vs crack motion direction (case 1)

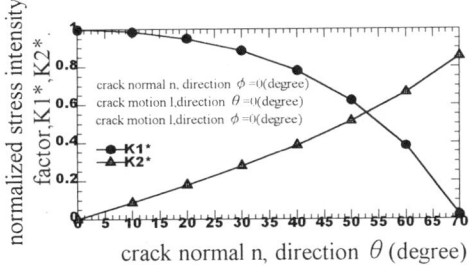

Figure 5(b) Numerical stress intensity factor vs. crack normal direction (case 2)

3 EXPERIMENT

3.1 Specimens

All specimens of dimension (10cm x 10cm x 40cm)

Table 1 Mechanical properties

	unit weight (kg/m³)				(cc)	(cm)	(%)	(MPa)		(GPa)	(m/s)
	W	C	S	G	air-entrained agent	slump	air	comp. strength	Poisson ratio	young modulus	velocity of P wave
Concrete	172	346	834	1021	104	8.0	5.0	52.8	0.24	32.5	4730
Mortar	342	570	1140					53.7	0.19	23.4	4130

were cast and moisture-cured in water for 28 days in the standard room (20℃). Mechanical properties were obtained from cylindrical specimens of concrete and mortar with 10cm diameter and 20cm height. These are summarized in table 1.

3.2 Fracture tests.

Three-point bending tests on notched beams were conducted. 3cm pre-cracked notch of 1 mm width was introduced in all specimens by sawing. They are a center-notched beam under center loading (type CC), and an off-center-notched beam under center loading (type OC). Loading speed applied to CC type specimen was 0.01 mm/min, while loading speed applied to OC type specimens was 0.02 mm/min. Experimental set-up is given in Fig. 6. The location of center-loading and off-center loading are indicated by a solid arrow and a broken arrow, respectively. Those of center notch and off-center notch are also given by solid line and broken line, respectively. In addition, as shown in the Fig. 6, six AE sensors numbered from 1 to 6, were employed. AE waveforms were detected, amplified, filtered, and recorded by using LOCAN-TRA system. Sensors are of wide-band type in the frequency range 200-1000kHz. From AE waveforms at six locations, moment tensor components were determined by the SiGMA procedure. Locations of source, crack types, and crack orientations were analyzed.

4 RESULTS AND DISCUSSION

4.1 SiGMA analysis

Some of results on crack kinematics are shown in Figs. 7. AE sources located are plotted at their location. These are classified into tensile cracks and shear cracks. Tensile cracks are indicated by arrow symbol. Shear and mixed-mode cracks are denoted by cross symbol. In both symbols, two direction indicate crack normal n and crack motion l. As can

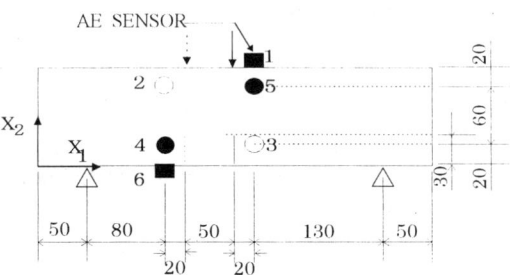

Figure 6 Experimental set-up

be seen in these figures, types of cracks are so complicated and mixed-up that simple explanation can not cover the generating mechanisms of final crack surfaces.

4.2 Shear ratio and stress intensity factor.

In order to classify the cracks, shear ratio was applied. The ratio is derived from the decomposition of eigenvalues of moment tensors (Ohtsu 1995). The crack of which the shear ratio is less than 40% is classified into a tensile crack. In the case that the shear ratio is greater than 40% and less than 60%, the crack is classified as mixed-mode. Over 60% of the shear ratio, cracks are classified into shear cracks. A relationship between the shear ratio and relative stress intensity factors is shown in Fig. 8.

From a crack normal vector determined from the eigenvectors of the moment tensor, relative stress intensity factors K_I^* and K_{II}^* were determined. To clarify the relation between shear ratio and the stress intensity factors, the case of mixed-mode cracks is omitted. From these figures it is obviously found that K_I^* is dominant in an AE event of which the shear ratio is less than 40% and K_{II}^* is dominant in the case that the shear ratio is greater than 60%. Thus, the criterion on crack-type classification in the SiGMA analysis is comparable to the dominant mode of stress intensity factors.

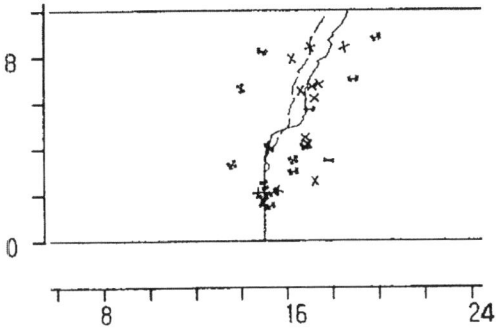

Figure 7(a) Results of SiGMA analysis, (OC type, Concrete specimen).

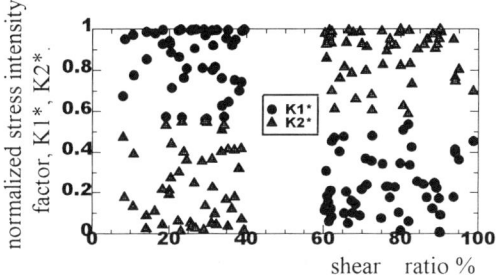

Figure 8(a) Stress intensity factor vs. shear ratio, (OC type, Concrete specimen).

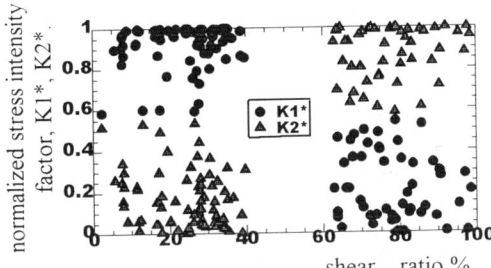

Figure 8(b) Stress intensity factor vs. shear ratio, (CC type, Mortar specimen).

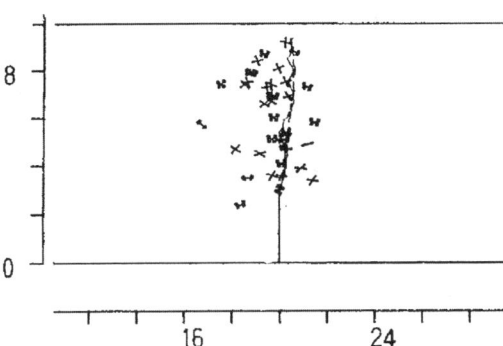

Figure 7(b) Results of SiGMA analysis, (CC type, Mortar specimen).

4.3 Cracking process

To study the process of cracking, the occurrence of AE events vs. relative stress intensity factors K_I^* and K_{II}^* are plotted. Fig. 9 (a) shows the results of concrete specimen of OC type. The horizontal axis corresponds to the loading stage. In the beginning of loading, AE events detected were not successfully analyzed. As a result the number of plotted data are few. At the intermediate stage, intensely data are plotted. Both modes of K_I^* and K_{II}^* dominant are observed so mixed-up as to suggest that the cracking mechanisms are complicated and any single mechanism is not dominant. In the final stage, it is observed that the K_{II}^* mode becomes dominant. In Fig. 9 (b), results of mortar specimen of CC type are plotted. Both mode are dominantly observed in all stages. It implies that both types of crack are generated even under center loading in the center-notched beam, although only tensile cracks are macroscopically observed.

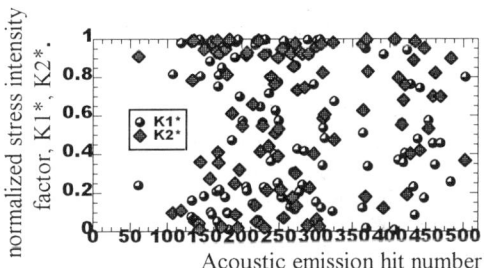

Figure 9(a) Stress intensity factor vs. acoustic, emission hit number (OC type, Concrete specimen).

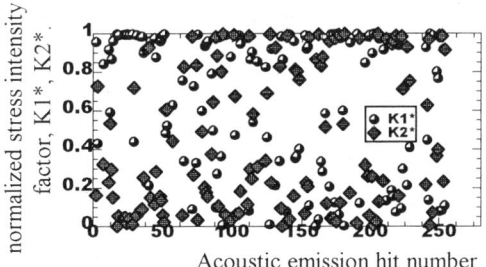

Figure 9(b) Stress intensity factor vs. acoustic, emission hit number (CC type, Mortar specimen).

5 CONCLUSION

This investigation was performed to determine relative stress intensity factors in three-point bending tests of notched concrete and mortar specimens from the moment tensor analysis. The following conclusions are obtained:

1. The procedure to determine K_I^* and K_{II}^* values from the eigenvectors of moment tensor is developed. According to numerical experiments, the ratios of K_I^* and K_{II}^* are varied, depending on the angles between the crack normal vector and crack motion vector.

2. The procedure is applied to the experimental data of notched concrete and mortar beams. Crack orientation and crack types are determined by the SiGMA analysis.

3. The relation between the shear ratio in the SiGMA analysis and the relative stress intensity factors is clarified. It confirm the applicability of the proposed criterion for crack classification in the SiGMA code.

4. The variation of dominant failure mode during the crack propagation is clarified from relative stress intensity factors.

REFERENCES

Carpinteri, A. 1986. Mechanical Damage and Crack Growth in Concrete: Plastic Collapse to Brittle Fracture, pp1-31.

Erdogan, F. & Sih, G. C. 1963. On the Crack Extension in Plates under Plane Loading and Transverse Shear. Journal of Basic Engineering, ASME, Vol.85, pp.519-527.

Kaplan, M. F. 1961. Crack Propagation and the Fracture of Concrete, ACI Journal, Vol.58, No.11.

Kim, K.Y. & Sachse, W. 1984. Characterization of AE Signals from Indentation Cracks in Glass. Progress in Acoustic Emission II, JSNDI, pp.163-172

Ohtsu, M. 1987. Determination of Crack Orientation by AE. Materials Evaluation, ASTM, Vol.45, No.9. pp.1070-1075.

Ohtsu, M. 1995. AE Theory for Moment Tensor Analysis. Research of Non-destructive Evaluation Vol.6, pp.169-184.

Ohtsu, M. 1996. International Workshop sponsored by the Max-Planck-Society on Materials Research with Advanced Acoustic Emission Techniques, Germany 1996.

Simulation of borehole breakout using fracture mechanics models

B. Shen
CSIRO Division of Exploration and Mining, Brisbane, Qld, Australia

X. Tan & C. Li
Department of Civil and Mining Engineering, Luleå University of Technology, Sweden

O. Stephansson
Department of Civil and Environmental Engineering, Royal Institute of Technology, Stockholm, Sweden

ABSTRACT: Borehole breakouts often occur as tensile spalling or shear fracturing. To simulate and explain the borehole breakout phenomena, two linear fracture mechanics approaches are applied, namely a tensile splitting model and a shear fracturing model. Both models predict the typical 'dog-ear' shaped breakout. The width and depth of breakouts are found to depend upon the magnitude and ratio of *in-situ* stresses. The results of modelling agree well with laboratory test results and field observations. Factors controlling the breakout mechanism are discussed.

1 INTRODUCTION

Borehole breakout, i.e. failure of the borehole wall due to stress concentrations, results in an elongation of the borehole cross section in the direction of minimum principal stress. An understanding of the breakout phenomena is important for determining the orientations of *in-situ* stresses. The relation between the magnitude of the *in-situ* stresses and the width and depth of the breakouts is of particular importance for stress measurement.

Observations and theoretical analyses of borehole breakouts indicate that failure of the borehole wall are of two different modes governed by either tensile spalling or shear fracturing (Vardoulakis et al., 1988 and Guenot, 1989). In the case of tensile spalling, the rock breakage starts in the vicinity of a borehole as a result of tensile crack initiation and propagation in the direction of the maximum principal stress. A series of subparallel cracks are formed and the coalescence of these tensile cracks forms a layer which may fall off from the hole wall. This phenomenon is typical for hard crystalline rocks such as granite under compression with no or small lateral confinement (see e.g. Ewy and Cook, 1990a, 1990b; Guenot, 1993; Lee and Haimson, 1993; Martin et al., 1994; Haimson and Lee, 1995). In the case of shear fracturing, shear failure along one or more shear bands extends from the hole wall into the rock. The shear fractures (or shear bands) can cause breakout when they intersect one another. This type of failure is often observed in soft and porous rocks, such as dolomite, limestone and sandstone (Zoback et al., 1985, Guenot, 1989) and even in hard rocks (Haimson and Lee, 1995). Both failure modes can result in 'dog-ear' shaped breakouts.

Theoretical studies have been conducted to understand and predict the two breakout mechanisms. Breakout by shear was assumed to follow a Mohr-Coulomb failure criterion (Zoback et al., 1985). This could explain the wide and shallow breakout sometimes observed in field, but not the formation of sharp-edged breakouts of 'dog-ear' type.

Extensile cracking has been observed in uni- or bi- axial borehole tests in the laboratory. Extensile cracking is attributed to the structural instability of the borehole wall (Vardoulakis et al., 1985). Zheng et al. (1989) used a compressive failure criterion with a numerical method and predicted a 'dog-ear' shaped breakout as a result of gradual failure. The results provided a good representation of the phenomenon, but could not explain the physical mechanism.

In this work, we study the two borehole failure modes by applying two different fracture mechanics models. First, we simulate the extensile breakout by using a splitting fracture model and then the shear induced breakout by applying a shear fracturing model. The growth of extensile cracks and shear fractures are simulated numerically by applying the two fracture models and the 'dog-ear' shaped breakouts are predicted numerically. The relationship between the *in-situ* stresses and the shape of the breakout is also examined.

2 BRIEF DESCRIPTION OF THE FRACTURE MODELS

In this study, the rock mass is considered as a linearly elastic, homogenous and isotropic medium loaded in plane strain. Two fracture models, i.e., the splitting fracture model and the shear fracture model, are applied.

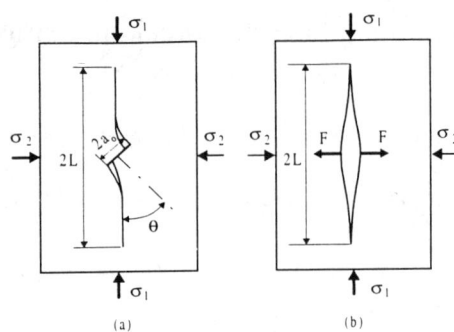

Figure 1. Splitting fracture model: a) failure of a single crack under compression, and b) simplified failure pattern (after Li and Nordlund, 1993).

2.1 *Splitting fracture model*

It is assumed that in the continuous elastic rock medium, there exist many small internal flaws or microcracks. At a certain stress state these microcracks can propagate and develop to become macrocracks.

In the splitting fracture model, wing cracks are initiated at the tips of the pre-existing cracks and propagate in the direction of major compressive stress, see Fig. 1. For simplicity, the propagating crack is treated as a tensile fracture driven by a pair of equivalent wedge forces, F, on the two opposing surfaces of the crack as

$$F = a_o [(\sigma_1 - \sigma_2) f(\theta, \phi) - 2 \sigma_2 \cos \theta \tan \phi] \quad (1)$$

where $f(\theta, \phi) = (1 + \cos 2\theta)(\sin \theta - \cos \theta \tan \phi)$; σ_1, σ_2 = the major and minor principal stresses, where compression is defined as positive; θ = the angle of the normal of the pre-existing crack surface with respect to the direction of σ_1; a_o = half of the pre-existing crack length; ϕ = frictional angle of the pre-existing fracture surface.

For a crack of length 2L subjected to a wedge force F and a lateral stress σ_2 (see Fig. 1b), the stress intensity factor K_I is given by

$$K_I = \frac{F}{\sqrt{\pi L}} - \sigma_2 \sqrt{\pi L} \quad (2)$$

When the wing cracks propagate the stress intensity factor is equal to the fracture toughness K_{IC}. Substituting K_{IC} into Eq. 2 gives the length of propagating crack as

$$L_a = \frac{1}{4\pi} \left[\frac{\sqrt{K_{IC}^2 + 4F\sigma_2} - K_{IC}}{\sigma_2} \right]^2 \quad (3)$$

where L_a = apparent length of the wing crack; K_{IC} = fracture toughness.

The true crack length is obtained by referring to the original length of the splitting crack as

$$L = L_a \frac{L_0}{L_{a0}} \quad (4)$$

where $L_0 = a_0 \sin\theta$, projection of the original crack along the direction of σ_1; a_0 = half length of original crack length; L_{a0} = apparent wing crack length obtained at critical load for initiation of wing crack.

Using these formulas, one can predict crack development for a given stress field and initial crack location. The longest cracks which are also oriented in a favourable direction in relation to the *in-situ* stress state will achieve the greatest propagation. The magnitude of stresses and the stress ratio control the failure pattern. The wing crack development involves complicated failure mechanisms in the microscale. For simplicity we do not look into in detail the process of cracking, only the final crack extension is provided.

2.2 *Shear fracture model*

In nature, rock fractures often initiate and extend in shear, which is not described by the classical mode I fracture criteria. Note that we use the term fracture here for rock discontinuities in macroscale. A modified fracture criterion, F-criterion, has been developed (Shen and Stephansson, 1994), based on the concept of energy release rate criterion (G-criterion). In this criterion not only the energy release associated with tensile fracturing, but also that associated with shear fracturing, influence the failure process. The direction of the critical condition for fracture propagation is determined by:

$$F(\theta)|_{\theta=\theta_0} = \frac{G_I(\theta)}{G_{IC}} + \frac{G_{II}(\theta)}{G_{IIC}} = F_{max} \geq 1 \quad (5)$$

where θ is the direction angle of the fictitious fracture tip to the face of an initial fracture (see Fig. 2); G_I and G_{II} represent the energy release rate by pure tension and pure shear at the fracture tip, respectively. The criterion is capable of predicting both mode I and mode II fracturing. The fracture propagation is simulated numerically by a DDM (Displacement Discontinuity Method) program implemented with the F-criterion (Shen, 1993).

The DDM for crack initiation and propagation
The DDM, one of the three boundary element techniques, is a very convenient tool for representing fractures. In this method a relative displacement between the two opposite surfaces of the fracture is allowed (Crouch, 1976). The solution of the system is very efficient in comparison to finite element method.

The displacement discontinuity, D_i, is defined as the difference in the displacements (u_i) between the two sides of a fracture element (Fig. 2)

$$\begin{aligned} D_s &= u_s^- - u_s^+ \\ D_n &= u_n^- - u_n^+ \end{aligned} \quad (6)$$

where s, n represent shear and normal directions respectively and $+$, $-$ signs denote the upper and lower surfaces respectively. A system of equations are constructed for D_i (i=s,n) with specified boundary conditions (Crouch, 1976) and the displacements and stresses can be calculated by solving the system of equations

$$\sigma_s^i = \sum_j \left(A_{ss}^{ij} D_s^j + A_{sn}^{ij} D_n^j \right)$$
$$\sigma_n^i = \sum_j \left(A_{ns}^{ij} D_s^j + A_{nn}^{ij} D_n^j \right) \quad (7)$$

where A_{ss}^{ij}, etc., are the boundary influence coefficients determined by the elastic properties of the materials and the element geometry. The stresses at the fracture elements meet one of the following conditions

i) $\sigma_s^i = \sigma_n^i = 0$ (open crack)

ii) $\sigma_s^i = K_s D_s^i$
$\sigma_n^i = K_n D_n^i$ (closed crack)

iii) $|\sigma_s^i| = \sigma_n^i \tan\phi$
$\sigma_n^i = K_n D_n^i$ (sliding crack)

where K_s, K_n are the fracture shear and normal stiffness, and ϕ is friction angle of rock.

The energy release rate used in Eq. 5 is calculated numerically by introducing a small crack tip, Δa, and is given by

$$G = -\frac{\Pi(a+\Delta a) - \Pi(a)}{\Delta a} \quad (8)$$

where Π is the system potential energy expressed as

$$\Pi(a) = -\frac{1}{2}\sum_{i=1}^{m_1} a^i (\sigma_s^i D_s^i + \sigma_n^i D_n^i) - \frac{1}{2}\sum_{i=m_1+1}^{m_1+m_2} a^i (\sigma_s^i u_s^i + \sigma_n^i u_n^i) \quad (9)$$

with m_1, m_2 = total numbers of fracture elements and the geometry boundary elements, respectively; a^i = length of the ith element.

3 BOREHOLE AND MODEL PARAMETERS

In this study, a borehole is assumed with a diameter a of 10 cm. The rock properties and model parameters used in the two models are listed in Table 1. They represent typical properties of hard rocks.

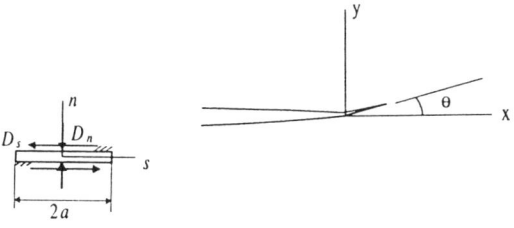

Figure 2. The DDM element and fracture model.

Table 1. Rock and model parameters.

Young's modulus, E (GPa)	60
Poisson's ratio, ν	0.25
Hole diameter (m)	0.1
Splitting fracture model:	
Fracture toughness, K_{IC} (MPa m$^{1/2}$)	1.0
Initial half crack length, a_0 (mm)	4
Frictional angle of existing cracks, ϕ (degree)	30
Shear fracture model:	
Critical energy release rates, G_{IC}, G_{IIC} (J/m^2)	17, 1700
Crack shear and normal stiffness, K_s, K_n (MPa/m)	10^{15}
Frictional angle of new fractures, ϕ (degree)	40

4 SIMULATION OF BOREHOLE BREAKOUT

4.1 *Simulation of splitting induced borehole breakout*

In the simulation of splitting induced breakouts, one quarter of the borehole and the surrounding rock is modelled due to symmetry. It is assumed that a certain distribution of original microcracks exists in the rock mass. For simplicity the pre-existing cracks are assumed to be uniformly distributed in the vicinity of the borehole. The crack centre is at the grid points shown in Fig. 3. The development of the cracks, which follow an extensile pattern and propagate in the direction of the principal compressive stress, will cause crack coalescence and hence cause spalling and hole breakout. The original crack oriented at an angle $\theta = 60$ degrees (see Fig.1) to σ_1 is considered as the most favourable initial crack, where maximum shearing exists on the crack surface.

The simulation was carried out with the following steps: 1) specify a far field state of stress; 2) solve for the local principal stresses, σ_1 and σ_2, at specified grid points around the borehole using a boundary element program; 3) examine if the wing crack can form from the original cracks using Eqs. 1 to 4.

The spalling or degradation of material from the borehole wall occurs when the splitting cracks

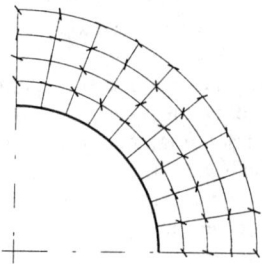

Figure 3. Arrangement of nodes deposited with original cracks as candidates for extensile cracking.

extend and coalesce. To simulate the spalling phenomenon we assume that spalling occurs when the wing crack length reaches a critical length L_c. If the density of the pre-existing microcracks is known, the critical length of wing cracks for spalling will be roughly equal to the average distance between cracks, which of course depends on the rock properties. In this study, L_c is chosen to be 3 mm.

The spalling occurs by gradual degradation of material, whereby the borehole geometry and hence the stresses are altered. This may influence the development of extensile cracking and the shape of breakouts. Once spalling is established, the failed part of the borehole wall is removed and the new hole geometry is then used to calculate whether the spalling progresses or stops. The spalling gradually alters the hole contour to reach the final stable state, and often gives a dog-ear shaped breakout.

Patterns of extensile cracking around a borehole
The results with stress ratio of the maximum horizontal principal stress to the minimum, $\sigma_H/\sigma_h = 3$ and $\sigma_H = 15$ MPa are shown in Fig. 4a. The wing cracks are drawn as straight lines for convenience. The wing cracks are initiated in a location close to the hole wall. The crack length varies around the hole wall due to different stresses at the various locations. The cracks are longer close to the hole wall and shorter farther into the wall. When a higher stress ratio is applied in the far field, say, $\sigma_H/\sigma_h = 4$ for the same σ_h magnitude, the cracked zone extends wider and deeper (see Fig. 4b). The cracks close to the wall may first coalescence and the rock chips spall off.

Shape of the hole breakout
With a stress ratio $\sigma_H/\sigma_h = 4$ ($\sigma_H = 20$ MPa), the gradual change of hole breakout is simulated. The

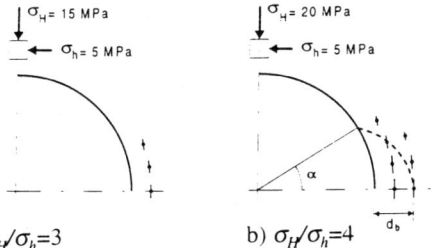

a) $\sigma_H/\sigma_h=3$ b) $\sigma_H/\sigma_h=4$

Figure 4. Extension of cracks under different stress ratios.

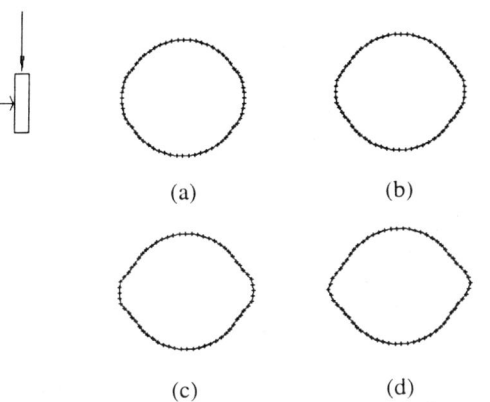

Figure 5. Gradual evolution of hole wall for stress ratio $\sigma_H/\sigma_h=4$ ($\sigma_H=20$ MPa). (a) Commencement of spalling; (b) and (c) further development of spalling; (d) final "dog-ear" shape.

evolution and the final stable "dog-ear" break-out shape are illustrated in Fig. 5. The gradual degradation of the material leads to a realistic contour of hole breakout.

Borehole breakout with further loading

With the *in-situ* stress σ_H increasing from 20 MPa to 22 MPa, the already existing 'dog-ear' shaped breakout extends further. The depth of the breakout is increased from 0.2 to 0.6×the borehole radius, but the angle of breakout, α, does not change (Fig. 6).

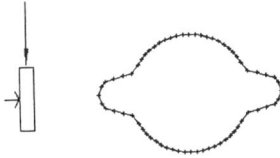

Figure 6. Change of hole wall contour with loading from $\sigma_H=20$ to 22 MPa.

The effect of in-situ stress ratio on hole breakout

Given an *in-situ* stress ratio $\sigma_H/\sigma_h = 5$ for the same σ_h value, the borehole breakout geometry by gradual degradation is calculated (Fig. 7). Comparing Figs. 5 to 7, we find that with a higher stress ratio, the breakout becomes wider on the hole wall and extends deeper into the wall. The former has a breakout-angle/depth-ratio 37°/0.2 and the latter 44°/0.7.

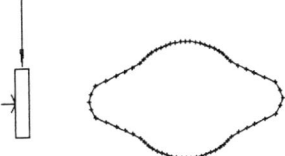

Figure 7. Borehole breakout at $\sigma_H/\sigma_h=5$ ($\sigma_H=25$ MPa).

4.2 Simulation of shear induced borehole breakout

In principle, borehole breakout can be generated by two different mechanisms: spalling and shear failure. The DDM code discussed in section 2.2 is used here to simulate borehole breakout due to shear failure. The mechanical properties of the rock are listed in Table 1.

Initial cracks and crack angle

Short cracks are created by a drilling bit during drilling. In the DDM simulation, the drilling induced cracks are treated as pre-existing cracks and it is investigated whether they propagate and form a breakout under different stress states. A borehole with a diameter of 10 cm is simulated. The length of the pre-existing crack at the borehole wall is assumed to be 1/20 of the hole diameter. The pre-existing cracks often have random orientations, but only those oriented in the most favourable direction can propagate and form breakouts. An initial study is conducted to look into the effect of crack angle (β) relative to the borehole wall, see Fig. 8a, as a function of the magnitude of stress when the crack starts to propagate. The results shown in Fig. 9 are for one single crack which is located at the wall with an arc angle $\alpha=20°$ (see Fig. 8a for the definition of α). The stress ratio σ_H/σ_h is 2.0. Four different crack angles β, ranging from 30° to 40°, are investigated. The results presented in Fig. 9 show that when the crack angle β is about 30°, the magnitude of stress

σ_H required to propagate the crack is the lowest. Because the accuracy of the DDM results drops considerably when the crack angle is less than 30° (the centre of a crack element is too close to the centre of a borehole element), no crack angle less than 30° is investigated. However, as the rock at the borehole wall is under almost uniaxial loading condition, shear failure is expected to occur along a plane of about 30° from the principle stress direction (see Fig. 8b). The most favourable crack angle for crack propagation, therefore, should be about 30°. This angle should not change significantly as the stress ratio σ_H/σ_h changes, because the almost uniaxial stress condition in the immediate borehole wall is unchanged.

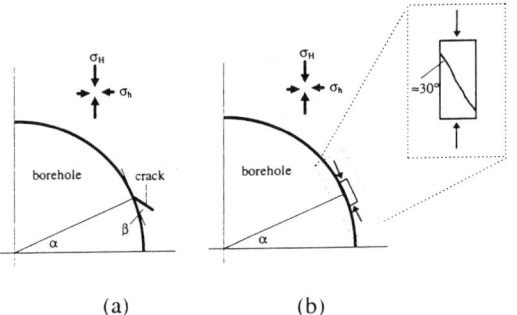

(a) (b)

Figure 8. Initial condition for generation of borehole breakout. (a) A single crack at the borehole wall which may propagate and form a breakout. (b) The uniaxial loading condition at the borehole wall can lead to shear fracturing in a direction about 30° from the borehole wall.

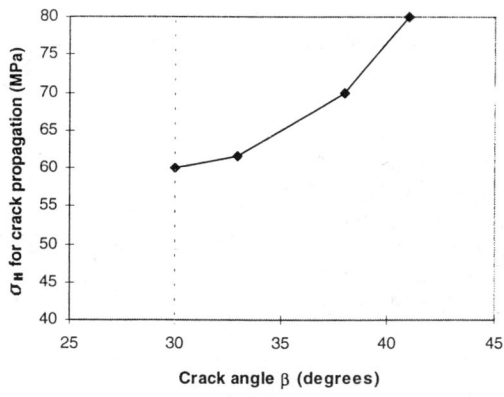

Figure 9. Effect of the initial crack angle (β) on the magnitude of maximum horizontal stresses (σ_H) at which the crack starts to propagate. Results are for stress ratio of $\sigma_H/\sigma_h = 2$.

Shape of borehole breakout

To simulate borehole breakout due to shear failure, three short pre-existing cracks (length = 1/20 of hole diameter) on each of the four quarters of borehole wall are considered, all of them having a crack angle (β) of 30°, i.e. the most favourable angle of crack propagation. The three cracks are located in different locations at arc angle α = 20°, 30° and 40°, respectively. Three different stress ratios are used, σ_H/σ_h = 4.0, 2.0 and 1.5.

During the DDM simulation, *in-situ* stresses with a given ratio are applied to the model with the twelve cracks. The code then calculates whether any of these twelve cracks (here only three due to symmetry) propagate. If no crack propagation is found, the magnitude of the applied stresses is increased automatically by 5% in each step until crack propagation initiates. The stress ratio is kept constant as the magnitude of the applied *in-situ* stress increases. When crack propagation is detected for any of the pre-existing cracks at a certain stress level, new elements will be added to the pre-existing crack tip(s) in the predicted direction of crack growth. This process is repeated until no further crack propagation occurs. In this way, the DDM code predicts both the critical load for borehole breakout and the breakout shape.

(a) Stress ratio $\sigma_H/\sigma_h = 4.0$

With this relatively high stress ratio, the cracks at the arc angle of $\alpha=20°$ are found to propagate when the maximum stress reaches $\sigma_H = 60$ MPa, while the pre-existing cracks at the arc angles of $\alpha=30°$ and 40° are stable. The crack propagation continues at the same stress level and follows a curved path to finally form a small breakout, see Fig. 10. The stress distribution in the vicinity of the hole and the breakout is shown in Fig. 11.

At higher stress levels, i.e., $\sigma_H = 73$MPa and 95MPa, respectively, the pre-existing cracks at the arc angles of 30° and 40°, respectively, start to

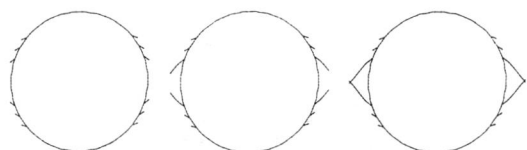

Figure 10. Formation of borehole breakout due to shear fracture propagation ($\sigma_H/\sigma_h = 4.0$, $\sigma_H = 60$MPa, $\alpha = 20°$, $d_b \approx 0.25 \times$ borehole radius).

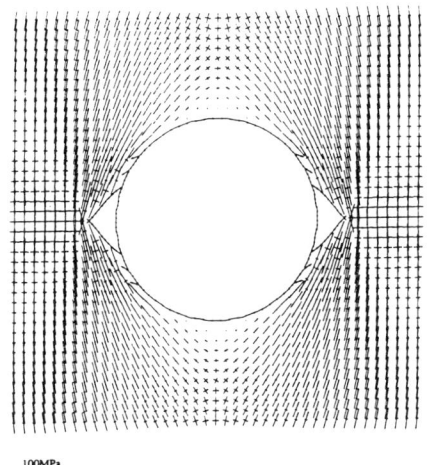

Figure 11. Stress distribution in the vicinity of the borehole and its breakout ($\sigma_H/\sigma_h = 4.0$, $\sigma_H = 60$MPa).

propagate as well. They form wider and deeper breakouts.

(b) Stress ratio $\sigma_H/\sigma_h = 2.0$

When the maximum stress reaches $\sigma_H = 70$MPa, crack propagation starts from the inner cracks ($\alpha=20°$), and a small breakout similar to that shown in Fig. 10 is formed. When the stress level is $\sigma_H = 78$MPa, the middle cracks ($\alpha=30°$) start to propagate and form a wider and deeper breakout, see Fig. 12. The stress level for the outer-most cracks ($\alpha=40°$) to propagate is $\sigma_H=91$MPa.

(c) Stress ratio $\sigma_H/\sigma_h = 1.5$

The propagation of the pre-existing cracks at the three arc angles $\alpha=20°, 30°$ and $40°$ starts when the applied maximum stress is $\sigma_H = 75$MPa, 82MPa and 86MPa, respectively. Fig. 13 shows the case where all the pre-existing cracks propagate when the

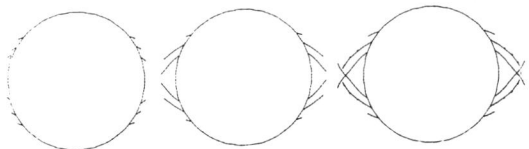

Figure 12. Formation of borehole breakout due to shear fracture propagation ($\sigma_H/\sigma_h = 2.0$, $\sigma_H = 78$MPa, $\alpha = 30°$, $d_b \approx 0.35\times$borehole radius).

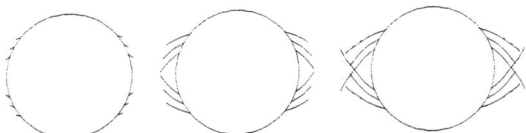

Figure 13. Formation of borehole breakout due to shear fracture propagation ($\sigma_H/\sigma_h = 1.5$, $\sigma_H = 86$MPa, $\alpha = 40°$, $d_b \approx 0.5\times$borehole radius. The solid lines with dots are the DDM results. The broken lines are idealised borders of the breakout).

applied stress $\sigma_H = 86$MPa. The final breakout is wide (angle $\alpha=40°$) and extends to about 50% of the hole radius into the wall. In the case where only the inner and middle cracks propagate at slightly lower stress, $\sigma_H = 75$MPa and 82MPa respectively, the shapes of the breakout are similar to those shown in Figs. 10 and 12, respectively. The stress ratio seems not to change the path of the propagation of shear fractures.

Effect of stress ratio on borehole breakout

The numerical results for breakout angle and depth are plotted in Fig. 14 against the magnitude of maximum stress σ_H for the three stress ratios ($\sigma_H/\sigma_h = 4.0, 2.0$ and 1.5). The following trends can be observed: (1) As the maximum stress increases, the width (arc angle α) and depth of the breakout increase for all three *in-situ* stress ratios. (2) In most

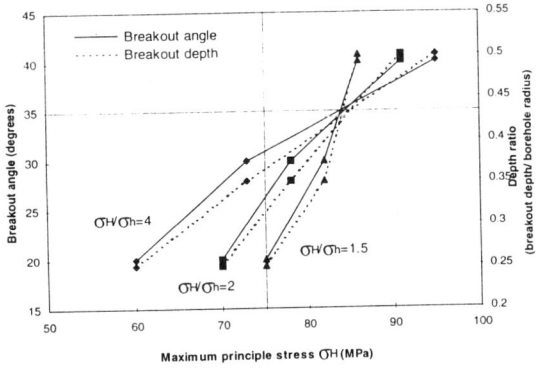

Figure 14. Variation of borehole breakout angle and depth ratio (breakout depth/borehole radius) with the magnitude of the maximum principle stress for three different stress ratios, DDM modelling results.

cases, for a given magnitude of the maximum stress, higher stress ratio results in wider and deeper breakouts. For instance, when the maximum stress is $\sigma_H=75$MPa, the breakout-angle / depth-ratio for the three stress ratios (σ_H/σ_h = 4.0, 2.0 and 1.5) are approximately 31°/0.37, 27°/0.31 and 20°/0.25. However, when the breakout-angle / depth-ratio reaches about 35°/0.43, higher stress ratio prevents extension of the breakouts. This can be understood as the highly mismatched stresses are likely to cause high stresses in some localised regions and low stress in other regions.

Breakout formed by randomly distributed initial cracks

In order to simulate a more realistic situation, a borehole with 36 random cracks (symmetric) is simulated using the DDM code for shear fracturing, see Fig. 15. The cracks all have a length of 1/20 of the hole diameter. The crack angle (α, see Fig. 8a) of each crack is generated randomly, varying from 25° to 155°. The stress ratio used for the randomly oriented cracks is σ_H/σ_h = 2.0.

Among the nine randomly oriented pre-existing cracks in each quarter of the borehole wall, the one with crack angle $\alpha \approx 40°$ and at the arc angle $\beta=40°$ is found to propagate at the stress $\sigma_H=73$ MPa. At the same stress level, this crack propagation is unstable and finally a deep and wide breakout is formed. The rest of the pre-existing cracks are stable, some experiencing only a small propagation and then stopping.

The results indicate that, among all the pre-existing cracks created by drilling, only those at the right location with a favourable orientation can propagate and form breakouts. The path of fracture propagation always follows the direction of least shear resistance, and therefore, the shape of the breakout is not much affected by the position and orientation of the pre-existing cracks.

5 DISCUSSION

The two fracture models are used to describe two mechanisms of stress induced borehole failure. The two models are valid for elastic material and give a fairly good simulation of the fracture phenomena during borehole breakouts. In the splitting model the stresses in the borehole wall are governed by the continuous, elastic medium without pre-existing cracks. The gradual degradation of rock on borehole wall is a way to obtain more realistic shape of hole breakout. In the shear fracturing simulation using DDM, the stresses in the borehole wall are changing with the development of shear fractures, which directly gives the stress release between the shear fractures and thus delineates the contour of the breakout.

In the simulation of extensile cracking, we used a network of grid points for the original cracks with favourable directions in the borehole wall and assumed that spalling will occur when the length of a tensile crack reaches a critical length L_c. L_c is associated with the crack density. To simulate real rock conditions, the number of grid points should be equal to the number of microcracks if the microcracks have some distribution in size and orientation.

The results of the simulations show that the breakout formed by the two mechanisms can have different shapes. Breakouts formed by extensile cracks are often shallow and have a smooth shape, while shear induced breakouts can be deep and often have sharp ends. The *in-situ* stress ratio is found to influence the breakout shape for spalling but not for shearing. A recent laboratory study by Haimson and Lee (1995) revealed distinct and sharp breakouts in specimens of Lac du Bonnet granite. The size of the breakout increases with σ_H and the shape of the breakout remains similar, independent of the state of the far-field stresses. The laboratory test results agree well with our numerical results predicted by

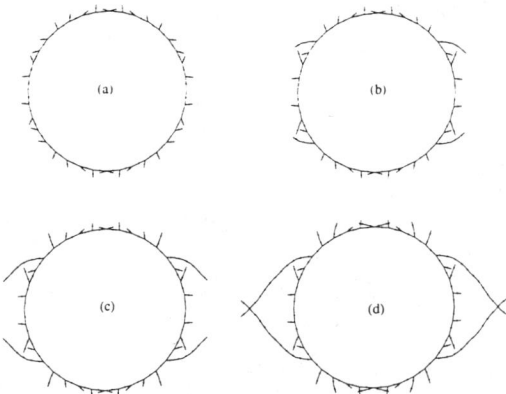

Figure 15. Formation of borehole breakout due to shear fracture propagation with randomly oriented initial cracks (σ_H/σ_h = 2.0, σ_H = 73MPa, α = 40°, $d_b \approx 0.75\times$borehole radius).

the shear fracturing model. The agreement suggests that shear fracturing is likely to be a common phenomenon for both microscale and macroscale failure mechanisms in hard rocks.

Obviously, borehole breakout can form either as tensile spalling or shear fracturing. Discussions are still ongoing about what controls the mechanism of a breakout - material behaviour, stress state or others? It is believed that, besides stress ratio, material behaviour is one of the most important factors to control the mechanism of borehole breakouts. Rocks can fail both in tension and shear. It is common knowledge that, in laboratory uniaxial tests, some rocks fail in splitting whereas some fail in shear. The failure mode in uniaxial testing is likely to decide the mechanism of borehole breakout in the same type of rock, since the rock in the wall of the borehole is under an almost uniaxial stress state (fluid pressure is not considered here).

It has been argued that the mode of breakout is associated with the ratio of compressive strength to tensile strength, σ_c/σ_t, and that shear fracturing occurs more easily in porous material (Vandoulakis et al., 1988; Guenot, 1989, Shen, 1993). Extensile cracking is inhibited under confined conditions (Horii and Nemat-Nasser, 1985; Li, 1993). The microstructure of rocks is often different, some rocks having densely packed particles or minerals and some having relatively loosely cemented particles. The size and distribution of microcracks or voids inside the rock play an important role in the formation of the failure and hence the breakout formation. Large but loose microcracks are more likely to exhibit splitting failure as they propagate in tension in the direction of maximum principle stress; small but dense microcracks (voids) tend to exhibit shear failure more easily as they coalesce in the direction of maximum shearing. This may explain why more shear-induced breakouts were observed in rock types such as sandstone (Rawlings et al, 1993; Kutter and Rehse, 1996).

6 CONCLUSIONS

The splitting model and shear fracturing model can be used to describe the borehole extensile cracking and shear fracturing of borehole wall, respectively. Both models predict breakouts of 'dog-ear' shape, whilst a more distinct and sharp breakout is found for the shear fracturing. Good agreement is obtained between numerical simulation and laboratory observations for the two failure modes.

Both simulations indicate that the width of borehole breakout varies with the magnitude of *in-situ* stresses. The breakout depth and the breakout angle increase with loading. A larger stress ratio makes more distinct and sharper breakouts when spalling is the dominating mechanism.

ACKNOWLEDGMENTS

B. Shen wishes to thank the Royal Institute of Technology (Sweden) for its financial support of this study.

REFERENCES

Crouch, S.L. 1976. Solution of plane elasticity problems by the Displacement Discontinuity Method, *Int. J. Num. Methods Engng.* 10: 301-343.

Ewy, R.T. & Cook, N.G.W. 1990a. Deformation and failure around cylindrical openings in rock—I. Observations and analysis of deformations. *Int. J. Rock Mech. Min. Sci. & Geomech. Abstr.* 27: 387-407.

Ewy, R.T. & Cook, N.G.W., 1990b. Deformation and failure around cylindrical openings in rock —II. Initiation, growth and interaction of fractures. *Int. J. Rock Mech. Min. Sci. & Geomech. Abstr.* 27: 409-427.

Guenot, A. 1989. Borehole breakouts and stress fields. *Int. J. Rock Mech. Min. Sci. & Geomech. Abstr.* 26: 185-195.

Haimson, B.C. & Song, I. 1993. Laboratory study of borehole breakouts in Cordova Cream: a case of shear failure mechanism. *Int. J. Rock Mech. Min. Sci. & Geomech. Abstr.* 30: 1047-1056.

Haimson, B.C. & Lee, M.Y. 1995. Estimating *in-situ* stress conditions from borehole breakouts and core disking—experimental results in granite. *Int. Workshop on Rock Stress Measurement at Great Depth.* Sept. 30, Tokyo, Japan, 19-24.

Horii, H. & Nemat-Nasser, S. 1985. Compression induced microcrack growth in brittle solids: axial splitting and shear failure. *J. Geophy. Res.* 90(B4): 3105-3125.

Lee, M.Y. and Haimson, B.C. 1993. Laboratory study of borehole breakouts in Lac du Bonnet granite: a case of extensile failure mechanism, *Int. J. Rock Mech. Min. Sci. & Geomech. Abstr.* 30: 1039-1045.

Li, C. & Nordlund, E. 1993. Deformation of brittle rocks under compression —with particular reference to micro cracks. *Mech. of Mater.* 15: 223-239.

Li, C. 1995. Micromechanics modelling for stress-strain behaviour of brittle rocks. *Int. J. for Num. & Anal. Meth. in Geomech.* 19:331-344.

Kutter, H.K. & Rehse, H. 1996. Laboratory investigation of factor affecting borehole breakouts. *Eurock'96, Barla (ed.),* Balkema, Rotterdam, 751-758.

Martin, C.D., Martino, J.B. & Dzik, E.J. 1994. Comparison of borehole breakouts from laboratory and field tests. *Eurock'94: SPE/ISBM Int. Conf. Rock Mech. in Petrol. Engng.* Delft, Netherlands, Aug. 29-31. Balkema, Rotterdam, 183-190.

Rawlings, C.G., Barton, N.R., Bandis, Addis, M.A. & Gutierrez, M.S. 1993. Laboratory and numerical discontinuum modelling of wellbore stability. *J. Pet. Technol.*, 45: 1086-1092.

Shen, B., 1993. *Mechanics of Fractures and Intervening Bridges in Hard Rocks.* Ph.D. Thesis, Royal Institute of Technology, Stockholm, Sweden.

Shen, B. & Stephansson O. 1993. Numerical analysis of Mode I and Mode II propagation of rock fractures. *Int. J. Rock Mech. Min. Sci. & Geomech. Abstr.* 30: 861-867.

Shen, B. & Stephansson O. 1994. Modification of the G-criterion for crack propagation subjected to compression. *Engng. Fract. Mech.* 47(2): 177-189.

Vardoulakis J., Sulem, J. & Guenot, A. 1988. Borehole instabilities as bifurcation phenomena. *Int. J. Rock Mech. Min. Sci. & Geomech. Abstr.* 25: 159-170.

Zheng, Z., Kemeny, J. & Cook, N.G.W. 1989. Analysis of borehole breakouts. *J. Geophy. Res.*, 94(B6): 7171-7182.

Zoback M.D., Mooss, D., Mastin, L. & Anderson R. 1985. Wellbore breakout and in situ stress. *J. Geophys. Res.* 90(B7): 5523-5530.

In-situ stresses in the North Sea from careful analysis of breakouts and fracturing data

A.S. Batchelor & K.A. Kwakwa
GeoScience Limited, Falmouth, UK

ABSTRACT: Stress assessments have been made by the authors for several fields in the North Sea for projects involving borehole stability, sand production and hydraulic fracturing performance. This paper presents stress orientation plots showing a strong correlation with the strike of major structural features mapped in the area. Composite plots of leakoff pressures are presented with over 100 data points from 500 m to 4000 m TVD and they show that the stress regime follows predictable patterns. An example of a hydraulic fracturing stress measurement using both breakout and fracturing pressure data is described for a location adjacent to a major fault. It is concluded that stresses in the North Sea are strongly anisotropic and that both the magnitudes and the orientation are controlled by structural features. It is argued that these results imply that the sedimentary formations are coupled closely to the basement and that the stresses are being transferred throughout the vertical section.

1 INTRODUCTION

The authors have undertaken various engineering design projects in the North Sea during the last ten years and most of the work has involved the assessment of the local in-situ stress field. The orientation and leakoff data from several fields are presented in this paper together with an example using both wellbore breakout and hydraulic fracturing data from a location just onshore in Scotland. The purpose of the paper is to show that the stress data obtained by the authors has proven reliable where it has been used for engineering purposes and it does correlate with the major structural features in the area.

2 ORIENTATION OF THE STRESSES

Figure 1 shows the base map of Klein and Barr (1986), with the data obtained by the authors superimposed. The authors' data is shown with a slightly larger symbol and a capital letter alongside. Some of these data have been fully reported in other papers but we have chosen not to distinguish between data sets. At first glance, there appears to be significant nonsystematic variation in direction, eg see points A, G and C. However, if the major structural features in the central area are superimposed, see Figure 2, a correlation with the strike direction of the faults is clear. Sites A and D also correlate with the main trend of the Central Graben.

2.1 *Example Stress Orientation at Station K*

Two holes to a maximum depth of 1250 m were drilled onshore with extensive testing and wireline logging. Visible breakout was seen on a borehole televiewer image. These features extended over more than 300 m of one hole and over a more limited distance in the other. A clear NW-SE breakout direction was evident from the shapes of the holes. The full description with figures and analysis was presented by Batchelor et al, 1995. The strict criteria used for the breakout analysis were those proposed by Plumb and Hickman (1985) and we have shown them to be reliable throughout this work.

A note of caution is necessary on all forms of oriented wireline log information. The authors have found that it is essential to make very considerable efforts to verify the orientation data by independent means. Typically this has involved comparison with hole survey data, locally known dip of key stratigraphic units and cross checking between orientation cartridges. Scanner logs, such as a televiewer, have been generally reoriented during processing to match data from the fixed pad tools. The

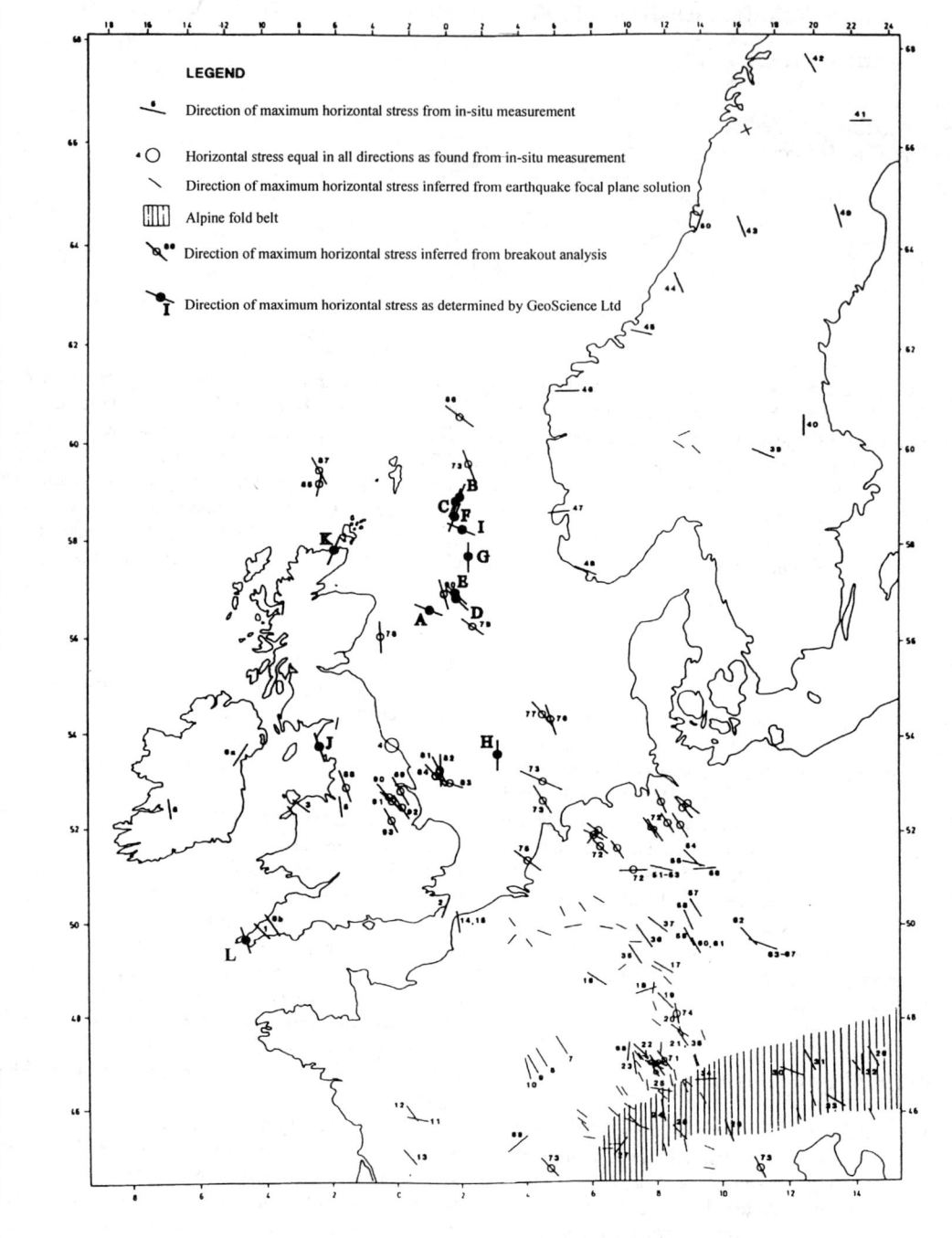

Figure 1　Orientation of maximum horizontal principal stress within Western Europe (Klein and Barr 1986), updated by GeoScience Ltd 1997

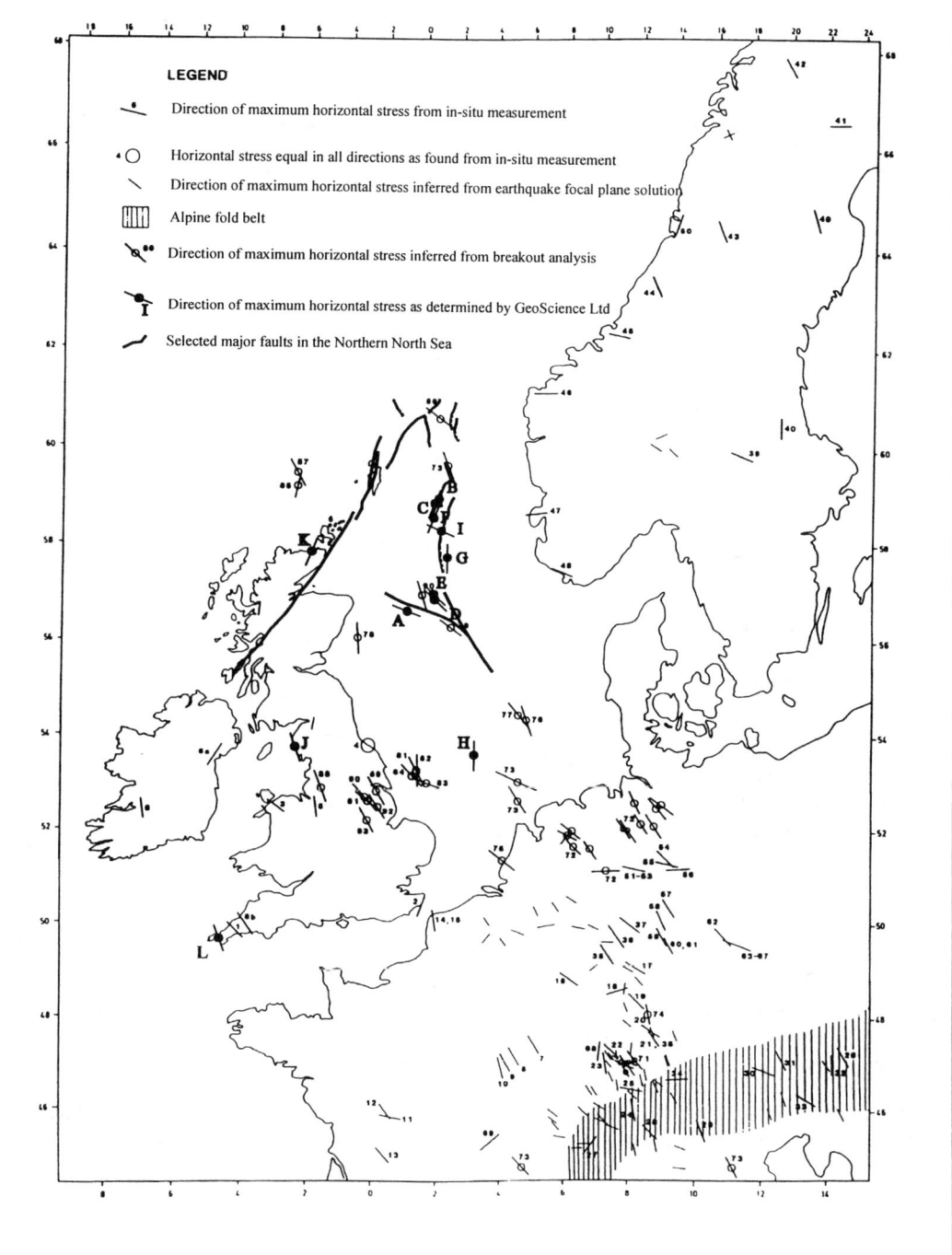

Figure 2 Orientation of maximum horizontal principal stress and major faults within Western Europe (Klein and Barr 1986), updated by GeoScience Ltd 1997

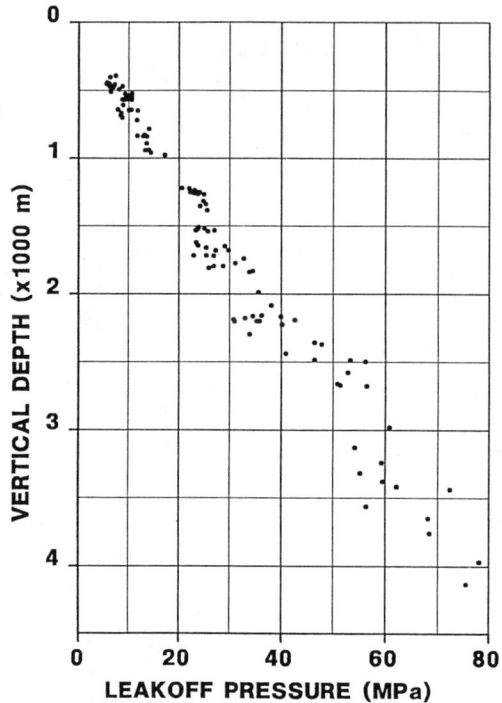

Figure 3 Leakoff data collected and analysed by GeoScience, 1985 to 1997

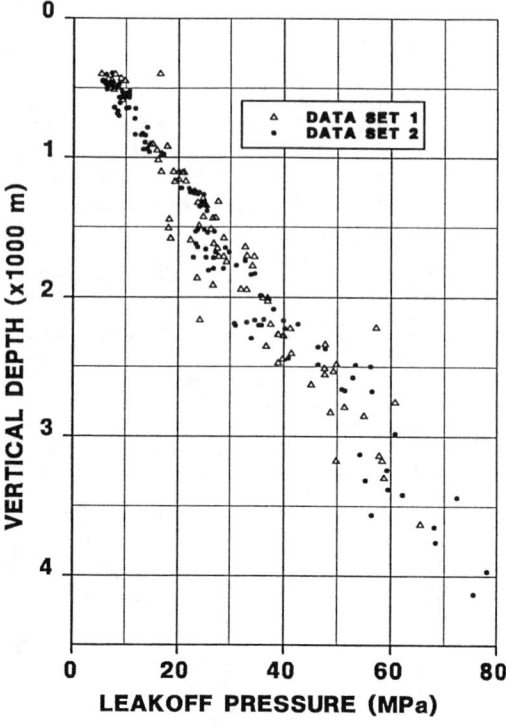

DATA 1 after Breckles and van Eekelen, 1982
DATA 2 after GeoScience Ltd

Figure 4 Leakoff data collected and analysed by GeoScience, 1985 to 1997, compared with data from Breckels and van Eekelen, 1982

intrinsically higher accuracy of the pad tools eliminates some of the orientation problems with the scanners.

It is believed that the extensive breakout had been caused when a partially inflated packer was tripped from the hole after testing. The effective pressure in the tight formation dropped by approximately 2.6 MPa (400 psi) (see later section) during this trip.

The wells were also pressurized to the point of fracturing prior to logging and these induced tensile fractures should be normal to the breakout direction if the above interpretation is correct. Careful examination showed that the fractures are indeed normal to the breakout. These patterns were identical in both holes and the direction of maximum principal stress was clearly 44° -> 224° in azimuth with an error of ±15°.

3 STRESS MAGNITUDES

Stress magnitudes have been estimated by the authors using both the breakout and induced tensile fractures to constrain the values. One of the key data items is reliable leakoff data and Figure 3 shows leakoff data values derived by the authors from 500 m to 4000 m TVD. A clear trend with some scatter is evident.

This data has been compared with that published by Breckels and van Eekelen (1982), see Figure 4, and the agreement is obvious. Breckels and van Eekelen estimated that the leakoff pressures were some 11% greater on average than the estimated least principal stress.

3.1 Example of Least Principal Stress Magnitudes at Station K

Batchelor et al, 1995 (op cit) presented a detailed analysis of the stress derivations at Station K. The methods we have used to derive stress magnitudes use the following steps:

(i) Derive the best estimates of the least horizontal stress from fracturing and injection data and define the range of uncertainty.

(ii) Compute a compatible range of maximum

Table 1 : Basic Measurement Data After Hydrofracturing

Observations to Match	MPa	psi	ppg
Peak Fracture Pressure	27.76	4025	19.6
Fracture Opening Pressure	23.01	337	16.3
Pore Pressure	12.00	1741	8.48
Least Well Pressure	9.21	1336	6.5
Rock Properties	Sc = 86.2 MPa (12500 psi) Im = 18 Is = 1 Tc = 4.77 MPa (692 psi)		

Table 2 : Estimates of Stress Magnitude

Results, at a depth of 1225 m		
	MPa	Ratio to Vertical Stress
Least Horizontal Stress	23.0	.74
Vertical Stress	31.3	
Maximum Horizontal Stress	34.0	1.09

horizontal stress values that match the observation of fracturing pressure, the existence of breakout, the inclination and direction of the well.

This approach is iterative and time consuming but does lead to reliable estimates of most probable values and their associated uncertainty.

In the case of Station K, Table 1 shows a summary of all the observed data that was available to constrain the stress values. The authors' estimated values are shown in Table 2. It should be noted that the ratio between the maximum and least stresses is 1.48 to 1 in total stress terms but 2 to 1 in effective stress terms.

The overall shape of the pressure breakdown curve is not uncommon for this area of the North Sea with pressures rising substantially after leakoff. On some occasions pressures as high as the inferred maximum principal stress have been seen. The authors believe that these shapes are due to the fact that the fracturing pressures are low because of the anisotropic nature of the in-situ stresses. The authors would welcome alternative interpretations of the observations.

4 COMMENT

Borgerud and Svare (1995), Dart et al (1995) and Fejerskov et al (1995) have all presented detailed analyses of stress direction and some magnitudes in the northern North sea and Barents Sea areas. Each paper makes reference to the influence of the major tectonic features and the general correlation of the direction of maximum principal stress and the strike direction of the structures.

We believe that the data show that the influence of major tectonic features in the North Sea (and elsewhere near the U.K., Morecambe Bay, Western Approaches) may dominate and control the stress orientation and magnitude.

5 CONCLUSIONS

The authors believe that their data shows:

- The stress regime in the North Sea is strongly anisotropic in the areas that they examined.

- There is strong evidence of correlation in the direction of the maximum in-situ stress and major fault structures known in the North Sea.

- The correlation with these major features can be taken to show that there is significant coupling between the basement and the overlying sediments.

- All of the authors' data has been tested in demanding engineering applications after the assessments have been made and has been found to have supported reliable predictions of performance. While this cannot be taken as proof that the data are correct, it does add confidence to the values presented.

The authors hope that further data of this type will be released for general publication in the fullness of time.

ACKNOWLEDGEMENTS

None of this data would be available but for the support of various clients of GeoScience, their support is acknowledged.

The authors acknowledge their colleagues at GeoScience for encouragement and constructive criticism on this topic. The views expressed in this paper are entirely those of the authors and are not the views of any other entity.

REFERENCES

Batchelor, A.S., Kwakwa, K.A., Pearson, R.A.P., Lanyon, G.W.L. and Thin, I.G.T. 1995. Stresses in the North Sea. Proc. Workshop on Rock Stresses in the North Sea, Trondheim, Norway, 13-14 Feb., pub. Sintef, Rock and Mineral Engineering, N-7034, Trondheim, Norway.

Borgerud, L. and Svare, E. 1995. In-situ stress field on the Norwegian Margin, 62°-67° north. Proc. Workshop on Rock Stresses in the North Sea, Trondheim, Norway, 13-14 Feb., pub. Sintef, Rock and Mineral Engineering, N-7034, Trondheim, Norway, pp. 165-178.

Breckels, I.M. and van Eekelen, H.A.M. 1982. Relationship between horizontal stress and depth in sedimentary basins. JPT, September, pp 2191-2199.

Dart, C., Inderhaug, O.H., Kløvjan and Ottesen, C. 1995. The present day stress regime in the Barents Sea from borehole breakout. Proc. Workshop on Rock Stresses in the North Sea, Trondheim, Norway, 13014 Feb., pub. Sintef, Rock and Mineral engineering, N-7034, Trondheim, Norway, pp. 179-190.

Fejerskov, M., Myrvang, A.M., Lindholm, C. and Bungum, H. 1995. In-situ rock stress pattern on the Norwegian Continental shelf and mainland. Proc. Workshop on Rock Stresses in the North Sea, Trondheim, Norway, 13-14 Feb., pub. Sintef, Rock and Mineral Engineering, N-7034, Trondheim, Norway, pp. 191-201.

Klein, R.J. and Barr, M.V. 1986. Regional state of stress in Western Europe. In Proc Int Symp. Rock Stress and Rock Stress Measurements, Stockholm, pp 33-44.

Plumb, R.A. and Hickman, S.H. 1985. Stress induced borehole elongation: A comparison between the four arm dipmeter and Borehole Televiewer in the Auburn Geothermal Well. J. Geophys. Res., 90, pp. 5513-5521.

Concrete structures cracking survey by video image processing

M.J. Rouis, M. Zairi & M.S. Bouhlel
Ecole Nationale d'Ingénieurs de Sfax, Tunisia

ABSTRACT: Concrete structures may present a cracks coming from stress exceed of their elastic limit. This cracking may be stabilised in time or developed by cracks opening and extension or also by new fissures generation. Surveying of this evolution in time and specially estimation of the rate of cracks volume increasing constitute the alone way to know if a structure has reached stability conditions or it continues in plastic strain.
The developed computer driven device consists of a video camera related to a digitisation card. This paper describes the image processing device and a simulation of a concrete column fissuring using this tool. Two specific case were examined: extension of an old fissure and the generation of a new ones. The results has shown the efficiency of the device to follow fissures evolution in time. Thus, the area covered by new cracks or by stretches due to extension of existing ones is automatically calculated for a fixed time period. Increasing of this area in time is represented on a graph, allowing an estimation of the velocity of phenomenon evolution.

1 INTRODUCTION

Non destructive control of various construction is actually very important and getting rapid progress.
Permanent surveying of concrete structures comes from the necessity to have detailed knowledge of it's global state. If we have an adequate instrumentation, it's possible to well describe the construction behaviour in order to verify if it's in accordance with which is predicted or calculated. The supervision must permit an early detection of eventual anomalies in the construction behaviour.

Civil engineering structures pose the problem of specific control which complexity depends on their extent, their geometry and their construction mode. The common point of civil engineering materials is their heterogeneity and anisotropy, these characteristics make difficult investigation data interpretation (Ballivy and Rhazi, 1993).
There is a lot of concrete fissuring surveying techniques (Mazars, 1981). They may be classified in two types, the firsts are indirect observation methods containinig wave propagation and acoustic emissions. The seconds are direct methods and contain microscopic and macroscopic observation. These surveying methods allow the location and the following of a concrete degradation in time. In this paper a second type surveying device is presented.

2 IMAGE PROCESSING PROCEDURE

The first stage in an image processing procedure is the image digitisation. A scanner or a digitising card related to a video camera may be used for this stage. The results are expressed as a numeric or digitiscd image. This consists of a transformation of light signals to a numeric values (Rimmer, 1993).

On figure 1 is presented a general layout of an image processing system. This last is mainly constituted by the analog processors, numeric image processors, mass memory and screen memory. These compounds are computer driven. In fact, the host computer role is the piloting of the image processing system, to collect the issued information in order to control the system constituents function. This is done by selecting the active camera when the system contains a lot and selecting the display screen and the video signal acquisition. The numeric image processors are composed of filtering processors and contours extraction ones. The mass and screen memory ensure the data saving and the screen display (Toumazet, 1987).

The video image processing device used in this work is essentially composed by a CCD sensors video camera related to a digitising card which serves a microcomputer.

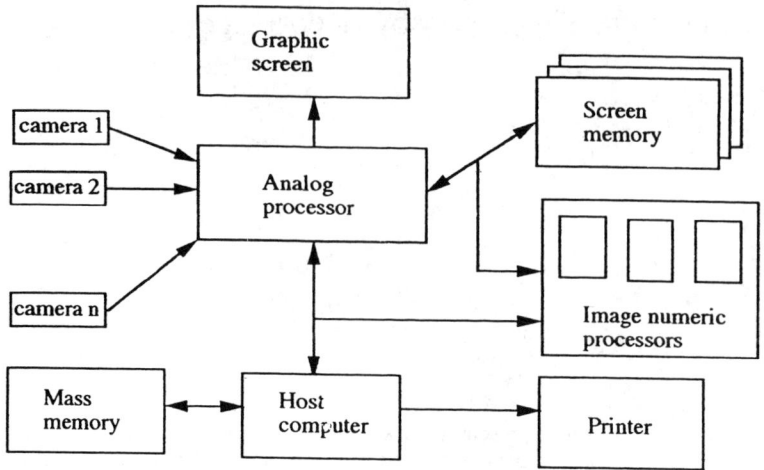

Figure 1 General layout of an image processing system.

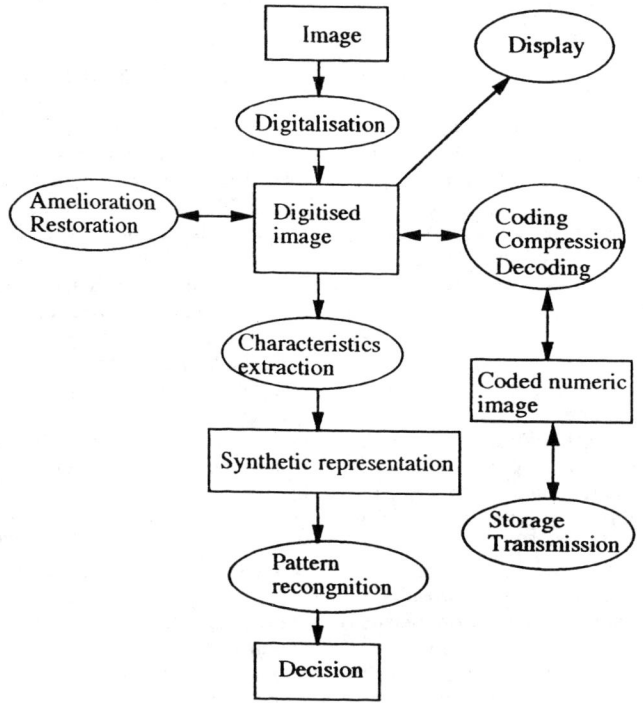

Figure 2 Main stages of image processing

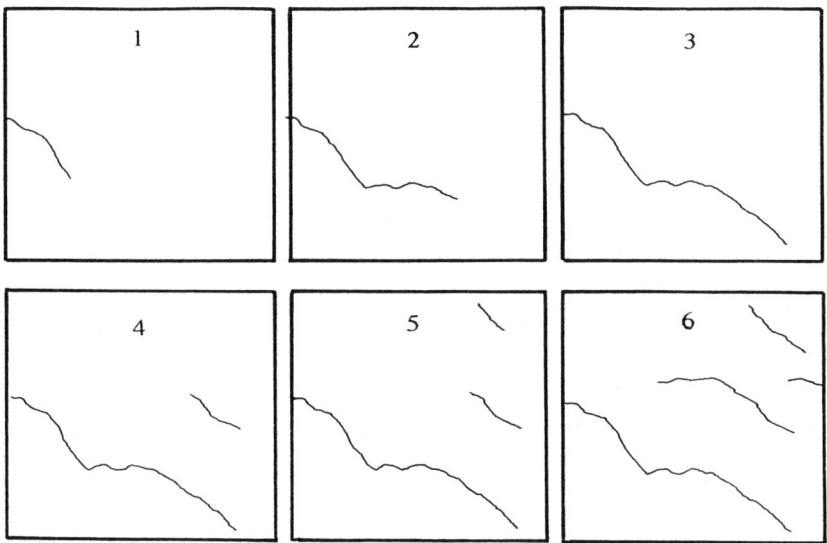

Figure 3 Images taken during the simulation of a concrete pile fissuring simulation.

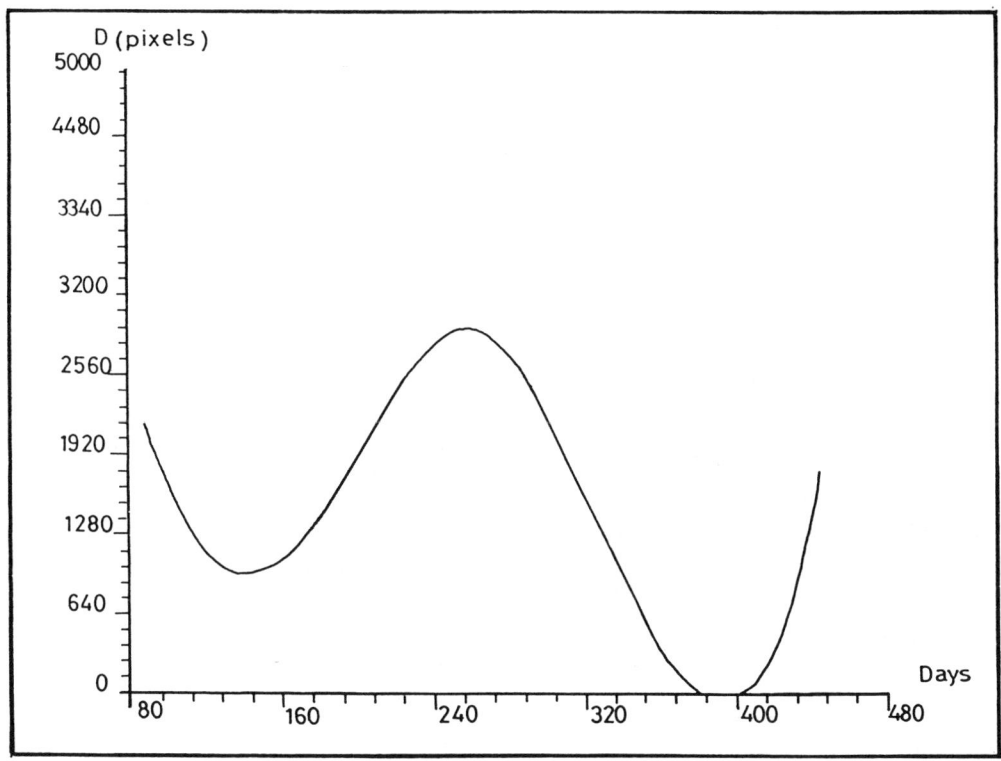

Figure 4 Time evolution of an image points differences.

3 IMAGE PROCESSING STAGES

The image processing process is mainly realised in five stages (figure 2). The first is the digitalisation which permits the obtaining of a digitised or numeric image by using a digitising card related an image acquisition device (for example a video camera). The amelioration - restoration stage is often necessary and groups all methods of increasing the visual quality of an image, such as centring, contrast, luminosity, sharpness and colours balance. In order to well conduct this stage, filtering techniques are often used. If the gradation process is known, we speak about restoration rather than amelioration.

It's very important, during the image processing, to display images on a screen, in order to visually test the efficiency of the used treatments. The fourth stage or coding - decoding stage allows firstly the coding of the image in order to reduce the memory necessary for it's storage and perhaps transmission through a network. A compression techniques is used in this stage. A decoding phase in this stage is necessary to realise the inverse process. The last stage is pattern recognition, it's usually begin by an image characteristics extraction phase using a variety of techniques such as, components number reduction, segmentation, contours follow-up and thinning down. All these techniques allow a synthetic representation of the interesting part of the treated image.

4 CONCRETE FISSURING EVOLUTION

The chosen application consists to follow a concrete structure fissuring. This application can't be realised in real time because it needs a very long observation time period. For the previous reasons, a simulation from a fissured structure is done. This simulation will reconstitute all stages of a fissures observation and cartography of their evolution.

The simulations are conducted on a fissured concrete pile. It consists of the covering of the fissures by paper sheets having the same colour as the pile paint. Fissures are then, progressively discovered in many stages in order to simulate the extension of a same fissure and a new fissure generation. Thus the following six images are taken (figure 3).
- the first image is a part of a fissure;
- the second is a partial prolongation of the same fissure;
- the third image represents the whole fissure;
- the fourth and the fifth show a new fissures generation;
- the sixth one represents the real state of the pile without any camouflage.

After the saving of these images on files, we proceeded to comparisons of images pairs, thus the difference between each two images is visualised on the video monitor. The number of points differences is also calculated. The problem encountered is the imprecision of this number. In fact, it's difficult to have the same conditions for image taking, the brightness and contrast are continually varying. The issue for this problem is to diminish the grey level during the difference calculation. All numbers of point of difference between two images are plotted on a graph. The time evolution of points of differences for an image taken several days is presented on a graph form on figure 4. No interpretation may be made from this representation because it's not corresponding to a real case coming from a real mechanical behaviour. In fact, a real case graph may be constant, linear or exponential. When the graph of the time evolution of points of differences is constant or linear, the fissure is not dangerous for short term. If the graph is exponential, the fissure become dangerous and the failure of the structure is near in time.

5 CONCLUSIONS

This case study has shown the ability of the device to pursue the evolution of the fissuring of concrete structures. Thus, the surface covered by a new fissures or by a portions of existing ones may automatically calculated for a fixed time periods. These surfaces increase is represented on a graph giving the phenomenon velocity and consequently allowing to make decisions depending on it's degree of aggravation.

REFERENCES

Ballivy G. and Rhazi J., Auscultation et ninstrumentation: problématique et devenir, Troisième *colloque sur la réfection des infrastructures de béton. Auscultation et instrumentation des ouvrages en service, Université de Sherbrooke,* Canada, 1993.

Mazars J., Evolution de la micro-fissuration dans les bétons, *cahier de l'AFB*, 183, 1981.

Rimmer S. , *Les images Bitmap*, 2ème édition, Dunod, 1993.

Toumazet J.J., *Traitement de l'image sur micro-ordinateur*, Sibex, 1987.

Rock Stress, Sugawara & Obara (eds) © 1997 Balkema, Rotterdam, ISBN 90 5410 901 7

Crack angle dependence of initial yield stress and stress concentration in rocks

Gyo-Cheol Jeong
Department of Geology, Andong National University, Korea

T. Seiki & Y. Ichikawa
Department of Geotechnical and Environmental Engineering, Nagoya University, Japan

ABSTRACT: To understand better the fundamental problems on crack angle dependence of yield stress and stress distribution in rock containing cracks, uniaxial compression tests of mortar specimens containing cracks inclined to the loading axis at an angle of 0°, 15°, 30°, 45°, 60°, 75°, 90° respectively were conducted under direct observation. Next, homogenization theory and finite element analysis were used to analyze the stress state of the vicinity of crack and initial shear and tensile yield stresses for each crack angle. The comparison of experimental data with prediction have shown that the analytical models are fairly sufficient to predict the effect of cracks on the mechanical response of rocks having cracks.

1 INTRODUCTION

Rock is a natural material with some pre-existing cracks and its yield stress is strongly dependent on cracks and cavities occurring during loading. The problem of the description of inelastic behavior of rock is essential for the solution of numerous boundary value problems in engineering geology and civil engineering (e.g., underground space development and radioactive waste disposal (Jeong 1994).

The development of underground space has been becoming an attractive option, particularly in/around the metropolitan cities such as Tokyo, Osaka in Japan (Seiki et. al. 1993). Therefore the ground conditions are great interest for the design and construction of underground structures. As underground structures are of large scale, the assessment of the stability of the structures is of paramount importance.

Failure of biotite-bearing rocks during complex loading could result from microstructures of the grain boundary, biotites and related cracks. That is, cleavage planes in biotite are generally those planes with the lowest bond density or strength, and lowest surface energy (Brace et. al. 1962). Thus strain energy stored in the grain as a result of applied stresses will tend to be relieved on those planes.

Our petrographic observations also show that low-angle cracks within quartz and feldspar grains granite samples deformed in compression are commonly associated with the ends of biotite grains inclined cleavage cracks (Figure 1), which reveals in the same experimental results of Gottschalk (1990) and Wong et al. (1985).

In this study we are concerned with the effects of yield stress by inclined cracks. For this purpose, we used specimens made of mortar with one crack set which has a constant length and same direction. Orientation of the set was varied with respect to the loading axis. Finally we analyzed our experiments by FEM and Homogenization theory.

2 EXPERIMENTS

The specimen size of rectangular prisms is 320 mm × 150 mm × 45 mm and all specimens were made of mortar by using an early age hardening portland cement and standard sand. For every batch we prepared three rectangular prism specimens. We varied crack angle from 0° to 90° by an increment of 15° (Figure 2). At first to make cracks in specimens we laid an ulethane sheet which is 5 mm thick to maintain the opening state of initial crack at the bottom side of it. And then after molding we inserted 18 steel strips, which are 26 mm wide, 0.5 mm thick and 60 mm deep and were fixed on an acrylic plate by screws. Finally after 4 hours later from casting they were pulled out.

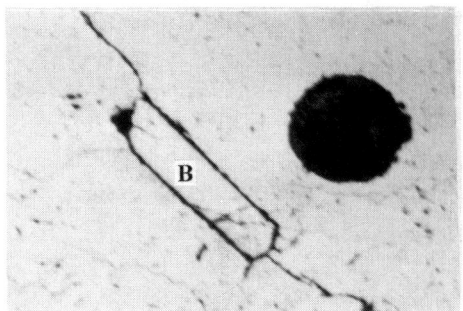

Figure 1. Geometrical relationships between biotite(B) with cracks and stress-induced cracks.

Uniaxial compression test was carried out by high stiffness compression testing machine which has 100 ton loading capacity and stiffness of 3.04×10^2 MN/m. The strain rate was 0.025 %/min. In experiments, axial stress, axial strain and lateral strain were measured (Figure 3).

3 DISCUSSION

3.1 *Mechanical properties*

From the relation between the peak strength and crack angle, it can be stated that the peak strength monotonically increases as the crack angle increases (Figure 4). This is different from the case of the normalized elastic modulus. It implies that the ratio may be different for elastic behavior from plastic behavior. Therefore, the peak strength is regarded as

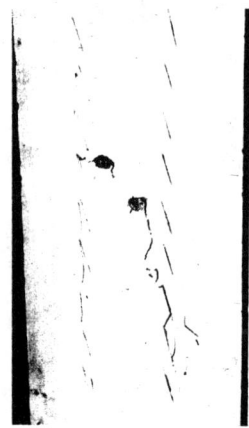

Figure 2. Cracked mortar specimen for experiments.

the strength of the remaining columns at the final stage of crack propagation. In the other words, at the peak state, it indicates that the larger the crack angle is, the wider the columns, which the load is supported, are.

3.2 *Crack propagation*

As seen Figure 3, it can be stated that the peak strength with increasing crack angle. It is obvious that the larger crack angle is, the smaller the projected section area of crack area in the loading direction. Therefore, stress increases in portion to the rotation of crack clockwise.

We attempted to determine an index for the initial

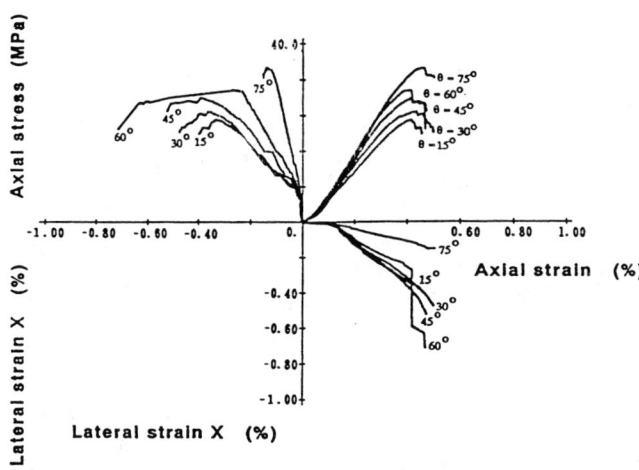

Figure 3. Axial stress, axial strain and lateral strain relation for each crack inclination.

yielding point from the crack initiation during the testing of specimens. Since the point of initiation depends on the visibility of cracks, it was difficult to do so. We determined the initial yielding point from X-direction response of the axial stress and lateral strain. If this index can be determined from the relation between the axial stress and axial strain, it is ideal index. As the marked variation can not be observed from the relation, we ultimately paid attention to the marked increase of lateral strain in X-direction occurred in tests. This marked variation can be seen in almost all tests. As a result we assumed this index as the point of crack initiation.

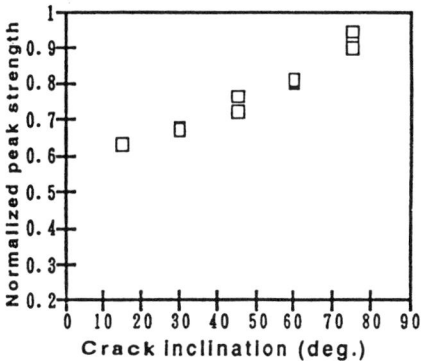

Figure 4. Relation between the normalized peak strength and crack inclination.

3.3 Numerical analysis

Theoretically, the initial yielding point must be associated with the crack initiation. Because of the assumed index to determine the crack initiation, it become obvious that observed crack initiation may or may not directly correspond to that determined from tests, and it is always not easy to see the initiation of cracks during tests. We made a plane strain finite element to have a fine picture of the stress state around cracks. Since the specimen have a periodic crack set, a unit cell having one crack was selected.

In general, the stress at crack tip must be calculated by using a special element in FEM or applying BEM (Washizu et al. 1983). In this study, our purpose is to predict the yield stress state around the crack rather than that at a crack tip. In FEM analysis the crack angle was varied from 0° to 90° by an increment of 15°. We used the mechanical properties given in Table 1.

The applied tractions were 5 Mpa and 10 Mpa to calculate the yielding around the crack. At first, we determined the element which has the minimum safety factors for shear yielding (SFS) and tension yielding (SFT). The minimum applied load at shear yielding for each crack inclination was determined by using the Mohr-Coulomb criterion. We predicted yield stress by shearing failure by using maximum principal stress and minimum principal stress which

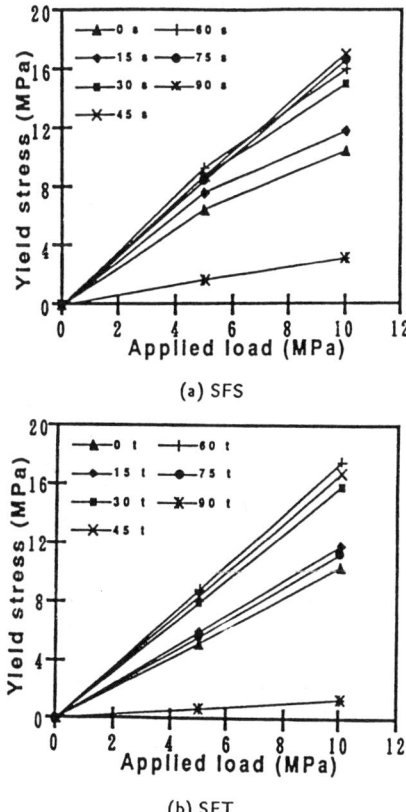

Figure 5. Relation between the applied load and initial yielding stress.

Table 1. Mechanical properties of mortar.

Elastic modulus E	(MPa)	1.432×10^4
Poisson's ratio ν		0.09
Internal friction angle ϕ	$(deg.)$	35.0
Cohesion c	(MPa)	9.567
Tensile strength σ_t	(MPa)	5.003

were selected by using the minimum SFS and material parameters. We also predicted the tensile yield stress by using tension-cut concept. The

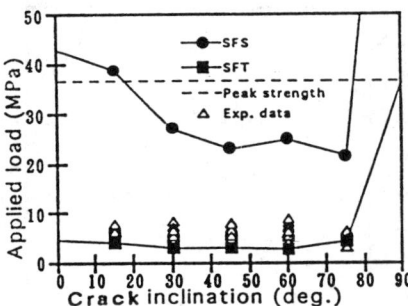

Figure 6. Relation between the applied load at initial yielding and crack inclinations.

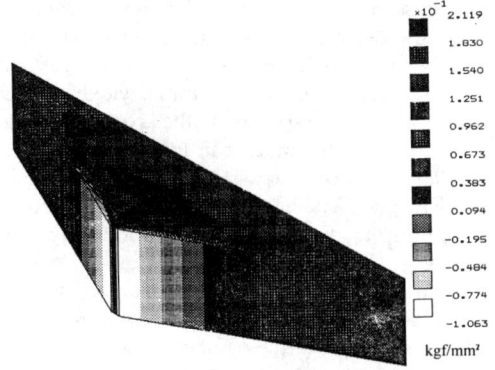

Figure 7. Stress concentration at crack tip.

relation between the applied load and the predicted initial shear and tensile yield stresses for each crack inclination is obtained as shown in Figure 5.

As expected, the selected element which has the minimum safety was almost located in the vicinity of crack tips except for 0° inclination. From these relations, we obtained a relation between the crack angle and the applied load at the time of initial yielding for shear and tension (Figure 6). As seen Figure 6, the failure may occur by tension for almost all crack inclinations. For inclination exceeding 75°, the applied load for the initial yielding becomes very large. This tendency was also supported by the observation on experiments. The relation between the applied stress and experimental data means that the initial yielding may occur mainly due to tensile stresses. Tensile stress distribution was calculated at crack tip by homogenization theory (Jeong 1993). Local values of the tensile stress normalized to the loading stress in the vicinity of crack tip are shown in Figure 7.

On the other hand, the yield stress by shearing failure is obviously different from experimental data. This does not mean that there is no relation between the initial yielding and shear failure. We can see that applied load by SFS has lower values than the peak strength for crack inclination from 30° to 75°. This means that the secondary yielding or secondary crack propagation may occur due to shearing.

4 CONCLUSIONS

A macroscopic continuum model based on the consideration of the mechanical effect of periodic cracks can fairly predict the averaged macroscopic mechanical properties. However, these models are not sufficient to predict the initial yielding. When a specimen having many cracks was tested under uniaxial compression, it is difficult monitor the crack propagation process. Nevertheless it is possible to observe the crack initiation and the orientation and length of cracks in relation to the stress-strain response. The initiation and propagation may be predicted by FEM and the stress concentration at the crack tip may be also calculated by homogenization theory. The comparison of experimental data and prediction have shown that the analytical models are fairly sufficient to predict the effect of crack inclinations on the initial yield stress in rocks having cracks.

REFERENCES

Brace, W. F. & J. B. Walsh 1962. Some direct measurements of the surface energy of quartz and orthoclase. *Am. Mineral.*, 47: 1111-1122.

Gottschalk, R. R., A. K. Kronenberg, J. E. Russel & J. Handin 1990. Mechanical anisotropy of gneiss: Failure criterion and sources of directional behavior. *J. Geophy. Res.*, 95: 21613-21634.

Jeong, G. -C. & Y. Ichikawa 1994. An experimental study on damage propagation of intact granite. *J. Society of Materials Sciences*, 43: 317-323.

Jeong, G. -C. & Y. Ichikawa 1993. An analysis of stress concentration in major minerals of granite by homogenization method. *Proc. of 7th Japan Computational Mechanics Symp.*, Tokyo, 229-236.

Seiki, T., Y. Ichikawa, O. Aydan & F. Ito 1993. Mechanical behavior and failure of rock masses having distributed sets of cracks of finite length. *Int. Symp. on Assessment and Prevention of*

Failure Phenomenon in Rock Engineering, Istanbul, Balkema, 181-186.

Washizu, H., H. Miyamoto, Y. Yamada, Y. Yamamoto & T. Kawai 1983. FEM handbook II Applied edition. Baifuukan, Tokyo.

Wong, T. F. & R. Biegal 1985. Effects of pressure on the micromrchanics of faulting in San Marcos gabbro. *J. Struct. Geol.*, 7: 737-747.

Effect of normal stiffness and strain rate on the shear strength of soft joints

Buddhima Indraratna & Asadul Haque
Department of Civil and Mining Engineering, University of Wollongong, N.S.W., Australia

ABSTRACT: The effects of normal stiffness and strain rate on the shear strength of soft simulated rock joints are investigated in the laboratory, using a large-scale Constant Normal Stiffness (CNS) apparatus. The shear strength of joints having an asperity angle of 9.5° (Type S1) is observed to increase with the increase in initial normal stress from 0.16 to 2.43 MPa, and also with the increase in normal stiffness from 0 to 8.5 kN/mm. Results of this study show that a bilinear shear strength envelope is appropriate for joints tested under zero normal stiffness condition, whereas a linear envelope is adequate for joints tested under a normal stiffness of 8.5 kN/mm. Test results show that the strain rate has a considerable effect on the shear behaviour of Type S2 joints having an asperity angle of 18.5°. The peak shear strength of joints increases together with the dilation and normal stress as the strain rate is increased from 0.35 to 1.70 mm/min.

1 INTRODUCTION

Shear tests are usually carried out in the past by using conventional direct shear apparatus where the normal stress during testing remains constant. It has been demonstrated by several researchers [Obert et al., 1974; Benmokrane and Ballivy, 1989; Johnstone and Lam, 1989; Archambault et al., 1990; Ohnishi and Dharmaratne, 1990; Skinas et al., 1990] that the shear behaviour of non-planar discontinuities may be explained more realistically by conducting shear tests under Constant Normal Stiffness (CNS) rather than under Constant Normal Load (CNL) condition. In the past, tests have been mainly conducted on harder rock joint surfaces. However, very little attention has been paid in relation to the shear behaviour of soft joints, especially under varying strain rates. In view of this, a large-scale CNS shear apparatus has been designed by the authors which can be used for testing soft joints under both CNS and CNL conditions. The effect of strain rate on the shear strength of sandstone, limestone and slate joints have been investigated by Donath et al. (1972) and Lama (1975) under CNL condition, where highly scattered or non-uniform results have been reported due to the difficulty in obtaining similar surface profiles and changing material property. The influence of strain rate on the specimens reproduced from controlled model material is easier to quantify as discussed by Lama (1975). It is pointed out by the authors that the shear stress of joints tested under low normal stress decreases with increasing shear strain rate due to the effect of dynamic friction. Also, the shear stress increases with enhanced strain rate under high normal stress due to the increased frictional resistance of the joint surfaces. Chong et al. (1987) have investigated the strain rate effect on mechanical properties of Western oil shale, where they observed an increase in Young's modulus (E) with higher strain rate and no significant change in the Poisson's ratio. However, the effect of normal stiffness and shear strain rate on the shear behaviour of soft joints has not been thoroughly investigated. Therefore, in this study, an attempt is made to investigate further, the effect of normal stiffness and strain rate on the shear behaviour of soft joints under CNS conditions.

2 EXPERIMENTAL STUDY

2.1 CNS shear apparatus

The shear apparatus consisted of (i) main frame that holds the shear boxes, (ii) strain controlled shear loading device and (iii) Constant Normal Stiffness spring assembly. The size of the top box is 250x75x150mm, and that of the bottom box is 250x75x100mm. The top box can move only in the vertical direction, whereas the bottom box can move along the shear direction. The shear load can be applied through the strain controlled device at a prefixed strain rate of 0.30 to 1.70 mm/min. The

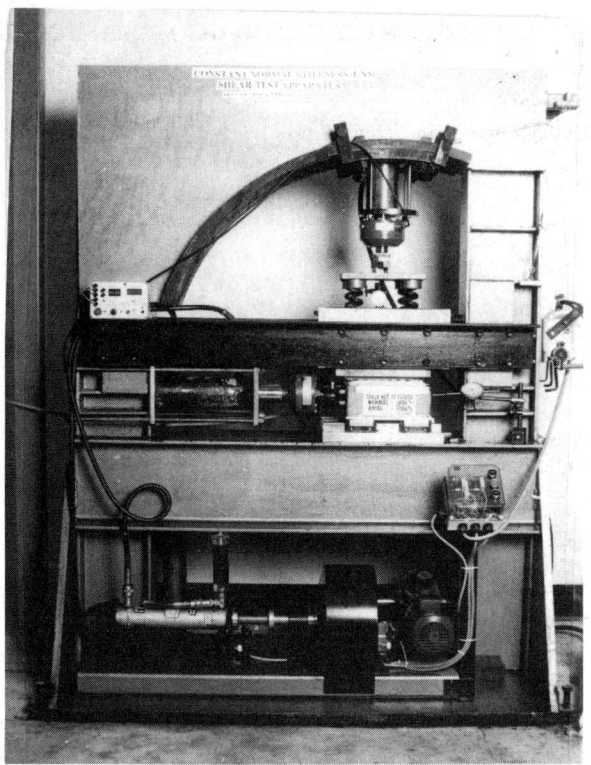

Figure 1. A close view of the large-scale CNS apparatus.

apparatus has maximum shear and normal load capacities of 120 kN and 180 kN, respectively. Springs of known stiffness (Figure 1) were used to simulate the normal stiffness of the surrounding rock mass applied over the shear plane. A special type of hydraulic jack (constant internal pressure) was used to maintain a normal stiffness of zero which refers to the k=0, CNL condition.

2.2 *Tests on unfilled soft joints*

Ordinary casting plaster (gypsum) was mixed with water in the ratio of 5:3 and then poured inside the specially designed shear box that contains the desired surface profile. The specimens were prepared inside the mould to ensure that the joint surfaces were fully mated. Regular saw-tooth profiles of inclinations of 9.5° (Type S1) and 18.5° (Type S2) were used during this investigation. The top specimen was cast over the bottom box and the moulds were stripped after an hour. A curing period of 14 days at an oven controlled temperature of 50° C were allowed for all specimens. The mechanical properties of the cured specimens were similar to those of many soft rocks [uniaxial compressive strength (σ_c)=11-13 MPa; Young's modulus (E) = 1.9-2.3 GPa; and Poisson's ratio (ν)=0.25].

Shear tests were performed on cured specimens for various normal stiffness (k) and shear strain rates. For each test, changes in normal stress and shear stress with horizontal displacement were recorded by digital strain meters. The vertical and horizontal displacements were recorded by dial gauges mounted on the top specimen and the side of the bottom box.

3 EFFECT OF NORMAL STIFFNESS

Tests were conducted on Type S1 interface for normal stiffness (k) of zero and 8.5 kN/mm, under initial normal stresses (σ_{no}) of 0.16 to 2.43 MPa. For each value of k, six specimens were tested for the above range of σ_{no} values and their effects on shear behaviour are discussed below:

3.1 *Variation of shear stress*

The shear stress is observed to increase with the horizontal displacement until the "peak to peak"

Table 1. Peak shear stress for different k values.

σ_{no} (MPa)	Peak shear stress (MPa)	
	k = 0	k = 8.5 kN/mm
0.16	0.214	0.483
0.30	0.369	0.661
0.56	0.665	1.026
1.10	1.295	1.539
1.63	1.770	1.833
2.43	2.472	2.732

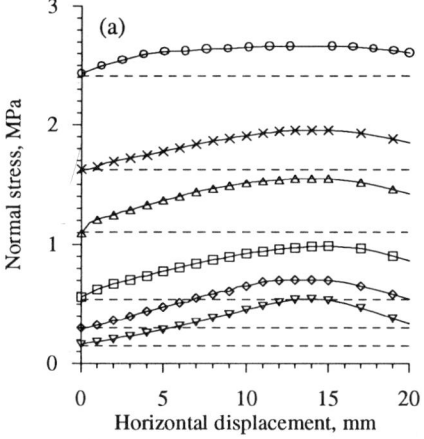

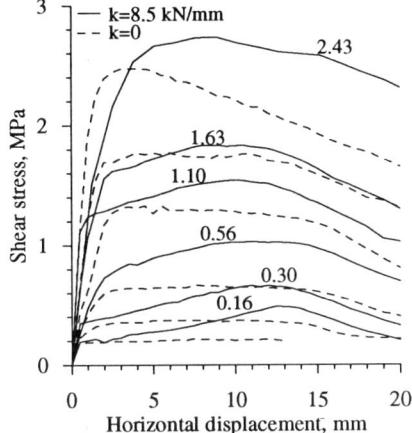

Figure 2. Effect of normal stiffness (k) on peak shear stress of S1 joints for various values of σ_{no}.

contact of the asperity is reached. At very low initial normal stresses (<0.56 MPa), the peak shear stress at normal stiffness of 8.5 kN/mm is more than twice that of the zero stiffness condition. However, this difference is less prominent at higher values of σ_{no} (>1.00 MPa), where the asperity degradation is inevitable (Table 1). Skinas et al. (1990) have observed similar results for the sand-barytes-cement hard joint surfaces. The variation of shear stress with horizontal displacement for Type S1 joints under normal stiffness of zero and 8.5 kN/mm is plotted in Figure 2 for comparison. It is evident that the shear stress of joint increases with the increase in initial normal stress and stiffness. The peak shear stress is attained more quickly as the value of the normal stiffness is reduced from 9.5 kN/mm to zero.

3.2 Variation of normal stress and dilation

The normal stress acting over the interface during shearing increases with the shear displacement for normal stiffness greater than zero (Figure 3a). In contrast, the normal stress remains almost the same when the constant normal stiffness is zero. As

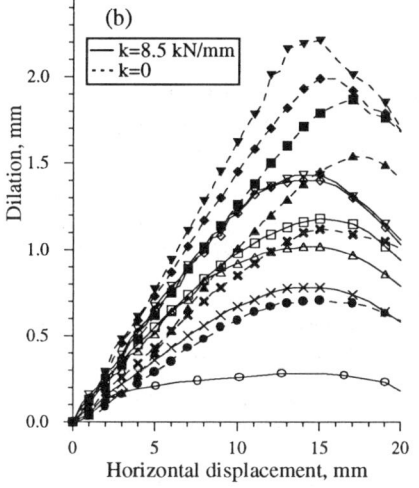

Figure 3. (a) Normal stress and (b) dilation against horizontal displacement for varying σ_{no}.

expected, the dilation of the joints decreases with the increase in normal stiffness (Figure 3b). The dilation of joints under k=0 condition is much greater than that associated with a normal stiffness of 8.5 kN/mm. This implies that the degradation of asperities at high initial normal stress is significant, and often results in reduced dilation of joints. The shape of the plots of normal stress and dilation against shear displacement at very low normal stress generally follow the initial shape of joint interfaces (Figure 3a). This is because no asperity breakage takes place at very low normal stress levels.

3.3 Peak strength envelopes

The shear stress corresponding to the normal stress

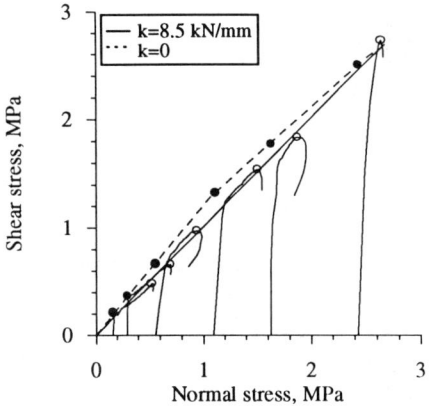

Figure 4. Shear stress vs normal stress plot for S1 profile.

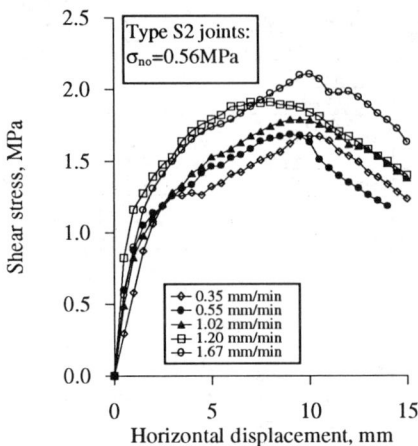

Figure 5. Shear stress vs horizontal displacement for Type S2 joints.

is plotted in Figure 4 to obtain the peak strength envelopes under the two stiffness conditions, k=0 and k=8.5 kN/mm. It is evident that the stress paths corresponding to low initial normal stress tend to propagate along the shear strength envelope (Figure 4). The bi-linear strength envelope obtained under zero stiffness condition represents the upper bound for the given surface profile, Type S1. However, a linear strength envelope seems to be more appropriate for the normal stiffness of 8.5 kN/mm. A non-linear envelope may be required to explain the shear behaviour of asperities having higher inclinations, where significant sliding and shearing through asperities occurs. Ohnishi & Dharmaratne (1990) have conducted tests on cement-sand joints having a Joint Roughness Coefficient (JRC) of 8 to 12 under normal stiffness of zero and 1437 kPa/mm. Their test results indicated that the envelope under zero stiffness may be considered as the upper bound. This observation is true for softer joints, based on the current study.

4 EFFECT OF SHEAR STRAIN RATE

Tests were conducted on Type S2 joints under varying strain rates of 0.35 to 1.67 mm/min. The initial normal stress (σ_{no}) and normal stiffness (k) were maintained at 0.56 MPa and 8.5 kN/mm, respectively, for all the tests.

4.1 *Effect of strain rate on shear stress of joints*

Initially, joints were sheared at a very low strain rate of 0.35 mm/min, and the changes in shear stress with horizontal displacements were recorded. The strain rate was then gradually increased and the variations of shear stress with horizontal displacement for all the tests were plotted together in Figure 5 for comparison. It is observed that the peak shear stress increases with the increase in strain rate from 0.35 to 1.67 mm/min under the given normal stress and stiffness conditions. As discussed earlier, the frictional resistance offered by the joint surface itself becomes greater as the strain rate is increased further, and thereby, increasing the overall shear strength of joints.

4.2 *Variations of normal stress and dilations*

The changes in normal stress and dilation with the horizontal displacements are plotted for varying strain rates in Figure 6. Both the normal stress and dilation are observed to increase with the horizontal displacements, as the strain rate is increased further. The normal stress is increased by at least 25% when the strain rate is increased from 0.35 mm/min to 1.67 mm/min (Figure 6a).

4.3 *Peak shear stress under varying strain rates*

Test results indicate that the rate of shear strain has a significant effect on the peak shear stress of soft joints. The variation of shear strength with different strain rates is plotted in Figure 7, and it is observed that the peak shear stress increases considerably with the increase in strain rate. Lama (1975) reported a similar behaviour for gypsum joints under constant normal load (σ_n=2 MPa) condition. In order to define the peak shear strength envelope of soft joints more precisely, the effect of strain rate on the shear

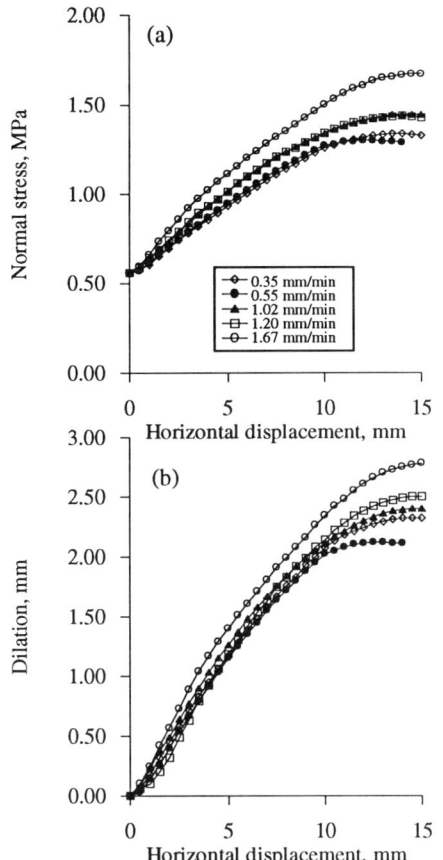

Figure 6. Normal stress and dilation against horizontal displacement for various strain rate of Type S2 joints.

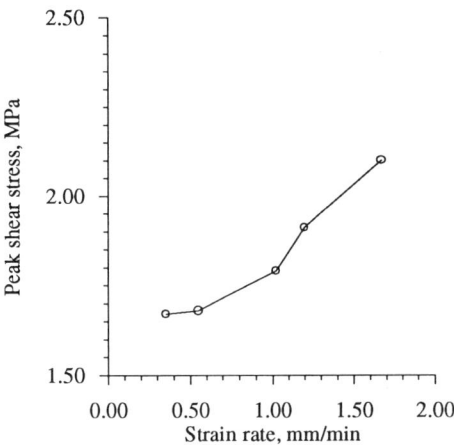

Figure 7. Effect of strain rate on the peak shear stress of S2 joints.

behaviour should be considered more carefully, based on both CNL and CNS testing.

5 CONCLUSIONS

Shear tests were conducted in the laboratory on soft synthetic joints under different normal stiffness conditions and varying shear strain rates. Results confirm that both the normal stiffness and strain rate have a significant effect on the shear behaviour of soft joints tested within the normal stress range of 0.16 to 2.43 MPa. The peak shear stress clearly increases with the increase in normal stiffness and this is particularly significant under high normal stress levels. In contrast, the increase in normal stress and dilation of joints become negligible at high initial normal stress levels due to shearing through joint asperities. The peak shear strength envelope under zero normal stiffness condition can be considered to be bi-linear, representing an upper bound for the measured data. However, a linear strength envelope is sufficient to explain the shear behaviour of joints tested under a normal stiffness of 8.5 kN/mm. This study also confirms that the shear strength of joints increases with the increase in the rate of shear strain, under CNS conditions.

6 REFERENCES

Archambault, G., Fortin, M., Gill, G.E., Aubertin, M. & Ladanyi, B. (1990). Experimental investigations for an algorithm simulating the effect of variable normal stiffness on discontinuities shear strength. Proc. *Int. Symp. Rock Joints*, Leon, (Barton & Stephansson eds.), Balkema Publishers, Rotterdam, pp. 141-148.

Barton, N. (1973). Review of a new shear strength criterion for rock joints. *Engineering Geology*, **7**, Elsevier, pp.287-332.

Benmokrane, B. and Ballivy, G. (1989). Laboratory study of shear behaviour of rock joints under constant normal stiffness conditions. *Proc. 30th U.S. Symp. Rock Mech.*, (Khair ed.), Balkema Publishers, Rotterdam, pp. 899-906.

Chong, K.P., Harkins, J.S., Kuruppu, M.D. and Leskinen, A.I. (1987). Strain rate dependent mechanical properties of Western oil shale. Proc. *28th US Symp. on Rock Mech.*, Tucson, 29 June-1 July, pp. 157-164.

Donath, F.A., Fruth, L.S. and Olsson, W.A. (1972).

Experimental study of frictional properties of faults. *Proc. 14th Symp. Rock Mech.*, Univ. Park, Penn., USA, pp. 189-222.

Johnstone, I.W. and Lam, T.S.K. (1989). Shear behaviour of regular triangular concrete/rock joints -- analysis. *J. Geotech. Eng.*, ASCE, Vol. 115, No.5, pp. 711-727.

Lama, R.D. (1975). *The concept of creep of jointed rocks and the status of research project A-6. SFB77*, Jahresbericht, 1974. Inst. Soil Mech. & Rock Mech., Univ. Karlsruhe, Karlsruhe.

Obert, L., Brady, B.T. and Schmechel, F.W. (1976). The effect of normal stiffness on the shear resistance of rock. *Rock Mechanics & Rock Engineering*, Vol.8/2, pp. 57-72.

Ohnishi, Y. and Dharmaratne, P.G.R. (1990). Shear behaviour of physical models of rock joints under constant normal stiffness conditions. *Proc. Int. Symp. on Rock Joints*, Leon, (Barton & Stephansson eds.), Balkema Publishers, Rotterdam, pp. 267-273.

Skinas, C.A., Bandis, S.C. and Demiris, C.A. (1990). Experimental investigations and modelling of rock joint behaviour under constant stiffness. *Proc. Int. Symp. Rock Joints*, Leon, (Barton & Stephansson eds.), Balkema Publishers, Rotterdam, pp. 301-308.

Effect of surface roughness on peak and residual shear stress of irregular rock joints

Shouji Du, Tetsuro Esaki & Yujing Jiang
Institute of Environmental Systems, Kyushu University, Fukuoka, Japan

Jun Sun
Faculty of Geotechnical Engineering, Tongji University, Shanghai, People's Republic of China

ABSTRACT: The correct evaluation of the shear strength of rock joints plays an important role in the design, construction and management of rock engineering. Based on the measurement of rough profiles of irregular rock joints and the results of shear tests under constant normal stresses for different surface roughness, a new method is developed for quantifying the surface roughness of rock joints. That is, surface roughness can be represented by the average roughness angle, which is calculated through the linear slope and the fractal parameters (amplitude and fractal dimension) of the several profiles on joint surfaces. And the empirical criterion is suggested for modeling and predicting the shear strength of irregular rock joints at low normal stresses.

1 INTRODUCTION

As various deep underground utilizations, such as radioactive waste disposal sites, have lately attracted considerable attention, it becomes more important to investigate the mechanical and hydraulic properties of jointed rock mass simultaneously. Strength, deformation behaviour and flow properties of rock joints are strongly dependent on the joint surface geometry, in particular, surface roughness. Therefore, it is important to characterize surface roughness quantitatively and to investigate the relation between shear strength and surface roughness.

By carrying out direct shear tests on the plaster specimens including artificial joint asperities, Patton (1966) found that the failure envelope for the joints can be approximated by two straight lines with different slopes. That is, a bilinear shear strength criterion has been used by combining the dilatant model for low normal stresses and the Coulomb linear criterion for high normal stresses. Ladanyi and Archambault (1970) developed a sophisticated strength model considering that the two modes of failure occur simultaneously. Although the concept of their model is excellent, it is difficult to determine the parameters used in the model. By introducing two parameters called JRC (joint roughness coefficient) and JCS (joint compressive strength), Barton (1973) proposed an empirical equation to estimate the shear strength of rock joints. Based on back-calculation using the equation, Barton and Choubey (1977) determined the values of JRC for ten typical profiles of rock joints, which are adopted in the suggested methods for the quantitative description of discontinuities in rock masses (ISRM, 1978). In order to determine JRC value of a profile in question, the profile must be visually compared with the ten typical profiles. As a result the estimate has been found to be subjective and unreliable. For the reason, some researches have investigated the correlation between JRC values and statistical parameters (Tse, 1979; Reeves, 1985; Maerz, 1990) or fractal dimension (Lee, 1990; Xie, 1992) of typical profiles. However, it is found that even for the same profile, controversial and anomalous estimates about fractal dimension or statistical parameters were made by different researchers or by employing different methods and scale parameters. On the other hand, JRC values, fractal dimension and statistical parameters can only describe the stationary roughness profiles of joints. They give no directional information.

In this paper, based on the measurement of rough profiles of irregular rock joints and the results of shear tests under constant normal stress for different surface roughness, a new method is developed for quantifying the surface roughness of irregular rock joints, and an empirical criterion is suggested for modeling the shear strength of irregular rock joints at low normal stress. Finally, it is stated that the criteria can be used to predict shear strength for different normal stress and surface roughness.

2 JOINT SHEAR BEHAVIOR UNDER CONSTANT NORMAL STRESS

2.1 Direct shear testing apparatus and specimens

A specially designed testing apparatus has been developed, as described in detail by Esaki et al.(1991). This system consists of a direct shear loading unit with a specially designed shear box, a control and data acquisition unit and an artificial joint creating unit. Using this apparatus, an artificial joint can be created in the rock specimen, and normal and shear stresses can be arbitrarily applied on the joint.

Hard granite specimens from Nangen of Korea are used in this study. The uniaxial compressive strength of granite is 190MPa. The size of specimens is 120mm length, 100mm width and 80mm height. Each specimen has a couple of saw cut slits (width 1mm, depth 10mm) at mid-height of the specimen for creating an artificial joint correctly and easily. Thus, the horizontal area of joint shear plane is 100mm × 80mm.

2.2 Testing procedure

This experiment was conducted under constant normal stress of 5MPa for different surface roughness. At first, a prescribed value of normal stress was loaded up on the jointed specimen of granite. And then shear displacement was controlled in steps at a rate of 0.1mm/sec until maximum shear displacement of 20mm in order to investigate shear behavior during the post-peak process. Finally, the normal stress was unloaded and the procedure was repeated in the reverse direction until the beginning point. The irregular rough surfaces of jointed specimens were measured by laser scanning instrument before and after each shear test.

2.3 Experimental results

Shear deformation curves under constant normal stress for granite joints, as an example, are shown in Fig.1. Here parameter α means the average roughness angle of irregular rock joints. In general, shear stress reaches a rather sharp peak at a relatively small shear displacement as approximate linear, and then down to a roughly constant residual value with increasing shear displacement. Peak and residual shear stress become larger with increasing surface roughness. Dilatancy will occur when shear stress approaches to peak. It increases at reduced rate with increasing shear displacement. Dilatancy becomes more large as surface roughness increases.

3 A NEW METHOD FOR QUANTIFYING SURFACE ROUGHNESS OF IRREGULAR JOINTS

In general, roughness profiles of irregular rock joints consist of non-stationary and stationary components. To quantify surface roughness in a certain shear direction, firstly, the non-stationary component may be represented by a linear function with a positive or a negative slope ϕ_0, as shown in Fig.2(a), which is estimated through regression analysis in measured profile heights (Kulatilake, 1995). Next, removal of the non-stationary component from actual profile obtains the stationary component of the roughness profile. And a new fractal model for quantifying stationary roughness has been proposed by Du et al. (1997). That is, the average roughness angle U(h) is defined as root mean square increment of the first derivation of two asperity heights separated by a lag distance h:

$$U(h) = \left\{ \frac{1}{(N-j)} \sum_{i=1}^{N-j} \left[\frac{Z(x_i+h)-Z(x_i)}{h} (\cos\phi_0)^2 - \frac{\sin 2\phi_0}{2} \right]^2 \right\}^{1/2} \quad (1)$$

The relation between U(h) and fractal parameters (B and D) can be written as:

$$U(h) = B\, h^{(1-D)} \quad (2)$$

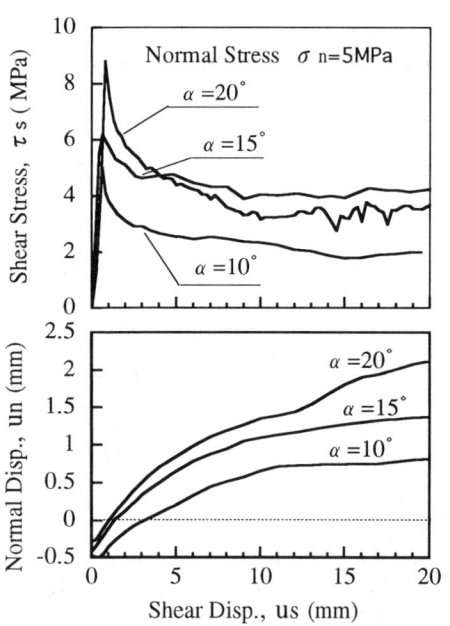

Fig. 1 Shear stress-displacement and normal-shear displacement (dilatancy) curves of granit joints for different surface roughness.

On a log-log plot of U(h) vs. lags h (Fig.2(b)), amplitude B is the intercept on U-axis, and (1-D) is the slope of the plot and D is the fractal dimension. It has been shown that fractal dimension D alone cannot quantify stationary roughness. But the combined fractal parameters (amplitude B and fractal dimension D) is able to quantify the stationary roughness in practice.

Moreover, since joint surface is three-dimensional, one of the approaches is therefore to select several parallel profiles on joint surface along a certain shear direction. At first, the asperity heights of the profiles are recorded at every (lag distance of) 0.05mm up to an accuracy of 0.001mm by laser scanning instrument along each line. Then, the slope (ϕ_0) and fractal parameters (B and D) of each profile are calculated from the above equations. Finally, the weighted average values of the slope (ϕ_0) and fractal parameters (B and D) of the several parallel profiles on joint surface are estimated. Therefore, the average roughness angle α of irregular rock joints can be given by the following form, which represents the surface roughness of non-stationary and stationary components.

$$\alpha = \phi_0 + U(h) = \phi_0 + B\, h_0^{(1-D)} \qquad (3)$$

4 THE RELATION BETWEEN SHEAR STRENGTH AND SURFACE ROUGHNESS

4.1 Suggested peak shear strength criterion

According to the measurement of rough profiles of joint surfaces, the fractal parameters (B, D and ϕ_0) are calculated by the new fractal model and the peak shear angles (ϕ_P) are obtained from the results of shear tests. As shown in Fig. 3, the peak shear angles (ϕ_P) increase with increasing the two fractal parameters (amplitude B and fractal dimension D). However, the correlation between ϕ_P and amplitude B is better than that between ϕ_P and fractal dimension D. It is represented that the effect of amplitude B on shear strength is more remarkable than that of fractal dimension D. It is also clear that fractal dimension D alone cannot quantify roughness. Fig. 4 shows the relation between the peak shear angles ϕ_P and average

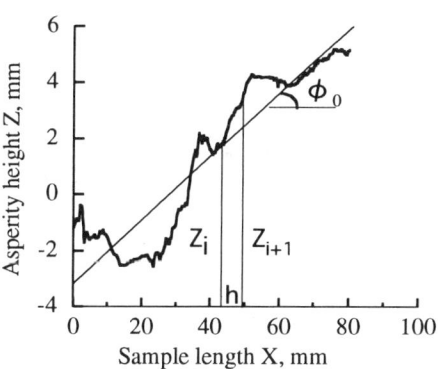

(a) The slope ϕ_0 for non-stationary roughness

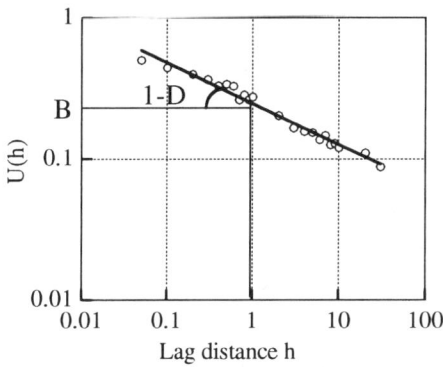

(b) The fractal parameters (B and D)

Fig. 2 The diagram used to calculate statistical and fractal parameters for joint profile.

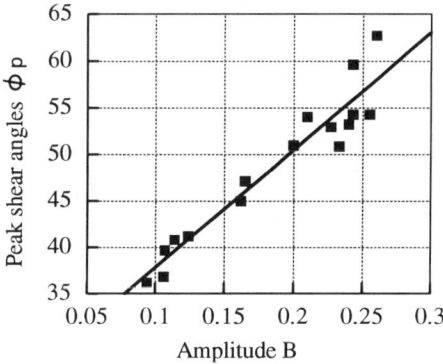

(a) The relation between peak shear angle and amplitude

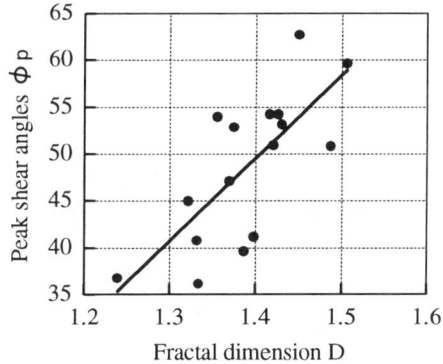

(b) The relation between peak shear angle and fractal dimension

Fig. 3 The distribution relation between peak shear angle and fractal dimensions (B and D).

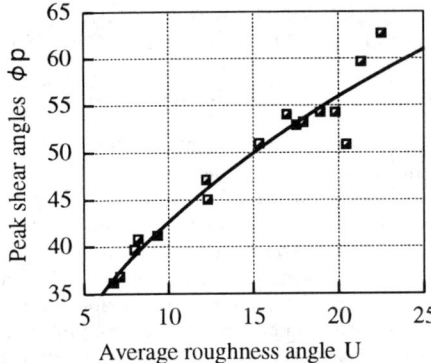

Fig. 4 The distribution relation between peak shear angle and average roughness angle for granite joints (normal stress $\sigma_n = 5MPa$).

Fig. 5 Relation between peak shear strength and normal stress for the different average roughness angle of granite joints.

roughness angle U. ϕ_p increases with increasing U and the two parameters have high correlation. It is very clear that the combination of B and D, i.e., the average roughness angle U can directly quantify stationary roughness of joint surfaces.

It has been shown in literature that the peak shear strength (τ_p) is principally governed by the surface roughness, normal stress (σ_n) and the wall compressive strength (σ_j). Therefore, the following equation is suggested to estimate peak shear strength of irregular rock joint under low normal stresses:

$$\tau_p = \sigma_n \tan\left\{a\, U^b \left[\log_{10}\left(\frac{\sigma_j}{\sigma_n}\right)\right]^d + \phi_0 + \phi_b\right\} \quad (4)$$

Where U, ϕ_0, and ϕ_b denote, respectively, the stationary roughness parameter (average roughness angle), the non-stationary roughness parameter (average inclination angle) and the basic friction angle. Coefficients a, b and d are determined by performing regression analysis on experimental data.

The peak shear strength data and the surface roughness parameters (U and ϕ_0) were used, for normal stress $\sigma_n = 5MPa$, and the wall compressive strength $\sigma_j = 137MPa$ and the basic friction angle $\phi_b = 21°$ of granite joints, to estimate the coefficients a, b and d values as 4.00, 0.71 and 0.14, respectively, by performing multiple linear regression analysis on the experimental results. The correlation coefficient is r=0.978.

It is important to note that, for smooth joint surfaces, the value of stationary roughness angle U becomes zero. Then the equation (4) reduces to following equation (5), which is applicable for smooth inclined joint surfaces.

$$\tau_p = \sigma_n \tan(\phi_b + \phi_0) \quad (5)$$

For horizontal smooth joint surfaces, non-stationary inclination angle (ϕ_0) is zero. This reduces equation (5) to equation (6), which is applicable for smooth horizontal joint surfaces.

$$\tau_p = \sigma_n \tan\phi_b \quad (6)$$

4.2 Prediction of peak shear strength

Fig. 5 shows the prediction of peak shear strength under the different average roughness angle α with the equation (4). The peak shear strength increases as a non-linear relation with increasing normal stress. On the other hand, for the same normal stress, the peak shear strength increases with increasing average roughness angle α.

4.3 The residual shear strength of rock joints

Goodman (1976) proposed the following model for the variation of the residual shear strength (τ_r) with the normal stress (σ_n).

$$\begin{aligned}\tau_r &= \tau_p\left(B_0 + (1-B_0)\frac{\sigma_n}{\sigma_T}\right) \quad \text{when} \quad \sigma_n < \sigma_T \\ \tau_r &= \tau_p \quad \text{when} \quad \sigma_n \geq \sigma_T\end{aligned} \quad (7)$$

In above equations, B_0 ($0 \leq B_0 \leq 1$) is the ratio of residual to peak shear strength at zero (or very low) normal stress and σ_T is a transitional stress. Goodman has suggested that uniaxial compressive strength of intact rock can be used as an estimate to σ_T. However, the estimate doesn't accord with reality. In fact, σ_T is treated as an independent material parameter of rock joint and its value can be estimated by the joint wall compressive strength (σ_j).

Fig. 6 shows the relation between residual and peak shear strength for the non-historical joints of granites. The residual shear strength (τ_r) increases linealy

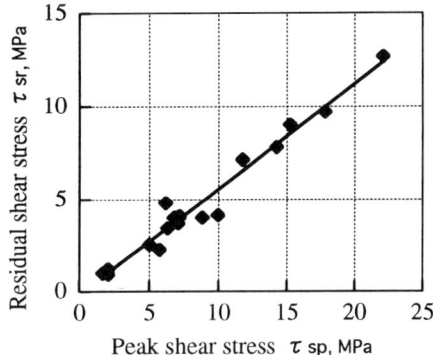

Fig. 6 The distribution relation between residual shear stress and peak shear stress for granite joints (normal stress $\sigma_n = 5 MPa$).

with increase of peak shear strength. Through performing linear regression analysis on experimental strength data, the coefficient B_0 is determined as 0.56.

5 CONCLUSIONS

In this study, based on the measurement of rough profiles of irregular rock joints and the results of shear tests under constant normal stress for different surface roughness, a new method was developed for quantifying the surface roughness of irregular rock joints, and the empirical criterion was suggested for modeling the shear strength of irregular rock joints at low normal stress. Some significant results are obtained below.

(1) Surface roughness of irregular rock joints can be represented by the average roughenss angle, which is calculated through the linear function with a positive or a negative slope (ϕ_0) and the fractal parameters (amplitude B and fractal dimension D) of the several profiles on joint surfaces.

(2) For two fractal parameters (amplitude B and fractal dimension D), the effect of amplitude B on shear strength is more remarkable than that of fractal dimension D. It is clear that fractal dimension D alone cannot quantify roughness. The peak shear angles (ϕ_p) and average roughness angle U have high correlation. The combination of B and D, i.e., the average roughness angle U can directly quantify the stationary roughness of joint surfaces.

(3) Based on the results of shear tests, an empirical criterion is suggested for modeling peak shear strength at low normal stress. Furthermore, it was stated that the criteria can also be used to predict shear strength for different normal stress and surface roughness of rock joints.

Acknowledgments. The authors wish to thank Mr. Y. Wada and K. Kobayashi for their cooperation in experimental works.

REFERENCES

Barton N., Review of a new shear strength criterion for rock joints, *Engineering Geology* 7, pp. 287-332, 1973.

Barton N. and Choubey V., The shear strength of rock joints in theory and practice, *Rock Mech*, 10, pp. 1-54, 1977.

Du S., Esaki T., Jiang Y. and Kobayashi K., The relation of fractal characteristics on the rough surface and shear strength of rock joints, *Proc. 28th Symp. Rock Mech., Tokyo, Japan*, pp. 167-173, 1997.

Esaki T., Hojo H., Kimula T. and Kameda N., Shear-flow coupling test on rock joints, *Proc. 7th Int. Congr. Rock Mech.*, pp. 389-392, 1991.

Goodman R. E., Methods of geological engineering in discontinuous rock, *West publishing company, West St Paul, Minnesota*, 1976.

ISRM, Suggested methods for the quantitative description of discontinuities in rock masses, *Int. J. Rock. Mech. Min. Sci*, 15 (6), 1978.

Kulatilake P. H. S. W., Shou G., Huang T. H. and Morgan R. M., New peak shear strength criteria for anisotropic rock joints, *Int. J. Rock. Mech. Min. Sci. & Geomech. Abstr.*, Vol. 32, No. 7, pp. 673-697, 1995.

Ladanyi B. and Archambault G., Simulation of shear behavior of a jointed rock mass. *Proc. 11th Symp. Rock Mech., AIME, New York*, pp. 105-125, 1970.

Lee Y. H., Carr J. R., Barr D. J. and Hass C. T., The fractal dimension as a measure of the roughness of rock discontinuity profiles. *Int. J. Rock. Mech. Min. Sci, Abstr.* 27 (6), pp. 453-464, 1990.

Maerz N. H. and Franklin J. A., Roughness scale and fractal dimension, Scale effect in rock masses, *Proc. 1st Int. Workshop on Scale Effects in Rock Masses (Edited by A.Pinto da Cunha)*, pp.121-126, Balkma, Rotterdam/Brookfield,1990.

Patton F. D., Multiple modes of shear failure in rock, In: *Proc., 1st Congress Int. Soc. Rock Mechanics, Lisbon*, 1, pp. 509-513, 1966.

Reeves M. J., Rock surface roughness and friction strength, *Int. J. Rock. Mech. Min. Sci, Abstr.* 22 (6), pp. 429-446, 1985.

Tse R. and Cruden D. M., Estimating joint roughness coefficients. *Int. J. Rock. Mech. Min. Sci, Abstr.* 16, pp. 303-307, 1979.

Xie H. and Pariseau W. G., Fractal dimension of joint roughness coefficients, *Preprints of fractured and jointed rock masses, Lake Tahoe*, pp. 132-139, 1992.

Relaxation of shear stress along rock discontinuity

N. H. Tubagus
Graduate School, Department of Geo-system Engineering, The University of Tokyo, Japan

K. Fukui & S. Okubo
Department of Geo-system Engineering, The University of Tokyo, Japan

ABSTRACT: Although several fundamental aspects of rock discontinuities have been resolved and widely accepted, most of them are based on either geologically-oriented research or mechanically-oriented research without paying proper attention to the time-dependent behaviour. These researches up to date are insufficient to describe the rheological properties of rock discontinuities. This paper presents some results from an ongoing experimental research aiming at a fundamental rheological or time-dependent behaviour of rock discontinuities. In order to investigate rheological aspect in the shear behaviour of rock discontinuities, relaxation tests in a direct shear testing machine were carried out on artificial rock discontinuity. It was found that shear behaviour of rock discontinuity is a kind of time-dependent behaviour and similar to the time-dependent behaviour of rock in uniaxial compression.

1. INTRODUCTION

It is known that a mine will easily drift when discontinuities exist in rock mass. This phenomenon is relating not only to mine but also to construction in civil engineering. Although a great number of studies on discontinuities were performed, however cohesion and coefficient of internal friction are often used for expressing mechanical behaviour of discontinuities [Sancio & Goodman 1979; Singh 1979]. It means that discontinuities in rock mass are considered to cause frictional sliding. According to the experience up to now, enlargement of displacement and deformation were observed frequently after excavation [Balthasar et al. 1987, Panet 1979]. In this case usually the discontinuities are in existence around the field. This is an analogue to interpret that deformation and displacement of discontinuities exhibit a time-dependent behaviour. Research on discontinuities from this point of view is hardly ever carried out [Warwersik 1974; Kaiser & Morgenstern 1987].

In this study, first, in order to investigate time dependent phenomena of shearing surface of rock, relaxation tests in a direct shearing experiment were conducted. Current direct shearing machine was improved and used as experiment equipment. It was found that paying close attention to the measurement of stress and displacement was important. So far relaxation test in shearing experiment was not performed, the experiment was started after the experiment method was well established. Moreover, for the purpose of comparison, relaxation tests were conducted under uniaxial compression and uniaxial tension using the same sample rock. Many studies on relaxation in uniaxial compressive tests were carried out [Fukui 1990], the experiment was brought to completion in a short time relatively. On the other hand, relaxation test under uniaxial tensile stress condition is hardly ever carried out, the study had to start from developing of experimental method. The experiment was conducted using simplified uniaxial tension testing method for complete stress-strain curves [Okubo & Fukui 1996].

This paper presents studies of relaxation under shearing stress condition, uniaxial compressive stress condition and uniaxial tensile condition. It is thought that the paper is the only one studies on relaxation under these 3 stress conditions.

2. EXPERIMENTAL SETUP AND PROCEDURE

The main features of the experimental equipment are illustrated in Fig. 1. The lower shear box is set to be fixed to the main frame. The upper shear box can be pulled back and forth by means of spanner and screw connected to the horizontal load cell which pushes the side bearing between the load cell and the shear box. The direction of the upper shear box is kept constant as it moves and the rotation of the shear box about the vertical axis is restricted. The normal stress is applied through a bearing on the upper surface of the upper shear box along a vertical fixed line. This stress is applied by hydraulic ram whose pressure is controlled by pressure-control valve in order to maintain the setting value. The basic design of the measuring system is depicted in Fig. 2. Electrical transducers (LVDTs) are used to measure normal and shear displacement, while load cells monitor stress. All the measurement data are transmitted by amplifiers set with 10 Hz filter to TEAC A/D converter equipment. The equipment records the data of load cells and transducers with 5 Hz sampling frequency on floppy disk digitally. In the experiment, a pen-recorder is also set for plotting normal, shear stress and displacement versus time curves.

Methods used to asses time dependent behaviour of rock discontinuity are based on results of creep test and relaxation tests performed on the samples in laboratory test. Having purpose on investigating viscoelastic phenomena, frequently creep tests are carried out and great deal of works have been completed for uniaxial compressive test [Fukui 1990]. In shear test, creep test is also representing time dependent testing method, unfortunately it is very difficult and needs special technique to satisfy creep condition in post-failure region of shearing test. This gives the authors reason to carry out relaxation test in the study.

After setting the sample in the shear box, shear test was run with initial value of normal stress 2 MPa. A relaxation test (constant normal, shear displacements) in pre-failure region was conducted for 1 hour when shear stress reached value of 4 MPa. Then shear test continued to develop discontinuity as failure progressed in shear plane. In post-failure region where the discontinuity was completely developed, relaxation tests were conducted 4 times for 1 hour each. Retrieving starting relaxation state, sample was pushed forward for about 100 μm before the next relaxation test started. The experiment was terminated when the last relaxation test finished. During the relaxation tests shear stress acting on predetermined plane (shear plane in pre-failure region and discontinuity in post-failure region) was measured as the experiment result.

The rock samples used in this study were bored from Japanese Tage tuff. The samples had a 50 mm diameter, 50 mm length, and were dried more than 1 month in room kept between 20 °C before the experiments. During the experiments, temperature and relative humidity were maintained 22±2°C and 60±15%.

Mechanical properties of the samples are given in table 1.

3. EXPERIMENT RESULTS

In order to investigate time-dependent behaviour of shearing surface, relaxation tests in post-failure region were performed. The stress data which is detected by load cell has possibility not expressing stress relaxation of discontinuity surface, but the whole part of sample. Neglecting this possibility, relaxation test in pre-failure region was conducted when shear stress reached 4 MPa which was greater then stress level of relaxation in post-failure region.

Table 1 Mechanical properties of Tage tuff

Compressive strength (MPa)	17
Tensile strength (MPa)	0.8
Shear strength (MPa)	7.2
Young's Modulus (GPa)	6.6
Specific gravity	1.8

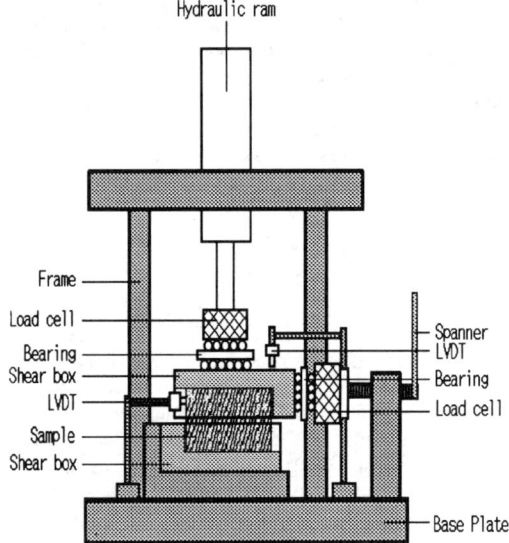

Fig.1 Experiment equipments for rock relaxation test under shearing condition

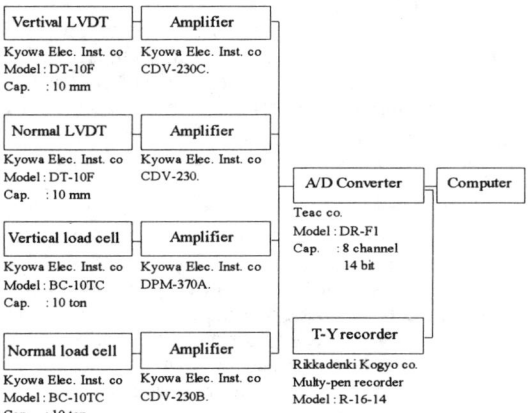

Fig.2 Measuring system design

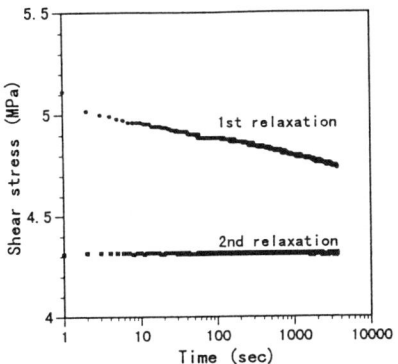

Fig.3 Preliminary test results

In post-failure region stress relaxation was negligible at the other part of sample after this higher level stress relaxation was conducted. To clear up this point a preliminary test was conducted.

Preliminary test

Two relaxation tests in pre-failure region of shearing test were performed. After loading the sample to 5 MPa, relaxation test was carried out for 1 hour. Then 0.5 MPa unloading was conducted before the 2nd relaxation test was started. Fig.3 showing the tests result approves that stress relaxation can not be detected after the higher level of stress relaxation is conducted.

Shearing test.

Fig. 4 shows the data obtained from 3 experiment results of the relaxation test in pre-failure region. Shear stress are plotted versus time, during the test. After the test was started, the stress decreased rapidly in 100 sec. The decreasing of stress became slower until it was too small to be measured after 2000 sec. Within a relaxation time of 1 hour, the stress dropped approximately 0.15 MPa. Relationship between the shear stress relaxation and log time is shown in Fig.5. The stress decreased along straight lines having the same inclination.

The shear stress relaxations which are observed in post-failure region result in a nearly uniform type of stress relaxation curves, as shown in Figs. 6 and 7. These curves represent the stress relaxation of discontinuity. In post-failure region, relaxation tests were conducted 4 times for 1 hour each. The stress dropped sharply in 100 sec then became slowly until it indicated very small change after 3000 seconds. The decreasing of stress came not up to about 0.4 MPa within the test duration amounting to 1 hour. The shear stress has a linear relation with log time as shown in Fig. 7, which can be expressed as

$$\tau = a - b\log(t) \qquad (1)$$

where a, b are constants relating to initial shear stress relaxation and t is time of relaxation test. It is apparent that the characteristics of the data resemble data obtained from relaxation test in compression.

In post-failure region, relaxation tests were repeated after the sample was pushed forward for about 100 μ m where discontinuity reached residual

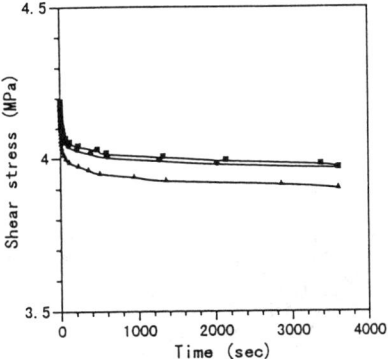

Fig.4 Shear stress versus time (pre-failure region)

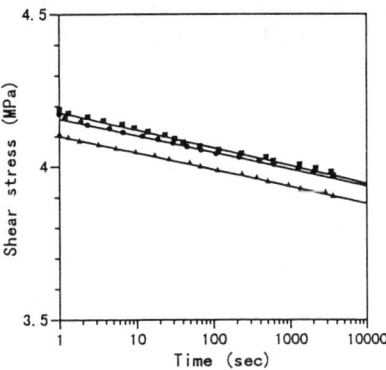

Fig.5 Shear stress versus time in semi-log scale (pre-failure region)

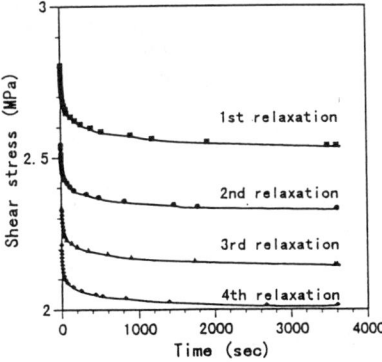

Fig.6 Shear stress versus time (post-failure region)

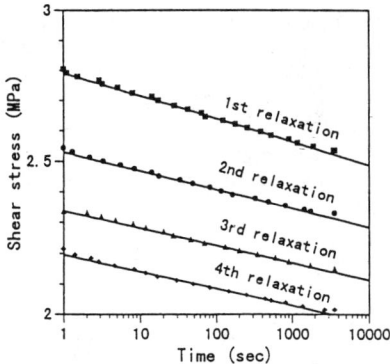

Fig.7 Shear stress versus time in semi-log scale (post-failure region)

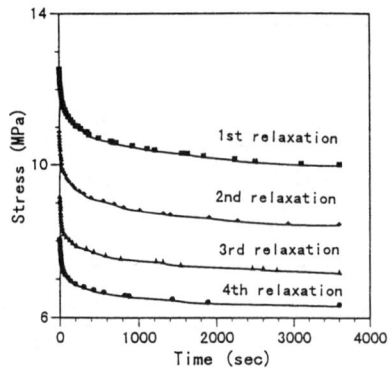

Fig. 9 Relaxation in compression (post-failure region)

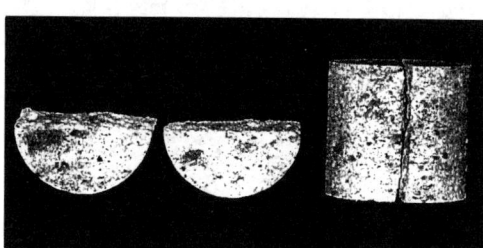

Fig.8 Photograph of the used samples

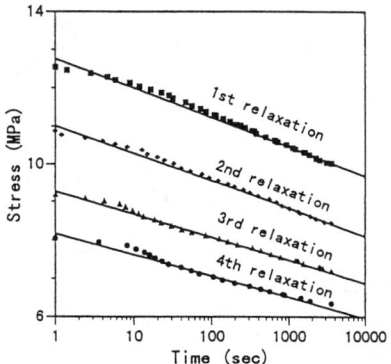

Fig. 10 Relaxation in compression in semi-log scale (post-failure region)

stress condition. The results (Figs. 6 and 7) also allow observation of the repeated relaxation effect on structure change of the sample with decreasing of initial stress since each relaxation is a response to the material properties at the given stress and strain condition. This phenomenon suggest that relaxation causes decreasing of residual stress of discontinuity.

Fig.8 is photograph of the used samples. The discontinuity surface was smoother than the expected.

Compression test

A closed-loop servo-controlled testing machine was used to carry out relaxation test in uniaxial compression test. The specifications of the machine are as follows: (i) loading capacity: 100 kN, (ii) stroke: ±0.01 m, (iii) maximum piston speed: 0.015 m/sec, (iv) oil pressure: 21 MPa, (v) maximum flow rate: 45 l/min, (vi) control method: digital.

The machine enables control of experimental variables automatically and precisely. A feedback signal representing some experimental condition is generated by transducers and compared with the program signal which represents the desired condition. If a difference exists, an error signal is generated and used to instigate corrective action.

Compression test was performed with 10^{-5}/sec strain rate. Relaxation tests were conducted in post-failure region 4 times for 1 hour each. After the last relaxation test was finished, the experiment was terminated.

Representative results of the relaxation tests are given in Fig. 9. The stress decreased linearly to the log time as shown in the Fig. 10. The inclinations of the stress drop are almost the same. The test result shows common tendency of relaxation test in compression. Decreasing of initial stress in relaxation following the number of test is more effected by increasing of strain than repeated relaxation as in the shearing test.

Tension test

The main specifications of the servo-controlled testing machine employed for uniaxial tension test are as follows: (I) capacity: 10 kN, (ii) frame stiffness: 1GN/m, (iii) maximum ram speed: 3 cm/sec, and (iv) system frequency: DC-100 Hz. Platen displacement and force are respectively, measured by a LVDT with 0.1 μm resolution and a strain gauge type of load cell.

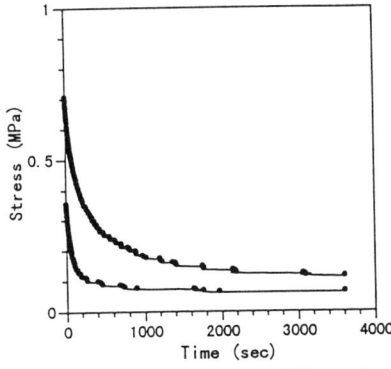

Fig. 11 Relaxation in tension (post-failure region)

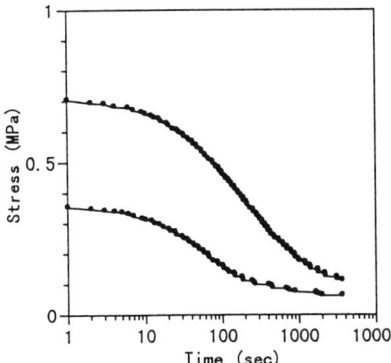

Fig. 12 Relaxation in tension in semi-log scale (post-failure region)

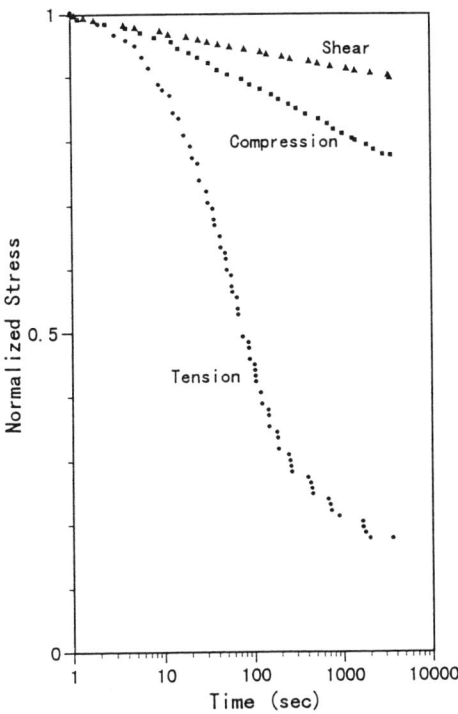

Fig. 13 Relaxation in post-failure region of shear test, compression and tension

Before uniaxial tension test is carried out, the experiment devices and specimen were prepared as follows. After liberally coating the top end of specimen with epoxy resin, it is affixed to the surface of upper platen (bolt head) and allowed to set for 24 hours. The bolt portion of the platen is then screwed into the ram head and the specimen's bottom end is correspondingly affixed to a similar in-place lower platen, after which a slight load (100 N) is placed on the specimen for 24 hours prior to tension. This test assembly has been acceptable alignment in the previous work [Okubo & Fukui 1996].

Tension tests were performed with 10^{-6}/sec loading rate. Sets of typical relaxation curves in tension are presented in Fig. 11. Relaxation test was performed 1 hour in post-failure region. The stress dropped sharply in 200 sec, then this decreasing of stress became slowly before it was too small to be measured in 3000 sec. Fig.12 shows stress relaxation versus time in semi-log scale. In contrast to tension never the inclination of stress in semi-log curve decreased in shear test and compression.

4. DISCUSSION AND CONCLUSION

It is found that discontinuity exhibits time-dependent behavior as indicated in Figs. 6 and 7. The relaxation stress of discontinuity may be represented by equation 1. Relaxation stress in post failure region of compression is also satisfied to equation 1.

In order to find the value of b in equation 1, relaxation data in the different stress conditions are compared quantitatively in Fig. 13. The stress were normalized by their initial values then plotted versus time in semi-log scale. This depiction illustrates stress curves of relaxation in shear test (post-failure region) has the slight different inclination from in compression. If only the linear part of relaxation in tension is considered, the values of b increase in turn of shear, compression, tension. Within 1 hour of the relaxation time, stress dropped approximately 10% in shearing test which is almost double compared with the value in compression.

In post-failure region of shear test, compression and tension, crack (or discontinuity) are in existence. In case of shearing test and compression it is thought that compressive stress work on crack perpendicularly restricting crack propagation and frictional force occur along the crack surface. This similar stress state condition in shearing test and compression cause similar tendency in relaxation behavior. In tension, tensile stress worked on crack accelerating crack propagation, thus the stress drop rapidly.

In this study, the experiments showed that discontinuity exhibits time-dependent behaviour and relaxation behaviour of discontinuity has a similar tendency to relaxation in compression.

ACKNOWLEDGMENTS

The authors wish to thank to Mr. M. Akiyama of the University of Tokyo for various aspects of preparation and experiment support.

REFERENCES

Balthasar, K., M. Haupt, Ch. Lempp, & O. Natau 1987. Stress relaxation behaviour of rock salt: comparison of in situ measurements and laboratory test result. Proceedings of the 6th International Congress on Rock Mechanics: 11-13.
Dieterich, J. H. 1972. Time-dependent friction in rocks. Journal of Geophysical Research. 77: 3690-3697.
Fukui K. 1990. Creep and retardation time of rock. Doctoral thesis, University of Tokyo.
Kaiser, P. K. & N. R. Morgenstern 1979. Time-dependent deformation of jointed rock near failure. Proceedings of the 4th International Congress on Rock Mechanics: 195-202.
Lembo, F. A., P. Tommasi & R.Ribacchi 1990. Sheared bedding joints in rocks engineering: two case histories in Italy. Proceedings of the 1st International Symposium on Rock joints: 83-90.
Natau, O., Ch. Lempp & G. Borm 1986. Stress relaxation monitoring prestresssed hard inclusions. Proceedings of the International Symposium on Rock stress and rock stress measurements: 509-514.
Okubo, S. & K. Fukui 1996. Simplified Uniaxial tension testing: complete stress-strain curves for various rock types. Int. J. Rock Mech. Min. Sci. & Geomech. Abstr. 33: 549-556.
Okubo, S., Y. Nishimatsu & C. He 1990. Loading rate dependence of class II rock behavior in uniaxial and triaxial compression tests: an application of proposed new control method. Int. J. Rock Mech. Min. Sci. & Geomech. Abstr. 27: 559-562.
Panet, M. 1979. Time-dependent deformations in underground works. Proceedings of the 4th International Congress on Rock Mechanics: 279-289.
Passaris, E. K. S 1979. The rheological behavior of rocksalt as determined in an in situ pressurized test cavity. Proceedings of the 4th International Congress on Rock Mechanics: 257-264.
Sancio, R. T. and R. E. Goodman 1979. Analysis of the stability of slopes in weathered rocks. Proceedings of the 4th International Congress on Rock Mechanics: 723-730.
Sigh, D. P. 1979. A study of frictional properties of rock. Proceedings of the 4th International Congress on Rock Mechanics: 301-305.
Warwersik W.R. 1974. Time-dependent behavior of rock in compression. Proceedings of the 3rd International Congress on Rock Mechanics: 357-363.

Penetration experiment of rocks by use of TBM roller bit with aiming the fast execution: Effect of bit shape

H. Takahashi, S. Suzuoki & N. Hatakeyama
Department of Geoscience and Technology, Tohoku University, Sendai, Japan

S. Nunomura & Y. Shimizu
Hitachi Zosen Corporation, Japan

ABSTRACT: This paper presents the effect of TBM roller bit shape on rock cutting under high thrust forces. As a fundamental study, the penetration experiment of rocks by use of TBM roller bit was carried out. Through the experiment, it was found that the round tip bit is useful for soft rock cutting. The chipping was observed quite often at high thrust forces, and the specific energy became small. On the other hand, the sharp tip bit is useful for hard rock cutting. The penetration distance was quite small when the round tip bit was used even if the thrust force was 40 ton. However, the chipping was observed when the sharp tip bit was used and specific energy was much smaller than that of round tip bit.

1 INTRODUCTION

Recently, Tunnel Boring Machine(TBM) has been used widely to construct the tunnel. Many studies have been already carried out to investigate the cutting mechanism of rocks by using the disc cutter, gauge cutter and roller bit. Although TBM is a useful machine, the bits and cutters installed on the cutting face of the machine are supported by the bearings which are not so strong for high thrust forces of the hydraulic cylinders. Therefore, previous studies dealt with the thrust forces less than about 20 ton per cylinder. However, a new bearing for high thrust forces has been developed recently. Therefore, the high thrust forces by the cylinder will be available in the near future, resulting in the fast execution. However, the cutting mechanism under high thrust forces is not made clear yet.

Therefore, the aims of this study are to examine the effect of the TBM roller bit shape on rock cutting behavior under high thrust forces up to 50 ton and to search the possibility of fast execution with increasing the thrust forces.

2 EXPERIMENTAL APPARATUS

Figure 1 shows the schematic diagram of the experimental apparatus. As shown in this figure, the servo-controlled testing machine was used. Since the aim of this experiment is to investigate the effect of bit shape on rock cutting mechanism through the penetration experiment, a part of the actual roller bit was made and fixed in the testing machine. The thrust forces were measured with the load cell. The penetration distance was measured with the displacement transducers. The signals from the load cell and displacement transducers were transmitted to the personal computer through a strain meter and an A/D converter. The sampling interval was 0.1 sec. Since it was difficult to control the loading speed automatically, it was controlled by hands. The approximate loading speed was 3 ton/sec.

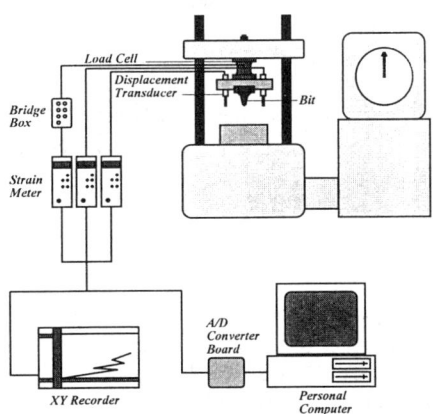

Fig.1 Schematic diagram of experimental apparatus

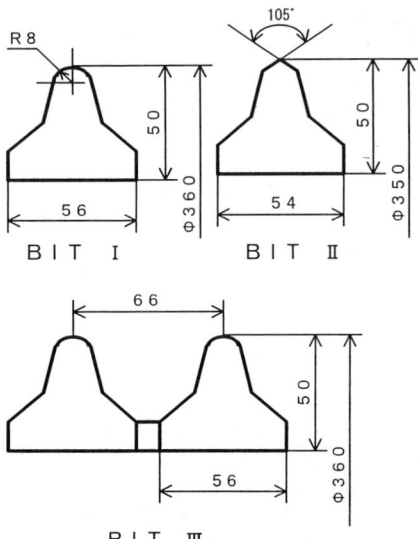

Fig.2 Shape of the bits used in this experiment

Table 1 Properties of rocks

Rock	Density [kg/m^3]	Uniaxial Compressive Strength [MPa]	Young's Modulus [Gpa]
Shirakawa welded tuff	2057	34.2	3.57
Iidate Granite	2635	226.6	31.18
Cement	2185	86.1	11.38

Figure 2 shows the schematic diagram of the bits used in this experiment. In the actual operation of TBM, the bits rotate and cut the rock. However, because this experiment is a penetration experiment, the bit does not need to rotate. Therefore, a part of the actual bit as shown in this figure were made and was used in the experiment. Two kinds of roller bit were used to investigate the effect of bit shape on the rock cutting mechanism. One is the bit whose tip is rather round (Type Ⅰ). The radius of the tip is 8mm. The other one is the bit whose tip is sharp (Type Ⅱ). The angle of the bit tip is 105 degree. Type Ⅲ is the bit which two Type Ⅰ bits are set with a distance of 66mm.

Two kinds of rocks were used in this experiment. One is Shirakawa welded tuff and the other one is Iidate granite. Furthermore, the cement was used to investigate the effect of uniaxial compressive strength of rocks. The size of rock sample is 200mm × 200mm × 150mm. The physical properties of the rocks are listed in Table 1.

3 EXPERIMENTAL RESULTS

Figure 3 and 4 show the relationship between the penetration distance of the bit and resistive forces for Shirakawa welded tuff and Iidate Granite, respectively. For Shirakawa welded tuff, the effect of chipping on the rock cutting is remarkable at higher thrust forces and penetration distance became very large when the Type Ⅰ bit was used. On the other hand, when Type Ⅱ bit was used, the chipping is not so remarkable and cutting volume of the rock was not so large. Since the rock is soft and the bit tip is sharp, the bit is easy to penetrate into the rock, but it does not work efficiently for breaking the rock.

For Iidate granite, since the rock is hard, the penetration distance of Type Ⅰ bit is very small and the chipping was not observed. Furthermore, the cutting volume of the rock is quite little. On the other hand, when the Type Ⅱ bit was used, the chipping

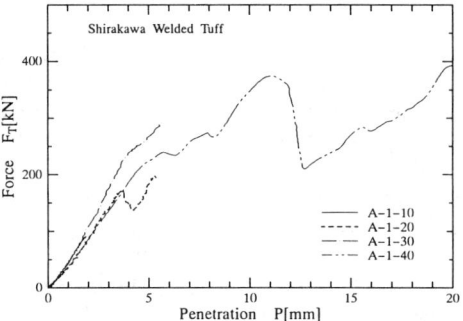

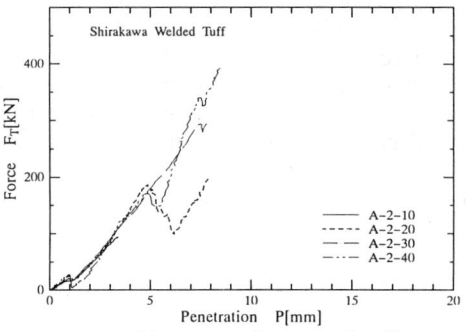

Fig.3 Relationship between the penetration distance and resistive forces for Shirakawa welded tuff

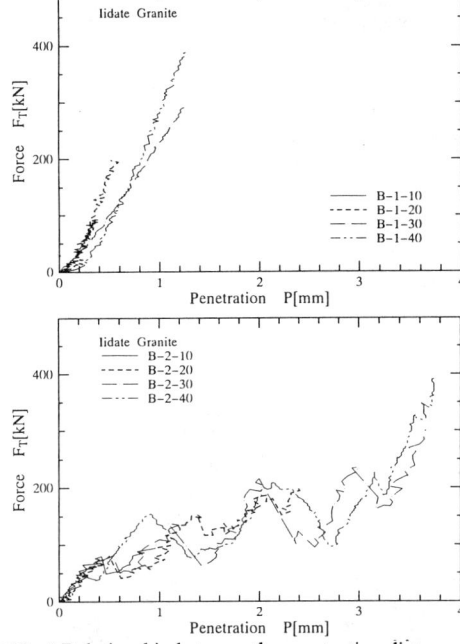

Fig.4 Relationship between the penetration distance and resistive forces for Iidate Granite

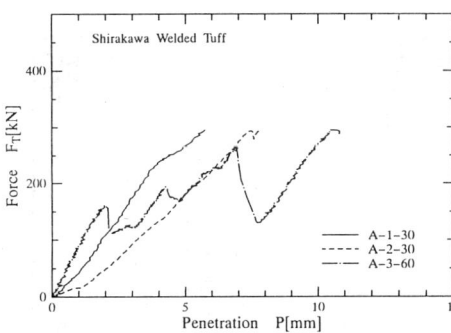

Fig.5 Effect of the bit shape on the rock cutting for Shirakawa welded tuff

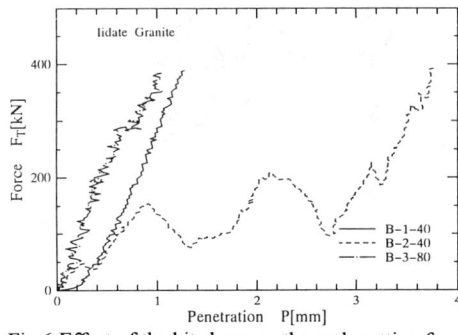

Fig.6 Effect of the bit shape on the rock cutting for Iidate granite

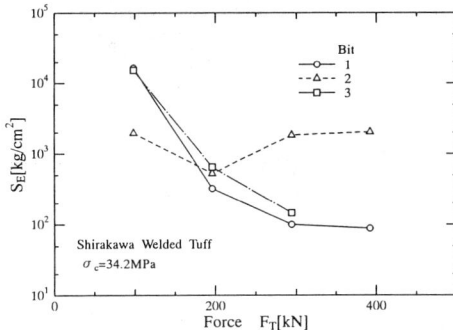

Fig.7 Specific energy of rock cutting for Shirakawa welded tuff

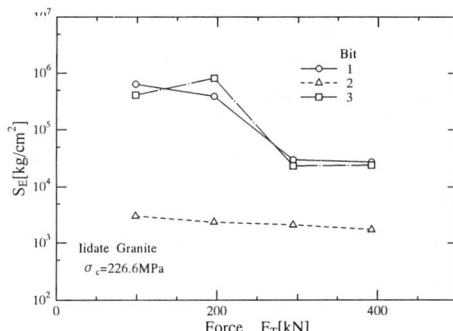

Fig.8 Specific energy of rock cutting for Iidate granite

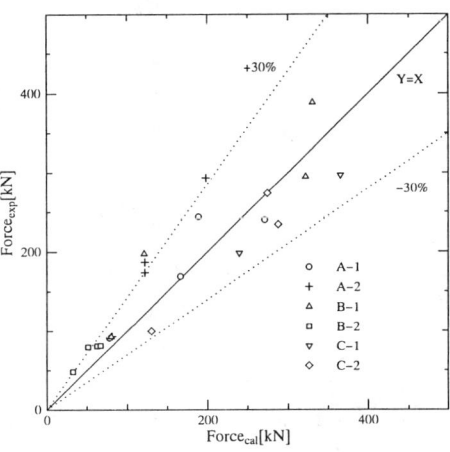

Fig.9 Comparison between calculated values and measured ones for resistive forces

was observed quite often at higher thrust forces and the penetration distance was larger compared to the one of Type I.

Figure 5 shows the effect of the bit shape on the

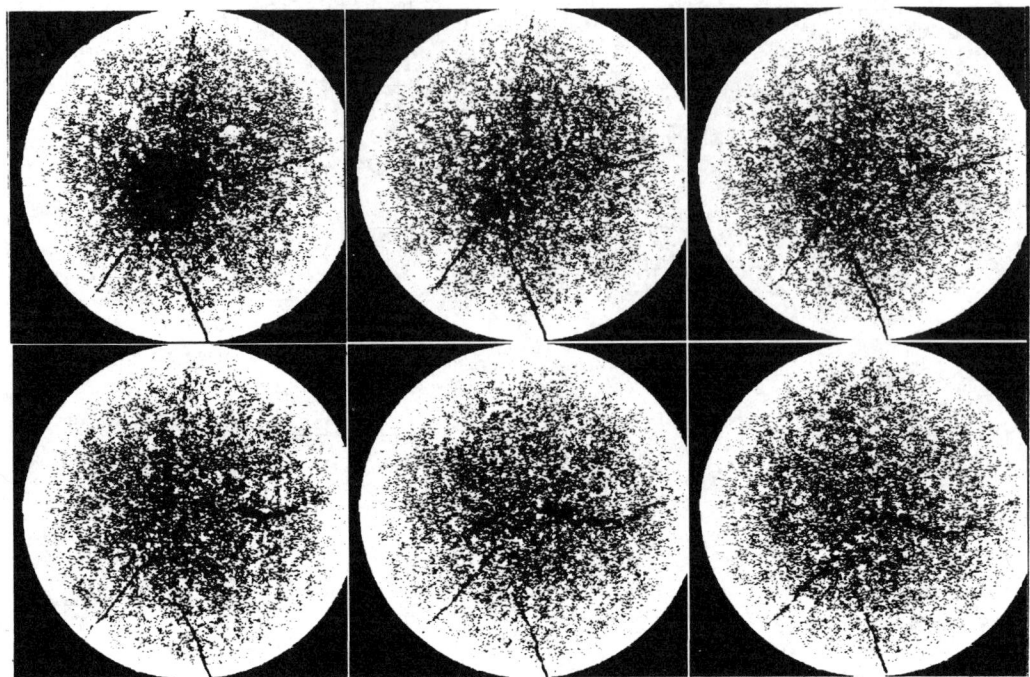
Iidate granite : Type I

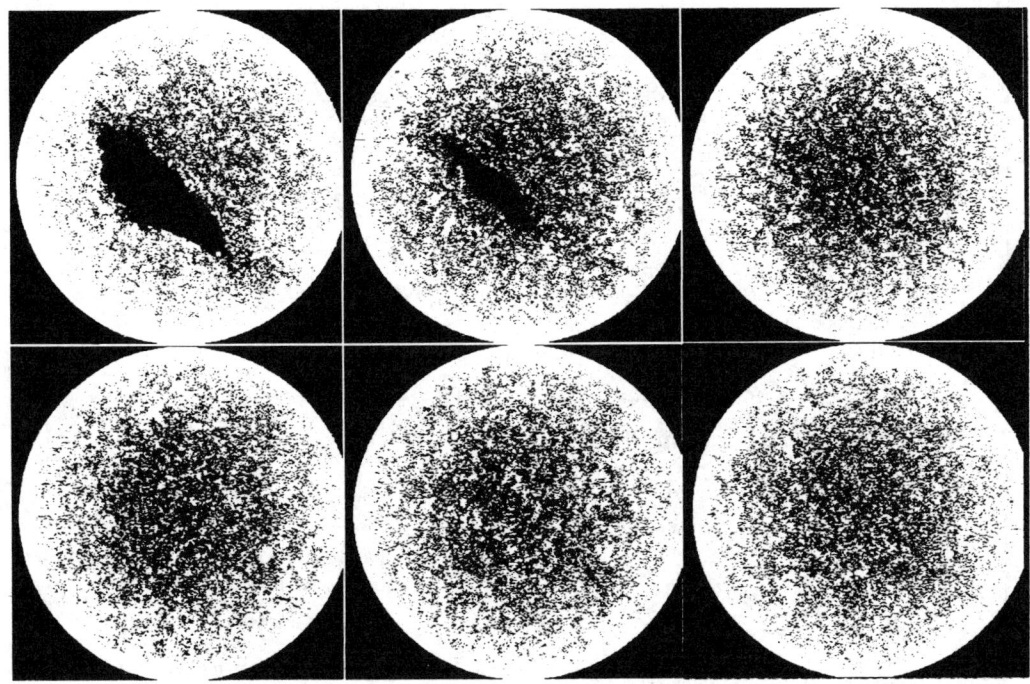
Iidate granite : Type II

Fig.10 Images of cross section of rocks after penetration experiment

rock cutting for Shirakawa welded tuff. The Type III bit shows the deepest penetration distance. It can be considered that this result is due to the effect of neighbor breaking between two bits.

Figure 6 shows the effect of the bit shape on the rock cutting for Iidate granite. The penetration distance of Type I and III bit is about 1mm. On the other hand, the penetration distance of Type II bit is about 4mm. This result shows that shape bit is much more effective for hard rock cutting.

Figure 7 and 8 shows the specific energy of rock cutting for Shirakawa welded tuff and Iidate granite, respectively. The specific energy is defined by the required energy to cut the unit volume of rocks, and is given by

$$S_E = \int_0^P F dP / W \quad (1)$$

Small specific energy means the high efficiency of rock cutting. For Shirakawa welded tuff, S_E of Type I and III bit is large at lower thrust forces. However, S_E of Type I and III bit decreases with increasing the thrust forces and it became smaller than that of Type II bit at higher thrust forces. For Iidate granite, S_E of Type I and III bit decreases with increasing the thrust forces, but it is much larger than that of Type II regardless of the thrust forces. This concludes that the round tip bit is useful for soft rock cutting and the sharp tip bit is useful for hard rock cutting.

It is reported that the relationship between the thrust forces and penetration distance until the first chipping occurs is expressed by the following equation:

$$F_T = a\sigma_c P^n \quad (2)$$

Here a is the coefficient and σ_c is the uniaxial compressive strength of rocks. Several values of n were reported by several researchers, but n is about within the range of 0.5-1.5. Since above equation is obtained at lower thrust forces, it is not made clear that above equation is applicable for the rock cutting at higher thrust forces. Therefore, a and n were obtained from the measure data by using the least square fittings. In result, n was about 1.12 regardless of the rocks and bit shape. The value of a depends on the bit shape and a=0.11 for Type I bit and a=0.061 for Type II bit.

Figure 9 shows the comparison between the measured thrust forces and calculated values from Eq.(2). It is found from this figure that agreement is satisfactory and Eq.(2) is applicable for rock cutting under high thrust forces.

4 OBSERVATION BY USE OF X-RAY SCANNER

Figure 10 shows the images of cross section of the rock after the penetration experiment. These images were obtained by X-ray image scanner. If the fracture exists, the part of fracture becomes black. Excavated parts are also shown with black in this image. When the Type I bit was used, the excavated part is quite little but some fractures exist inside of the rock. On the other hand, when the Type II bit was used, excavated part is large, but any fractures are not observed inside of the rock. In this experiment, the bit does not rotate. If the bit rotates and the fractures which exist inside of the rock are connected with each other, the chipping is expected. This result shows that the possibility to use the round tip bit for hard rock cutting is not very low if the fractures are made inside of the rock by the penetration of the bit into the rock.

5 CONCLUSIONS

In this study, the effect of the bit shape on rock cutting was experimentally investigated under high thrust forces with aiming the fast execution.
(1) When the rock is not so hard, the round tip bit is useful for rock cutting. The chipping was observed quite often at thigh thrust forces, and the specific energy became small.
(2) When the rock is hard, the sharp tip bit is much more useful for rock cutting. The chipping was observed when the sharp tip bit was used and specific energy was much smaller than that of round tip bit. On the other hand, the penetration distance was quite small when the round tip bit was used even if the thrust force was 40 ton. However, it was observed that some fractures exist inside of the rock. This result shows the possibility to use the round tip bit for hard rock cutting.

REFERENCES

Y.Nishimatsu, N.Okuno and Y.Hirasawa 1975. The rock cuttings with roller cutters, *J. of Mining and*

Metallurgical Institute of Japan, 91, 653-658.

G.Fangming, K.Sato and H.Asai 1992. Tool force acting on a disc cutter during circular rock cutting, *J. of Mining and Material Processing Institute of Japan*, 108, 557-562.

G.Fangming, K.Sato and H.Asai 1992. Optimal cutting condition and Maximum tool force in circular rock cutting, *J. of Mining and Material Processing Institute of Japan*, 108, 557-562.

G.Fangming, K.Sato and C.Uchiumi 1994. Tool force and twist acting on TBM gauge cutters, *J. of Mining and Material Processing Institute of Japan*, 110, 277-282.

G.Fangming, K.Sato and C.Uchiumi 1994. Design criterion for restricting tool force exerted on TBM gauge cutters, *J. of Mining and Material Processing Institute of Japan*, 110, 851-856.

G.Fangming, K.Sato and H.Asai 1994. External load imposed on a disc cutter and reaction force excerted at bearing assemblies, *J. of Mining and Material Processing Institute of Japan*, 110, 1133-1138.

G.Fangming, K.Sato and T.Goto 1995. Penetration experiment of rocks by means of disc cutter, *J. of Mining and Material Processing Institute of Japan*, 111, 617-622.

R.A.Snowdon, M.D.Ryley and J.Temporal 1982. A study of disc cutting in selected British rocks, *Int. J. Rock Mech. Min. Sci. & Geomech. Abstr.* 19, 107-121.

F.F.Roxborough and H.R.Phillips 1975. Rock excavation by disc cutter, *Int. J. Rock Mech. Min. Sci. & Geomech. Abstr.* 12, 361-366.

H.P.Sanio 1985. Prediction of the performance of disc cutters in Anistropic rock, *Int. J. Rock Mech. Min. Sci. & Geomech. Abstr.* 22, 153-161.

EX. A-2-30 means as follows:
sample : Shirakawa welded tuff
bit used in the experiment : Type II
maximum thrust forces : 30 ton

APPENDIX

F : resistive force   [kN]
n : power index   [-]
P : penetration distance of the bit   [mm]
S : specific energy   [kg/cm^2]
W : the weight of broken rocks   [kg]

From Fig.3 to Fig.8
  A : Shirakawa welded tuff
  B : Iidate Granite
  1,2,3 : Bit I, II, III
  numbers : maximum thrust forces [ton]

Borehole instability – New drilling tool technology for stability control

J.C. Rowley
Pajarito Enterprises Consulting Services, Los Alamos, N.Mex., USA

ABSTRACT: This paper provides background information on borehole instability encountered for geoscientific projects. These deep core-drilling projects have attempted to use conventional methods of weighted drilling fluids for stability control. In crystalline rocks these measures have often failed. Procedures and new tools for positive borehole stability control have been developed.

1 BACKGROUND AND INTRODUCTION

Several recent ultra-deep geoscientific core drilling projects have experienced borehole instability problems that could not be controlled with the usual method of weighting the drilling fluid.

1.1 *The German KTB project*

The recent ultra-deep geoscientific project in Germany (Chur, et al., 1995) experienced severe borehole breakouts and instability. The Kontinentale Tiefbohrprogramm der Bundesrepublik Deutschland (KTB) project attempted to use weighting of the drill fluid to control these problems. Hoffers & Rischmuller (1991) has provided the basic rock mechanics background for the KTB ultra-deep corehole drilling project. For the crystalline rocks encountered it was noted (Hoffers, et al., 1994 & Haimson, 1996) intrusion of free water into gneiss and amphibolite rocks and speculated that this strategy probably enhanced the borehole instability tendencies.

1.2 *An example from oil and gas drilling*

A recent report (Hogg & Boyle 1997) on drilling of deep oil wells in an overthrust geology in Columbia illustrates the problem of instability of boreholes. The use of water based drilling fluids led to severe borehole instability. Use of air and foam drilling completely relieved the problem in the crystalline rock overthrust geologic setting.

2 NEW METHODS AND TOOLS

Severe borehole instabilities encountered in some geologic conditions, when the conventional weighted fluid method fails, has led to the development of improved methods and new tools. Some of these are new and innovative in approach, while others are well proven and have been in service for several years. Some methods rely on rock mechanics (Wong, et al., 1994) testing of cores. Others are expandable linings that provide mechanical supporting materials cemented in place with fiber reinforced cements. These latter methods and tools resemble the lining and ground control techniques common in tunneling and shaft drilling.

2.1 *Use of pilot coring and on site rock mechanics testing*

It has been suggested (Rowley, et al., 1996) that the use of pilot core-ahead and ream-out techniques could provide the potential for predicting borehole instability. This concept is illustrated in Fig. 1. Recently the Italian petroleum drilling industry has adopted a similar methodology and procedures (Zousa, et al., 1997).

For the proposed pilot coreahead method, a large diameter reaming bit with a hollow center has a wireline core barrel and bit that extends through the reaming bit. Cores from the pilot core hole are rapidly tested with appropriate rock mechanics tests (Chevenert & Amanullah, 1997) in an on-site laboratory. Therefore, a prediction of the stability or instability of the main, large diameter hole can be made before the reaming step is continued. Then by selection of the appropriate drilling fluid to be used for the reaming operation the borehole stability can be maintained.

Alternatively, rock property measurements in the pilot core hole can be used to predict stability (Mizzoni, et al., 1997). Both methods are being employed in oil and gas drilling. Ewy, et al., (1994) illustrates the early configuration changes and the nature of the crack initiation in the borehole wall, Fig. 2, as borehole breakouts start to occur. Such crack initiation patterns should be detectable with properly devised sensors within the pilot core hole.

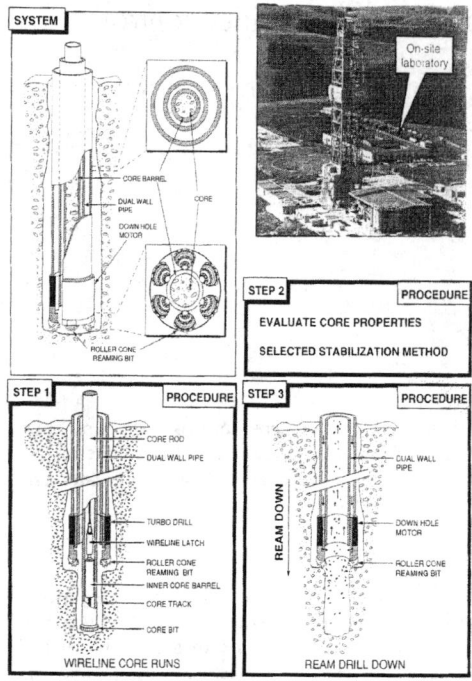

Figure 1. Pilot core drilling strategy & on-site core testing to predict & mitigate borehole instability.

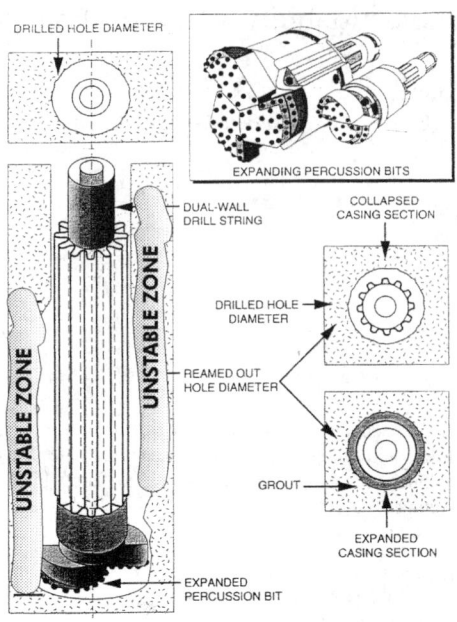

Figure 3. Illustration of conceptual design of tool for borehole stability control, uses an expandable, corrugated tube.

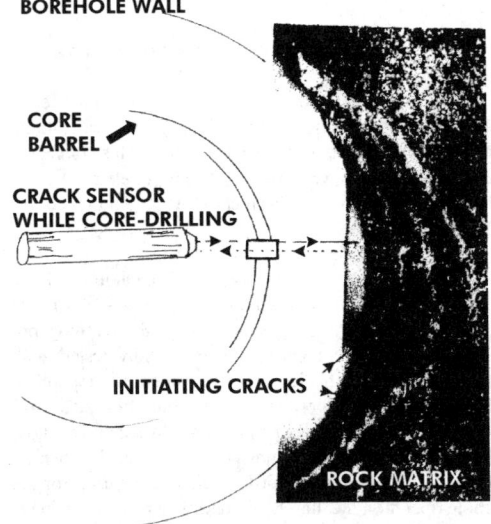

Figure 2. Liquid metal enhanced indications of initiation of borehole breakout; an illustration of potential for measurements while coring.

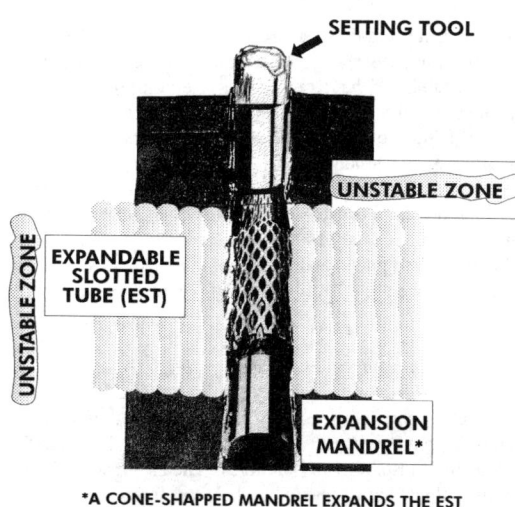

Figure 4. Example of an expandable tool for borehole stabilization, available from Shell E. & P. Int'l.

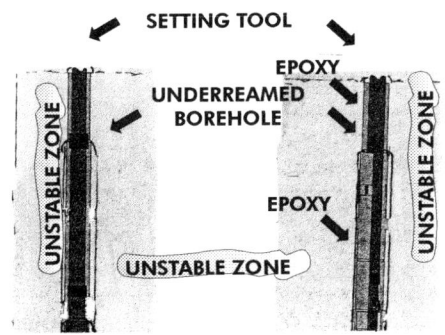

| UNDERREAMING | PRESSURE EXPANSION OF ISOLASION PROFILE LINER |

EXPANDABLE ISOLATION PROFILE
LINER COVERS UNSTABLE ZONES

Courtesy: The TatNIPIneft Institute,
Bugulma, Tatarstan

Figure 5. Expanding tube with epoxy glue; available commercially from Tatarstan.

These approaches require a considerable collaboration between the scientists in the on-site laboratory and the drilling technologist. Rapid and real-time tests and drilling fluid changes are required.

In addition rock property measurements on core or out-crop samples can be tested before the ultra-deep core drilling is initiated, if such samples can be obtained.

2.2 *Borehole lining tools*

Three new tools have been proposed or are in use in oil and gas drilling to support severely unstable zones in a wellbore.

Rowley, et al., (1996) suggests that an expandable percussion hammer can be used to ream an unstable zone and a laterally corrugated liner-patch expanded into the zone and cemented in place with an appropriate epoxy, Fig. 3. This concept is based on a very successful existing casing patch tool.

There are two expandable patches that can be used in a reamed-out zone. The patch is cemented in place using cement re-enforced with specially selected fibers. Fig. 4 shows an expandable mesh technique (Gill, et al., 1995) offered by the Shell Co. In addition, Fig. 5 (Abdaklmanov, et al., 1995) illustrates a Tatarstan technique for placement and expoxy cementing of an expandable section of tubing into a reamed-out unstable zone.

3. CONCLUSIONS

The above suggested approach can provide an advance warning of the potential bore stability problems that may be encountered by ultra-deep geoscientific core-drilling projects. One such project is being planned and studied in Japan. This project is projected to require depths greater than 10 km and will penetrate rather young geologic age rocks (Urabe, 1994). Therefore, this project, named Japan Ultra-Deep Geoscientific Experiment (JUDGE) should be alert to the need for the perfection and development of the methods and techniques described here.

It is apparent that suitable current methods in rock mechanics testing, core analyses, and downhole measurements can be devised. This will ensure that borehole instability will not compromise nor limit the depth or technical sampling of the inter-plate zone between the Pacific and Philippines Sea plates as envisaged by the authors of the JUDGE project.

Early and intense work will be required by scientists, rock mechanics experts, and drilling engineers if the potential borehole instability problems for projects such as the JUDGE project are to be solved.

REFERENCES

Abdaklmanov, G. S., B. Roberson & B. Powel 1995. "Isolation Profile Liner Helps Stabilize Problem Well Bores", Oil & Gas Jour., 50-52, Sept., Tulsa OK USA.

Chenevert, M. E. & Amanullah 1997. "Shale Preservation and Testing Techniques for Borehole Stability studies", Proceedings of the SP/IADC Drilling Conference, 863-868, Amsterdam, Netherlands.

Chur, C.B., T. Bendzko, B. Engesser, A. Sperber, T. V. Trach, & L. Wohlgemuth 1995."KTB-4 Year's Experience at the Limits of Drilling Technology", Proceedings of the SPE/IADC Drilling Conference, 673-686, Amsterdam, Netherlands.

Ewy, R. T., L. R. Myer & N. G. W. Cook 1994. "Investigation of Stress-induced Borehole Enlargement Mechanisms by a Liquid Metal Saturation Technique", J. Spe Drilling & Completions Engrg., 65-72, March, Richardson TX USA.

Gill, D. S. & W. C. M. Lohbeck 1996. "Expandable Tube Is Novel Tool for Difficult Completions, Drilling", Oil & Gas Jour., 37-40, June, Tulsa OK USA.

Haimson, B. G. 1996. "Improved In Situ Stress Determination in the KTB Ultra-Deep Hole From Logged Breakouts and a Truely Tri-Axial Strength Criterion", Proceedings of the VIIIth International Symposium on the Observation of the Continental Crust Through Drilling, 194-203, Tsukuba, Japan.

Hoffers, B., B. Engeser & H. Rischmuller 1994. "Wellbore Stability of a Superdeep Bore hole in Crystalline Rock", Proceedings SPE/ISRM International Conference, SPE 28073, 371-378, Delft, Netherlands.

Hoffers, B., & H. Rischmuller 1991. "Borehole Stability of a Large Diameter Borehole in Hard Rock - First Results of Continental Deep-Drilling Project", Proceedings of the 7th International Soc. of Rock Mechanics Congress, 1639-1644, Aachen, Germany, Balkema, Rotterdam, Netherlands.

Hogg, R. W., & J. Boyle 1997. "Columbian Underbalanced

Drilling Operations - Start-Up Experience", Proceedings of the SPE/IADC Drilling Conference, 891-900, Amsterdam, Netherlands.

Mizzoni, R., T. Wahdan, A. Bassem & C. D. Ward 1997. "Real-Time Pore and Fracture Pressure Prediction FEWD in the Nile Delta", Proceedings of the SPE/IADC Drilling Conference, 825-836, Amsterdam, Netherlands.

Moody, F. & A. H. Hale 1993. "Bore-Hole Stability Model the Mechanics and Chemistry Drilling Fluids/Shale Interactions", SPE Jour. Pet. Engrg., 1093-1104, November, Richardson TX USA.

Rowley, J.C., R. Long, S. Saito & T. Ito 1996. "Ultra-Deep Core-Drilling Strategy and System Concepts", Proceedings of the VIIIth International Symposium on the Observation of the Contentinal Crust Through Drilling, 316-321, Tsukuba, Japan.

Urabe, T., 1994. "Ultra-Deep Drilling into the Subduction Plate Boundary in the Japanese Island Arc (JUDGE Project)" Proceedings V the VIIth Int'l. Symposium on the Observation of the Continental Crust Through Drilling, 225-228, Santa Fe NM USA.

Wong, S.W., C. A. M. Veekam & C. J. Kentner 1994. "The Rock-Mechanical Aspects of Drilling a North Sea Horizontal Well", J. SPE Drilling & Completion Engrg., March, Richardson TX USA.

Zousa, F., 1. Civil+oni, M. Brignoll & F. Sontraelli 1997. "Real-Time Wellbore-Stability Analysis at the Rigsite" Conference, 837-846, Amsterdam, Netherlands.

A tensile principal stress analysis for estimating three-dimensional in-situ stresses from core discing

K. Matsuki, K. Hongo & K. Sakaguchi
Department of Geoscience and Technology, Tohoku University, Sendai, Japan

ABSTRACT: The direction and magnitude of tensile principal stresses within and below a long HQ core stub were analyzed using a finite element method for 77 in-situ stress conditions. Core discing was considered to be likely to occur under 26 of these stress conditions. A criterion for core discing was then proposed by evaluating the maximum tensile principal stress which is necessary for the contour plane to be formed throughout a cross-section of the core. Summarizing the results obtained by an analysis of the distribution of the direction of the tensile principal stress, a procedure for determining the direction of principal in-situ stress from the geometry of a disc was proposed, based upon the symmetry of the end surfaces, the normal direction in the central part of the end surfaces and the direction of the concave or convex axes in the end surfaces.

1 INTRODUCTION

Several researchers have tried to use core discing to obtain information about in-situ stresses (Jaeger and Cook 1963, Obert and Stephenson 1965, Durelli et al. 1968, Sugawara et al. 1978, Stacey 1982, Haimson and Lee 1995). Most of these previous investigations, excluding a few (Dyke 1989), were based on the incorrect assumption that one of the principal in-situ stresses is always in the direction of the core axis. In particular, this assumption is not applicable to an inclined well bore. Recently, it was shown that the directions of the maximum and intermediate principal stresses could be determined from a so-called saddle-shaped disc (Dyke 1989, Haimson and Lee 1995). However, the effects of the direction of principal in-situ stress on the shape of a disc are not well understood, particularly when the principal in-situ stresses are inclined relative to the core axis.

In this study, to develop a method for estimating three-dimensional in-situ stress from core discing, a tensile principal stress analysis was carried out based on the assumption that core discing occurs due to tensile stress. The magnitude and direction of tensile principal stress were analyzed with a finite element method for a region within and below a long HQ core stub, which is bored in a general state of in-situ stress. In-situ stress conditions under which core discing is likely to occur were identified by examining the direction of tensile principal stress. A criterion for core discing was proposed by evaluating the maximum tensile stress which is necessary for the contour plane to be formed throughout a cross-section of the core, and was compared to previous experimental results. By analyzing the distributions of the direction of the tensile principal stress in detail, a procedure for determining the direction of principal in-situ stress from the geometry of a disc was proposed.

2 FINITE ELEMENT ANALYSIS

A finite element code for an axisymmetric body subjected to nonaxisymmetric boundary conditions (Wilson 1965, Sugawara et al. 1978) was used to calculate the stress in the model shown in Figure 1. The core was an HQ (core radius/borehole radius = 0.6612) which had a length of 8 times the core radius (R). The whole model was composed of 957 6-point and 8-point elements with 2688 nodes. A tensile principal stress analysis was carried out for a region within and below the core stub, shown by thick lines in Figure 1(b) and referred to as the analyzed region below. A cross-section of the analyzed region was divided into 168 equal area elements (7 for the radial direction x 24 for the circumferential direction), and stresses at the gravity center of each element were analyzed.

If all of the principal in-situ stresses are in compression, the maximum (σ_1) and intermediate (σ_2) principal stresses normalized by the mean stress (σ_m) should lie within the triangular area shown in Figure 2. To consider general in-situ stress conditions, 11 sets of the normalized principal stress magnitudes (from (1) to (11)) were adopted for the analysis, as shown in Figure 2. The direction of σ_1

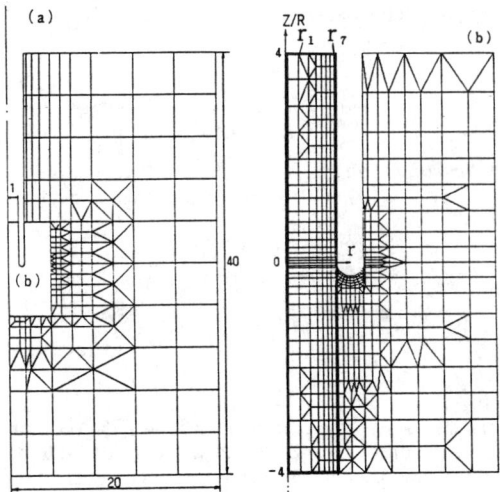

Figure 1. A mesh diagram for a long HQ core model.

was restricted within the XZ-plane, where the Z-axis is the core axis, and the inclination angle of σ_1 from the core axis (ϕ_1) was varied from 0° to 90° in steps of 30°. The direction of σ_2 was varied in the plane perpendicular to σ_1 by increasing the angle from the Y-axis towards the X-axis from 0° to 90° in steps of 30°. As a result, the analysis was performed for 77 in-situ stress conditions.

3 RANGE OF IN-SITU STRESSES FOR CORE DISCING

Core discing is believed to occur due to tensile stress within or below a core stub (Jaeger and Cook 1963, Sugawara et al. 1978). The tensile principal stress analysis in this study was performed based upon this belief. Therefore, the direction of tensile principal stress within or below a core stub must be nearly within the core axis if core discing occurs. Figure 3 shows the relationship between the inclination angle of the maximum tensile principal stress relative to the

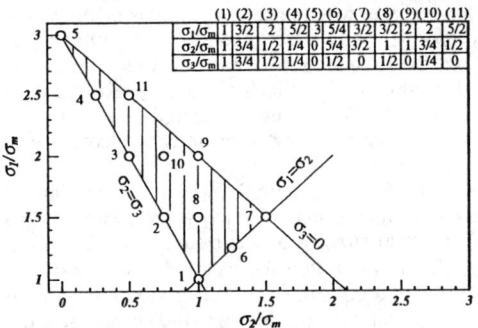

Figure 2. Magnitudes of principal in-situ stresses used for analysis.

core axis (ϕ_{tmax}) in the central part ($r=r_1$) and that in the outermost part ($r=r_7$) of the analyzed region for all of the in-situ stress conditions ($r_1/R=0.251$ and $r_7/R=0.961$; see Fig. 1). The in-situ stress conditions are clearly divided into two groups. In one group, the maximum tensile principal stress in the central part is greatly inclined relative to the core axis; in most cases it is nearly perpendicular to the core axis. Accordingly, core discing does not occur under these in-situ stress conditions. On the other hand, in the group surrounded by thick lines in Figure 3, the inclination angle (ϕ_{tmax}) in the central part is less than 30°, while that in the outermost part is less than 45°. The maximum tensile stress in the outermost part is always greater than that in the central part. However, the difference between these values is small in the latter group, suggesting that a tensile fracture that initiates from the periphery of the core grows more easily to the central part in the latter group. Thus, core discing was considered to be likely to occur under the in-situ stress conditions in the latter group. This group included 26 stress conditions.

This group was further divided into 5 sub-groups with regard to direction, as shown in Figure 4 (upper hemisphere). The magnitudes of the principal stresses in each sub-group are shown in Table 1. These stress conditions are consistent with previous studies, since core discing is more likely to occur when both the maximum and intermediate principal stresses are perpendicular to the core axis (Obert and Stephenson 1965, Sugawara et al. 1978). However, Figure 4 also shows that core discing could occur when the minimum principal in-situ stress is inclined relative to the core axis or when the maximum and/or intermediate principal stresses are inclined relative to the direction perpendicular to the core axis. A further analysis of tensile principal stresses was performed only for this stress group.

4 CRITERION FOR CORE DISCING

Core discing is a phenomenon in which a tensile fracture propagates throughout a cross-section of a core. In this study, a simple assumption was used to obtain a criterion for core discing. Figure 5 shows schematic cross-sectional views of a tensile principal stress contour plane within and below a core stub. When the tensile principal stress is low (Fig. 5(a)), two contour planes exist, and therefore there is greater tensile stress in the region between the contour planes. As the tensile principal stress increases, the two contour planes approach each other until eventually there are no contour planes which penetrate throughout the core (Fig. 5(c)). This tensile principal stress cannot produce a fracture propagated throughout a cross-section of the core. Thus, the tensile principal stress which makes the two contour planes contact each other at a point (Fig. 5(b)), called the critical tensile stress (σ_{tc}), is the maximum tensile

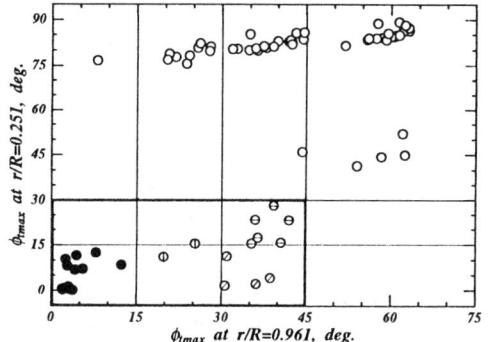

Figure 3. The relationship between the inclination angle of the maximum principal stress (ϕ_{tmax}) in the central part ($r=r_1$) and that in the outermost part ($r=r_7$).

Table 1. The magunitudes of in-situ stresses under which core discing is likely to occur.

Magnitude	Sub-group
(1)	None
(2)	2
(3)	2
(4)	2
(5)	2
(6)	2, 1A
(7)	2, 1A
(8)	2, 1A, 1B, 1C1
(9)	2, 1A, 1B, 1C1
(10)	2, 1A, 1B, 1C1, 1C2
(11)	2, 1A, 1B, 1C1, 1C2

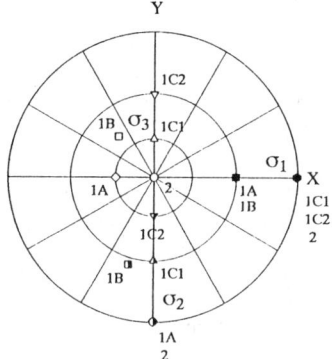

Figure 4. The directions of principal in-situ stresses under which core discing is likely to occur (upper hemishere).

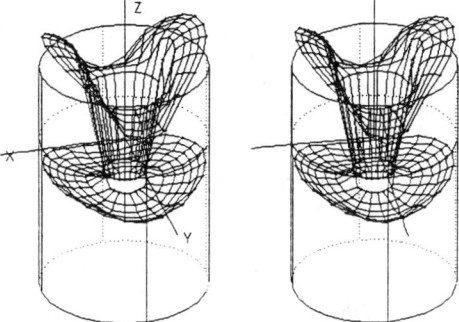

Figure 6. A stereogram of the critical tensile stress contour planes (stress sub-group 2 and magnitude (2)).

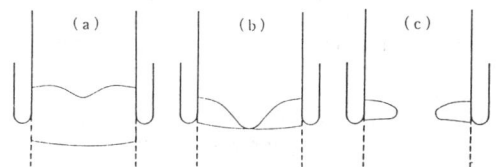

Figure 5. Schematic cross-sectional views of a tensile principal stress contour plane.

stress which can produce core discing. A stereogram of the contour planes of the critical tensile stress is shown in Figure 6. The critical tensile stress is the minimum of the maximum tensile stresses determined with respect to the Z-coordinate for each position in a cross-section.

Figure 7 shows the relationship between the normalized critical tensile stress (σ_{tc}/σ_m) and the normalized normal in-situ stress parallel to the core axis (σ_Z/σ_m). Solid symbols show the stress conditions for which σ_Z is equal to the minimum principal stress (σ_3). The relationship is linear when

$\sigma_3 = \sigma_Z$. The deviation of the critical tensile stress from this line increases linearly with the difference between σ_3 and σ_Z. Thus, the critical tensile stress is given by:

$$\sigma_{tc} = 0.302\sigma_m - 0.340\sigma_Z + 0.0910(\sigma_Z - \sigma_3) \quad (1)$$

where the third term expresses the effects of the difference between σ_3 and σ_Z. By assuming that core discing occurs when the critical tensile stress reaches the tensile strength of the rock (S_t), the following criterion for core discing of a long core was obtained:

$$S_t = 0.302\sigma_m - 0.340\sigma_Z + 0.0910(\sigma_Z - \sigma_3) \quad (2)$$

To examine the validity of the above criterion, the stress conditions under which core discing occurred were estimated from eq. (2) for the experiment by Sugawara et al. (1978), and compared to their experimental results. In their experiment, the disc was long, the tensile strength of the rock was 7.97 MPa, $\sigma_3 = \sigma_Z = 0$ and $\sigma_1 = \sigma_2 = \sigma_X = \sigma_Y$. The estimated values of $\sigma_X = \sigma_Y$ was 39.6 MPa, which is very similar to the stress of 39.2 MPa, under which

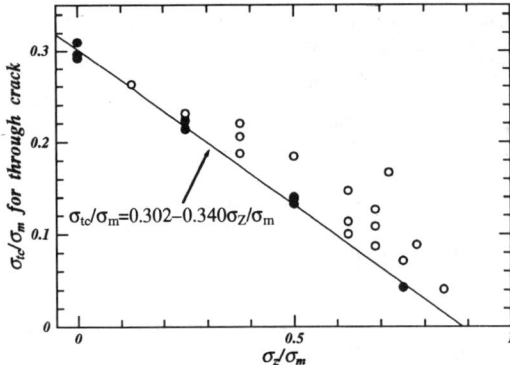

Figure 7. The relationship between normalized critical tensile stress (σ_{tc}/σ_m) and normalized normal in-situ stress in the direction of the core axis (σ_Z/σ_m).

core discing occurred. Thus, the criterion for core discing is consistent with the experimental results, although the stress conditions compared are far from a general state.

5 EFFECTS OF IN-SITU STRESSES ON THE SHAPE OF A DISC

A local tensile stress produces a local fracture perpendicular to the tensile stress. Therefore, the distributions of the direction of tensile principal stress within and below the core must be analyzed to clarify the effects of in-situ stress on the shape of a disc. For that purpose, the height (the Z-coordinate) at which the tensile principal stress is maximum was determined as a representative height for radii of r_1 and r_7 (see Fig. 1). These heights were below the core stub for r_1 and above the bottom of the core for r_7.

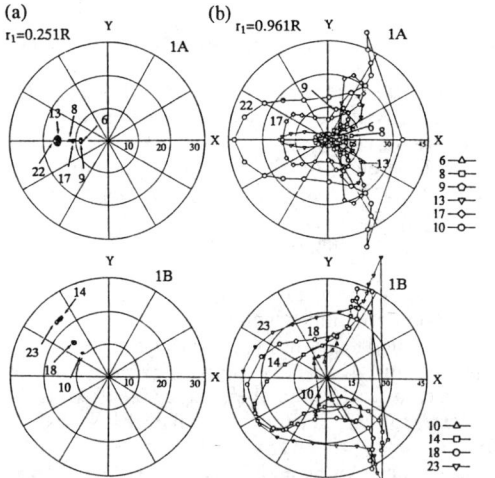

Figure 8. Examples of a stereo-plot of the tensile principal stress directions at (a) $r=r_1$ and (b) $r=r_7$.

Figure 8 shows examples of a stereo-plotted variation with the circumferential coordinate of the direction of the tensile principal stress at the representative height for r_1 and r_7. Numerals show each in-situ stress condition. Note that the great circle corresponds to an inclination angle of 30° for r_1 and 45° for r_7. The variation in the direction of the principal tensile stress is very small in the central part, while it is large in the outermost part. This suggests that the end surfaces of a disc are almost planar in the central part while those near the periphery of the disc are not so simple.

The direction of the mean tensile principal stress at ($r=r_1$, Z=the representative height) is shown in Figure 9 for all 26 of the in-situ stress conditions. The notations are the same as those in Figure 4. The direction of the mean tensile principal stress at $r=r_2$ is almost the same as that at $r=r_1$, which suggests that the direction of the tensile principal stress is uniform over a wide area of the central part. Comparison of Figure 9 with Figure 4 shows that the azimuth of the minimum principal in-situ stress approximately coincides with that of the mean tensile principal stress in the central part. On the other hand, the inclination angle (ϕ_m) of the mean tensile principal stress in the central part is approximately one third that of σ_3 (the average value is 1/2.65). As shown in Figure 9, ϕ_m is zero when $\sigma_3 = \sigma_Z$. Therefore, ϕ_m depends on the difference between them (σ_Z-σ_3). Figure 10 shows the relationship between ϕ_m and (σ_Z-σ_3)/σ_m. Using the least squares method, the following regression curve was determined for the relationship:

$$\phi_m = 3.09\xi^3 - 3.28\xi^2 + 1.34\xi. \tag{3}$$

where ξ is (σ_Z-σ_3)/σ_m, ϕ_m is given in radians, and two data points which were far from the mean relation were excluded.

If the tensile strength of the rock is measured and if the inclination angle of the normal direction in the central part of the end surfaces of the disc, which is identical to ϕ_m, is measured, two equations are obtained for determining three in-situ stresses (σ_Z, σ_3 and σ_m). Accordingly, if one of these stresses is

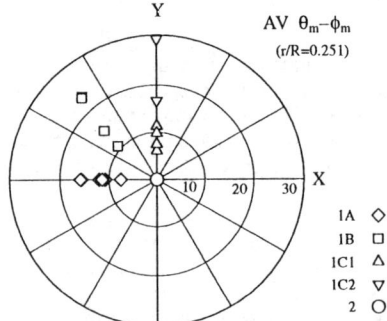

Figure 9. The directions of the mean tensile principal stress at $r=r_1$ for 26 in-situ stress conditions (upper hemishere).

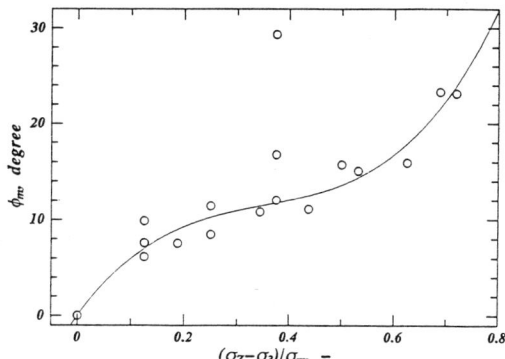

Figure 10. The relationship between ϕ_m and $(\sigma_Z-\sigma_3)/\sigma_m$ for $r=r_1$.

determined or estimated by another method, the others can be determined. If the core axis is vertical, σ_Z may be assumed to be the overburden stress.

To determine the inclination angle of σ_3 accurately, the following equation was obtained by the least squares method for the relationship between $(\phi_3-\phi_m)/\phi_m$ and $(\sigma_Z-\sigma_3)/\sigma_m$:

$$\phi_3-\phi_m=\phi_3(0.817-0.518\xi). \tag{4}$$

By diminishing ξ from eqs. (3) and (4), ϕ_3 can be determined from ϕ_m. An error of 23 % was estimated for this method by comparing the estimated values to the results obtained in the calculation.

As described previously, the geometry of end surfaces near the periphery of a disc is influenced by the large variation in the direction of the tensile principal stress. To identify a general tendency, the mean inclination of the tensile principal stress in the outward radial direction was analyzed for the X- and Y-directions in the outermost part of the analyzed region ($r=r_7$). Figure 11 shows the relationships between the mean inclination angle (ϕ_r) and (σ_1-σ_2)/σ_m for (a) the X-direction and (b) the Y-direction. Note that σ_1 lies within the XZ-plane. As the difference between σ_1 and σ_2 increases, outward (positive) inclination increases in the X-direction while inward (negative) inclination increases in the Y-direction. As schematically shown in Figure 11, a concave surface is created by outward inclination and a convex surface is created by inward inclination of the tensile principal stress. Accordingly, it can be said that a concave axis is approximately in the direction of σ_1 and a convex axis is approximately in the direction of σ_2. The end surfaces of the disc are more concave or more convex at the periphery as the difference in stress (σ_1-σ_2) increases. Discs of this geometry are called "saddle-shaped", and have been observed both in the laboratory and in the field (Paillet and Kim 1987, Perreau et al. 1989, Haimson and Lee 1995). On the other hand, radial inclination is very small if (σ_1-σ_2) is small. Under these stress conditions, a disc with almost flat end surfaces may be produced.

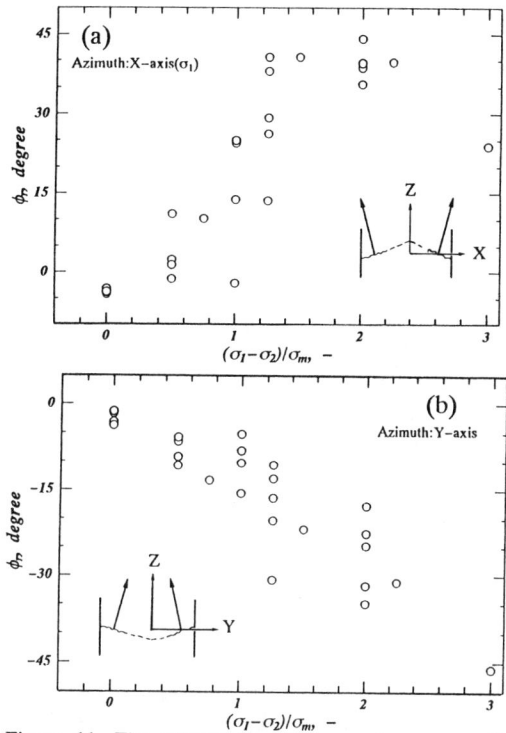

Figure 11. The relationships between the mean radial inclination angle (ϕ_r) and (σ_1-σ_2)/σ_m for (a) the X-direction and (b) the Y-direction.

In the above analysis, the asymmetry in the distributions of the tensile principal stress is ignored to determine the average tendency. However, as shown in Figure 8(b), the distribution of the direction of the tensile principal stress is not always symmetric with respect to the X-, Y- and Z-axes in the core. A disc with an asymmetric geometry may be created when σ_3 is not in the direction of the core axis. Therefore, the conclusions regarding the directions of the concave and convex axes in the end surfaces of a disc, described above, do not apply if σ_3 is not in the direction of the core axis.

Obviously, the symmetry of the disc geometry with regard to the axes in the core is identical to that of the in-situ stresses. Therefore, the symmetry of the in-situ stresses can be determined from that of the disc geometry. Furthermore, by examining the directions of the concave and convex axes in the end surfaces of a disc for all 26 of the in-situ stress conditions, we concluded that the concave axis is perpendicular to σ_2 when the directions of in-situ principal stresses are included in sub-group 1A, and that the convex axis is perpendicular to σ_1 when the directions of in-situ principal stresses are included in sub-groups 1C1 and 1C2 (see Figure 4).

Summarizing the results described above, a

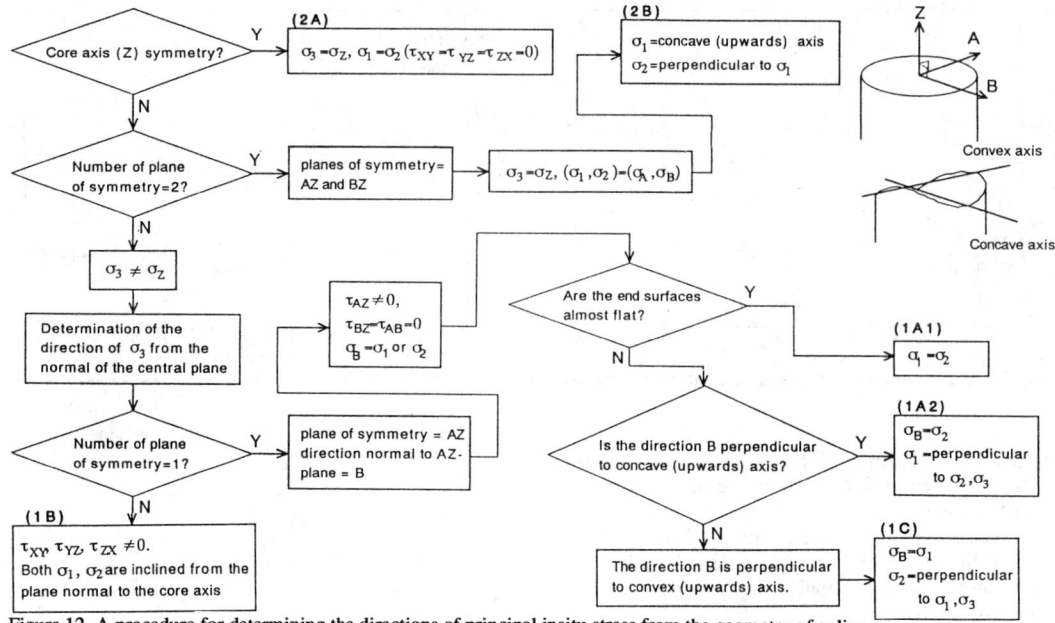

Figure 12. A procedure for determining the directions of principal insitu stress from the geometry of a disc.

procedure for determining the directions of principal in-situ stress was proposed as shown in Figure 12. If one of the principal in-situ stresses is in the core axis or perpendicular to the core axis, all of the directions can be determined from the geometry of the disc, based upon the symmetry of the end surfaces, the normal direction in the central part of the end surfaces and the direction of the concave or convex axes in the end surfaces.

6 CONCLUSION

The direction and magnitude of tensile principal stresses within and below a long HQ core stub were analyzed for 77 in-situ stress conditions which covered all possible conditions at intervals. Core discing was considered to be likely to occur under 26 of these stress conditions. A criterion for core discing was proposed by evaluating the maximum tensile stress at which a contour plane could be formed throughout a cross-section of the core. By analyzing the distributions of the direction of the tensile principal stress in detail, a procedure for determining the directions of principal in-situ stresses from the geometry of a disc was proposed.

Acknowledgements: This work was supported by a Grant-in-Aid for scientific research (No. 08405066) from the Ministry of Education, Japan.

REFERENCES

Durelli, A.J., Obert, L. and Parks, V.J. 1968. Stress required to initiate core discing, *Trans. SME*, 241: 269-276.

Dyke, C.G. 1989. Core disking: its potential as an indicator of principal in-situ stress directions, *Rock at Great Depth*, Maury & Fourmaintraux (eds.): 1057-1064. Rotterdam, Balkema.

Haimson, B.C. and Lee, M.Y. 1995. Estimating in-situ stress conditions from borehole breakouts and core disking experimental results in graniteranite, *Proc. Int. Workshop on Rock Stress Measurement at Great Depth*: 19-24.

Jaeger, J.C. and Cook, N.G.W. 1963. Pinching off and discing of rocks, *J. Geophy. Res.* 68: 1759-1765.

Obert, L. and Stephenson, D.E. 1965. Stress conditions under which core discing occurs, *Trans. SME*, 232: 227-235.

Paillet, F.L. and Kim, K. 1987. Character and distribution of borehole breakouts and their relationship to in situ stresses in deep Columbia River basalts, *J. Geophy. Res.* 92: 6223-6234.

Perreau, P.J., Heugas, O. and Santarelli, F.J. 1989. Tests of ASR, DSCA, and core discing analyses to evaluate in-situ stresses, *SPE* 17960 : 325-336.

Stacey, T.R. 1982. Contribution to the mechanism of core discing, *J. South Afr. Inst. Min. Metall.* 17:269-274.

Sugawara, K. et al. 1978. A study on core discing of rock, *J. Min. Metall. Inst. Japan*, 94: 797-803.(Japanese with English abstract)

Wilson, E.L. 1965. Structural analysis of axi-symmetric solids, *AIAA J.*, 3: 2269-2274.

State of stress in the earth's crust

Stress measurements by the hydraulic fracturing in the 1995 Hyogoken-nanbu earthquake source region

H. Ito, Y. Kuwahara & O. Nishizawa
Geological Survey of Japan, Tsukuba, Japan

ABSTRACT : We conducted hydraulic fracturing stress measurements in three wells drilled after the 1995 Hyogoken-nanbu earthquake in the vicinity of the Nojima fault (at Ikuha) and the Arima-Takatsuki tectonic line (at Takarazuka and Ikeda). The Ikuha site is located at the end of the movement of the Nojima fault, and the Takarazuka site is at the intersection of the aftershock zone and the Arima-Takatsuki tectonic line. At Takarazuka, we observed high differential stress, which is consistent with the observation of borehole breakouts and core disking in the Takarazuka well. The stress state is rather hydrostatic at Ikuha and Ikeda. The maximum principal stress direction at Ikuha estimated from borehole breakouts is almost normal to the surface strike of the Nojima earthquake fault.

1. INTRODUCTION

The Hyogo-ken Nanbu earthquake of January 17, 1995 (M_{JMA} 7.2), was the most damaging to hit Japan since the 1923 great Kanto earthquake that destroyed large parts of Tokyo and Yokohama. The earthquake epicenter was located about 20 km southwest of Kobe and just northeast of Awaji Island, and occurred along the fault network of the Rokko Mountains near Kobe and to the southwest along the Nojima fault on Awaji Island. A 10.5 km long surface break on the Nojima fault displayed offsets up to approximately 2 m (Awata et al., 1996).

We drilled five boreholes at various site of the fault movement along the Nojima fault and the Arima-Takatsuki tectonic line (Fig. 1). Ikuha (1,000 m deep; IKH) is located at the southwest end of the Nojima fault. At Hirabayashi (747 m; HRB), the maximum displacement was observed and considered as the site where the fault smoothly slipped. Tarumi (300 m; TRM) is also the site where the fault smoothly slipped. The Takarazuka site (1,000 m; TKZ) is at the intersection of the aftershock zone and the Arima-Takatsuki tectonic line. Ikeda (800 m; IKD) is along the Arima-Takatsuki tectonic line.

We made core stress measurements (AE/DR, DSCA and ASR) for the cores from these wells (Ito et al., 1996; Ito et al., 1997; Kudo et al., 1997) and also conducted hydraulic fracturing stress measurements in the three wells; Ikuha, Takarazuka and Ikeda. We also observed borehole breakouts at Takarazuka and Ikuha, and core disking at Takarazuka.

2. HYDRAULIC FRACTURING STRESS MEASUREMENTS

We conducted hydraulic fracturing stress measurements in the three wells; Ikuha, Takarazuka and Ikeda. We used straddle packers with the packer interval of about 1 m, and applied water with the flow rate of about 10-20 l/min. The maximum principal stress S_H and the minimum principal stress S_h were obtained

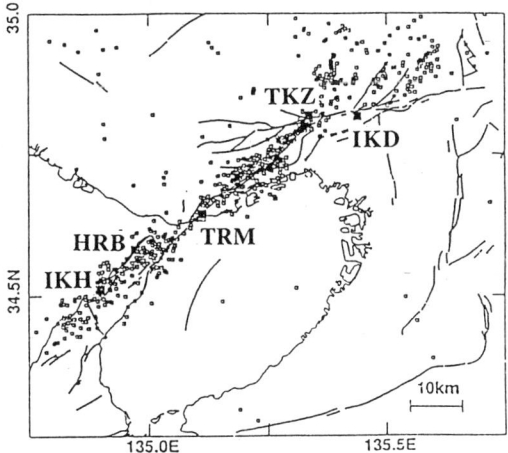

Fig. 1 The location of the boreholes and aftershock distribution.

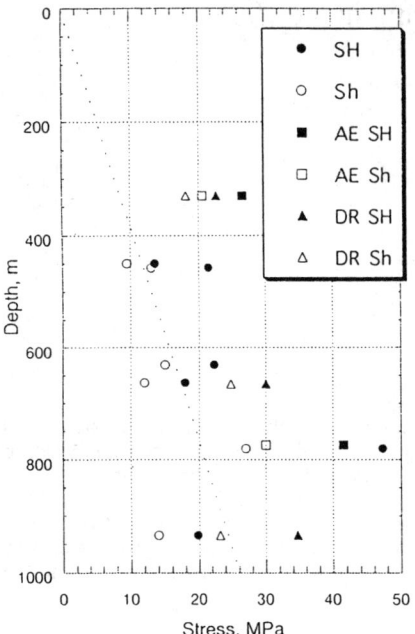

Fig. 2 Stresses in the Takarazuka borehole.

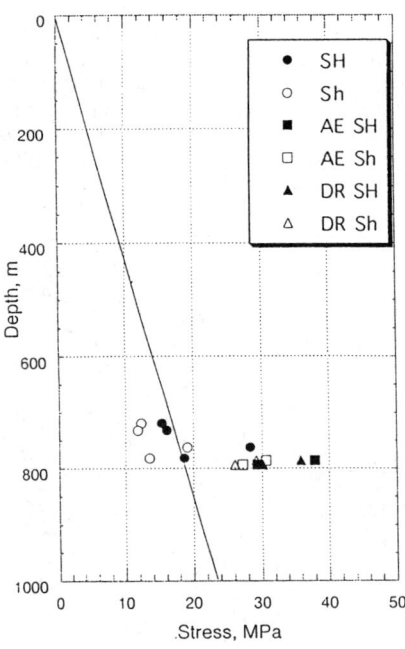

Fig. 3 Stresses in the Ikeda borehole.

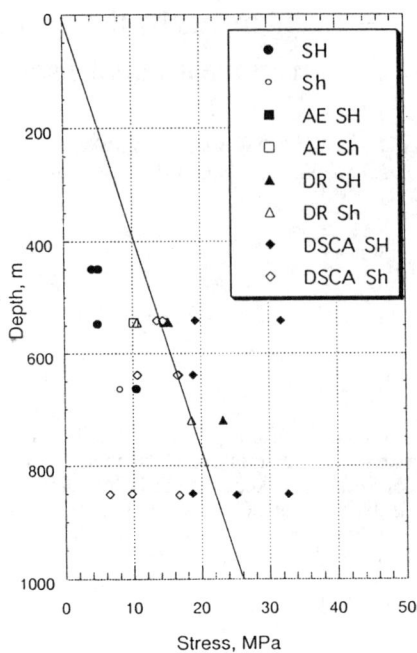

Fig. 4 Stresses in the Ikuha borehole.

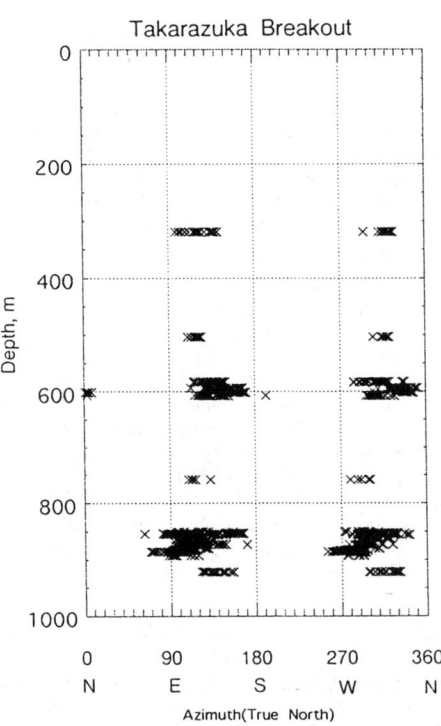

Fig. 5 Borehole breakouts orientation in the Takarazuka borehole.

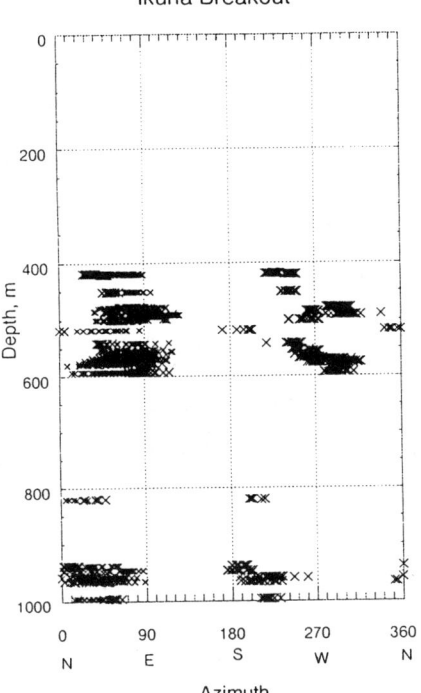

Fig. 6 Borehole breakouts orientation in the Ikuha borehole.

from the following equation;

$$P_b(T=0) = 3S_h - S_H - P_p$$

where $P_b(T=0)$ is the fracture re-opening pressure obtained on the second or later pumping cycle, and P_p is the pore pressure. The minimum principal stress S_h was calculated from the instantaneous shut-in pressure. The Cauculated resulta are shown in Fig. 2, 3 4. The orientation of the maximum principal stress was estimated from the azimuth of the induced hydraulic fractures detected by ultrasonic BHTV or impression packer.

3. BOREHOLE BREAKOUTS

Borehole breakouts are the failure at borehole wall due to the stress concentration at the azimuth of least horizontal principal stress. Stress -induced borehole breakouts is an important indicator of horizontal stress direction (Bell and Gough, 1979; Zoback and Zoback, 1980; Shamir and Zoback, 1992). Borehole breakouts were observed in the Takarazuka and Ikuha wells. The azimuth of the borehole breakouts was determined from the digital image of the ultrasonic borehole televiewer data (Ito, 1995). Fig. 5 and 6 show the azimuth of the borehole breakouts in the Takarazuka and Ikuha wells.

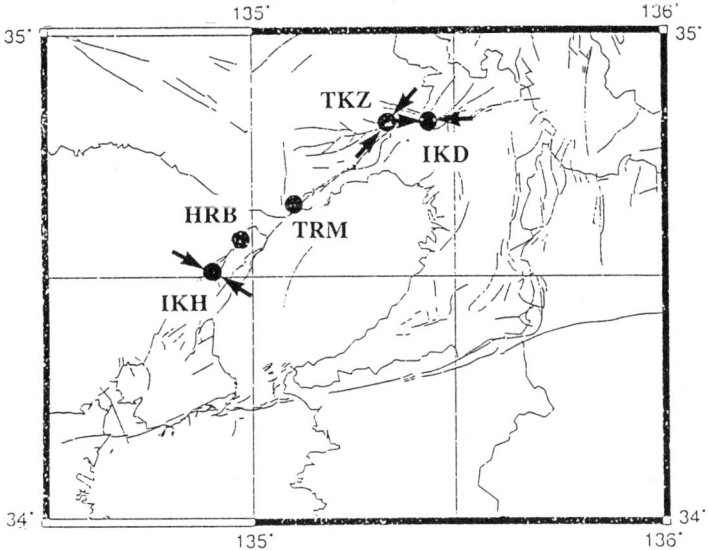

Fig. 7 Summary of stress orientation by borehole breakouts (Takarazuka and Ikuha) and hydraulic fracturing (Ikeda).

4. DISCUSSION

The principal stress values from hydraulic fracturing at Takarazuka (Fig. 2) show the strong differential stress ($S_v < S_h < S_H$), whereas the results at Ikeda is rather isotropic (Fig. 3). At Ikuha, the stress values from the hydraulic fracturing is much smaller than S_v. This is probably due to the altered condition of the formation of the Ikuha borehole. Judging from the occurrence of borehole breakouts in the Ikuha borehole, the stress state at Ikuha has large differential stress. The strong differential stress at Takarazuka is also confirmed by the occurrence of borehole breakouts and core disking. The core disking is believed to be generated under extremely high differential stress (Stacey, 1982; Dyke, 1989; Maury, 1988). Although we did not make hydraulic fracturing stress measurements at Tarumi and Hirabayashi, the results of core stress measurements show rather isotropic stress state in both boreholes.

The results generally show that the stress state at the both ends of the faults system (Ikuha and Takarazuka) has large differential stress and that close to the main event (Tarumi and Hirabayashi) is isotropic.

The maximum horizontal principal stress orientation at Ikuha is almost perpendicular to the extent of strike of the Nojima fault (Awata et al., 1996). At Ikuha, there was no surface rupture of the Nojima fault associated with the 1995 Hyogo-ken Nanbu Earthquake, the drilling results show that there is a fault at about 670 m depth. The maximum horizontal principal stress perpendicular to the Nojima fault implies that the Nojima fault can not sustain shear stress.

The maximum horizontal principal stress orientation at Takarazuka is not consistent with the right lateral fault movement of the Arima-takatsuki tectonic line, wheares the east-west stress orientation at Ikeda is consistent with that. One of the reason of the diecrepancy at Takarazuka is strong local stress heterogneity at the edge of the fault system.

REFERENCES

Awata, Y., K. Mizuno, Y. Sugiyama, R. Imura, K. Shimokawa, K. Okumura, E. Tsukuda and K. Kimura, Surface fault ruptures on the northwest coast of Awaji Island associated with the Hyogo-ken Nanbu earthquake of 1995, Japan, Zisin, Suppl. 2, 49, 113-124, 1996.

Bell, J. S., and D. I. Gough, Northeast-southwest compressive stress in Alberta: Evidense from oil wells, Earth Planet. Sci. Lett., 45, 475-482, 1979.

Dyke, C. G., Core discing: its potential as an indicator of principal in situ stress directions, In: Maury, V. and D. Fourmaintraux (eds), Rock at Great Depth, Balkema, Rotterdam. 1057-1064, 1989.

Ito, H., Development of a borehole televiewer digital data acquisition system and fracture system observed in the Tanna Basin, Rept. Geol. Surv. Japan, No. 282, 297-316, 1995.

Ito, H., Y. Kuwahara, O. Nishizawa, K. Yamamoto, O. Sano, T. Yokoyama, R. Kudo and Z. Xue, Stress State in Hanshin Awaji area, The Japan Society of Engineering Geology, Oct 31-Nov.1, 1996.

Ito, H., O. Nishizawa, Z. Xue, O. Sano, Estimation of In-situ Stresses from ASR and DSCA Measurements on Drilled Cores in the 1995 Hyogokennanbu Earthquake Source Region, RS Kumamoto, 1997.

Maury, V., F. J. Santarelli and J. P. Henry, Core discing: a review, Proc. Ist African Conf. Rock Mech., Swaziland, 221-231, 1988.

Shamir, G. and M. D. Zoback, Stress orientation profile to 3.5 km depth near San Andreas Fault at Cajon Pass, California, J. Geophys. Res., 97, 5059-5080, 1992.

Stacey, T. R., Contribution to the mechanism of core discing, J South Afr. Inst. Min. Metall., 83, 269-274, 1982

Zoback, M. L., and M. D. Zoback, Tectonic stress in the conterminous United States, J. Geophys. Res., 85, 6113-6156, 1980.

Estimation of in-situ stresses from ASR and DSCA measurements on drilled cores in the 1995 Hyogoken-nanbu earthquake source region

H. Ito & O. Nishizawa
Geological Survey of Japan, Tsukuba, Japan

Ziqiu Xue
Kiso-Jiban Consultants Co., Ltd, Japan

O. Sano
Yamaguchi University, Japan

ABSTRACT: Anelastic strain and differential strain measurements performed on two freshly drilled cores were used to determine in situ stresses. Both techniques, ASR(Anelastic Strain Recovery) and DSCA (Differential Strain Curve Analysis) rely on the development of preferentially oriented strain distribution in a piece of core due to relief of the stress field. Cores retrieved from depth about 600m have exhibted similar relaxation behavior, and distinctive patteren have been observed. Directions of the three principal strains determined by each sample have been definitive and results have agreed within acceptable magnitude. Results obtained from ASR and DSCA methods, have suggested that the maximum principal stress acting in the horizontal plane which perpendicular to borehole axis. Stress induced borehole breakouts at that depth, have close relation with the large deviated stresses in the horizontal plane.

1. INTRODUCTION

Strain relaxation methods, which have been used primarily to determine stress orientation, rely on the development of a preferentially oriented strain distribution (believed to be due to microcracks) in a piece of core due to relief of the in situ stress at the time of drilling. Two methods; Anelastic Strain Recovery (ASR) and Differential Strain Curve Analysis (DSCA) are used for this purpose (Blanton, 1983; Ren and Roegiers, 1983; Warpinski and Teufel, 1986).

ASR techniques measure the relaxation of the core with displacement gages immediately upon retrieval from the core barrel. The core needs to be retrieved in several hours, instrumented quickly, and then monitored for one and three days. DSCA measures the of the rock to laboratory-applied stress fields. From the strain behavior during loading, some eastimates of the stress field can be obtained. Both ASR and DSCA cannot be used if a microcrack fabric exists at depth due to tectonic or other causes. Both of these techniques can provide information on the stress magnitudes if a valid constitutive model can be developed.

Although the ASR is a convenient and economical method to estimate stress, it is still necessary to compare ASR, DSCA and in-situ stress to confirm the validity of the ASR method.

In this paper, we discuss the results obtained using ASR and DSCA methods for the same cores extracted from the Takaraduka well that was drilled just after the 1995 Hyogoken-nanbu earthquake to compare the results from ASR and DSCA, and with the in-situ stress measurements and regional tectonics.

2. EXPERIMENTAL METHODS

Anelastic strain Recovery techniques (ASR) measure the relaxation of the core immediately upon retrieval from the core barrel. The core needs to be instrumented quickly, and then monitored for one to three days. Strain gages were mounted directly on the surface of the core, with the core covered in film wrapping to prevent moisture loss. The instrumented cores were set inside a container, and we kept the air conditioner running for minimising changes of the room temperature. In order to monitor the temperature

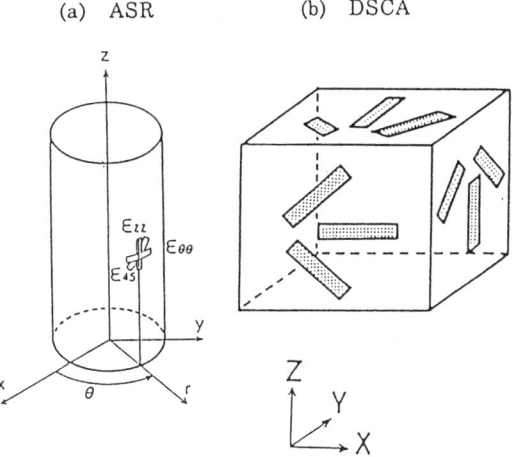

Fig. 1 Strain gages for ASR and DSCA.

a platinum temperature probe is placed directly on the surface of the core. Strain and temperature were measured by a portable data acquisition system, and data can be every ten minutes foe periods of several weeks at a time without attendance.

Differential Strain Curve Analysis (DSCA) techniques measure the response of the rock under hydrostatic pressure. A cubic oriented sample is cut from the ASR measurement core, with a 'scribe line' marked on the position for gage #1, and all measurements and calculations are made relative to this line. Strain gages are mounted to the surface of the sample, and the entire sample is sealed with silicon rubber as an impermeable jacket. The data analysis method used in this study is similar to that described by Dey and Brown (1986).

Three core samples were selected from the depth about 600m of the well. Samples are 57 mm in diameter. Sample preparations are shown in Fig.1. The z axis is always taken parallel to the vertical axis of the core and the x and y axes are aligned with respect to the gage#1.

3. Experimental Results

Sample TDA-1

Core depth is 591m and core length is about 11 cm. Recovery behavior of the TDA-1 is showed in Fig. 2. The results show both expansion and contraction during the first several hours. By comparing strains for three directions(ε_{zz}, $\varepsilon_{\theta\theta}$, ε_{45}), it is seen that the strain in the vertical direction(ε_{zz}) is much less than those in the other directions, except for the gage #1. Strains of gage #1 in direction ZZ and gage #5 in

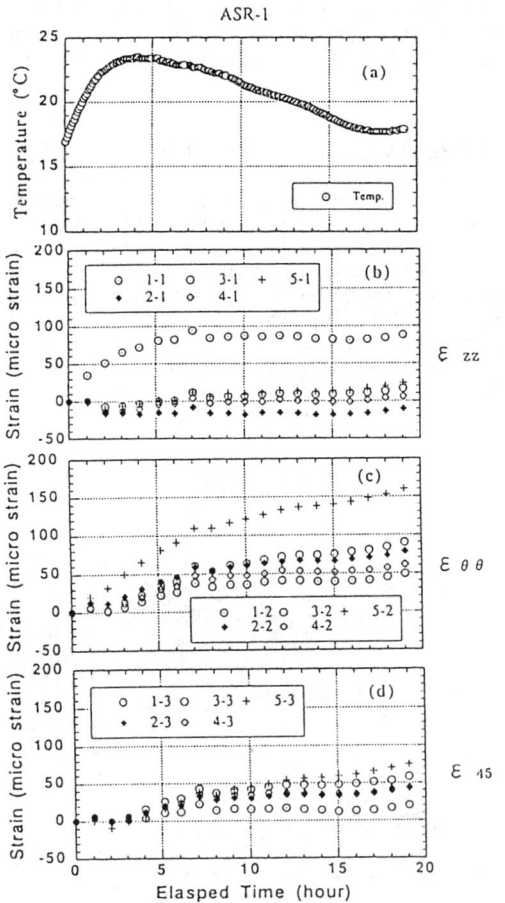

Fig. 2 Temperature and anelastic strain changes with time for the sample TDA-1.

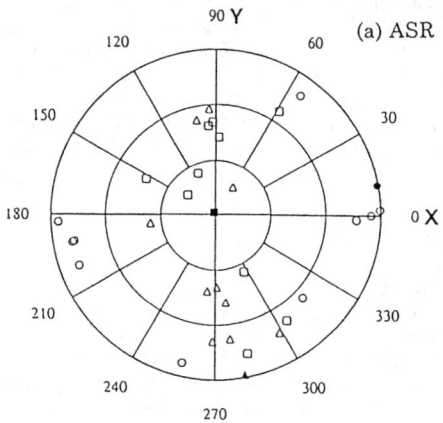

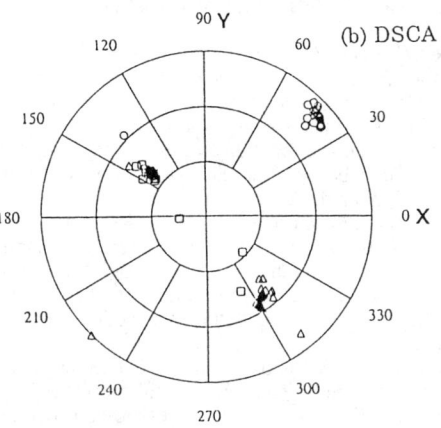

Fig. 3. Direction of principal strains (upper hemisphere) for the TDA-1. The maximum; ε_{11} (shown by open circles), the intermediate; ε_{22} (shown by open triangles), the minimum; ε_{33} (shown by open squares).

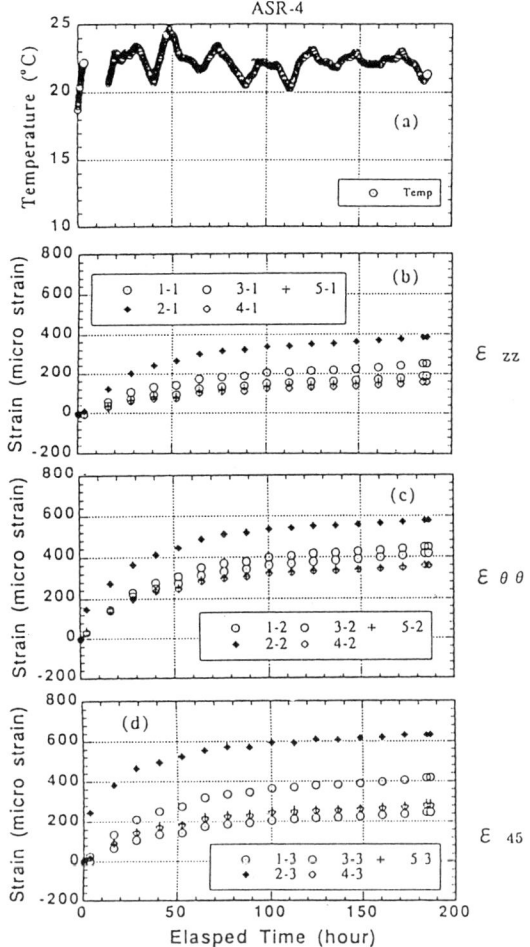

Fig. 4 Temperature and anelastic strain changes with time for the sample TDA-4.

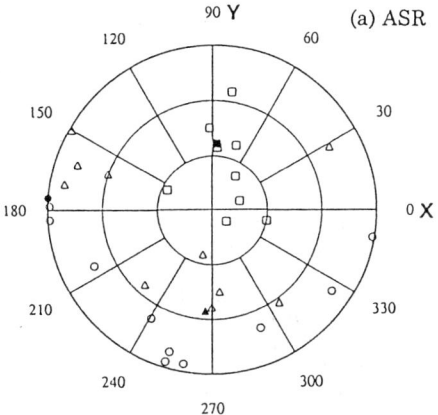

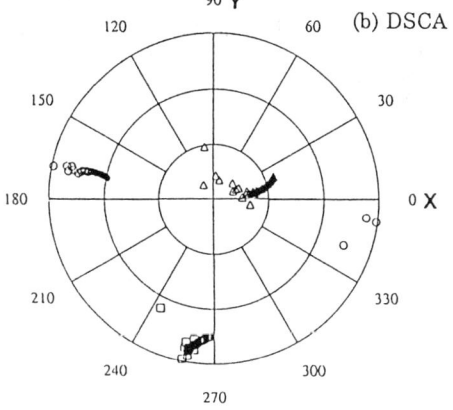

Fig. 5 Direction of principal strains (upper hemisphere) for the TDA-1.

direction $\theta\theta$ showed drastic increase during the first 5 hours, and then increased gradually with time.

The direction of the principal strains (the maximum; ε_{11}, the intermediate; ε_{22}, the minimum; ε_{33}) are shown in Fig. 3.

ASR as well as DSCA indicate the same orientation for the major deformation. This orientation is perpendicular to the principal major stress.

Sample TDA-4

Core depth is 602m and core length is about 33 cm. Recovery behavior of the TDA-1 is showed in Fig. 4. Because we found the measured time for the TDA-1 sample was not long enough to obtain the stable strain values, we measured the strain recovery for several days. The strain is several times larger than that of TDA-1, altough the sample depth and lithology is almost the same.

The direction of the principal strains (the maximum; ε_{11}, the intermediate; ε_{22}, the minimum; ε_{33}) are shown in Fig. 5. The results by ASR and DSCA did not agree.

4. DISCUSSION

To estimate stress by DSCA method, we need two assumptions; 1) the cracks associated with strain relief are perpendicular to the maximum principal stress and 2) the effect of preexisting cracks on the strain is negilibly small compared with that by cracks associated with strain relief. Both the results for TDA-1 and TDA-4 samples seem to cinfirm that the assumption 1 is valid.

Both the results for TDA-1 and TDA-4 samples show that the direction of the maximum principal strain is in the horizontal plane. This is consistent with the occurrence of the borehole breakouts in the Takarazuka borehole, because the stress induced borehole breakouts is considered to be generated under large diffrential stress.

REFERENCES

Blanton, The relation between recovery deformation and in-situ stress magnitude, SPE/DOE, 11624, 213-218,1983.

Dey, T. N. and D. W. Brown, Stress measurements in a deep granitic rock mass using hydraulic fracturing and differential strain curve analysis, Int. Sympo. Rock Stress and Rock Stress Measurements, 351-358, 1986.

Warpinski and Teufel, A viscoelastic constitutive model for determining in-situ stress magnitudes from anelastic strain recovery of core, SPE 15368, 1986.

Ren, N. K., and J. C. Roegiers, Differential strain curve analysis - A new method for determining the pre-existing in situ stress state from rock core measurements, Proc. 5Th Int. Conf. Int. Soc. Rock Mech., Melbourne, Australia, F117-F128, 1983.

Stress measurements with core samples by AE-DRA methods in the 1995 Hyogoken-nanbu earthquake source region

R. Kudo & T. Yokoyama
Oyo Corporation, Ohmiya, Japan

H. Ito, Y. Kuwahara & O. Nishizawa
Geological Survey of Japan, Tsukuba, Japan

K. Yamamoto
Tohoku University, Japan

ABSTRACT: In this study, we estimated in-situ stresses in the area of the 1995 Hyogoken-nanbu Earthquake by means of the methods of acoustic emission (AE) and deformation rate analysis (DRA). In the present experiments, the AE and deformation rate were measured simultaneously for the same specimen. Test specimens were obtained from the boring cores of five different depths at Hirabayashi site on the Nojima fault. The experimental results indicate that the state of both vertical stresses and horizontal stresses were changed across the fault zone along the Nojima fault.

1 INTRODUCTION

The Hyogo-ken Nanbu earthquake (M 7.2) took place in the southern part of Hyogo Prefecture on January 17 in 1995. The epicenter of the earthquake was located at about 14 km southwest from Kobe in the northeast end of Awaji Island.

Geological Survey of Japan has performed several drilling near the end of the earthquake rupture (Takarazuka site: 1000 m depth, Ikuha site: 1000 m depth), on the Arima - Takathuki tectonic line (Ikeda: 800 m depth), close to the epicenter (Tarumi site: 300 m depth) and on the Nojima fault where the maximum surface displacements were observed (Hirabayashi site: 747 m depth) as shown in Figure 1. They have conducted many geophysical and geological investigations, in-situ experiments including hydraulic fracturing stress measurements, and downhole monitoring activities by using these boreholes and obtained boring cores.

To know the stress condition around the fault, we applied deformation rate analysis (DRA) and acoustic emission (AE) to the boring core samples obtained from these five areas. In this paper, we describe about the experimental results and the stress condition at Hirabayashi site on the Nojima fault.

2 OUTLINE OF THE TEST

All the boring core samples at Hirabayashi site consist of granodiorite. In these cores, a deformed zone is recognized between 557 m to 713 m, with distinct clay gouges between 623.4 m and 625.4 m

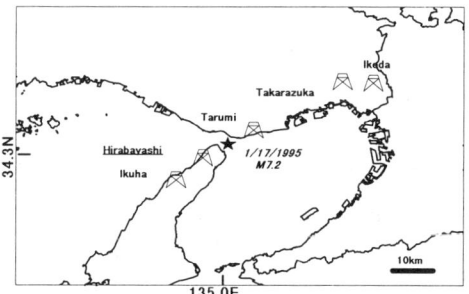

Figure 1. Location of the drilling sites and the epicenter of the 1995 Hyogoken-nanbu Earthquake.

(Ito et al., 1996). In this study, stress measurements were conducted using the core samples retrieved from 255 m, 350 m, 470 m, 530 m (above the deformed zone) and 735 m (below the deformed zone). The physical properties are listed in Table 1 and the uniaxial compressive strength is larger than 130 MPa.

To estimate vertical stress and principle stresses in a horizontal plane, test specimens were cut out from boring core samples in the directions shown in Figure 2. The specimens to estimate horizontal principle stresses were cut out in directions at an interval of 45° in azimuth. In this study, about 15 specimens were tested for each depth. The specimens were rectangular in shape 25×25×50mm and opposite faces were formed paralleled in an accuracy of 0.05mm. The ends of a specimen were affixed to endpieces made of stainless steel with epoxy cement.

The loading pattern used in this study is shown in Figure 3. All loading processes in these tests were controlled under a constant displacement rate ranging between 0.004 MPa/min. and 0.06 MPa/min. by the servo-controlled apparatus. In the experiments, a spherical seating was put on the top of the specimen in order to keep an uniform stress in the specimen. The maximum load was decided to be twice to 4 times of the overburden pressure corresponding to the each depth where core samples were recovered. The loading and unloading were repeated more than 4 times to obtain the strained difference function.

The schematic diagram of the AE and strain measuring system is shown in Figure 4. For AE measurements, a pair of AE transducers was attached on two opposite sides of the test specimen for ringdown count, and the other pair of transducers was attached on the top and the bottom of the specimen to locate AE sources. The AE transducers of piezo electric type with resonance frequency of 200 kHz, 500 kHz, 1 MHz, and that of wide range type (which has high sensitivities between 100 kHz and 2 MHz) were used in this experiment. AE signals were amplified with a gain of 40 dB by the pre-amplifiers and filtered by high pass filters of 100 kHz and amplified further with a gain of 40 dB by main amplifiers. All AE signals over threshold level were detected by a pair of AE transducers attached on the sides of the specimen, on the other hand, the AE signals generated only inside of the rock specimen were detected by the transducers attached on the top and the bottom of the specimen by means of a coincident processor. This processor removes noise from the AE signals by taking the difference in arrival times to the transducers. AE parameters such as AE generation time, ringdown count, event count, duration, risetime etc. were recorded in the data chamber (NF-9640A) as digital data. In the relation between the cumulative AE event-count and applied stress, in-situ stress was estimated in the point where a remarkable sudden increase of AE events in the first loading was appeared.

For DRA, four strain gauges (10 mm length) were glued on opposite sides of the specimen on which AE transducers were not attached and other four gauges were glued on a dummy specimen for compensation of temperature influence. The output signals in voltage from two full bridge circuits of gauges are amplified by dynamic strain amplifier and differential amplifier. Finally, direct strain and differential strain were converted in digital data and recorded in a hard disk of PC9801. After the experiments, we estimated in-situ stresses by regarding the bending point on the strain difference function for all cyclic loading except the first loading as the value of in-situ stress.

Table 1. Physical properties of rock core samples.

depth (m)	density (g/cm³)	Vp (km/s)	E (Gpa)
255	2.70	4.43	59.9
350	2.71	4.94	55.5
470	2.61	4.08	38.6
530	2.61	3.95	32.1
735	2.64	4.44	54.0

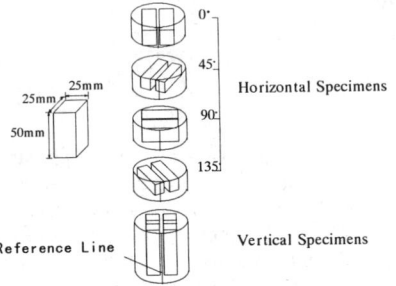

Figure 2. Typical orientation of specimens cut out from core samples.

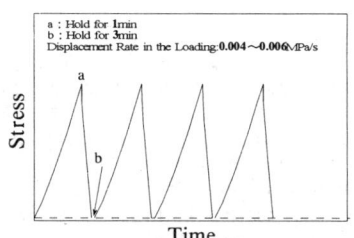

Figure 3. Loading diagram.

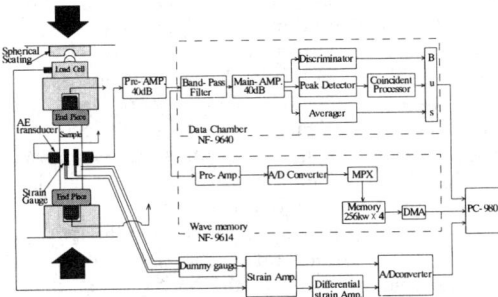

Figure 4. A schematic diagram of the measuring system.

3. RESULTS AND DISCUSSION

3.1 Experimental results

In the AE method, the observed features related between the stress and the accumulated ringdown

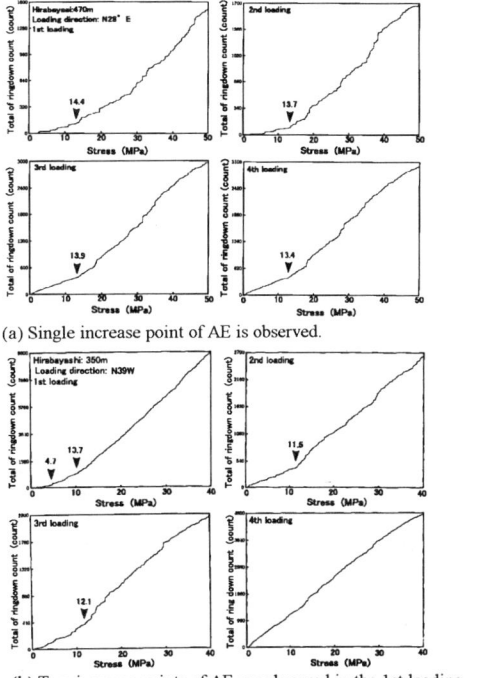

(a) Single increase point of AE is observed.

(b) Two increase points of AE are observed in the 1st loading.

Figure 5. Examples of the experimental results by the AE method.

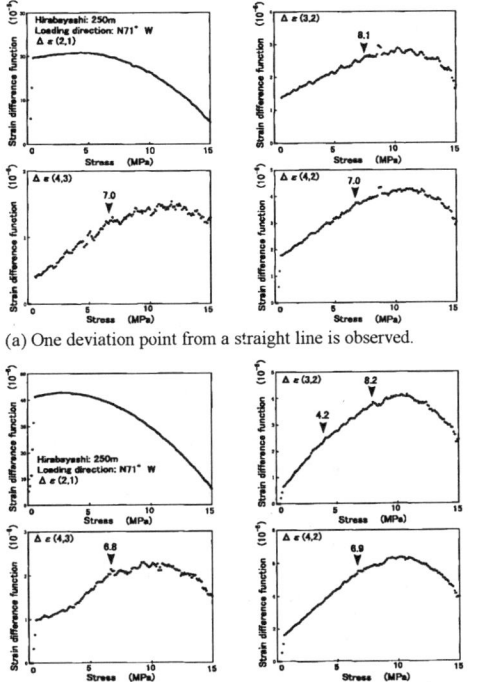

(a) One deviation point from a straight line is observed.

(b) Two bending points of straight line are observed in $\Delta \varepsilon (3,2)$.

Figure 6. Examples of the experimental results by the DRA method.

count in the first loading were classified into three patterns as follows: one increase point of AE was observed, two increase points of AE were observed, and Kaiser effect was not recognized. The experimental results on a specimen from 470 m depth showing single increase point of AE is presented in Figure 5(a). Kaiser effect was recognized on about 14 MPa not only in the first loading, but also in the second to fourth loading. Figure 5(b) shows the experimental result on a specimen from 350 m depth. This specimen was characterized by two increase points of AE in the first loading, however only one increase point of AE was recognized in the following loading. Note that the relation between stress and AE mentioned above characterize neither the depth of the retrieve core samples nor the loading direction. These characteristics seem to depend on the condition of the individual specimen. In AE method, we could not estimate in-situ stresses at depth of 530 m and 735 m, because Kaiser effect was not recognized clearly in some loading directions.

In DRA, we estimated in-situ stress regarding the stress point at which the strain difference function was deviated from a straight line as in-situ stress. The features of the strain difference function observed on core samples from Hirabayashi site were classified into three patterns as same as the results of AE measurement: the strain difference function has one deviation point from a straight line, the strain difference function has more than two deviation point from a straight line, and the strain difference function curved from the initial low stress level and no bending point or deviation point from a straight line was found. Figure 6(a) and Figure 6(b) show the experimental results on the specimens from 255 m depth. The specimen shown in Figure 6(a) revealed clear one deviation point from a straight line of the strain difference function, however another specimen had two bending point of straight line of the strain difference function as shown in Figure 6(b). Similar to the results of the AE method, these features of the strain difference function did not characterize the depth from which core samples were retrieved or the heterogeneity of the rocks at a depth. Core samples from 470 m, 530 m, and 735 m depth had the tendency that the strain difference function behaved as a curved line and had no deviation point from a straight line. On the other hand, core samples from 255 m and 350 m showed clear deviation points from a straight line.

3.2 Estimation of stress condition at Hirabayashi site

The estimated state of stress by AE and DRA at each depth are shown in Figure 7. Figure 8 shows the direction of the maximum horizontal principal stress at each depth.

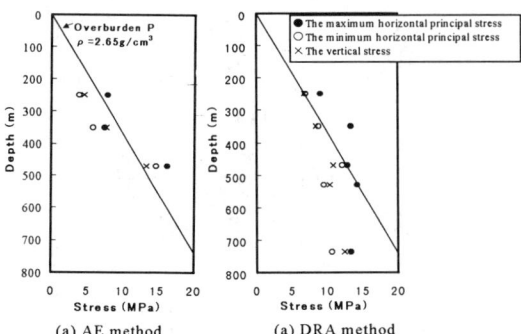

(a) AE method   (a) DRA method

Figure 7. The relation between the estimated stresses and the depth.

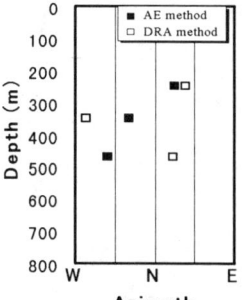

Figure 8. The relation between the direction of the maximum horizontal principal stresses and the depth.

The experimental results of the AE method showed that vertical stresses were consistent with the overburden pressures calculated from the rock density data at 250 m, 350 m, and 470 m. In horizontal plane, both the minimum and maximum stresses became large with depth, while the state of stress became isotropic with depth. The directions of maximum horizontal principal stresses differed with depths as shown in Figure 8, e.g. N21.5° E at 255 m, N29.2° W at 350 m, and N54° W at 470 m.

In the results of DRA method, the estimated vertical stresses at 250 m, 350 m, and 470 m were consistent with the overburden pressures as well as the results of AE method. However, those at 530 m and 735 m were recognized to be small compared to the overburden pressures as shown as Figure 7. Estimated vertical stresses at these depths were equivalent to 73% and 63% of the overburden pressures respectively. Average of horizontal principal stresses conducted same trend with the vertical stresses, with an average increased with depth to 470 m, although those at 530 m and 735 m did not have increasing trend and became small compared to those of shallower depth. It is the characteristics that average horizontal principal stresses were larger than vertical stresses at the 250 m, 350 m, 470 m, and 530 m, while vertical stress was larger than average horizontal stress at 735 m depth located beneath the deformed zone. Differential horizontal stresses had a trend to decrease slightly with depth and the ratio of maximum to minimum horizontal stress were likely to be close to 1. The directions of the maximum horizontal principal stresses were N34.0° E at 250 m, N77.6° W at 350 m, and N20.0° E at 470 m. There were some inconsistency with the estimated directions by AE method. On the other hand, those at 530 m and 735 m were unknown because the orientations of the core samples were not measured.

As mentioned above, the state of stress in this site were found to be varied across the fault zone. This experimental results suggest that the present state of stress in Hirabayashi site have been influenced strongly by the 1995 Hyogoken-nanbu Earthquake.

4. CONCLUSIONS

The state of stress at Hirabayashi site were estimated using retrieved core samples from five depths by the AE and DRA methods. The experimental results indicate that vertical stresses were consistent with the overburden pressures to the depth of 470 m (above the fault zone), although those at 530 m and 735 m depth (within the fault zone) were small compared with the overburden pressures. Also, average horizontal stresses increased with depth to 470 m, while those did not increase and had a constant value at 530 m and 735 m. The direction of maximum horizontal principal stress pointed different orientations at each depth. The state of stress in Hirabayashi site were found to be changed across the fault zone along the Nojima fault.

REFERENCES

Ito H., Y. Kuwahara, T.i Miyazaki, O,Nishizawa, T.u Kiguchi, Ko.o Fujimoto, T.i Ohtani, H. Tanaka, T.

Higuchi, S. Agar, A.Brie and H. Yamamoto, 1996: Structure and physical properties of the Nojima Fault by the Active fault Drilling, *Buthuri-tansa*, 49, 522-535.

Kanagawa T. and K. Shin, 1990: A study on Kaiser effect for Geo-Stress measurement -Acoustic emission, deformation rate and acoustic elasticity method, *Proc. 22nd symp. On Rock Mech*, 431-435.

Yamamoto K.,Y.Kuwahara, N.Kato and T.Hieasawa, 1990: Deformation rate analysis: A new method for in situ stress estination from inelastic deformation of rock samples under uniaxial compressions, *Tohoku Geophys. J.*, 33, 127-147.

Yoshikawa S. and K. Mogi, 1981: A new method for estimation of the crustal stress from cored rock samples: Laboratory study in thecase of uniaxial compression, *Tectonophysics*, 74, 323-339.

Zang A., C.F.Wagner and G. Dresen, 1996: Acoustic emission, microstructure, and damage model of dry and wet sandstone stressed to failure, *J.Geophys. Res.*, 101, 17,507-17,521.

A geomechanical model of crustal waveguides dynamics

Yu. I. Kuznetsov
Joint-Stock Research Industrial Company GERS, Moscow, Russia

A. V. Karakin
All-Russian Scientific-Research Geosystems Institute, Russia

ABSTRACT: The analysis of geophysical data show that continental crust is divided with many cracked layers (waveguides) filled with mineralized fluids. This paper presents some mechanism of fluid movement in these waveguides which can produce self-exited oscillation regime providing the state of dynamical equilibrium. The model includes two-layer system. The upper layer is elastic. In the lower, second layer, two regimes - compaction and dilatation competing with themselves are existing. We expect that this mechanism is mainly responsible for stress state and fluid regime in the continental crust during geological times corresponding waveguide size scale. This mechanism is important for understanding human-life valuable processes: earthquakes and hydrocarbons transportation from mother-rocks to the deposits.

1. INTRODUCTION

The volume of crustal water is commensurable with that of the world ocean and amounts to about 4% of the crust volume. Such an amount of the crustal water has a considerable influence on all geologic processes occurring in the crust. It is natural to anticipate the maximum influence of the fluids in fractured, high-permeability layers, which also include crustal waveguides.

The results of drilling the Kola superdeep well, interpretation of deep seismic sounding data (Krasnopevtseva, 1978; Seismic Models ..., 1980) and magnetotelluric data (Vanian, 1984; Feldman, 1976) show that the crust has a complex layered structure and resembles a sandwich of alternating hard, seismically transparent and opaque layers. The experimental data accumulated since 1960s suggest that, at depths of 15 to 20 km, the above zones are most probably caused by the presence of electrically conductive fluids. The fluid volume content in the high-conductivity layers reaches several per cent. This porosity value seems reasonable to be taken as an original porosity value in the waveguide.

It has been shown (Nikolayevskii, 1996) that only destruction mode changes with depth, whereas the destruction itself can be observed quite deep – possibly, to the crust bottom. In the upper crust, the destruction surfaces are represented by subvertical fractures and main ruptures. Then, with depth, a system of inclined fractures and small fracturing appear and occupy a certain finite volume. When the Coulomb friction force reaches the ultimate strength, the destruction along the main fractures becomes essentially impossible, the entire medium becomes brittle, and the deformation occurs in the cataclastic flow state. The given concept identifies the crustal waveguides with an unsteady destruction zone which ends at the Conrad boundary.

The overlying layers can move along the waveguide as if in a lubricant. This suggestion agrees with the tectonic stratification concept and the idea about two-stage platform tectonics based on the latter (Lobkovski, 1988). In accordance with these schemes, the Earth crust consists of the layers sharply different in their viscosity. The upper, hardest crust is divided into macroplates which move relative to each other in the way similar to that in the classical scheme of plate tectonics. The latter concept can also solve the problem of the tectonic forces moving the system as a whole. They are the forces which cause the intraplate deformations and upper layers motion against the lower ones. The global motion energy transforms into that of regional microplate motion.

A two-layer geomechanical model for the crustal waveguide is suggested. It is the further development of the model proposed in a work by Karakin (1990). This work presents the model as individual horizontally homogeneous blocks. The process was phase-shifted in different blocks compared to neighboring ones. In this model, the layers are horizontally continuous and slightly heterogeneous. The latter means that values change much more vertically than horizontally.

2. VALIDATION PROCEDURE AND SOLUTION

Depending on the pore pressure and porosity values, the crustal waveguide medium can exist in two states: compaction and dilatation. Assume the waveguide medium is linear-viscous, with its shear and volume viscosities η_1 and η_2 respectively, in the compaction state. Its viscocity state occurs when the spherical component of the effective stresses tensor is less than a certain limit caused by physical properties of the medium. The full stresses are determined by the geodynamical situation, which changes little within a wave period. Therefore, the effective stresses change mostly due to the deviation of the pore pressure p^a from its geostatic component (determined from the formula $p = p^a - \rho g z + const$). Here, the z axis is directed vertically upwards. Consequently, the viscous state takes place for $p<\sigma_*$, $m_0<m<m_*$, where σ_* is the critical value of the sphere component of the effective stresses tensor. From the reason of the problem, $\sigma_* <0$. When $m = m_0$, the pores are being closed, so their further reduction is impossible. When $m = m_*$, the matrix is being destroyed in the dilatation state and transition to the viscous state occurs, in which only porosity is being decreased. Fig. 2 shows the state diagram for the plane (p,m).

Introduce a coordinate system (x,z) on a vertical plane. From the reason of the problem, the wave moves in the positive direction of the x axis. In a steady-state wave, all values depend on the argument $y = x - vt$. In a moving coordinate system, the wave phase coordinates are distributed as follows. When $y_1<y<y_2$, a dilatation phase occurs, and when $y_2<y<y_3$, a compaction one takes place. The normal stress σ in the upper layer can be set at the start point

$$\sigma = \sigma_0 \quad \text{at} \quad y = y_1. \tag{1}$$

This stress can be divided into two components corresponding to the tangential forces increments at each of the phases, $\sigma_0 = \sigma_1 + \sigma_2$. Here, σ_1 and σ_2 are the normal stresses corresponding to the dilatation and compaction phases, respectively. At the boundary of both phases, there is the following condition for the normal stress:

$$\sigma = \sigma_2 \quad \text{at} \quad y = y_2. \tag{2}$$

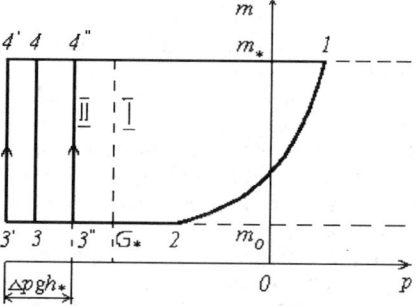

Fig. 2. Waveguide medium state diagram. The display point motion along the closed contour in the phase plane (p,m) corresponds to the wave process oscillation cycle for two points of the waveguide which are placed at the waveguide top and bottom and, at the same time, on the same vertical line. One and two strokes mark the trajectory intervals corresponding to the waveguide bottom and top. The other trajectory intervals are the same for all points located on the same vertical line. The display point motion along the closed contour on the diagram (the direction is indicated by the arrow) represents an oscillation cycle. The display point on the diagram corresponds to some points of the crustal waveguide. In the compaction mode, all points of the waveguide's vertical line correspond to a single display point on this diagram.

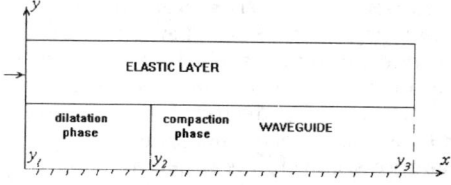

Fig. 1. Schematic diagram of two-layer waveguide model. The arrow points to the tectonic forces direction.

2.1. Solution for dilatation zone

The dilatation state in the lower layer (Fig. 1) can be described by Rice equations (Rice, 1980)

$$d\gamma = d^p\gamma - d\tau/G_e,$$
$$d^p\gamma = [d\tau - \mu(d\sigma - dp)]/G_p,$$
$$d\theta = d^p\theta - [d\sigma - (1 - K/K_s)dp]/K,$$
$$d^p\theta = \frac{\beta}{E}[d\tau - \mu(d\sigma - dp)]$$

Here, γ and θ are the shear and volume deformations in this layer, index p is the plastic component of deformation, G_e and K are the porous medium shear and volume elastic moduli, τ and σ are the shear stress and pressure in the porous medium, G_p is the nonelastic tangential deformation modulus, β and μ are the friction and dilatation factors. It is assumed that the nonelastic volume and shear deformations are rather great compared to the elastic ones ($d\gamma \cong d^p\gamma$, $d\theta \cong d^p\theta$). Therefore, the dilatation equation system can be simplified and, after some elementary integration, reduced to the simple kinematic relations ($d\theta = \beta d\gamma$, $m - m_0 = \beta\gamma$), i.e., with increasing shear deformations in the waveguide zone porosity increases from m_0 to its critical value m_*, which results in transition into the viscous phase. It means that the following relations hold for the dilatation and compaction zones boundary: $m = m_0$ and $\tau = \tau_0$ at $y = y_1$; $m = m_*$ and $\tau = \tau_*$ at $y = y_2$; $m = m_0$ and $\tau = \tau_0$ at $y = y_3$. Here, τ_0 and τ_* are the minimum and maximum values of the tangential stress. The porosity value $m = m_*$ is an initial value for the compaction phase.

In the upper elastic layer 1, because of the assumptions made, a one dimension stressed and strained state occurs which can be described by the relation $\sigma = E\varepsilon$, where ε is the horizontal deformations, and E is the Young's modulus in this layer. At the moment of the dilatation phase start, the shear deformation in the lower layer is equal to zero. Its further rise is connected with the upper layer deformation by the kinematic relation

$$\frac{du}{dx} = \varepsilon, \quad u = h_2\gamma.$$

So, we have evident relations resulting from the condition of forces balance and previous reasoning. These relations connect the normal stress in the upper layer, the tangential stress in the lower one, and porosity:

$$h_1\frac{d\sigma}{dx} = \tau, \quad \sigma = \frac{Eh_2}{\beta}\frac{dm}{dx}. \quad (3)$$

Combining (3) and transformating to the moving coordinate system, i.e., to the argument, $y = x - vt$, we can derive the equation

$$\frac{d^2m}{dy^2} = \alpha^2(m - m_0), \quad \alpha^2 = \frac{G_p}{h_1 h_2 E}. \quad (4)$$

Solving Eq. (4) with the corresponding boundary conditions can yield

$$m - m_0 = (m_* - m_0)\frac{Sh\alpha(y - y_1)}{Sh\alpha(y_2 - y_1)}. \quad (5)$$

Note that $\alpha(y_2 - y_1) \sim 1$. Since $E \gg G_p$, then the dilatation phase length $(y_2 - y_1)$ is much greater than the layer thicknesses h_1 and h_2.

Using (1), (3) and (5), we can find the full normal stress

$$\sigma_0 = \frac{\alpha Eh_2(m_* - m_0)}{\beta Sh\alpha(y_2 - y_1)} \quad (6)$$

and the component of the normal stresses which corresponds to the dilatation phase,

$$\sigma_1 = \frac{\alpha Eh_2(m_* - m_0)(1 - Ch\alpha(y_2 - y_1))}{\beta Sh\alpha(y_2 - y_1)}.$$

From that, the normal stress σ_2 value for the compaction phase can be found:

$$\sigma_2 = \frac{\alpha Eh_2(m_* - m_0)Ch\alpha(y_2 - y_1)}{\beta Sh\alpha(y_2 - y_1)}. \quad (7)$$

This expression allows evaluation of the dilatation phase length, since the normal stress σ_0 can be determined from the boundary condition (1).

2.2. Solution for compaction zone

We accept linear rheological equations for the viscous phase. Therefore, the shear and volume deformations occur independently from each other. The volume viscous deformations when $m \ll 1$, the same way as in the earlier work (Karakin, 1990), can be described by the following compaction equations:

$$\frac{\partial}{\partial z}\left(\eta\frac{\partial j}{\partial z}\right) = \delta j - \Delta\rho g, \quad \frac{\partial m}{\partial t} + \frac{\partial j}{\partial z} = 0,$$

$$\rho = -\eta \frac{\partial j}{\partial z}, \qquad \eta = \eta_2 + \frac{4}{3}\eta_1, \qquad (8)$$
$$t > 0, \qquad -h(x,t) < z < 0.$$

Here, j – the filtration flow, δ – the hydraulic resistance factor, and the z axis is directed vertically upwards. As mentioned above, the main difference from the work cited is that the compaction layer thickness (as well as other model parameters) is not constant and depends on the horizontal coordinate x as a parameter.

The lower boundary G_1 of the viscous consolidation zone can be either movable or stationary depending on its porosity value. In the nonstationary situation, different motion modes are possible on it. In particular, it is stationary and impermeable when $m > m_0$.

When porosity at that boundary reaches the m_0 value, the boundary begins moving upwards up to its contact with the boundary G_2. If the stationary wave moves, then the only situation possible is when we have a receding front condition on the lower boundary G_1

$$j = 0, \qquad m = m_0. \qquad (9)$$

The upper boundary G_2 of the waveguide is stationary. There is a porous layer with an elastic matrix above the boundary. For this layer, it is necessary to solve an edge problem of piezoconduction (elastic consolidation problem) and "join" the solution obtained and the waveguide solution. However, for the purpose of a qualitative research, the joining condition may be replaced with a simpler one G_2:

$$p - \sigma_* = bj. \qquad (10)$$

The constant b can be expressed via geometric and filtration characteristics of the elastic matrix zone located over the waveguide. The edge conditions system also includes the start condition

$$m = m_* \quad \text{at} \quad t = 0 \qquad (11)$$

which is determined by the porosity at the moment of transition from the dilatation to compaction mode. For each oscillation cycle, the starting moment of time is matched with the beginning of the compaction phase. Since the shear and volume deformation equations split, then time exists independently in each of these equation groups. The edge problem (8) – (11) was solved numerically. Combination of the solutions in each of the phases allowed construction of a full wave solution and evaluation of all its parameters.

2.3. Major consequence of this model

This mechanism is suggested to be one of the major factors determining the stressed state and dynamic fluid mode of the continental crust in geologic time scale at the distances corresponding to the waveguide sizes. In particular, it is a component of two natural processes important to mankind – earthquakes and hydrocarbon transfer from oil origin rocks to oil and gas fields. The knowledge of the fluid flow direction for geologic time scale seems to be of interest from the viewpoint of choosing the place for radioactive waste burial.

3. CONCLUSION

1. A flat two-layer self-excited oscillation model for the crustal waveguide has been constructed.
2. A wave solution of the model equations which agree with the fact of the dynamic equilibrium state of the Earth crust's fractured saturated layers has been found.
3. The wave solution results in periodic vertical movements of fluids into and from the waveguide.
4. This model allows explanation of some geologic phenomena: closed water reservoir and subsoil water level fluctuations, periodical seismic mode, ore and hydrocarbon deposit origin processes, etc.
5. The model consequences (directional fluid motion in the crust) can be used for choosing optimum places to bury industrial and radioactive wastes.

REFERENCES

Vanian L.L. 1984. Conductivity of the Earth Crust in View of Its Fluid Regime. In: *Crustal Anomalies of Conductivity*: 27-34. Leningrad: Nauka.

Karakin A.V. 1990. Model of Fluid Movement in Geological Time Spans. *Mathematical Modeling*, 2 (3): 31-42.

Krasnopevtseva G.V. 1978. Geological and Geophysical Peculiarities of Structures of Layers with Reduced Velocities in the Earth Crust. In: *Regional, Exploration and Field Geophysics*: Moscow: VIEMS: 40.

Lobkovsky L.I. 1988. *Geodynamics of Spreading, Subduction Zones and Two-Stage Plate Tectonics*. Moscow: Nauka: 252.

Seismic Models of Lithosphere of the Major Geostructures of the U.S.S.R. Territory. 1980. Moscow: Nauka: 184.

Nikolaevskii V.N. 1990. *Mechanics of Porous and Fractured Media.* Singapore: World Scientific: 472.

Feldman I.S. 1976. On the nature of conductive layers in the Earth's crust and upper mantle. *Geoelec. and Geotherm.* In: Stud. KAPG Geophys. Monogr. Bp.: 721-745.

Rice J. R., 1980. Mechanics of Earthquake Rupture. In: Dziewonski & Bosch (ed.) *Physics of the Earth's Interior. Proceedings of the International School of Physics Enrico Fermi Course 78, 1979.* Amsterdam: Italian Physical Society: 555-649.

The general characteristics of the stress state in the various parts of the earth's crust

Ömer Aydan
Department of Marine Civil Engineering, Tokai University, Shimizu, Japan

Toshikazu Kawamoto
Department of Civil Engineering, Aichi Institute of Technology, Toyota, Japan

ABSTRACT: The stress state of the earth's crust is of paramount importance in geomechanics as well as in geophysics. Particularly, the stress state in the earth's crust before the excavation of structures is of great interest in mining and civil engineering since their stability is very much influenced by that. The stress state of the crust is also of great interest in geophysics in association with understanding the mechanism and prediction of earthquakes. Data on in-situ stress measurements carried in the various parts of the earth's crust have been complied in a data-base called *ISMEAS*. In this paper, a brief outline of the data-base system is given and the results of data processing on the general characteristics of the stress state in the earth's crust are described in detail and discussed.

1 INTRODUCTION

The stress state of the earth is of paramount importance in geomechanics and geophysics. Particularly, the virgin stress state in the earth's crust is of great interest in mining and civil engineering since the stability of excavations is very much influenced by that. Geophysicians are also concerned with the stress state of the crust in association with understanding the earthquake mechanism and predicting earthquakes. The general tendency among geophysicians is that the stress state in the earth is almost hydrostatic and many existing formulations for the stress state in the earth is based on that concept (Heim 1878, Jeffrey and Bullen 1940, Anderson and Hart 1976).

The measurements of in-situ stresses in various engineering projects showed that this was not always the case (Hast 1969, Brown and Hoek 1978). Furthermore, many measurements indicated that horizontal stresses could be several times vertical stresses in shields such as Canadian or Scandinivian shields (Herget 1986, Stephanson et al. 1986). In association with the excavations in mining and civil engineering fields and earthquake prediction projects, stress measurements in the earth crust have been undertaken over last 30 years. Most of the measurements are restricted to a depth below 5000 m.

The authors have complied data on in-situ stress measurements carried in the various parts of the earth's crust through a data-base called *ISMEAS*. The general characteristics of the stress state in the earth's crust are deduced from this data-base system. The authors first give a brief outline of the data-base system and describe the results of data processing on the general characteristics of the stress state in the earth's crust in detail.

2 A DATA BASE SYSTEM

In this section, a brief outline of a data-base system is first described and then results of in-situ measurements in various countries by using this data-base system are given. The integrated data-base system consists of two sub-systems: i) Data-base sub-system: *ISMEAS*, ii) Data Processing sub-system. They are briefly explained in the following sub-sections.

2.1 Data-base and Data Gathering

The items of the data-base involve type, mechanical characteristics of rock, geometrical characteristics of test, their location and reference, metho of measurement, overburden pressure and vertical and horizontal stresses and principal stresses and their orientations. The data-base covers in-situ stress measurements in many countries on 5 continents.

The data-base was coded by using soft-wear called *dBASE* and it is run on MS-DOS environment. However, it can be upgraded to run on WINDOWS environement. The data-base is called **ISMEAS** which stands for **IN-SITU STRESS MEAS**URMENTS.

Data were gathered from the author own sources and publications available in literature. An entry form is prepared for gathering and compiling data. Figure 1 shows an actual example of entries on the screen of the data-base. Presently the number of entries in the data-base is more than 700.

2.2 Interrelational Data Processing

A data processing sub-system was developed for studying interrelations among the items of the data-base. This sub-system consists of creating of data-files for given conditions and the graphical presentation of chosen items and establishing empirical relations. The data files for chosen items for a given condition is created by a program coded in *BASIC* programming language. Figure 2 shows an interactive screen of this system. The conditions available in the program can be expanded or changed as required. Once a data-file is created, a soft-wear called *NGRAPH* is used for graphical presentation of data and developing empirical relations. This soft-wear is preferred as it has a user-friendly interface and superior output quality of graphics. Examples are given in the next section.

3 STRESS STATE IN VARIOUS PARTS OF THE EARTH'S CRUST

A brief summary of stress measurements in various countries are outlined in the followings. The discussion is concentrated upon the characteristics of horizontal and vertical stresses in this particular summary.

3.1 Stress Measurements in Australia

Fig. 3 shows plots of vertical stresses and horizontal stresses. Most of these data are gathered in mining projects. It seems that the vertical stress near the ground surface is larger than the overburden pressure plotted by a solid line by assuming a unit density of 26 kN/m^3. On the other hand, it tends to be less than the overburden pressure as the depth increases. The horizontal stresses remain to be greater than the vertical stresses.

Fig. 3 also shows the ratio of horizontal stress to the vertical stress. The ratio is always greater

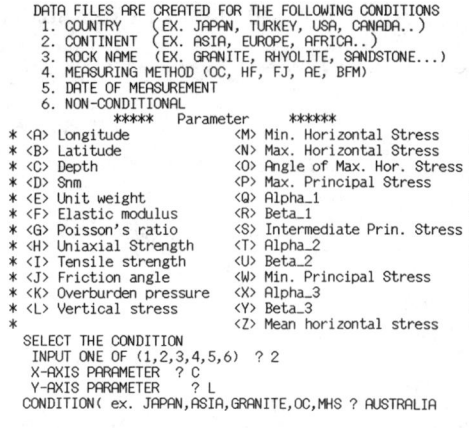

Fig. 1 An input screen of database ISMEAS

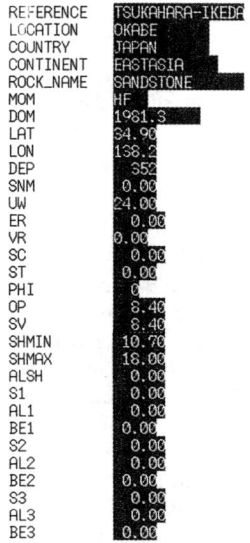

Fig. 2 An interactive screen of data processing subsystem

near the ground surface. The range varies between once to four times the vertical stress. The ratio tends to converge to a value of 1 as the depth increases.

3.2 Stress Measurements in East Asia

The data plotted in Figure 4 are those obtained in Japan and Korea, mainly. Since the published data of China is very limited and unreliable, they are excluded in the figure. The vertical stress almost coincide with the predicted overburden pres-

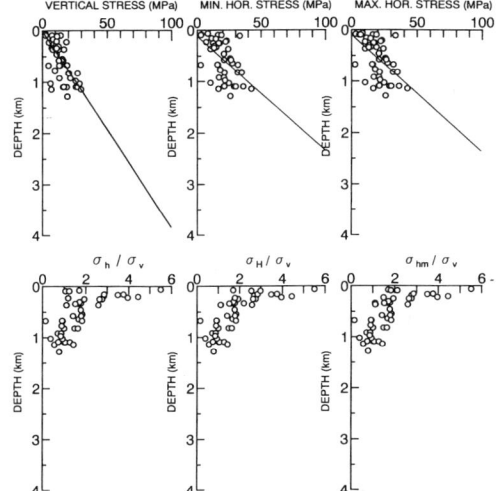

Fig. 3 Variation of vertical and horizontal stresses and lateral stress coefficients with depth in Australia

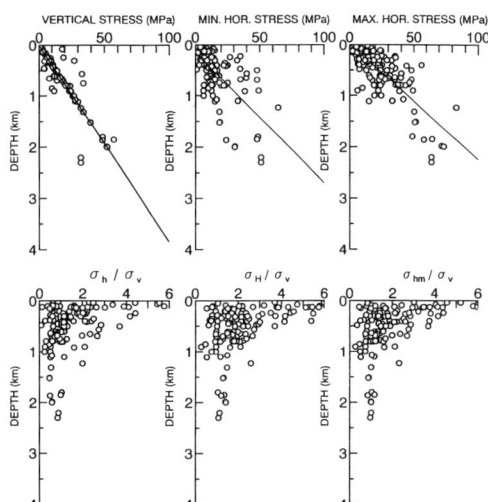

Fig. 5 Variation of vertical and horizontal stresses and lateral stress coefficients with depth in Europe

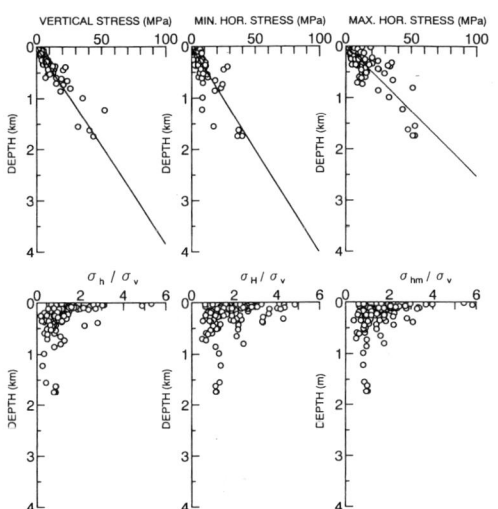

Fig. 4 Variation of vertical and horizontal stresses and lateral stress coefficients with depth in East Asia

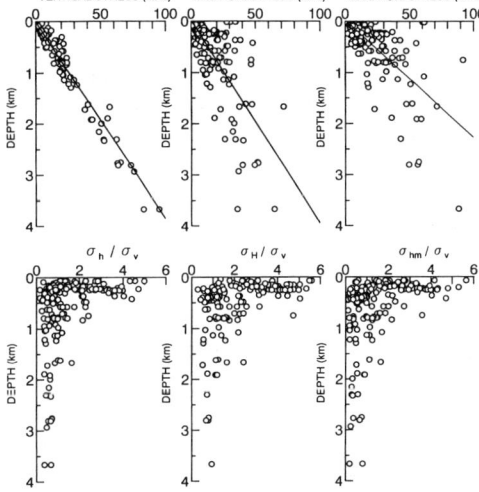

Fig. 6 Variation of vertical and horizontal stresses and lateral stress coefficients with depth in North America

sure. It seems that the vertical stress in these countries is the intermediate one. The ratio of the horizontal stress to the vertical stress near the ground surface varies between 1 to 3 and it tends to converge to unity as the depth increases.

3.3 Stress Measurements in Europe

The data shown in Figure 4 cover a number of countries (Italy, France, Sweden, Norway, Spain, Austria, Switzerland and Germany, UK). However, the data of Germany is very few since it is very difficult to find any reliable publication in english lit-

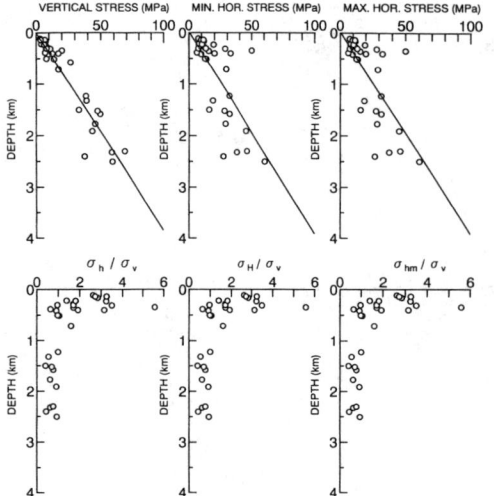

Fig. 7 Variation of vertical and horizontal stresses and lateral stress coefficients with depth in Africa

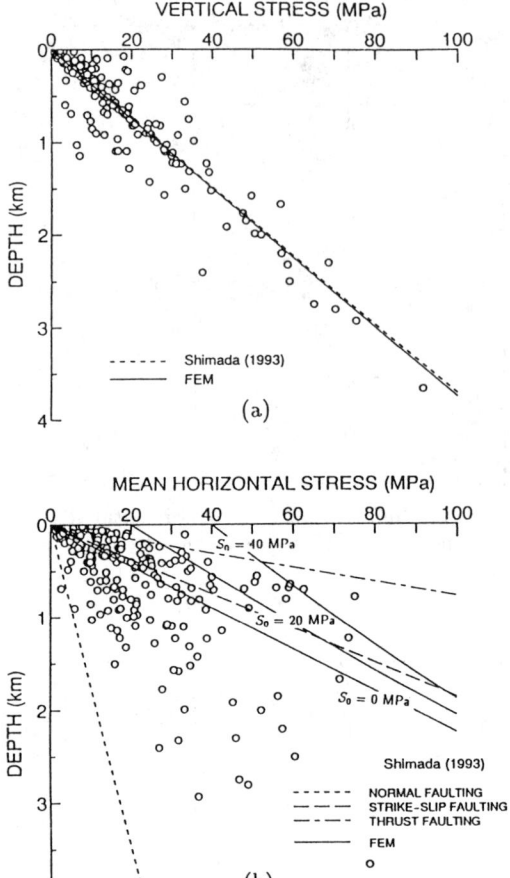

erature about measurements in that country. Most of the data on the vertical stresses are close to the overburden pressure. Once again we note that the vertical stress is an intermediate one. The maximum shear stress tends to zero as the depth increases. The ratio of the horizontal stress to the vertical stress varies between 1 to 5 near the ground surface and it tends to converge a value of 1 as the depth is greater than 1 km.

3.4 Stress Measurements in North America

Figure 6 shows the stress measurement results in Canada and USA. The reported stress measurements in USA and Canada are numerous and they are probably most usefull to understand the present stress state of the earth and its crust. The comments on stresses in North America are also similar to those made in previous summaries. It is worth noting that the maximum shear stress tends to zero as the depth becomes greater than 1 km. Except very high values of the ratio of horizontal to vertical stresses particularly in Canadian Shield, the value of the ratio varies between 1 to and it tends to become equal to unity or less than that.

3.5 Stress Measurements in Africa

Figure 7 shows the measurements in Zambia, Rhodesia and South Africa. Again most of the measurements are associated with mining projects. Although there are few reports on measurements in South Africa in recent years, the South Africa

Fig. 8 Comparison of distributions of horizontal and vertical stresses and lateral stress coefficient for different values of the strength S_0 of Earth's crust with in-situ measurements and predictions by Shimada (1993)

was one of the poineers in stress measurements in sixties and seventies. Similar conclusions could be stated for the measurements in Africa.

4 COMPARISONS AND DISCUSSIONS

Aydan (1995) caried out a series of parameteric studies by using the finite element method and he draw the following conclusions:

i-) If the sphericity of the earth is taken into account, it is possible to explain the large horizontal stresses near ground surface.

ii-) For a spherical symmetric earth, the tangential stress (lateral stress) is the maximum principal stress and radial stress (vertical stress) is minimum.

iii-) The crust and mantle are already in plastic state which has some important implications in rock mechanics and rock engineering.

He computed the distributions of stresses and the ratio of tangential stress to radial stress together which are shown in Figure 8 together with in-situ observations and predictions by Shimada (1993) for a depth of 4 km in the earth's crust. In the computations, the behaviour of materials was assumed to be thermo-elasto-plastic and the uniaxial compressive strength was varied from 0 MPa to 40 MPa by an increment of 20 MPa. The radial stress (vertical stress) almost coincided with each other. They are almost equal to the vertical stress calculated from $\rho g H$ (Shimada 1993) and it is a good fit to in-situ measurements.

The tangential stresses (horizontal stress) for each value of S_0 fit fairly well to in-situ measurements for a depth of 1 km from the ground surface (Fig. 8(b)). However, finite element computations overestimate the tangential stresses at depths greater than 1 km.

The ratio of tangential stress to radial stress for each value of S_0 provide upper bounds for insitu measurements. The discrepancy between computed and measured values may be eliminated if a thermo-elasto-visco plastic constitutive law is employed in finite element analysis.

CONCLUSIONS

The most striking feature from these results is that the ratio of horizontal stress over the vertical stress is very large near the ground surface and then it decreases as the depth increases. Furthermore, the horizontal stresses are not equal. Investigations show that the orientation of the maximum horizontal stress differ from region to region. Nevertheless, it may be said that the largest horizontal stress is aligned with the direction of the earth rotation. The ratio seems to converge to a value of 1.0. In addition, the range of the ratio for a given depth is very wide.

REFERENCES

Anderson, L.D. and R.S. Hart 1976. An earth model based on free oscillations and body waves. J. Geophysical Res., 81(8), 1461-1475.

Aydan, Ö., 1995. The stress state of the earth and the earth's crust due to the gravitational pull. 35th US Rock Mechnanics Symp., Lake Tahoe,

Brown, E.T. and E. Hoek 1978. Trends in relationships between measured in-situ stresses and depth. Int. J. Rock Mech. Min. Sci., 15(4), 211-215.

Hast, N. 1969. The state of stress in the upper part of the Earth's crust. Tectonophysics, 8, 169-211.

Heim, A. 1878. Mechanismus der Gebirgsbildung, Bale.

Herget, G. 1986. Changes of ground stresses with depth in the Canadian Shield. Proc. Int. Symp. on Rock Stress and Rock Stress Measurements, Stockholm, 61-68.

Jeffreys, H. and K.E. Bullen 1940. *Seismological Tables*. British Association for the Advancement of Science, London.

Shimada, M. 1993. Two types of brittle fracture of silicate rocks and scale effect on rock strength: their implications in the earth crust. Proc. of Scale Effects in Rock Masses, Lisbon, 55-62.

Stephanson, O, P. Sarkka and A. Myrvang 1986. State of stress in Fennoscandia. Proc. Int. Symp. on Rock Stress and Rock Stress Measurements, Stockholm, 21-32.

Tanaka, Y. 1986. State of crustal stress inferred from in-situ stress measurements, J. Phys. Earth, 34, 557-570.

Relation of in-situ stress field to seismic activity as inferred from the stresses measured on core samples

Kiyohiko Yamamoto & Yasuo Yabe
Faculty of Science, Tohoku University, Sendai, Japan

Hidekazu Yamamoto
Faculty of Engineering, Iwate University, Japan

ABSTRACT: *In-situ* stresses are estimated from rock specimens to be compared with seismic activity. The conditions for earthquake occurrence suggested by the comparison are as follows; 1) the ratio of shear stress to normal stress larger than a critical value of about 0.3, 2) the concentration rate larger than the relaxation rate of stress, and 3) external and/or internal disturbances to make stress field nonuniform.

1 INTRODUCTION

The Byerlee's law or the Coulomb's criterion of failure states that shear failure occurs when shear stress on a plane exceeds the strength which is determined by the normal stress and the coefficient of friction for the plane (Byerlee, 1978). Recently, this criterion is often employed to estimate the regional stresses, to discuss on the potential of the crust for generating earthquakes and to investigate frictional strength of faults (*e. g.* Gephart and Forsyth, 1984, King *et al.*, 1994, Iio, 1997).

The criterion was established by laboratory experiments, which were performed on homogeneous specimens of finite sizes subjected to uniform stresses from the macroscopic viewpoint. The criterion is thus represented in terms of the average stresses over the specimen. In such experiments, when fracturing or sliding occurs on a specimen, shear stress drop takes place uniformly in the specimen in order to turn the stress field toward an isotropic state. The criterion holds thus under the condition that applied shear stress is permitted to change by failure.

On the other hand, the shear faulting which generates an earthquake appears to occur in an infinite heterogeneous continuum. Let us consider the shear faulting which occurs in an area of continuum subjected to constant anisotropic (or nonlithostatic) stresses. The shear stress drop due to the faulting should increase the stresses in other parts, even if the stress field near the fault turns toward an isotropic state. The strain energy in an elastic material generally increases with an increase in nonuniformity of stress and strain fields under constant applied stresses. It is thus logically concluded that faulting brings about the increase in the strain energy in the area under the constant stresses.

It seems to be doubtful that earthquakes occurs in order to increase strain energy as suggested by the above conclusion. The conclusion rather suggests that faulting occurs in order to turn the stress field toward not an isotropic but a uniform state under the anisotropic stress condition. If this is true, large average shear stress may not be a unique condition for earthquake occurrence. This has been suggested from *in-situ* stress data by Tanaka (1987). It is not axiomatic thus that the Coulomb's criterion is applicable to the faulting in the crust as well as the failure in laboratory. This is the reason for investigating the conditions imposed on the stress field to generate earthquakes in this study.

In order to reveal the conditions, *in-situ* stresses estimated in an area of high seismic activity will be compared with those of low activity in the present paper. *In-situ* stresses have been estimated at four sites in the vicinity of the inferred fault of a shallow intraplate earthquake of M=6.8 by Yamamoto *et al.* (1994). The sites are located in an area of high seismic activity. The results of the estimation will be reviewed as the representative of the stress field in the active area. On the other hand, Kitakami province in northeast Honshu, Japan, is known of low seismic activity. *In-situ* stresses at three sites in the province are newly estimated. The results together with the existing stress data will be compared with those for the active area in order to derive the conditions on the stress field for earthquake occurrence.

2 IN-SITU STRESS ESTIMATION

2.1 *Deformation Rate Analysis*

All stress estimations in the present paper are performed by the method of deformation rate analysis (DRA). DRA was developed as a method for estimating *in-situ* stresses from inelastic strain behavior

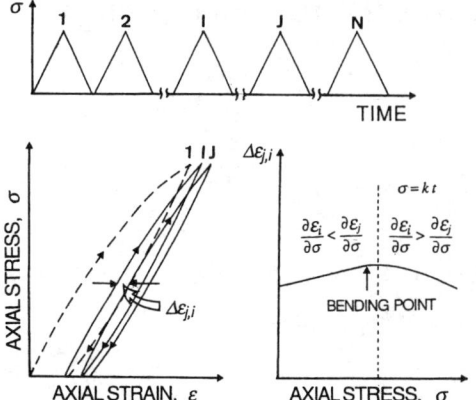

Fig. 1 Schematic illustration for deformation rate analysis (DRA). The upper figure shows loading history for the stress measurement. The vertical axis represents applied axial stress σ and the horizontal one does time t. The lower illustrates the definitions of strain difference function $\Delta\varepsilon_{i,j}(\sigma)$ and bending point. Bending point stress σ_0 is defined to be the value of σ corresponding to the bending point.

of rock specimens under uniaxial loading of compression by Yamamoto et al. (1983, 1990).

When uniaxial loading of compression is performed on a rock specimen, many acoustic emissions (AE) are generated by microfracturing. According to Kuwahara et al. (1990), microfracturing brings about an additional increase in inelastic strain. Therefore, the change in AE activity should be observed as the change in the increasing rate of inelastic strain. The rate change is detected by using the strain difference function $\Delta\varepsilon_{i,j}(\sigma)$ obtained by cyclic loading of compression to a specimen. The function is defined by

$$\Delta\varepsilon_{i,j}(\sigma) = \varepsilon_j(\sigma) - \varepsilon_i(\sigma), \quad j > i, \quad (1)$$

where $\varepsilon_i(\sigma)$ is axial strain of a specimen at an applied stress σ for the i-th loading. This function mainly represents the difference in inelastic strain between the i-th and the j-th loading. When contraction and compression are defined to be positive in sign, negative derivative of $\Delta\varepsilon_{i,j}(\sigma)$ with respect to σ means that inelastic strain rate is larger in the i-th than in the j-th loading.

Strain difference function is schematically illustrated in Fig. 1. Bending point means the point in the function at which the continuous decrease in its derivative starts. Bending stress or stress of memory is the axial stress at the bending point which is observed as the memory of previous stress, where the memory means the trace of the stress previously applied to specimens. Yamamoto, et al. (1990, 1995) have shown that the memory of *in-situ* stress is observed as the bending point and the axial stress at the bending point is identical to the magnitude of the *in-situ* stress, when no artificial stress has been applied to the specimen before the measurement. The mechanism of the *in-situ* stress memory is discussed also by Yamamoto (1995). Here, the *in-situ* stress means the normal component of *in-situ* stress in the direction of loading axis.

It has been empirically known that *in-situ* stress memory is found in the strain difference functions from the pair of loading cycles after the first cycle in many cases (Yamamoto et al., 1995). For this reason, uniaxial loading of three to five cycles was performed on each specimen for DRA.

2.2 Strain Measurement

Specimens used for the stress estimation are of rectangular prism in shape of about 15 x 15 x 38 (mm) or about 10 x 10 x 25 (mm) in size. They are sawed from boring cores in the vertical and the four horizontal directions at an interval of 45 degrees. Uniaxial stress of compression is cyclically applied in the direction of the longer axis for DRA. The largest and the smallest horizontal stress are calculated from the bending stresses observed for the horizontal specimens. Two or three specimens are used for estimating the stress in each direction.

Cyclic uniaxial loading is performed at a constant stress rate between 4 and 5 MPa a minute using a

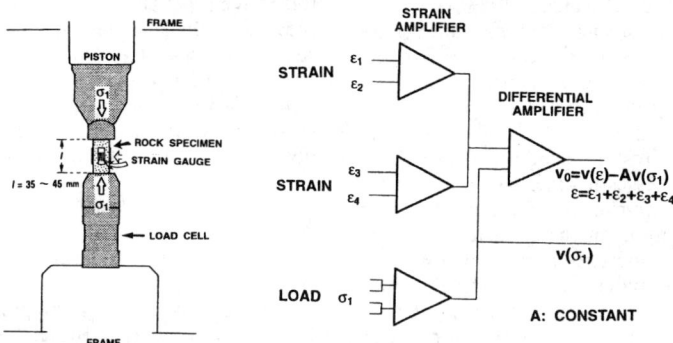

Fig. 2 Setup for uniaxial loading (left) and instrumentation for measurement of reduced strain (right). A strain gauge is pasted on each side of specimen.

servo-controlled apparatus. The peak applied stress is usually taken to be 1.5 to 2.5 times of the target stress. The setup for the axial strain measurement is illustrated in Fig. 2. The strain is measured with four strain gauges pasted on the sides of a specimen. In the case of hard rock specimens, the strain is required to be measured with a resolution better than 10^{-7} strain in order to identify the stress memory. The outputs of the four strain gauges are averaged to reduce the noises for the axial strain and the linear trend is removed from the relation between the stress and the averaged strain in the way as shown in Fig. 2. The residual strain thus obtained is called reduced strain. Strain difference functions are calculated using the amplified reduced strains.

2.3 *Analysis of Data*

If the bending points corresponding to *in-situ* stress memory are correctly specified for horizontal specimens, the azimuthal dependence of their bending stresses should be expressed by a sinusoidal function of azimuth as follows;

$$\sigma_0(\theta)=(\tau_{xx}+\tau_{yy})/2+(\tau_{xx}-\tau_{yy})\cos2\theta/2+\tau_{xy}\sin2\theta, \quad (2)$$

where $\sigma_0(\theta)$ is the bending stress or the normal component of *in-situ* stress to the plane perpendicular to the loading direction, θ is the azimuth and τ_{xx}, τ_{yy} and τ_{xy} are the stresses when x and y axes are taken in a horizontal plane. The maximum and the minimum horizontal stress are obtained by fitting a sinusoidal function to the observed relationship between bending stress and azimuth.

Here define a parameter r as follows;

$$r = (\sigma_1 - \sigma_3)/(\sigma_1 + \sigma_3), \quad (3)$$

according to Tanaka(1987), where σ_1 and σ_3 are the maximum and the minimum principal stress of compression. Usually, the frictional strength on a fault is expressed by the product of the coefficient of friction and the stress normal to the plane. Thus, r may be thought as an index for the shear stress level to the frictional strength. The parameter r is here called by relative shear stress. In the present paper, r is used to characterize the stress field to be compared with seismic activity, assuming that one of the principal direction is in the vertical.

3 STRESSES AROUND AN ACTIVE FAULT

3.1 *Sampling Sites of Cores for Measurement*

In-situ stresses around the inferred fault of the Nagano-ken Seibu earthquake ($M_{JMA} = 6.8$) have been estimated by Yamamoto *et al*. (1994). Their results are briefly reviewed in this section.

The earthquake took place in Nagano Prefecture, central Honshu, Japan, on September 14 in 1984. Focal depth was estimated at 2 km by Japan Meteorological Agency (JMA, 1985). The faulting process was revealed from geodetic data by Yamashina and Tada (1986) and from seismic data together with the geodetic data by Yoshida and Koketsu (1990). These studies show that the fault length is ten and a few km and the strike-slip component dominates in displacement. This fault is located at the foot of an active volcano which has erupted in 1979. Earthquake swarm had already begun at 1978 in the area around the fault (Aoki, 1987).

Yamamoto (1994) estimated *in-situ* stresses at four sites, OT-2, OT-3, OT-4 and OT-5 in Fig. 3 by DRA. The sites are at distances smaller than 5 km from the inferred fault and are about 2 to 6 km apart from one another. The boring cores used for the estimation were obtained from the depths between 331 and 722 m by New Energy Development Organization (NEDO). The boring was carried out in 1985 and 1986 and the stress estimation in 1989 and 1990.

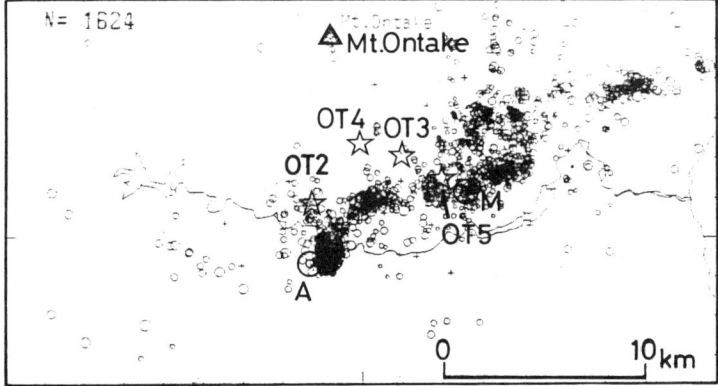

Fig. 3 The sites of core sampling for the stress estimation. The sites are marked with stars on the epicenter distribution of aftershocks of the 1984 Naganoken-Seibu earthquake (9/1/1983-10/22/1983) determined by Horiuchi *et al*. (1992). Double circles with M and A are the epicenters of the main shock and the largest aftershock determined by JMA (1985).

The stresses estimation three or four years after the boring may yield the stresses before the earthquake which occurred one or two years before the boring.

3.2 Results of Measurement

Table 1 shows the estimated values of the largest and the smallest horizontal stress and the vertical stress together with the r-value defined by (3). The last column of the table denotes the heat flow values reported by NEDO (1988). The stress orientation is unknown, because the cores have not been oriented. It is seen in Table 1 that the sites are in the field of strike-slip regime. This is consistent with the slip on the fault seismologically and geodetically estimated. The r-value varies site by site and ranges from about 0.15 to 0.44. This suggests that the stress field near active faults is strongly nonuniform.

As seen in Fig.3, no epicenters were determined around OT-4, while many epicenters crowd near OT-5 and OT-2. This suggests the correlation between the r-value and the seismic activity. The activity is very low in the area where r is smaller than 0.3, and *vice versa*. The value of about 0.3 seems to be critical for the seismic activity. The other importance is that the r-value is low at the site of high heat flow. This may suggest that the nonuniformity of the stress field is the reflection of the thermal state, that is, the nonuniformity is caused by the nonuniform relaxation rate of stresses.

4 STRESS FIELD OF AN INACTIVE AREA

4.1 Sampling Sites of Cores for Measurement

In Kitakami province in northeast Honshu, Japan, the stresses are newly measured at three sites, Hashikami (HSK), Fudai (FDI) and Tono (KGJ). The stresses at these sites are presented in this section together with the stresses already measured at Esashi and Kamaishi (KAM) in the province. Figure 4 shows the locations of these sites on the map of the epicenter distribution of shallow micro-earthquakes ($h < 30$ km) determined by Tohoku University.

In Kitakami province, the seismic activity in the southern part is higher than that in the northern part. The activity in the southern part is comparable to that in the other provinces in northeast Honshu. Although the activity is not especially low in the southern part, microearthquakes uniformly occur over the wide areas in the province. Further, no area where the epicenters crowd is found. This is one of the characteristics of seismic activity in Kitakami province. Another is that no large earthquake of the magnitude larger than 6.0 is known to occur after 1885 except for the earthquake of $M=6.5$ in the southern part. In the present paper, HSK and FDI are classified as the sites located in the northern part, and KGJ, KAM and Esashi as those in the southern part.

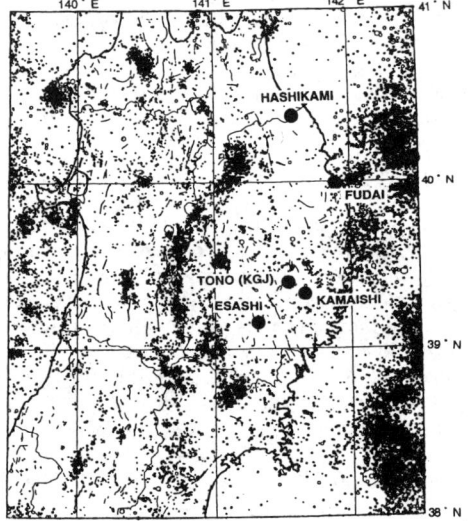

Fig. 4 The sampling sites of the rocks for the stress estimation in Kitakami province. The sites are shown together with the epiceters of shallow micro-earthquakes of depth less than 30 km (4/1/1974-10/31/1993). The epicenter are determined by Tohoku University.

Table 1. Estimated in situ stresses, r-value and average heat flow.

Site	Depth m	σ_{hmx} MPa	σ_{hmn} MPa	σ_v MPa	r	Average heat flow mW/m^2 (HFU)
OT-2	331	15.0±1.0	6.6±1.0	9.1±0.7	0.39	63 (1.5)
	448	15.4±0.6	6.4±0.6	11.7±0.1	0.41	(70 - 1203 m)
	547	17.3±0.9	7.4±0.9	12.5±1.0	0.40	
	722	25.8±1.1	12.1±1.1	19.5±1.0	0.36	
OT-3	376	12.9±0.5	6.2±0.5	10.0±0.6	0.35	143 (3.4)
	600	20.8±0.6	12.8±0.6	15.6±0.1	0.24	(110 - 1203 m)
OT-4	705	24.1±0.5	17.7±0.5	20.8±0.8	0.15	143 (3.4)
						(190 - 1002 m)
OT-5	470	17.3±1.1	7.1±1.1	12.8±1.3	0.42	59 (1.4)
	475	16.6±0.7	6.4±0.7	13.5±0.9	0.44	(160 - 502 m)

σ_{hmx}; Largest horizontal stress: σ_{hmn}; Least horizontal stress:
σ_v ; Vertical stress: r is defined by $r=(\sigma_1-\sigma_3)/(\sigma_1+\sigma_3)$; $\sigma_1 > \sigma_2 > \sigma_3$.
Data of average heat flow after NEDO (1988).

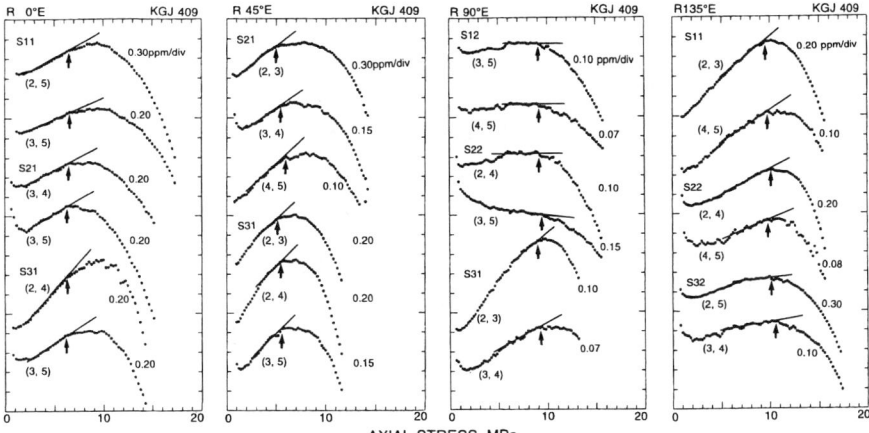

Fig. 5 Strain difference functions $\Delta\varepsilon_{i,j}(\sigma)$ for the horizontal specimens of 409 m depth at Tono (KGJ). R 0 E, R 45 E, R 90 E, R135 E, respectively, mean the data from the horizontal specimens of 0, 45, 90 and 135 degree clockwise from an arbitrary reference direction R. Arrows point the bending points determined by eye. Solid and dash lines are drawn in order to emphasize the gradient change of the function. Symbol 'S-n' means the specimen of the number n. Notation (i, j) stands for $\Delta\varepsilon_{i,j}(\sigma)$. Sensitivity of strain difference is indicated near the respective curves in 10⁻⁶ a division (ppm/div).

The sampling depths of the cores used for this stress estimation are equal to or more than about 400 m except for about 70 and 100 m at Esashi, as seen in Table 2. The samples at KAM were obtained from the depth of about 9.5 m in a horizontal hole drilled from the wall of a tunnel of about 3 m in width. Specimens at one of depths for each site are oriented except for those for Esashi.

4.2 Examples of Strain Difference Functions

Figure 5 shows the strain difference functions for the horizontal specimens of about 409 m in depth at KGJ (KGJ 409), for example. The functions are obtained from two or three specimens an azimuth and are shown in a frame for each azimuth. The azimuth is measured east from an arbitrary reference denoted by R. In this case the azimuth of R is 25 degree east from the magnetic north.

The bending points marked with arrows are found to have the nearly same value of bending stress for the specimens of the same direction. It can be confirmed even by eye that the stresses have azimuthal dependence with the period of 180 degrees and that the directions of the largest bending stress lie between 90 and 135 degree east from R.

4.3 Results of Measurement

The largest and the smallest horizontal stress are tabulated together with the vertical stresses in Table 2 for each site. The last column is the relative shear stress r_v in the vertical plane. The definition is put in the footnote to the table. It is seen that all the sites except for Esashi is in the stress field of the normal fault regime. The largest horizontal stress is close to the vertical one in magnitude. The direction of the smallest horizontal stress lie between the N-S and

Table 2. The vertical stress, the largest and the smallest horizontal stress and relative shear stress at sites in Kitakami province.

Site	Depth m	σ_v MPa	σ_{hmx} MPa	σ_{hmn} MPa	θ_{hmx} (N to E) deg.	r	r_v
Hashikami	398~400	10.7±0.2	10.0±0.4	7.6±0.4	105.1±4.3	0.17	0.14
	499~500	12.9±0.4	13.5±0.3	9.3±0.3		0.18	0.18
Fudai	405~406	--	9.0±0.2	4.7±0.2	92.3±1.9	(0.35)	(0.31)
	418~419	10.1±0.1	8.3±0.4	4.8±0.4		0.35	0.27
	495~496	12.1±0.2	11.0±0.5	6.4±0.5		0.31	0.26
Tono (KGJ)	409~410	9.8±0.2	10.5±0.2	5.2±0.2	113.0±0.7	0.34	0.34
	488~489	11.4±0.4	11.3±0.5	7.2±0.5		0.23	0.22
Kamaishi	about 650	16.1±1.4	17.1±1.0	9.1±1.0	136.4±3.5	0.31	0.31
EsashiI	73~74	1.7±0.2	2.2±0.1	0.9±0.1		0.42	0.42
	100~101	2.8±0.2	3.2±0.1	1.9±0.1		0.25	0.25

σ_v; Vertical stress: σ_{hmx} and σ_{hmn}; The largest and the smallest horizontal stress:
θ_{hmx}; Azimuth of the largest horizontal stress: r and r_h; Relative shear stresses defined by
$r = (\sigma_1 - \sigma_3)/(\sigma_1 + \sigma_3)$, $\sigma_1 > \sigma_2 > \sigma_3$: $r_v = (\sigma_{hmx} - \sigma_{hmn})/(\sigma_{hmx} + \sigma_{hmn})$

the NE-SW direction.

It is inferred from this result that the horizontal crustal deformation is predominant in extension in the N-S and the NE-SW direction. This expectation is consistent with the horizontal crustal strain during about 75 years measured by Geographical Survey Institute (1985). The strike-slip regime at Esashi may suggest that the field changes from the normal to the strike-slip fault regime toward inland.

The relative shear stress r is about 0.3 in the southern part. This value is not particularly small compared with those in other provinces in Japan, as seen in the data used by Tanaka (1987). In the northern part, although r is not small at FDI, the r_v-value of about 0.26 is small. The r_v-value appears slightly smaller in the northern part than the southern part.

5 DISCUSSIONS AND SUMMARY

The northern part of Kitakami province is lower in seismic activity than the southern part. The r-value appears slightly smaller than 0.3 in the northern part and about 0.3 in the southern part. These suggest that r of about 0.3 is critical for earthquake occurrence in Kitakami province as well as in the area around the fault of the Nagano-ken Seibu earthquake. It may be concluded with some uncertainties that the microearthquake activity is observable in the area where r is larger than about 0.3.

The seismic activity around the inferred fault of the Nagano-ken Seibu earthquake is obviously higher than that in Kitakami province on an average. The nonuniformity of the stress field is also seen to be stronger around the fault than in Kitakami province. The nonuniformity of stress field appears thus to be another condition for earthquake occurrence. If the stress relaxation means that the stress field turns toward a uniform state, the nonuniformity of stress field implies the stress concentration progressing at a higher rate than the relaxation.

The stress field of Kitakami province is supposed to be disturbed predominantly in the E-W direction due to the interaction of northeast Honshu to the Pacific ocean plate. The disturbance may be more effective on generating earthquakes in the southern part, because r_v is critical in the part. This may be a possible explanation for the relatively high seismic activity in the southern part.

As the summary, the requirements for the earthquake occurrence suggested in this study are 1) the relative shear stress larger than a critical value of about 0.3, 2) the concentration rate larger than the relaxation rate of stress, and 3) the external and/or internal disturbance to make stress field nonuniform.

ACKNOWLEDGEMENT: This study was partly supported by Grant-in-Aid for Scientific Research (C), Nos. 04640396 and 07640542.

REFERENCES

Aoki, H. 1987. The 1984 Western Nagano Prefecture Earthquake. *Proc. Earhq. Predic. Res. Symp.*, 1987. 109-114.

Byerlee, J. 1978. Friction of rocks. *Pure and Appl. Geophys.* 116: 615-626.

Geographical Survey Institute 1985. *The horizontal crustal strain in Japan.*

Gephart, J.W. and D.W. Forsyth 1984. An improved method for determining the regional stress tensor using earthquake focal mechanism data: Application to the San Fernando Earthquake sequence. *J. Geophys. Res.* 89: 9,305-9,320.

Horiuch, S., T. Matsuzawa, and A. Hasegawa 1992. A realtime processing system of seismic wave using personal computer. *J. Phys. Earth.* 40: 395-406.

Iio, Y. 1997. Frictional coefficient on faults in a seismogenic region inferred from earthquake mechanism solutions. *J. Geophys. Res.*. 102: 5,403-5,412.

Japan Meteorological Agency 1985. *The seismological bulletin of the Japan Meteorological Agency for September* 1984.

Japan Meteorological Agency 1986. Report on the Nagano-ken-Seibu earthquake, 1984. *Tech. Rep. Jpn. Meteoro. Agency.* 107: 1-46, (in Japanese).

King, G.C.P., R.S. Stein, J. Lin 1994. Static Stress Changes and the triggering of earthquakes. *Bul. Seis. Soc. Am..* 84: 935-953.

Kuwahara, Y., K. Yamamoto and T. Hirasawa 1990. An experimental and theoretical study of inelastic deformation of brittle rocks under cyclic uniaxial loading. *Tohoku Geophys. J. (Sci. Rep. Tohoku Univ., Ser 5)*. 33: 1-21.

New Energy Development Organization (NEDO) 1988. *Report for development and promotion of geothermal energy*, No. 17.

Tanaka, Y. 1987. Crustal stress measurements in Japan - Research trends and problems -. *Proc. Earthq. Predict. Res. Symp.* (1987): 199-212, (in Japanese with English abstract).

Yamamoto, H., K. Yamamoto, N. Kato, T. Hirasawa and Y. Iio 1994. Estimation of *n situ* stresses in the epicentral area of the Naganoken-Seibu earthquake of 1984. In K. Yamamoto (ed.), *Experimental study on uniformity of stresses in the crust* (Report for Grant-in-Aid for Scientific Reseach (C), No. 04640396). 47-82.

Yamamoto, K. 1995, The rock property of in-situ stress memory: Discussions on its mechanism. In Matsuki & Sugawara (eds.), *Proc. Int. Work Shop on Rock Stress Meas. at Great Depth*, Tokyo, 1995: 46-51.

Yamamoto, K., Y. Kuwahara and T. Hirasawa 1983. Discrimination of previously applied stress by deformation rate analysis: Application of the method to estimation of in situ stress. *Prog. Abst. Seism. Soc. Japan*, 1983. 2: 104.

Yamamoto, K., Y. Kuwahara, N. Kato and T. Hirasawa 1990. Deformation rate analysis: A new method for in situ stress estimation from inelastic deformation of rock samples under uni-axial compressions. *Tohoku Geophys. J (Sci. Rep. Tohoku Univ., Ser 5)*. 33: 127-147.

Yamamoto, K., H. Yamamoto, N. Kato and T. Hirasawa 1995. Deformation rate analysis for in situ stress estimation. In H. R. Hardy, Jr. (ed.), *Acoustic Emission V*, Trans Tech Pub., 243-255.

Yamashina, K. and T. Tada 1985. A fault model of the 1984 western Nagano Prefecture earthquake based on the distance change of trilateration points, *Bull. Earthq. Res. Inst.*, Univ. Tokyo. 60: 221-230 (in Japanese with English abstract).

Yoshida, S. and K. Koketsu 1990. Simultaneous inversion of waveform and geodetic data for the rupture process of the 1984 Naganoken-Seibu, Japan, earthquake. *Geophys. J. Int.* 103:355-362.

Statistical models of geomechanical processes in multiscale cracked geological media

A. V. Karakin
All-Russian Scientific-Research Geosystems Institute, Russia

Yu. I. Kuznetsov
Joint-Stock Research Industrial Company GERS, Moscow, Russia

ABSTRACT: The new statistical approach to a problem of averaging of heterogeneous media and development of mathematical models for various geomechanical processes in geological media (elastic and poroelastic) is offered.

1. INTRODUCTION

The main difficulty of the statistical continuum theory for heterogeneous media is that in this media the phases parameters form not random fields, but only the discrete random variables. Therefore for heterogeneous media there is the necessity in more details to consider a procedure of the probability density inference. This approach is applied to all heterogeneous media: to composites with various phases rheology, saturated and deformable cracked-porous materials, magnetic and conductive media and etc. However in the given work these ideas was realized for a dry cracked-porous media with an elastic skeleton, being in a static state.

General principles of the statistical continuum mechanics are stated in the monographs (Beran, 1968; Shermergor, 1977). The mathematical questions, concerning of the averaging methods in this media, are covered in the works (Sanchez-Palencia, 1980; Bakhvalov, Panasenko, 1984). As for the multiscale media, this direction is represented mainly heuristic approaches to modeling of heterogeneous media without the rigorous mathematical analysis (Bruggeman, 1935; Salganic, 1973; Vavakin, Salganic, 1975; Budiansky, O'Connel, 1976; Hashin, 1988). The publications of the last years (Chesnokov et. Al., 1991; Bayuk et. Al., 1991;) do not contain principal changes, concerning the theoretic-probabilistic approach. In the present work the function of distribution is found following those principles, which are founded on the Kolmogorov's definition of the elementary events space.

2. BASIC DEFINITIONS

We consider a random heterogeneous medium with some microstructure, for example, the cracks. In space between the cracks the static equations of the linear theory of elasticity are satisfied. We assume that the cracks are not crossed and do not touch each other. In particular the cracks can have the form of thin round disks, described in parameters $L = \{l, \theta, \varphi\}$, where l – the diameter, θ and φ – the angles of the spherical coordinate system giving a normal direction to a crack plane. Each crack is attributed to that space point, in which there is its geometrical center. The parameters of these cracks are random variables. The diameters of cracks lay in limits from the minimum size l_{min} up to maximum l_{max}.

We introduce a concept of an elementary volume ΔV (for simplicity let it has the cubic form) as of some volume of this medium having the following properties. The linear sizes of any crack and average distance between cracks is much less than this cube edge. Number of cracks inside cube is sufficiently great so the statistical samples on the cracks parameters are representative. Boundary conditions on the cube boundaries are homogeneous. Let us assume, that there are N_s of cubes, which were formed under similar physical conditions. We shall name them as "realizations". Each realization is described in term of the cracks parameters and their number N, which are random variables. Let us allow that cracks numbers in all realizations are identical formally and equal to their maximum number. In that realizations, where the cracks number is less than their maximum number, we shall add by their cracks with the zero size, which correspond to continuous medium in the given point. Under mathematical operations they does not differ from cracks with the finite size and can be considered formally as real objects. The Ψ_N space of the cracks parameters $(\vec{y}_1, \vec{y}_2, ..., \vec{y}_N, \vec{l}_1, \vec{l}_2, ..., \vec{l}_N)$ (where $\vec{y}_k$ - coordinate of the geometrical center of the k-th crack, $\vec{l}_k$ - the of variables describing its form, size and orientation, and the cracks number N is constant parameter) we shall name "as phase space". Formally the dimension of this phase space with round cracks is equal $6N$. In a general case the parameters of the cracks form are added to the coordinates of this space yet. In the phase space a each point corresponds to a realization.

Let us choose inside these elementary volumes any point and define a procedure of averaging in this point of the interesting us random additive fields (stresses, deformations, displacements, etc.) on an ensemble of realizations. For nonadditive fields (elastic moduli) the ensemble averaging is not meaningful. The probability density P_N, expressed through the phase space coordinates

$$P_N = P_N(\vec{y}, \vec{y}_1, \vec{y}_2, ..., \vec{y}_N; \vec{l}_1, \vec{l}_2, ..., \vec{l}_N),$$

takes the form

$$P_N = \frac{1}{N}\sum_{k=1}^{N}\delta(\vec{y}-\vec{y}_k)R_N(\vec{y}_1, \vec{y}_2, ..., \vec{y}_N; \vec{l}_1, \vec{l}_2, ..., \vec{l}_N). \quad (1)$$

This function satisfies to the conditions of homogeneity, isotropy and symmetry relatively of the cracks permutations.

We make an ergodic hypothesis

$$\overline{\varphi} = <<\varphi>>, \quad \overline{\varphi} = \frac{1}{\Delta V}\int_{\Delta V}\varphi d\vec{x}, \quad <<\varphi>> \equiv \int_{\Psi_N}\varphi P d\Psi_N,$$

where φ – any additive field, $\overline{\varphi}$ – the its average over an elementary volume ΔV, $<<\varphi>>$ – the ensemble average. It is supposed, that the stresses and strains increments in averaged medium are described by the linear equations, and the stress state does not change its homogeneity and isotropy properties.

We consider the realizations set as Ω set of elementary events. Following to the usual scheme let us consider set **F** of measurable subsets of this set, which forms a σ - algebra, and the subsets refer to random events. A probabilistic measure is introduced on set **F**. It is supposed, that in each concrete case there is the way of probabilistic measure determination. Thus the whole space of elementary events (Ω**FP**) is defined. Some stress state corresponds to an each random event.

Accordingly our definition in the monoscale heterogeneous media the microheterogeneity sizes vary in limits of one order. In multiscale media the microheterogeneity sizes vary on a some orders, but a probabilistic measure of various scales is one order. It is possible only if the probability density for one crack contains the nonintegrable singularity of a type

$$P_N \sim \frac{B}{A(l)},$$

where $A(l) = l^3, l^2, l$ – correspondingly in 3-D, 2-D, 1-D cases, and B – the function (which remains finite at $l = 0$) of all parameters of a crack. This condition can be considered as the multiscale medium definition. This is a principal difficulty of multiscale media.

Let us notice that the cracks influence on additive fields with volumes occupied by them but not their number. Though a crack occupies a vanishingly small volume, the volume of a stress state area for this crack is about l^3. We shall attribute this conditional volume (for brevity only volume) to each crack. The summary cracks volume, in general, can exceed the real volume, because of influence areas of cracks can be crossed. The factor $A(l)$, representing distribution of cracks volumes, enters into the expression for any additive field. Therefore we can make transformation of probability density and additive variables

$$\widetilde{P}_N \equiv A(l)P_N, \quad \widetilde{\varphi} \equiv \frac{\varphi}{A(l)}, \quad (2)$$

which keeps the averages of these variables the same

$$<<\varphi>> = \int_{\Psi_N}\widetilde{\varphi}\widetilde{P}_N d\Psi_N. \quad (3)$$

The factor $A(l)$ provides the convergence of integrals in the expressions for mathematical expectations and the finite specific variables. Thus the probability density is limited and there is the corresponding distribution function. Let us notice, that nonadditive fields does not contain a factor $A(l)$. That is why for the multiscale media the integrals (3) for nonadditive fields diverge. The transformation (2), (3) is applicable also for monoscale media. For them both definitions of the probability density are equivalent.

By changing the probabilistic measure, we should change also the space of elementary events. In this connection let us introduce the notion of a self-consistent crack and make partial averaging of the strain and stress tensors

$$<\varepsilon_{ij}(\vec{l}_1,\vec{y})> \equiv \int \varepsilon_{ij}(\vec{l}_1,\vec{y}) \times$$
$$\times Q_{N-2}(\vec{l}_1,\vec{y},\vec{y}_2,...,\vec{y}_N;\vec{l}_2,...,\vec{l}_N) d\vec{y}_3...d\vec{y}_N d\vec{l}_2...d\vec{l}_N \quad (4)$$
$$<\sigma_{ij}(\vec{l}_1,\vec{y})> \equiv \int \sigma_{ij}(\vec{l}_1,\vec{y}) \times$$
$$\times Q_{N-2}(\vec{l}_1,\vec{y},\vec{y}_2,...,\vec{y}_N;\vec{l}_2,...,\vec{l}_N) d\vec{y}_3...d\vec{y}_N d\vec{l}_2...d\vec{l}_N,$$

with the probability density of self-consistent cracks, which is given by expression

$$Q_{N-2}(\vec{l}_1,\vec{y},\vec{y}_2,...,\vec{y}_N;\vec{l}_2,...,\vec{l}_N) \equiv$$
$$\equiv P_N(\vec{y},0,\vec{y}_3-\vec{y}_2,...,\vec{y}_N-\vec{y}_2;\vec{l}_1,...,\vec{l}_N),$$
$$\vec{y} \equiv \vec{y}_1 - \vec{y}_2,$$

The variables $<\varepsilon_{ij}(\vec{l}_1,\vec{y})>$ and $<\sigma_{ij}(\vec{l}_1,\vec{y})>$ are self-consistent fields of the strain and stress for the given chosen crack. One can notice, that the contributions to a distant field (and hence to all expressions for averaged variables) of the true and self-consistent cracks are identical. The distinctions take place in a near field only, i.e. in a near vicinity of the chosen crack. This conclusion follows also from a Saint-Venant principle actually. For this reason in our consideration the true cracks can be replaced with the self-consistent cracks, which can be considered as elementary events. In above mentioned definition the set of elementary events the each realization can be represented as a sum of some more elementary events formed with the N self-consistent cracks. Thus in new definition the set of elementary events is formed by self-consistent cracks.

3. AVERAGING SCHEME

Averaging ε_{ij} and σ_{ij} over an elementary volume in limits of an elastic matrix, we get the known expressions (Salganic, 1973; Shermergor, 1977)

$$\bar{\varepsilon}_{ij} = \bar{\varepsilon}_{ij}^{(0)} + \bar{\varepsilon}_{ij}^{(1)}, \quad \bar{\theta} = \bar{\theta}^{(0)} + \bar{\theta}^{(1)},$$
$$\bar{\sigma}_{ij} = 2\mu(\bar{\varepsilon}_{ij} - \bar{\varepsilon}_{ij}^{(1)}) + \lambda(\bar{\theta} - \bar{\theta}^{(1)})\delta_{ij}, \quad (5)$$

where u_i – displacement, λ and μ – the Lame parameters of the continuous solid, $\bar{\varepsilon}_{ij}$ – the observable strain tensor equal to a difference of displacements on the opposite boundaries of an elementary volume, $\bar{\varepsilon}_{ij}^{(0)}$ and $\bar{\varepsilon}_{ij}^{(1)}$ – the parts tensor $\bar{\varepsilon}_{ij}$, caused accordingly with deformations of the continuos solid between the cracks and displacements of cracks boundaries. In other words the variable $\bar{\varepsilon}_{ij}^{(1)}$ is defined by cracks parameters $(\vec{x}_1,\vec{x}_2,...,\vec{x}_N;\vec{l}_1,\vec{l}_2,...,\vec{l}_N)$, being a sum over all cracks. Analogous expressions can be get for the local variables $\vec{u}$ and ε_{ij}

$$\vec{u} = \vec{u}^{(0)} + \vec{u}^{(1)}, \quad \bar{\varepsilon}_{ij} = \bar{\varepsilon}_{ij}^{(0)} + \bar{\varepsilon}_{ij}^{(1)}. \quad (6)$$

By definition the proportionality coefficients between tensors $<<\sigma_{ij}(\vec{x})>>$ and $<<\varepsilon_{ij}(\vec{x})>>$ are effective moduli

$$<<\sigma_{ij}(\vec{x})>> =$$
$$= 2\mu^* <<\varepsilon_{ij}(\vec{x})>> + \lambda^* <<\theta>> \delta_{ij} \quad (7)$$

Combining (5) and (7), we get

$$<<\varepsilon_{ij}>> = \frac{\mu}{\mu - \mu^*} <<\varepsilon_{ij}^{(1)}>>,$$
$$<<\theta>> = \frac{\lambda}{\lambda - \lambda^*} <<\theta^{(1)}>>, \quad (8)$$

The equation of forces equilibrium

$$\frac{\partial}{\partial x_j} \sigma_{ij} = 0,$$

is satisfied everywhere in the skeleton. It can be expressed in displacements

$$\mu \nabla^2 u_i^{(0)} + (\lambda + \mu) \nabla_i \theta^{(0)} = 0.$$

Substituting for $u_i^{(0)}$ accordingly (6) in here, we receive the equation of forces equilibrium in displacements

$$\mu \nabla^2 u_i + (\lambda + \mu) \nabla_i \theta = f_i,$$
$$f_i = \mu \nabla^2 u_i^{(1)} + (\lambda + \mu) \nabla_i \theta^{(1)}. \quad (9)$$

The decision of eq. (9) can be expressed into the Green function of a continuos elastic medium

$$u_i(\vec{x}) = \int_{\Delta V} G_{ij}^u(\vec{x} - \vec{y}) f_j(\vec{y}) d\vec{y},$$
$$\varepsilon_{ij} = \int_{\Delta V} G_{ijk}^\varepsilon(\vec{x} - \vec{y}) f_k(\vec{y}) d\vec{y}, \quad (10)$$
$$G_{ijk}^\varepsilon(\vec{x} - \vec{y}) = \frac{1}{2}\left(\frac{\partial}{\partial x_k} G_{ij}^u(\vec{x} - \vec{y}) + \frac{\partial}{\partial x_i} G_{kj}^u(\vec{x} - \vec{y})\right).$$

One can average the expressions (10)

$$<<\varepsilon_{ij}(\vec{x})>> =$$
$$= \int G_{ijm}^\varepsilon(\vec{y} - \vec{x}) f_m(\vec{y}) P_1(\vec{l}) d\vec{y} d\vec{l}. \quad (11)$$

Calculating the integral in (11), we get a formula, connecting variables $<<\varepsilon_{ij}(\vec{x})>>$ and $<<\varepsilon_{ij}^{(1)}>>$. Then with the help (8) we find effective moduli.

One can make ensemble averaging of eq. (9) for a self-consistent crack with parameters $\vec{x}_1, \vec{l}_1$ accordingly (4).

$$< \mu \nabla^2 u_i > + <(\lambda + \mu)\nabla_i \theta >=$$
$$=< \mu \nabla^2 \widetilde{u}_i^{(1)} > + <(\lambda + \mu)\nabla_i \widetilde{\theta}^{(1)} > + P_1(\vec{x}_1 \vec{l}_1)f_i. \quad (12)$$

The variables $< \mu \nabla^2 \widetilde{u}_i^{(1)} >$ and $<(\lambda + \mu)\widetilde{\theta}^{(1)} >$ are result of averaging over all cracks (except chosen one). The formulae (8) are valid not only for uniform averaged fields, but also for non-uniform fields in a vicinity of a self-consistent crack. If the parameters of various cracks are statistically independent, the functions $P_N(\vec{x}_1, \vec{x}_2,...,\vec{x}_N; \vec{l}_1, \vec{l}_2,...,\vec{l}_N)$ and $Q_1(\vec{y}, \vec{x}; \vec{l})$ are reduced to product of one-crack functions. Then one can show with help (4), that media are homogeneous and isotropic everywhere including a the vicinity of a chosen crack. In this case taking into account (4) and (12) we get the equation with constant effective moduli for a self-consistent crack

$$\mu^* \nabla^2 << u_i >> +(\lambda^* + \mu^*)\nabla_i << \theta >>=$$
$$= P_1(\vec{x}_1 \vec{l}_1)f_i \quad (13)$$

The decision of this equation is subject of various versions of the self- consistent field method. If the parameters of various cracks are statistically dependent, in a vicinity of a chosen crack the medium are not homogeneous and isotorpic already. In this case instead of the equation (13) it is necessary to consider a similar problem with the unisotorpic and nonuniform effective moduli C^*_{iklm}. Omitting the elementary calculations we have the final equation

$$C^*_{iklm} \nabla_k \varepsilon^{(1)}_{lm} = P_1(\vec{x}_1 \vec{l}_1)f_i,$$

which in the distance from a chosen crack is reduced to eq. (13) with the isotorpic and uniform moduli.

4. CONCLUSION

1. The statistical theory of heterogeneous media on the basis of Kolmogorov's definition of space of elementary events is offered.
2. The probability density function for self-consistent cracks is obtained from primary principles.
3. This theory is generalized for multiscale random cracked of media.

REFERENCES

Bakhvalov N.S. & G.P. Panasenko 1984. *Averaging of processes in the periodic media.* Moscow: Nauka (Science), (in Russian).

Vavakin A.S. & R.L. Salganic 1975. About the effective characteristics of non-uniform media with the isolated heterogeneities. *Mechanika tverdogo tela (The solid mechanics)* 3: 65-75 (in Russian).

Salganic R.L. 1973. The solid mechanics of bodies with large number of cracks. *Mechanika tverdogo tela (The solid mechanics).* 4: 149-158 (in Russian).

Shermergor T.D. 1977. The elasticity theory of the micro-heterogeneous media. Moscow: Nauka (Science), (in Russian).

Bayuk I.O., R.M. Nasimov, V.A. Kalinin & A.L. Levykin 1991. Elastic moduli and ultrasonic wave velocities in a two-phase medium under high pressure. *Acta Geod. Geophys. Mont. Hung.* 26: 77-87,

Beran M. J. 1968. *Statistical Continuum Theories.* New-York – London – Sydney: Wiley & Sons.

Budiansky B. & R.J. O'Connel 1976. Elastic moduli of a cracked solids. *Int. J. Solids Structures.* 12: 81-97.

Bruggeman D.A.G. 1935. Berechnung verschiedener physikalischer Konstanten von Heterogenen Substanzen. *Ann. Der Physik.* 24(7): 636.

Chesnokov E. & S. Zatsepin 1991. Effects of applied stress on effective elastic anisotropy in cracked solids. *Geophys. J. Int.* 107: 563-569.

Hashin Z. 1988. The differential scheme and its application to cracked material. *J. Mech. Phys. Solids.* 36(6): 719-734.

Sanchez-Palencia E. 1980. *Non-homogeneous media and vibration theory.* New-York: Springer-Verlag.

The relation between geological features and the stress state of the earth's crust in Central Japan

Takafumi Seiki
Department of Geotechnical and Environmental Engineering, Nagoya University, Japan

Ömer Aydan
Department of Marine Civil Engineering, Tokai University, Shimizu, Japan

Toshikazu Kawamoto
Department of Civil Engineering, Aichi Institute of Technology, Toyota, Japan

ABSTRACT: The stability assessment of any rock excavation requires information on the stress state of the site existing before excavation. For this purpose, in-situ stress measurements are commonly performed. Because of high cost involved in-situ tests, these tests are only performed for structures of great importance. Therefore, it is of great importance to develop a technique which can be easily used for inferring the stress state in the respective site. In this study, an attempt is made to develop a technique, which utilize the geological features, tectonic straining and seismicity, for inferring the stress state in the earth's crust. The validity of predictions by this technique at several sites in Central Japan are compared with actual measurements at those sites and its practical applicability is discussed.

1 INTRODUCTION

The virgin stress state in the earth's crust is of great interest in mining and civil engineering since the stability of excavations is very much influenced by that. The measurements of in-situ stresses in the earth's crust have been undertaken over last 30 years. Most of the measurements are restricted to a depth below 5000 m. Nevertheless, these measurements can not be easily carried out because of high cost, and measurements are performed if the stucture in question is of great importance. Therefore, there is an urgent necessity to develop a technique through which the stress state on site can be easily, rapidly and cheaply inferred.

It is well known that geological features such as faulting, folding, kinking dyke intrusions in the earth's crust are caused by the stress state in the past. They may be also indicative of its present stress state.

Measurements of plate motions by land and geo-space surveying become very common in recent years. From these measurements, relative horizontal straining of the earth's crust can be easily obtained.

Seismic networks in relation to earthquakes are widely established in many countries to locate earthquakes as well as to measure their characteristics. Focal plane solutions obtained from these networks yield the faulting mechanism and the directions of principal strains.

An attempt is made herein to develop a technique for inferring the stress state of the earth's crust by utilising the geological features, global straining and ongoing seismic activities in a given site. This technique is applied to several sites in Central Japan to infer their stress state and predictions are compared with actual measurements. In this paper, this technique is described and its applications to sites in Central Japan are presented. The validity and applicability of the technique is checked and discussed in the lights of actual in-situ measurements in the respective sites.

2 GEOLOGICAL FEATURES AND ASSOCIATED STRESS STATES

In this section, geological features and associated stress states are briefly explained.

2.1 Faulting

Faults or fracture zones found in the earth's crust are generally classified into three groups, namely (Anderson 1951) (Figure 1(a)):

1) Normal faults
2) Reverse faults, and
3) Strike slip faults.

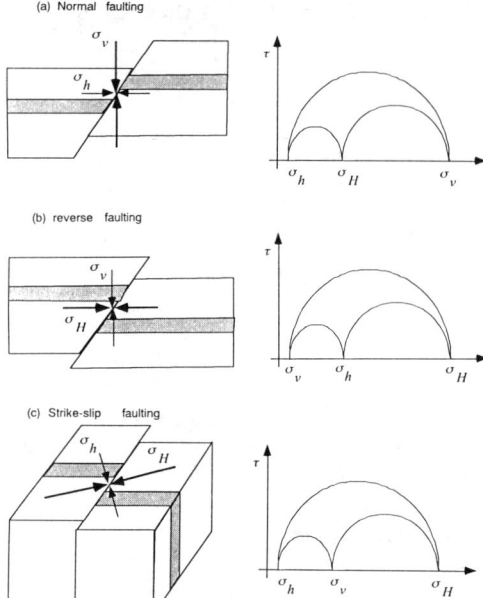

Fig. 1 Fault types and associated stress states

Taking into account the findings from the numerical analyses by Aydan (1996) on the stress state of earth's crust and interior of the earth, vertical stress σ_v, minimum horizontal stress σ_h and maximum horizontal stress σ_H may be assumed to be principal stresses. On the basis of this assumption, the stress state in the vicinity of each fault type may be contemplated as shown in Figure 1(b). It is very common that the yield function for rocks is a function of hydrostatic stress and deviatoric stress. As the pressure and temperature increase, the yield criterion can be represented by a function of deviatoric stress like metals. At depths near the earth's surface, Mohr-Coulomb yield function may be adopted. With such an assumption, the following relations may be written for each fault type as

$$\sigma_v = q\sigma_h + \sigma_c \quad \text{for normal faulting} \quad (1)$$

$$\sigma_H = q\sigma_v + \sigma_c \quad \text{Reverse faulting} \quad (2)$$

$$\sigma_H = q\sigma_v + \sigma_c \quad \text{Strike-slip faulting} \quad (3)$$

where σ_c is uniaxial strength of the crust and

$$q = \frac{1 + \sin\phi}{1 - \sin\phi}$$

As it is noted from above relations, the intermediate stress component is unkown. There is a tendency to assume the intermediate stress component as a mean of summed other two stress components. Another approach could be the use of Drucker-Prager yield criterion together with Mohr-Coulomb yield criterion.

The vertical stress component is assumed to be equal to overburden pressure, given by:

$$\sigma_v = \gamma h \quad (4)$$

where γ is unit weight of rock and h is overburden. This assumption has been both validated by in-situ stress measurements and numerical studies by Aydan (1995).

The uniaxial strength of the crust is a cause of controversy. Taking into account the findings from numerical analyses by Aydan (1996), the earth's crust must be in plastic state. If its behaviour is strain hardening type, then it should have a certain strength. On the other hand, if its behaviour strain-softening, then its strength should be the residual one which would be generally taken nill. However, taking into account re-cementation and pressure solutions mechanism of minerals, it may have a finite value. In the lights of in-situ stress measurements, this value could not be more than 40 MPa. However, it can be assumed to be almost nil in inferring stress state from fault types.

2.2 Folding

Folding is generally associated with sedimentary rocks in nature. Its mechanism is similar to buckling known in structural mechanics (Figure 2). This process in nature takes very slowly and many buckles with certain wave length occur. The folding is generally caused by the maximum horizontal stress and fold axes are generally perpendicular to that. During folding layers breaks and flexural slip occurs among layers. As a result, tensile stresses in layers are dissipated by fracturing layers. Once folding developes and driving force is still present, the folds gradually grow and in many cases result in mountain building. Therefore, the maximum horizontal stress is likely to be perpendicular to the principal fold axis while the vertical stress would be the least principal stress except the locations near the mountain crests. The minimum horizontal stress is likely to be the intermediate stress. In many cases, compressive fracturing takes place in the plane of horizontal stresses. The stress state in folded structures in synclines would be similar to that of reverse faulting while it may be similar to that of normal faullts except at anticlines

2.3 Schistosity

Schistosity is a characteristics of metamorphic rocks and it is generally well developed when parent rock is subjected to dynamic or thermo-dynamic metamorphism (Figure 3). The schistosity plane developes perpendicular to the maximum principal stress. Due to subsequent tectonic movements,

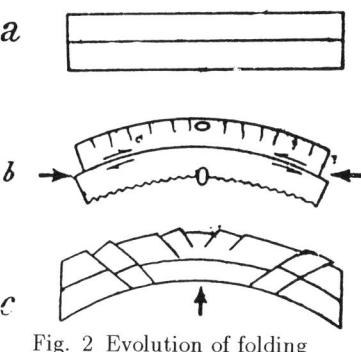

Fig. 2 Evolution of folding

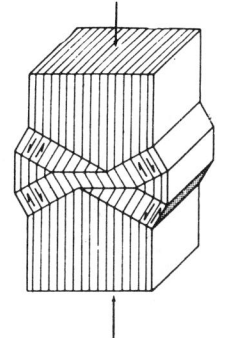

Fig. 4 Kink band formation

the dip of schistosity plane may be different from its initial position. Nevertheless, it is very likely that the direction of the strike of schistosity plane remains almost the same unless the principal driving force changes its direction.

2.4 Kinking

Kinking may be observed in both sedimentary rocks and dynamically metamorphised rocks in nature. Its mechanism is less understood. Kinking generally takes place when the maximum principal stress acts almost parallel to schistosity plane or layering and develops in the plane of the maximum and the minimum principal stresses (Figure 4). The angle between the kink band and the maximum principal stress is roughly equal to

$$\alpha = 45 + \frac{\phi}{2}$$

The yield criterion of rocks which fail in kinking mode would be also similar to the Mohr-Coulomb yield criterion. The stress state can be estimated from the procedure used in faulting.

2.5 Dyke Intrusions

Dyke intrusion is a very complex geological phenomenon. It may occur due to stretching or bending of the earth's crust in large scale. If one of the horizontal stress components is the minimum one among all stress components, the dyke intrusions may occur perpendicular to that in the earth's crust undergoing stretching. When the crust is subjected to high compression horizontally and the least horizontal stress is the minimum stress component, dyke intrusions may take place parallel to the maximum horizontal stress (Figure 5). This phenomenon is associated with the dilation of rock under compression as observed in laboratory tests. If the dyke is vertical and the plastic behaviour of rock obeys the Mohr-Coulomb yield criterion, the stress state can be assumed to be similar to that of strike-slip faulting.

3 LAND AND GEO-SPACE SURVEYING

The advance in space technology and surveying engineering has made possible to measure crust deformations (Figure 6). From these measurements

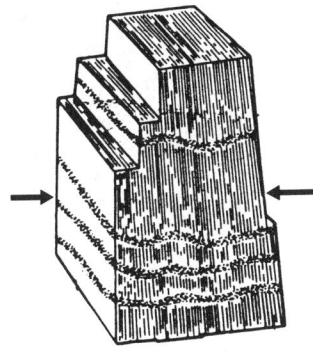

Fig. 3 Schistosity and associated stress state

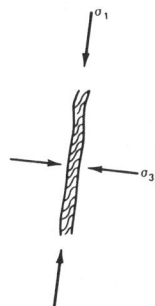

Fig. 5 Dyke intrusion and associated stress state

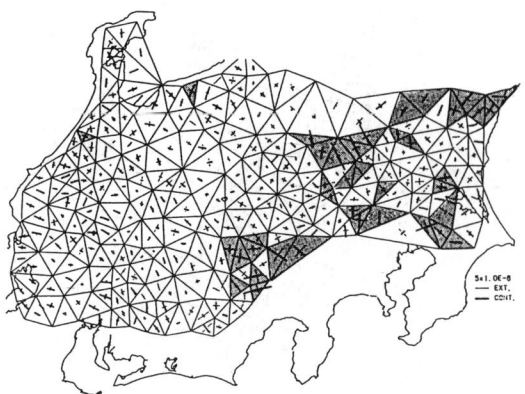

Fig. 6 Triangulation of Central Japan

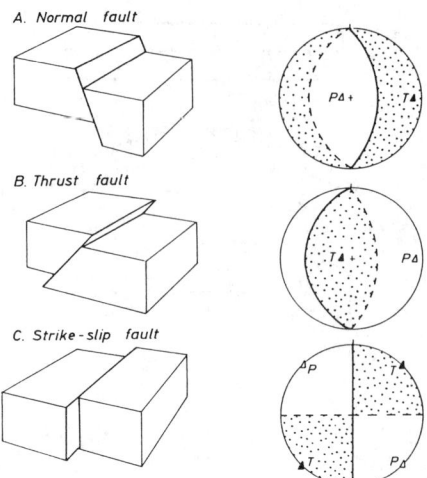

Fig. 7 Focal plane solutions

one can easily compute the crustal strains in the plane tangential to the earth's surface. These strains are relative and they are indicative of ongoing tangential straining in the crust. If there is no reversal of straining, it is most likely that the ratio of strain increments will be proportional to the stress state acting in the crust. From these measurements one may also infer the directions of horizontal stresses and their ratio. Nevertheless, their magnitude could not be determined.

4 SEISMIC ACTIVITY AND FOCAL PLANE SOLUTIONS

It is well known that 4 different kinds of waves are generated from any seismic incident. P waves are generally used to obtain its faulting mechanism and focal plane solutions are prepared (Figure 7). In this focal plane solutions, P and T axes correspond to compressive and stretching type straining. If a couple of shear stress is assumed to cause sliding along the fault, the P-axis correspond to the maximum compressive stress component while T-axis corresponds to the minimum tensile stress component. On the other hand, if a compressive normal stress acts on the fault plane, T-axis may also correspond to the minimum compressive stress. Therefore, P and T axes may be taken as the directions of the maximum and minimum principal stresses in the earth's crust. This information from the focal plane solutions will only provide that directions of the maximum and minimum principal stresses and the sense of faulting.

5 METHODOLOGY FOR INFERRING STRESS STATE

In the absence of in-situ stress measurement for a given site, the stress state in the crust can be inferred using information on

1) Geological features,
2) Land or geospace surveying, and
3) Focal plane solutions.

The stress states inferred from each method must be compared and the one, which satisy three methods, must be chosen. The basic steps of the methodology is as follows:

1) Gather data on type and geometrical characteristics of geological features, physical and mechaical characteristics of rocks, frictional properties of faults.

2) Set up a structural geological model of the site and compute the stress state by assuming the vertical stress is given by Eq. (4).

3) Check and compare with the relative horizontal straining data of the site if such data are available with an emphasis on the principal orientations of relative horizontal strains and their ratio.

4) Check and compare with the computed horizontal stress directions and information on directions of P-T axes and sense of faulting from focal plane solutions, and

5) Modify the structural geological model if there is any significant discrepancy among the geological model and tectonic model.

6 APPLICATIONS TO CENTRAL JAPAN

In this section, the applications of the methodology to sites in Central Japan, where in-situ stress measurements are available, are given and compared with the actual measurements. The main geological features such as large scale folding axes, active faults, metamorphic belts and active faults in Central Japan are presented as shown in Figure 8(a,b). Figure 8(c) shows the P-axis distribution of shallow earthquakes (depth less than 30 km). Figure (8d) shows the relative horizontal crustal straining between 1883 and 1993. Figure 9 shows the in-situ stress measurements in the Central Japan reported by Tanaka (1986). It is of great interest that the general directional tendency of the maximum and minimum horizontal stresses almost coincide with each other. Figure 10 shows that the variation of vertical stress, minimum and maximum horizontal stresses with depth. The general trend of the vertical stress can be closely predicted by Eq. (4) by assuming the unit weight of rock is 26 kN/m^3. In interpreting the horizontal stresses, the predictions from equations presented for faulting modes are also plotted in the same figure. The friction coefficient was assumed to 0.85 (Byerlee 1978). As seen from the figure, the horizontal stresses in Central Japan between bounds for strike slip faulting (SSF) and reverse faulting (RF) as expected from the tectonic model for this region of Japan.

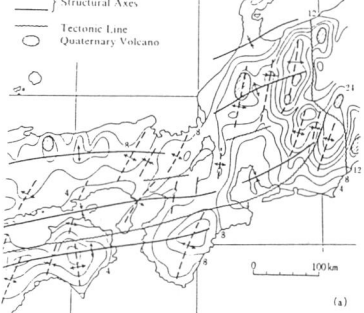
(a) Faults

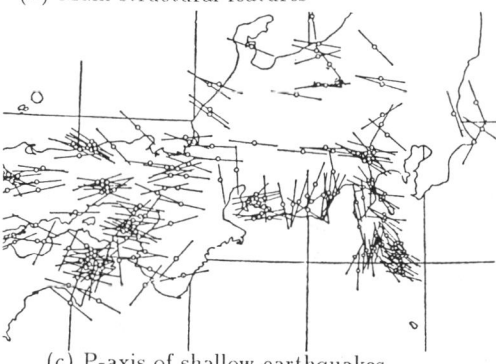
(b) Main structural features

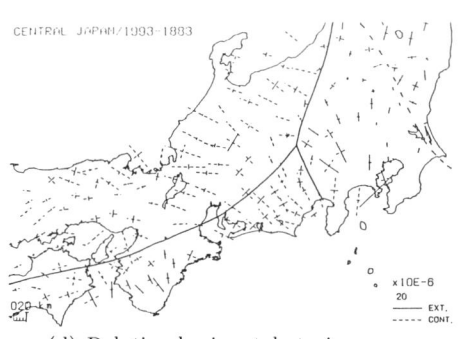
(c) P-axis of shallow earthquakes

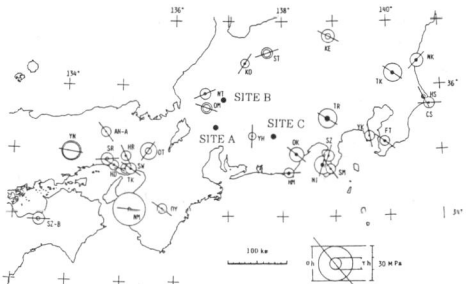
Fig. 9 Stress measurements (after Tanaka 1986)

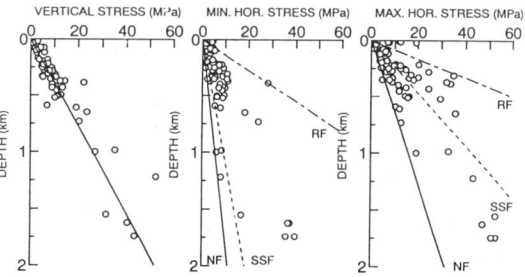
(d) Relative horizontal strains
Fig. 8

Fig. 10 Variation of vertical stress and minimum and maximum horizontal stresses with depth

389

Table 1 Comparison of inferred stress states with measurements (Site B)

Method	σ_v MPa	σ_h/σ_v	σ_H/σ_v	σ_H^{mean}/σ_v
NFM	8.71	0.30	0.65	0.47
RFM	8.71	2.20	3.39	2.80
SSFM	8.71	0.46	1.54	1.01
TEP-FEM	8.71	1.76	1.76	1.76
MEASURED	10.7	0.36	1.50	0.93

Table 2 Comparison of inferred stress states with measurements (Site C)

Method	σ_v MPa	σ_h MPa	σ_H MPa
SSFM	0.29	0.10	0.78
MEASURED	0.29	0.00	1.10

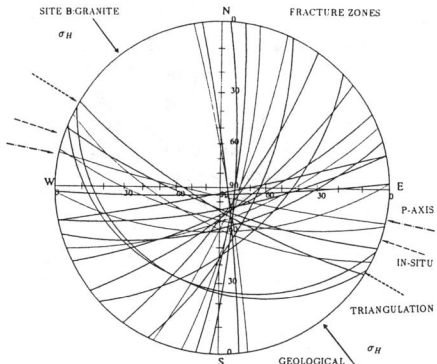

Fig. 11 Orientations of fracture zones together with inferred directions of the maximum horizontal stress from different methods

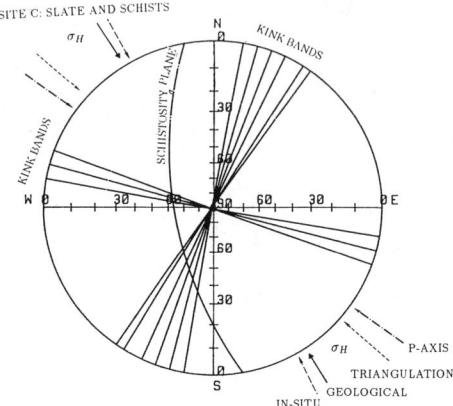

Fig. 12 Orientations of fracture zones together with inferred directions of the maximum horizontal stress from different methods

Next the stress states at Site B and Site C inferred by using the method described in this paper are compared with actual in-situ stress measurements. The depth of Site B is 335 m. The tilting tests on samples having slickensided surfaces yielded the friction angle as 35°. In the close vicinity of Site A a well-known fault exists. Figure 11 shows the fracture zone orientations on a lower hemisphere streo net together with maximum horizontal stress orientations from different approaches. Table 1 compares the inferred stress components with in-situ stress measurements. As seen from the table, the stress state inferred from strike-slip faulting model is very close to that measured. This is also in good agreement with focal plane solutions of earthquakes near this site.

Site C is a schistose rock where kink bands were observed. Figure 12 shows the orientations of kink bands on a lower hemisphere streo net together with maximum horizontal stress orientations from different approaches. There was not in-situ stress measurements near this site. The nearest in-situ stress measurement location with similar geology was selected and the stress states inferred are given in Table 2 together with in-situ stress measurements. The depth was 11 m and friction angle was chosen as 40° obtained from laboratory tests. As seen from the table, the stress state inferred is very close to that measured although the nearest site is about 40 km far away.

CONCLUSIONS

A technique, which utilize the geological features, tectonic straining and seismicity is proposed for inferring the stress state in the earth's crust. The validity of predictions by this technique at several sites in Central Japan are compared with actual measurements at those sites. Although it is still under development, it is very promising and it may be of great help to engineers during the feasibility studies for selecteing sites of rock engineering structures.

REFERENCES

Anderson, E.M. 1951. The Dynamics of Faulting and Dyke Formation with Applications to Britain. 2nd edn., Edinburgh, Oliver and Boyd.

Aydan, Ö., 1995. The stress state of the earth and the earth's crust due to the gravitational pull. 35th US Rock Mechnanics Symp., Lake Tahoe,

Tanaka, Y. 1986. State of crustal stress inferred from in-situ stress measurements, J. Phys. Earth, 34, 557-570.

Rock stress measurements in the Hong Kong region

H. H. Choy, C. F. Chan, W. K. Pun & L. S. Cheung
Geotechnical Engineering Office, Hong Kong Government, Kowloon, People's Republic of China

ABSTRACT : The state of insitu stress within the territory of Hong Kong was largely unknown before 1990. In the past six years a total of 145 shallow rock stress measurements were performed in drillholes for 8 rock cavern and tunnelling projects. These tests were carried out at depths ranging from less than 10 m to over 200 m by employing the SSPB overcoring or the hydrofracture method. The stress measurement data are variable, but largely conform to the regional trend in South China. The stress regime is $S_v \leq S_h < S_H$ above 170 m and $S_h < S_v < S_H$ below 170 m. The maximum horizontal stress orientation generally falls in the range of N100°±21° which is consistent with what is known about regional lithospheric plate movements, the crustal stress derived from South China and, borehole breakout analyses in the Pearl River Mouth Basin.

1 INTRODUCTION

The state of insitu rock stresses was largely unknown in the Hong Kong region prior to 1990 despite a long tradition of hard rock tunnelling since 1889 (Vail, 1989). Rock stresses were not measured because stress-induced failures such as spalling or rock burst were uncommon. This is due to the small span and shallow depth of the earlier tunnels and the favourable geology.

In the last decade, a number of large span rock caverns and deep tunnel systems were planned to solve the land shortage, transportation and environmental problems in the mountainous terrain of Hong Kong. Some of these projects are now complete. The information provided in this paper was gathered from the shallow rock stress measurements performed during the ground investigation for these civil engineering projects from 1990 up to the present.

2 GEOLOGY

The oldest rocks in Hong Kong are Devonian sandstones and conglomerates that crop out in the NE part of the New Territories. However, the most widespread rock types are the Jurassic/Cretaceous ash and lava tuffs and the intrusive granitoids comprising mainly granite and some granodiorite, syenite and porphyritic dyke rocks. The tuffs and granitoids are generally very strong with unconfined compressive strength of 100 - 200 MPa when fresh and well-jointed with spacing varying from 20 mm - 600 mm in volcanic tuffs and 600 mm - 1000 mm in the granitoids. They formed excellent media for underground rock excavation (Barton, 1989). The weathered mantle in the tuffs and granitoids varies from a few metres to over 100 m deep. Limited Cretaceous-Tertiary siltstones and mudstones are exposed in the Mirs Bay area in north-eastern part of Hong Kong. Quaternary deposits of colluvium and alluvium are widespread but are commonly less than 20 m deep.

Geological structures of varying width and inclination are found in Hong Kong. The major faults trend NE to ENE and NW to NNW (Lai & Langford, 1996). Many of the NE- to ENE-trending faults are persistent and can be traced into the Guangdong Province. The NW- to NNW-trending faults are generally less persistent and are often displaced by the NE-trending set.

A simplified geological map of Hong Kong showing the distribution of major rock types and geological structures is shown in Figure 1.

3 SHALLOW ROCK STRESS MEASUREMENTS

Before 1990, the only known stress measurements in Hong Kong were carried out during the construction of the 8.9 m diameter, twin dual lanes Aberdeen rock tunnel (Twist and Tonge, 1979). The maximum depth of the tunnel is about 250 m below ground level. The insitu stresses were evaluated at 3 sections in a pilot tunnel by 9 flat jack tests supplemented by

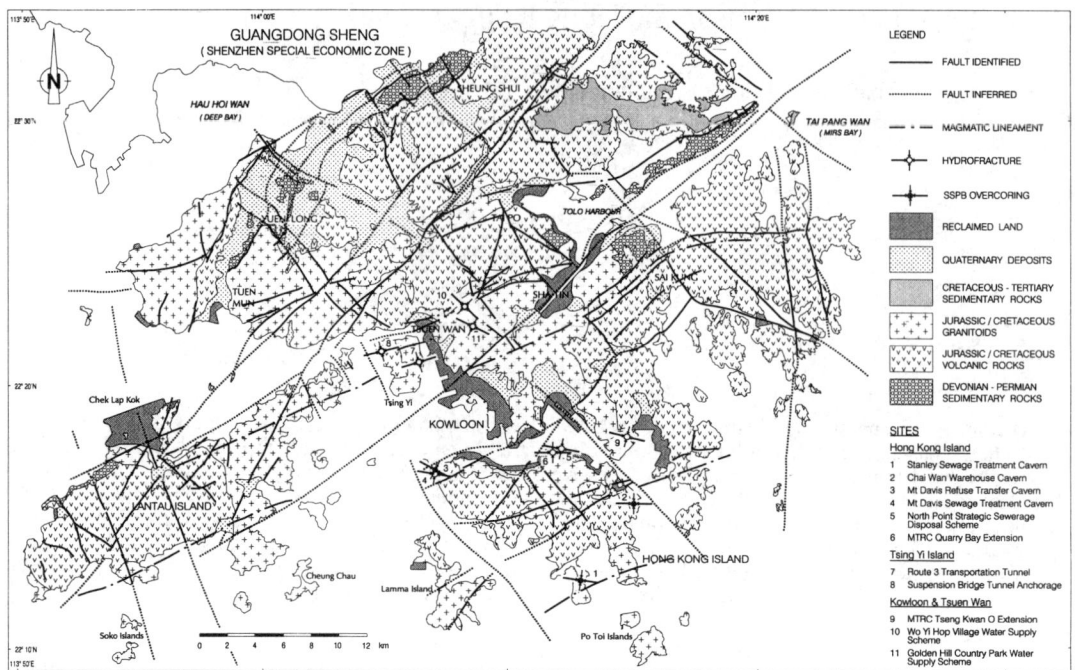

Figure 1. Simplified geology map of Hong Kong showing sites of stress measurement & maximum horizontal stress orientation. (Geology after Hong Kong Geological Survey)

the overcoring method using Leeman cells. The 9 Leeman cells indicated the horizontal stress was generally twice the vertical stress in magnitude. The measured insitu stress towards the northern portal was greater than the computed overburden stress, while 300 m from the northern portal at about 65 m below ground, the insitu stress was lower than the computed overburden stress and the horizontal stress was equal to the vertical stress.

Hong Kong built its first generation of rock caverns between 1982 to 1985. Three caverns were constructed, of which the 24 m span Tai Koo Mass Transit Railway Station was the largest. These caverns were heavily lined with reinforced concrete. The state of insitu stresses was not measured during the investigation or construction of these caverns.

In 1988, the Hong Kong Government, inspired by the municipal use of rock caverns in Scandinavia, carefully studied the feasibility of rock caverns for urban development. Some of these 'second generation' rock caverns constructed after 1988 were described in Malone and Chan (1993) and Roberts et al (1996).

Rock stress measurements using overcoring and hydrofracture methods were introduced to Hong Kong during ground investigation to determine the suitability of ground conditions for rock caverns projects after 1990. The hydrofracture method was also adopted by tunnelling projects. At present, a total of 15 overcoring measurements in 3 sites and 130 hydrofracture measurements in 8 sites were carried out for 8 projects. These results are gathered by the Geotechnical Engineering Office (GEO) of the Hong Kong Government.

4 OVERCORING METHOD

Due to the thick weathered rock mantle in Hong Kong, investigation drillholes over 100 m deep were often sunk during the feasibility stage of cavern and tunnel projects. The SSPB method (Hiltscher, 1979) was employed as tests can be performed in deep drillholes down to several hundred metres. Other methods such as the USBM or CSIRO may be limited to depths less than 50 m (ISRM, 1986).

Three proposed cavern projects were investigated by the SSPB method between 1990-1991 in the Hong Kong Island (Figure 1). These projects were described in Malone & Chan (1993). A total of 15 tests in 6 drillholes at 3 sites were performed including :

a. 6 tests in 2 inclined drillholes S17N & S20 in medium-grained granite in the Stanley sewage treatment cavern,

b. 5 tests in 2 inclined drillholes CW1 & CW4 in coarse-ash tuff in the proposed Chai Wan warehouse cavern, and

c. 4 tests in 2 inclined drillholes MD2 & MD3 in coarse-ash tuff in the Mt Davis refuse transfer cavern.

The mean values of the overcoring test results are tabulated in Table 1. The test results which show large variations in both magnitude and direction are likely to be influenced by localised discontinuities and the steep site topography. The measured vertical stress ($S_{v'}$) is generally lower than the theoretical values. The maximum horizontal stress (S_H) to measured vertical stress ($S_{v'}$) ratio (k) is greater than unity as expected.

The limited Hong Kong experience in SSPB overcoring method shows that up to half of the test attempts failed because of close-joint spacing in the volcanic tuffs. The typical instrumental error suggests this method should not be attempted at depth less than 100 m in general Hong Kong conditions unless a large number of tests are performed.

5 HYDROFRACTURE METHOD

The hydrofracture method was introduced to Hong Kong in the late 1990 using a wireline hydrofrac equipment PERFRAC II. It is the most popular method employed in Hong Kong now as tests can be performed in both shallow and deep drillholes. The interpretation of this method assumes the alignment of the drillholes to be parallel to a known principal stress, the overburden. Due to the low porosity and permeability of granitoids and volcanic tuffs in Hong Kong, stress analyses were carried out using the Hubbert and Willis method without considering the poroelastic effect.

A total 130 hydrofracture tests in 16 drillholes were carried out between 1990-1996 covering 8 sites in 5 projects (Figure 1). These include :

a. 35 tests in 4 drillholes CV-1, 2, 3 & 4 in coarse-ash tuff in Mt Davis and 10 tests in a drillhole III/NP/STW/S1 in medium-grained granite in North Point for the deep Strategic Sewage Disposal Scheme comprising a cavern and a deep tunnel system,

b. 25 tests in 4 drillholes HY/90/07/11, 12, 13 & 18 in medium-grained granite intruded by feldsparphyric rhyolite dykes for Route 3 project, which is a 3-lane, 17 m span dual transportation rock tunnel in Tsing Yi Island,

c. 18 tests in 2 drillholes 5T 45&46 in coarse-ash tuff intruded by basaltic dykes for a proposed suspension bridge anchorage in Tsing Yi Island,

d. 17 tests in 2 drillholes 660/TKE/DO15 & 17 in medium-grained granite in Tseung Kwan O and 8 tests in drillhole 660/QBE/DO53 in medium-grained granite in Quarry Bay for the extension of the Mass Transit Railway (MTRC) system, and

e. 7 tests in drillhole DH-205 in Golden Hill Country Park and 6 tests in drillhole DH-208 in Wo Yi Hop Village with both sites in medium-grained granite for a water supply scheme.

The mean value of the hydrofracture results are tabulated in Table 2. The results also show a fair degree of variability both in magnitude and direction. In general, the shallow stress data above 170 m is a thrust faulting stress regime with $S_v \leq S_h < S_H$ while the deeper data suggest a strike-slip faulting regime with $S_h < S_v < S_H$. The overall direction of the maximum principal stress varies from N090° to N134° with the exception of Tsing Yi Island which shows a consistent N073° to N076° direction. It seems that Tsing Yi Island has a local and independent stress regime that separates the island by the major faults to the NW and SE.

A linear regression of the stress-depth relations for all hyfrofracture tests are as follows :

$$S_h(MPa) = 0.0179 \cdot Z(m) + 1.844 \quad (1)$$

$$S_H(MPa) = 0.0347 \cdot Z(m) + 2.734 \quad (2)$$

$$S_v(MPa) = 0.0265 \cdot Z(m) \quad (3)$$

where: S_v is the theoretical vertical stress,
Z(m) is depth in metres
rock density equals 2.65 gm/cm^3.

6 DISCUSSION ON THE SHALLOW STRESS MEASUREMENT RESULTS

The shallow rock stress measurement data by SSPB overcoring method and hydrofracture method

Table 1. Mean values of SSPB overcoring method.

Site Location	No. of Drillholes	No. of Tests	Depth (m)	$S_{v'}$ (MPa)	S_H (MPa)	S_h (MPa)	Bearing of S_H
Stanley	2	6	43-51	1.30±2.70	3.88±3.16	0.35±0.64	N098°±60°
Chai Wan	2	5	87-124	2.16±1.97	5.06±3.30	0.86±0.90	N091°±31°
Mt Davis	2	4	94-131	3.10±2.24	3.98±1.81	2.58±0.90	N118°±34°

Table 2. Mean values of hydrofracture method.

Site Location	No. of Drillholes	No. of Tests	Depth (m)	S_v (MPa)	S_H (MPa)	S_h (MPa)	Bearing of S_H
Mt. Davis	4	26	67-147	2.80	6.89±3.37	4.17±1.74	N099°±33°
North Point	1	10	68-146	2.71	6.03±2.26	3.55±1.09	N100°±19°
Tsing Yi (Route 3)	4	24	9-50	0.73	2.31±1.22	1.63±0.62	N073°±23°
Golden Hill Park	1	7	22.5-68	1.20	6.79±0.38	4.30±0.28	N116°±14°
Wo Yi Hop Village	1	6	18-43	0.75	3.46±0.88	2.07±0.49	N134°±08°
Tsing Yi (Anchorage)	2	2	51-67	1.56	3.95±0.21	2.35±0.07	N076°±02°
Tseng Kwan O	2	17	72-205	3.55	8.17±0.67	4.47±0.27	N104°±04°
Quarry Bay	1	8	21-42	0.77	5.26±0.30	2.62±0.11	N090°±03°

gathered in Hong Kong show significant variations in magnitude and direction. Such variations are expected when considering:

a. most tests were performed at shallow depth with only a few hydrofracture tests exceeding 150 m,

b. the tests were carried out in closely- to widely-jointed rocks of granite and volcanic tuffs, some of which are intruded by dyke rocks, and

c. most tests were performed in sites of high topographic relief.

However, the overall direction of the maximum principal stress is rather consistent and the trend of the stress-depth relation is considered reasonable. All the shallow stress measurement data carried out in Hong Kong are plotted graphically in Figure 2 and can be summarized by:

$$k_h = S_h/S_v = 59.5/Z(m) + 0.664 \quad (4)$$

$$k_H = S_H/S_v = 86.6/Z(m) + 1.234 \quad (5)$$

The maximum principal stress direction varies from N073° to N134° with a mean of N100°± 21° or WNW. The plot of maximum horizontal stress orientation (Figure 1) suggests some rotation from N075° in Tsing Yi Island to N099° in Hong Kong Island and N118° in Kowloon and Tsuen Wan areas. The uncertainties of the stress magnitude and orientation at shallow depths may deviate as much as 100% or more. It is advisable for design optimization purposes that independent stress measurements on site should be obtained for major shallow engineering structures.

7 BOREHOLE BREAKOUTS

In late 70's to the early 80's, borehole breakout was recognised as a reliable indicator of the orientation of principal horizontal insitu stresses. In the World Stress Map Project (Zoback, 1992), borehole breakout data comprises a significant 28% of the data base and is an important source of stress orientation data in relatively aseismic areas.

With the help of BP Exploration and British Geological Survey, borehole dipmeter data was obtained from the Nanhai East Oil Corporation (Shenzhen). Borehole breakout analysis was carried out on 3 hydrocarbon exploration wells located in the Pearl River Mouth Basin approximately 220 km directly south of Hong Kong (Whittaker et al, 1992).

Calliper and resistivity eccentricity rose diagrams were analysed for the 3 boreholes. In general, the calliper eccentricity rose diagram shows a distinct unimodal trend while the resistivity eccentricity rose diagram showed a more bimodal trend with the main orientation being aligned with the calliper data. The bimodal trend can be explained by the presence of hydraulic fracturing traces that were induced in the direction of the maximum principal stress due to the weight of the heavy drilling mud. These induced fractures are orthogonal to the breakout direction.

A summary of the breakout analysis is given in Table 3. In PY 27-2-1, there is an overall breakout direction change at about -3800 mPD, therefore two independent zones were analyses in addition to an overall analysis. In EP 17-3-1 and PY 33-1-1, the breakout direction for each hole is rather uniform with depth and thus one overall direction is presented.

In general, local variability in principal horizontal stress orientations is to be expected. The breakout analyses showed the maximum horizontal stress orientation is consistent with the shallow stress measurement in Hong Kong.

8 SUMMARY AND DISCUSSION

The shallow stress measurement data obtained by SSPB overcoring and hydrofracture methods in Hong Kong show significant variability. This usually represents the effect of localised fracturing

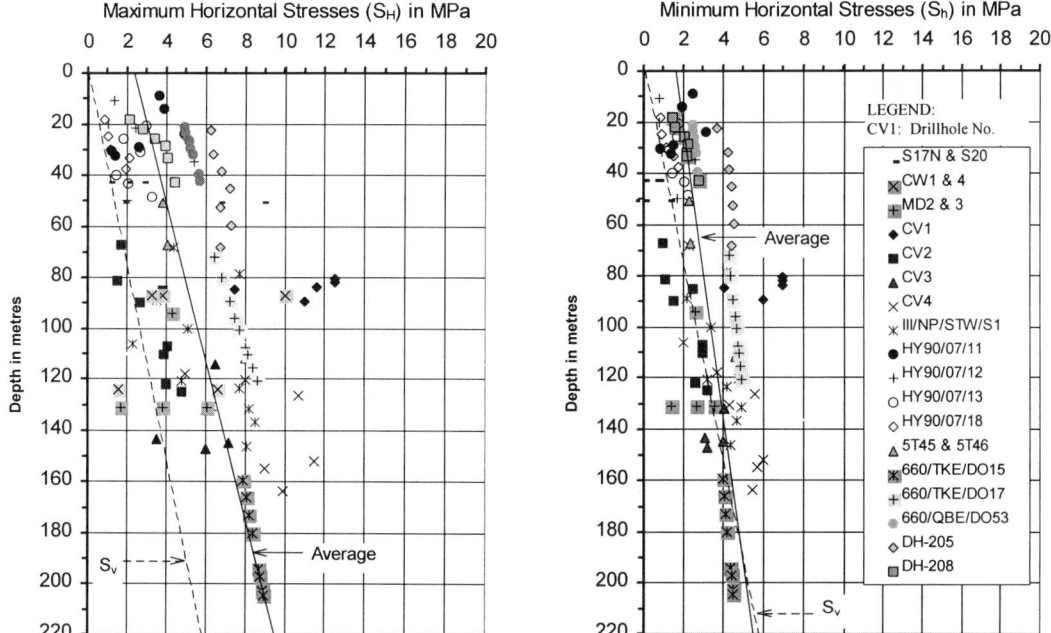

Figure 2   Plot of S_H and S_h horizontal stresses with depth by SSPB overcoring and hydrofracture methods.

Table 3. Summary of borehole breakout analysis (After Whittaker et al, 1992).

Area	Enping	Panyu		Panyu
Borehole No.	EP 17-3-1	PY 27-2-1		PY 33-1-1
Latitude	20 32 11.67N	20 14 32.63N		20 05 17.51N
Longitude	113 45 27.06E	114 27 54.03E		114 22 21.35E
Depth (mPD)	-2098 to -4682	-2596 to -3800	-3800 to -4794	-229 to -3809
S_H Orientation	N122°	N087° (Overall N104°)	N108°	N092°

and the rugged topography. The correlations of maximum and minimum horizontal stress with depth (Figure 2) give no indications of high or low localised stress regimes. The stress data can be described by equations (4) & (5). In general, the stress field above 170 m is characterised by a thrust faulting regime with $S_v \leq S_h < S_H$ while the deeper data suggest a strike-slip faulting stress regime with $S_h < S_v < S_H$. The high horizontal stress at shallow depth derived in Hong Kong largely conforms to the regional trend in South China.

The N100°±21° mean orientation of the maximum horizontal stress derived from the shallow rock stress measurements is consistent with the borehole breakout analyses from 3 boreholes in the Pearl River Mouth Basin which give maximum horizontal stress orientations of N092°, N104° and N122°. Other evidence to support this general NW to WNW orientation of the maximum horizontal compressive stress field in the vicinity of Hong Kong include :

a. the general direction of motion of both the Pacific and the Philippine plates is NW and this would be expected to give rise to compressive stresses in southeast part of China with an overall NW-SE regional orientation,

b. the results from about 1000 near surface measurements obtained since 1964 and a few deeper hydrofracture and borehole breakout measurements (Ding & Zhang, 1988) suggested that the principal horizontal compressive stress in South China is dominantly NW-SE,

c. based on focal mechanism solutions, Yan et al (1979) reported a South China regional stress field of WNW and Ding & Zhang (1988) also reported an overall orientation of NW-SE in South China,

d. the NW to WNW orientation of the maximum horizontal stress field in Taiwan and South China fault block is nearly perpendicular to the NE- to

NNE-trending regional tectonic belt (Yan et al, 1979), and

e. Zhang (1994) reported that a series of analyses and surveys such as stress measurements, simulation experiment and stress field analysis between 1985-1987 showed the maximum principal stress in Shenzhen Special Economic Zone immediately north of Hong Kong is essentially horizontal and is oriented in the NW-SE direction.

ACKNOWLEDGEMENT

This paper is published by permission of the Director of Civil Engineering of the Hong Kong Government. The authors are most grateful to the encouragement and advice of Prof. Dr. F. Rummel of MeSy in the preparation of this paper, and to the Mass Transit Railway Corporation for the permission to publish their hydrofracture data.

REFERENCES

Barton, N.R. 1989. Cavern design for Hong Kong rocks. *Proceedings of the Seminar Rock Cavern - Hong Kong*, edited by A.W. Malone & P.G.D. Whiteside. The Institution of Mining and Metallurgy :179-202,

Ding, X. & Zhang, W. 1988. State of modern tectonic stress field in East China mainland. *Acta Seismologica Sinica*, 2-1 : 26-44.

Hiltscher, R., Martna, J. & Strindell, L. 1979. The measurement of triaxial rock stresses in deep boreholes and the use of rock stress measurements in the design and construction of rock openings. *Proceedings of the Fourth International Congress on Rock Mechanics*, Mortreux, Switzerland, vol. 2 : 227-234. ISRM, Lisbon.

ISRM 1986. Suggested methods for stress determination. *International Journal of Rock Mechanics, Mining Science and Geomechanics Abstracts*, vol. 24 : 53-73.

Lai K.W. & Langford R.L. 1996. Spatial and temporal characteristics of major faults of Hong Kong. *Geological Society of Hong Kong* Bulletin 5: 72-84.

Malone A.W. & Chan C.F. 1993. Rock cavern development in Hong Kong. *Proceedings of the NTU-PWD Seminar on Rock Caverns for Underground Space Utilization*, Singapore : 23-32.

Roberts K.J., Choy H.H. & Martin R.P. 1996. Preliminary geotechnical assessment of the potential for underground space development in Hong Kong. *Proceedings of the 30th International Geological Congress, Beijing*, in press.

Twist, D.W.L. & Tonge, W.W. 1979. Planning and design of the Aberdeen Tunnel. *Hong Kong Engineer*, vol. 7-3 : 13-30.

Vail, A.J. 1989. Underground work in Hong Kong. *Proceedings of the Seminar Rock Cavern - Hong Kong*, edited by A.W. Malone & P.G.D. Whiteside. The Institution of Mining and Metallurgy : 1-6.

Whittaker A., Musson R.M.W., Bereton N.R., Busby J.P., Evans C.D.R. & Evans C.J. 1992. A review of the crustal structure and seismotectonic pertinent to Hong Kong. *British Geological Survey* Technical Report WC/92/17 International Geology Series.

Yan, J., Shi, Z., Wang, S. & Huan W. 1979. Some features of the recent tectonic stress of China and environs. *Acta Seismologica Sinica*, 1-1.

Zhang J. 1994. Geostress state and regional stability assessment in Shenzhen. *Bulletin of the Chinese Academy of Geotechnical Science* No. 29, 17-26.

Zoback, M.L. 1992. First and second-order pattern of stress in the lithosphere : the world stress map sheet. *Journal of Geophysical Research*, vol. 97-B8 : 11.703-11.728.

Influence of a fault and a dyke on stress distribution at two project sites in India

S. Sengupta, D. Joseph, C. Nagaraj & A. Kar
National Institute of Rock Mechanics, Kolar Gold Fields, Karnataka, India

ABSTRACT: Rotation of horizontal stress (σ_H) orientations relative to the regional horizontal stress (R_H) orientations, near two typical geological structures are noted at two project sites while measuring in-situ stresses by hydraulic fracture method. In the first case a fault at a hydroelectric project in Himalayas seems to have rotated horizontal stress (σ_H) by 75° and in the second case the measurement inside a dyke at a mining project has revealed a horizontal stress rotation by 65°. To understand factors responsible for the rotations, the fault and the dyke are simulated using a two dimensional Distinct Element Method incorporating Mohr-Coulomb model. The parametric study revealed that the elastic properties contrast between the geological structure and the surrounding rock, character of the geological structural contact, orientation of σ_H with respect to the geological structure, and the ratios of the magnitudes of the regional stresses are the prime factors responsible for rotation phenomena of the horizontal stresses.

1 INTRODUCTION

Based on the data available from different stress indicators like earthquake focal mechanism, borehole breakouts and in-situ stress measuring devices like hydrofracture method, two orders of stress distributions are identified; first-order or regional stresses and second-order or local perturbation of the regional stresses (Zoback et al., 1989; Zoback, 1992). There are many instances all over the world where regional stresses are found to have perturbed near geological structures like fold fault and the intrusives. These structures bring about local heterogeneities in rocks, thus leading to refraction and/or deflection of stress trajectories (changing orientation of bedding in folds, fault zones in which the mechanical rock properties differ from those in the surrounding media). From many construction sites from all over the world a large number of observations implicating the rotation of stress orientation as much as by 90° near geological structures are reported.

Anderson et al. (1951) cited reorientation of principal stress trajectories due to primary fault formation and postulated that reorientation of the stress trajectories takes place only at the ends of the principal fault. He also noted that dykes occupy fractures that form perpendicular to the least principal stress axis when the stress difference exceeds a critical value. Ez (1962) measured stresses around a network of strike slip faults in the principal anticline of the Donetz coal basin, and found reorientation of regional stress by almost 90° around the longitudinal faults in the core of the anticline.

Adams and Bell (1991) suggested that the stress trajectory rotation in case of Peace River Arch in western Canada is due to contrast in the elastic properties between the Arch and the surrounding area. A numerical simulation by them indicates rotation of 10° to 20°. Stephansson et al. (1991) analysed stress reorientation in a two dimensional distinct element model of a 6 by 4 Km rock mass using UDEC programme. The model gives an idea of how stress concentration takes place at the intersection of faults and how directions of principal stresses reorient them near the fault.

Zoback (1992) presumed that a strength contrast between a low frictional resistance fault inside a strong crust is responsible for rotation of σ_H in the San Andreas fault in central California.

We have encountered the stress rotational phenomena at Uri hydroelectric project in Himalayas where a small fault at the vicinity of the measurement site seems to have rotated the σ_H direction by 75°, and at Rajpura Dariba mines in the Aravalli mountain system where measurement inside a dyke shows a σ_H direction deflected by 65° from the regional stress direction.

Due to the proximity to these perturbed stresses to the underground structures it is expected that these stresses will have a greater impact on the overall stability of the underground structures rather than regional stress. Thus stress perturbations due to local geological structures at the site of hydroelectric or mining projects must be clearly understood before stress values are taken as an input parameter for design of any structure.

We tried to understand this σ_H rotational phenomena by numerical modelling using 2D-UDEC code. The model calculations indicate that the elastic properties contrast, friction angle of fault contact, angle between geological structure, regional horizontal stress, and the ratios of the magnitudes of the regional stresses are the prime factors responsible for rotation phenomena of the horizontal stresses.

2 DESCRIPTION OF THE PROJECT SITES

2.1 *Uri hydroelectric project, Jammu & Kashmir (North-West Himalayas)*

2.1.1 *Introduction*

Uri hydroelectric project is located at around 70 Km west of Srinagar, the state Capital of Jammu and Kashmir.

The project envisages construction of a 20 m high barrage across river Jhelum. The head water will be diverted initially into 1.2 km long power channel and then into 10.4 km long power tunnel, into the underground power house, through two numbers of pressure shafts. The power station will house four units of turbines of 120 MW each to have a total generating capacity of 480 MW. A programme of in-situ stress measurement by hydrofracture method was carried out to determine the stress regime acting around the tunnel as an input parameter for design and stability studies of the underground caverns.

2.1.2 *Regional stress province*

The project area is located at latitude 34°N and longitude 74°E in the North Western Himalayas. The nearest focal mechanism solutions with primary axis azimuths are as follows:

Table 1. Direction of R_H by focal mechanism.

Latitude	Longitude	Azimuth	Reference
1) 33.9°N	74.7°E	055° (235°)	Chandra (1978)
2) 33.7°N	75.3°E	046°	Chandra (1978)

2.1.3 *Local perturbed stress province*

A local fault zone of 10 m width trending N85°E and dipping 70° towards north with appreciable movement along it is the closest major discontinuity to the testing area. The perturbed stress was measured by hydrofracture method inside four boreholes at the vicinity of the fault zone.

Table 2. The stress tensors calculated by GENSIM.

In-situ stresses:	
Minimum Horizontal Stress (σ_h)	= 2.29 MPa
Maximum Horizontal Stress (σ_H)	= 9.16 MPa
Vertical Stress (σ_V)	= 8.84 MPa
Direction of σ_H	= 130°
The vertical stress corresponds to an overburden of 310 m and density of rock	= 2.91 gm/cm^3

Thus the following observations are made:
1) The direction of the regional maximum horizontal compression R_H by focal mechanism = 055°.
2) The direction of the perturbed maximum horizontal compression σ_H near the fault = 130°.
3) The total rotation of the maximum horizontal compression = 075°.

Figure 1 shows the regional and local perturbed maximum horizontal stresses.

2.2 *Rajpura Dariba lead-zinc mines, Rajasthan (Aravallis)*

2.2.1 *Introduction*

Rajpura Dariba mines are located 76 Km north east of the city of Udaipur in the state of Rajasthan. The leased area is demarcated by two ore zones, namely the main lode and the east lode. The main lode has a strike length of 1700 m, which is subdivided into north and south lodes. These lodes are separated by

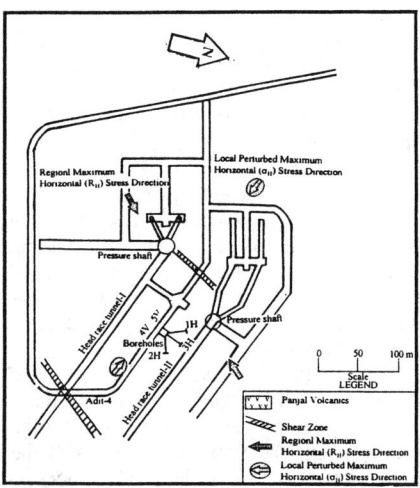

Figure 1. Plan showing the orientations of the regional and local perturbed maximum horizontal stresses, Uri hydroelectric project.

a barren zone having a strike length of 300 m. The south lode is currently being mined by cut and fill method above 300 MRL and by vertical retreat method (VRM) in between 200 MRL and 300 MRL.

2.2.2 *Regional stress province*

The Aravalli mountain range has a general trend of NE-SW extending from latitude 24°N to 28°N and longitude 73°E to 79°E. The Aravallis are known to be a horst-type feature, bounded by steeply dipping faults.

The regional stress at and around the study area is considered between 24°25'N latitude and 74°09'E longitude at Dariba Mines and latitude 25°03'N and longitude 74°09'E' at Bamnia. The regional stress is based on the measurements by hydrofracture method at a depth of 500 m and with a strike length of 450 m at Dariba mines (Sengupta et al., 1994) and at a depth of 210 m at Bamnia (Srirama Rao et al., 1990). The direction of maximum horizontal compression in the former case is N20°E and in the later case it is N30°E. Thus the regional maximum horizontal compression can be taken as N20°E - N30°E.

2.2.3 *Local perturbed stress province*

An eleven meter thick dolerite dyke has intersected the country rock (Calc-biotite schist) at the study area. The dyke is dipping 80° towards north. The perturbed stress was measured by hydrofracture method inside two boreholes inside the dyke.

Table 3. The stress tensors calculated by GENSIM.

In-situ stresses:	
Minimum Horizontal Stress (σ_h)	= 08.35 MPa
Maximum Horizontal Stress (σ_H)	= 16.17 MPa
Vertical Stress (σ_V)	= 11.09 MPa
Direction of σ_H	= 320°
The vertical stress corresponds to an overburden of 310 m and density of rock	= 2.80 gm/cm^3

Thus the following observations are made:
1) The direction of the regional maximum horizontal compression R_H hydrofracture method = 025°.
2) The direction of the perturbed maximum horizontal compression σ_H near the dyke = 320°.
3) The total rotation of the maximum horizontal compression inside the fault = 065°.

Figure 2 shows the regional and local perturbed maximum horizontal stresses.

3 NUMERICAL ANALYSES

Both the case histories are simulated by a two dimensional DEM programme, UDEC. In the analyses the following assumptions are made:

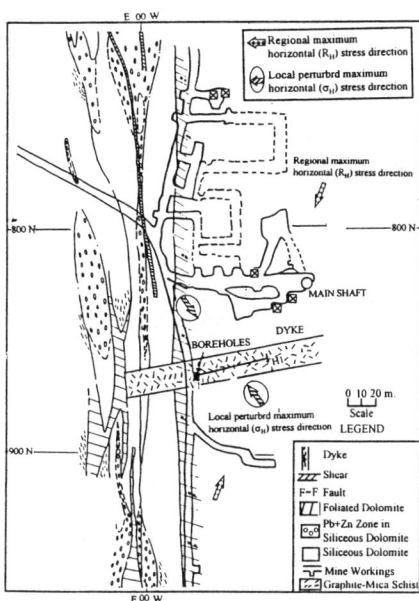

Figure 2. Plan showing the orientations of the regional and local perturbed maximum horizontal stresses, Rajpura-Dariba lead-zinc mines.

1) Plane strain conditions applied in the model.
2) The intact rock blocks are assumed to behave as non linear elastic/plastic material.
3) Joint area contacts as elastic/plastic with Coulomb slip failure.
4) Measured maximum compression direction and magnitude are assumed to be the perturbed stress direction and magnitude in and around the discontinuity.
5) The fault and the dyke are modelled as low or high moduli materials respectively relative to their surrounding material.
6) Regional stress directions are assumed to be the boundary stress directions.
7) Magnitudes of the boundary stresses (unknown) are manipulated systematically so as to achieve the horizontal stresses in around the discontinuity close to the measured stresses.

3.1 *Geometry and boundary conditions*

The 2-dimensional computational model is used which consists of a block with an intersecting fault or dyke. It is subjected to a bilateral tectonic stress field. The configuration, the dimensions and the initial boundary conditions for different cases are taken in accordance with the field conditions.

3.2 Modelling strategy

Different models are tried by varying the following parameters:
1) bulk moduli (K) and shear moduli (G) of both intact rock and the discontinuity.
2) cohesion (C) and friction angle (ϕ) of intact rock, discontinuity and the discontinuity contact.
3) normal stiffness (K_n) and shear stiffness (K_s) of the discontinuity contact.
4) angle (α) between the boundary stress direction and the strike of the discontinuity.
5) ratio of boundary stress magnitudes (K_0).

Table 4. The rock properties assumed are as follows.

	Uri H.E. project	Rajpura Dariba lead-zinc mines
Country rock:	Volcanics	Calc-biotite schist
Geological structure:	Fault	Dyke
Regional stress:		
R_H	9.2 MPa	16.85 MPa
R_h	1.1 MPa	01.50 MPa
R_H direction	055°	025°
Perturbed stress:		
σ_H	9.16 MPa	16.17 MPa
σ_h	2.29 MPa	08.35 MPa
σ_H direction	130°	320°
Deflection	75°	65°
Density (ρ Kg/m^3):		
Country rock	2910	2650
Fault/dyke	2060	2795
Bulk modulus (K in Pa):		
Country rock	8.33 x 10^9	17.90 x 10^9
Fault/dyke	1.66 x 10^9	21.30 x 10^9
Shear modulus (G in Pa):		
Country rock	6.25 x 10^9	10.20 x 10^9
Fault/dyke	1.25 x 10^9	12.24 x 10^9
Cohesion (C in Pa):		
Country rock	15 x 10^6	9.7 x 10^6
Fault/dyke	1 x 10^5	1 x 10^5
Fault contact	0	1 x 10^5
Friction angle (ϕ in degrees):		
Country rock	40°	45°
Fault/dyke	35°	20°
Fault contact	18°	30°

a) Material properties for Uri project taken from the report prepared by Department of Soil & Rock Mechanics Royal Institute of Technology, Stockholm, for the project authority.
b) Material Properties for Rajpura Dariba Mines taken from the report prepared by INCO. TECH, Canada, for the project authority.

3.3 Simulation results

Angle (α) between boundary stress direction and the geological structure is kept in accordance with the field conditions. The magnitudes of the regional stresses (R_H/R_h ratios) are varied systematically to achieve the stress magnitudes as close as possible to the measured stress magnitudes.

The fault is treated as a low modulus material with definite boundary surrounded with high modulus isotropic material. Along the fault contacts with zero cohesion, only slippage is allowed but not block rotation as in that case the angle between regional stress and the geological structure would not have represented the true field condition. Both the actual location (outside the fault) in the field and the measured stress magnitudes are considered while selecting the segment in the model to study the deflection of the stress direction in simulated condition.

The dyke is treated as a high modulus material inside a lower modulus matrix. No slippage is allowed against its contacts. Both the actual location (inside the dyke) in the field and the measured stress magnitudes are considered while selecting the segment in the model to study the deflection of the stress direction in simulated condition.

3.3.1 Effects of fault on stress trajectory

Figure 3 shows stress tensors along with the shear stress contours in and around the fault model.
Around the fault σ_H has rotated up to 33° in some of the segments as against 75° measured in the field. Inside the fault the deflection is 20°. Regarding the

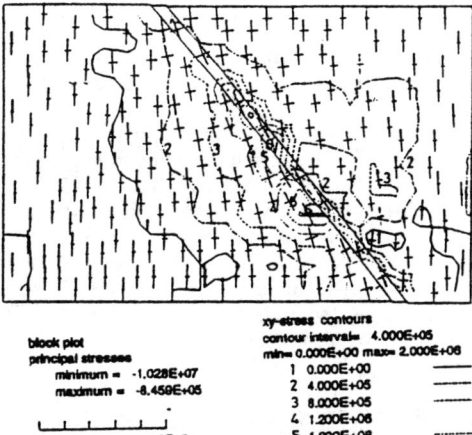

Figure 3. Effects of the fault on horizontal stress orientations with shear stress contours.

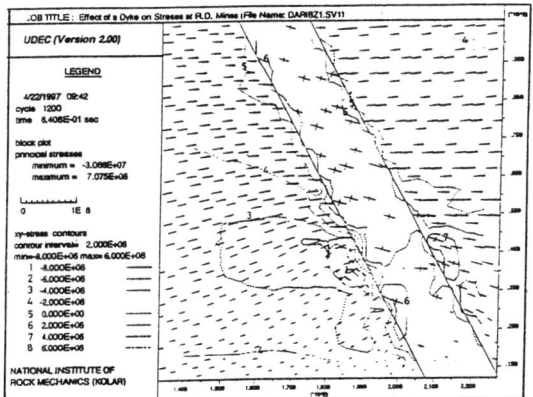

Figure 4. Effects of the dyke on horizontal stress orientations with shear stress contours.

stress magnitudes the simulated σ_H (9.32 MPa) matches well with the field (9.16 MPa) but the simulated σ_h magnitude (4.78 MPa) does not match well with that measured in the field (2.29 MPa).

Figure 4 shows stress tensors along with the shear stress contours in and around the dyke. Inside the dyke σ_H has rotated upto 35° in some of the segments as against 65° measured in the field. Around the dyke the deflection is negligible which is well supported by field observation.

Regarding the magnitudes, the simulated σ_H (16.5 MPa) and σ_h (8.95 MPa) match well with the field (16.28 MPa and 8.35 MPa).

4 PARAMETRIC STUDY

To check the factors influencing the stress deflections a systematic parametric study is carried out and 1) moduli values (G, K), 2) angle of friction (ϕ) and cohesion (C), 3) boundary stress ratio (K_0) and 4) the angle (α) between regional stress and the geological structures are taken in to consideration along with other factors.

The results of the parametric study are as follows:
1) A low friction angle to the fault contact deflects the stress direction by a higher degree.
2) A higher stress ratio between two horizontal stresses deflects the stress more.
3) There is significant deflection of stresses due the variations in elastic moduli between geological structure and the surrounding rocks.
4) The maximum deflection of stress orientation is noted when the angle between regional stress and the geological structures is around 40° in case of the fault and 10° in case of the dyke.

From the parametric study it can be concluded that a moduli difference alone between two materials can not deflect the stress direction beyond 22° when other parameters are kept constant in different models. The same is true with the friction angle and the cohesion.

The angle (α) between the geological structure and the R_H direction found to have the maximum influence on the stress deflection followed by the ratio of magnitudes of two regional stresses R_H and R_h. In a biaxial condition two directions of maximum shear stress lie at 45^0 to the α_1 and α_3. The deflection of the stress depend on the shear stress, it is obvious that the maximum deflection will be in such regions where shear stresses are high.

5 DISCUSSION AND CONCLUSIONS

Both the models and the parametric study give an idea regarding stress perturbation in and around the fault and the intrusive and the likely causes of such perturbations.

In case of Uri project the simulated σ_H deflection is 33° in some segments compared to 75° as measured in the field. Figure 3 reveals development of very high shear stresses around the fault with a gradual decrease in shear stresses on both sides of the fault. There is a general development of higher shear stresses on the left side of the fault as compared to the right side. The degree of rotation is higher for higher shear stress region. In case of biaxial condition, two directions of maximum shear stress lie at 45° to the σ_1 and σ_3. Figure 5 shows the effect of α (angle between regional horizontal stress direction and the strike of the geological structure) on the degree of horizontal stress deflection (β) due to the fault. Maximum deflection of 33.21° is attained with $\alpha=40°$.

In case of Rajpura Dariba mines the simulated σ_H

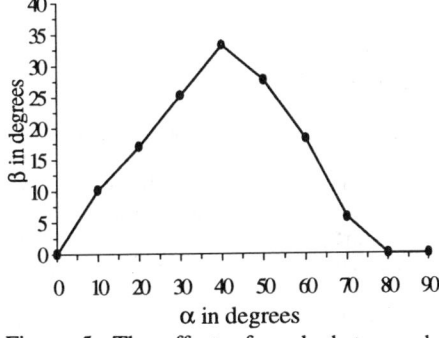

Figure 5. The effect of angle between horizontal stress direction and the strike of the geological structure (α) on the degree of horizontal stress deflection (β).

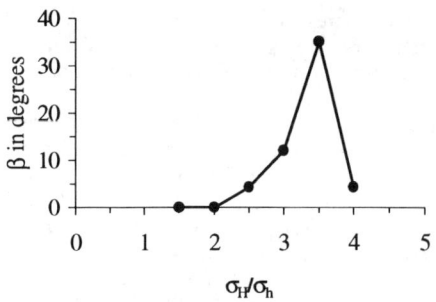

Figure 6 shows the effect stress ratio (K_0) on the degree of horizontal stress deflection (β) due to the dyke.

deflection is only 35° compared to 65° as measured in the field. Figure 6 reveals development of high shear stresses inside the dyke with a steep decrease in shear stresses on both sides of the dyke.

The higher deflection of σ_H in the field compared to the simulated conditions can be attributed to (1) Scale effect (2) anisotropic characters of both geological structures and the surrounding rocks in actual field condition against isotropic condition taken for simulations and may be (3) topographic effect in case of Uri project in Himalayas.

But we can conclude that the σ_H rotation due to a fault and a dyke is significant even not taking consideration of the above factors in simulated condition. The causes for stress deflection can be attributed to both moduli contrast between geological structure/country rock surrounding it and the regional stresses around it. Zhang et al., (1994) have demonstrated that it is not only moduli differences between two corresponding materials but moduli differences in two directions (x and y) of a single material will enhance the rotation of stresses. The inclusion of such data in a 3-D model may give stress rotation in simulated condition close to the field observations.

ACKNOWLEDGEMENTS

We are thankful to the Director National Institute of Rock Mechanics (NIRM), KGF, India, for permission to publish this paper. Mr. N.Reddy of NIRM is also thankfully acknowledged for his extensive support during numerical modelling. Thanks are also due to the all technical staffs of Uri hydroelectric project and Rajpura Dariba mines for rendering help during field measurements.

REFERENCES

Adams, J. & Bell, J.S. 1991. Crustal stresses in Canada. In D.B.Slemmons, E.R.Engdahi, M.D.Zoback & D.D.blackwell (eds.), *Neotectonics of North America. Geol.Soc.Am.Decade.Map. 1:367-386.* Colorado: Boulder.

Anderson, E.M. 1951. The dynamics of faulting and dyke formation with applications to Britain. *Oliver and Boyd.* London: Edinburgh.

Chandra, U. 1981. Seismicity, earthquake mechanisms and tectonics along the Himalayan mountain range and vicinity. *Phy. Earth and Planet. In*: 16: 109-131

Ez, V.V. 1962. Influence of Hercynian folding on the structure of the Caledonian structural stage in the Karatau mountain ridge and storeyed nature of folding. *In: Skladchatye deformatisii zemmoi kory, ikh tipy mekhanism o brazovaniya.* Moscow.

Rao, Srirama & Gowd, T.N. 1990. In-situ permeability of rocks and tectonic stresses at Bamnia-Kalan village, near R.D. mines Rajasthan, India. *NGRI project report (Unpublished).* India: Hyderabad.

Sengupta, S., Chavan, A.S., Joseph, D & Raju, N.M. 1994. In-situ stress measurement by hydrofracture method at R.D. mines, Rajasthan. *NIRM. Project Report (Unpublished)* India: KGF.

Stephansson, O., Ljunggren, C.& Jing, L. 1991. Stress measurements and tectonic implications for Fennoscandia. *Tectonophysics.* 189: 317-322.

Zhang, Y.Z., Dusseault, M.B., Yasir, N.A. 1994. Effects of rock anisotropy and heterogeneity on stress distribution at selected sites in North America. *J. Eng. Geol.* 37: 181-197.

Zoback, M.L. & Zoback, M.D., 1989. Tectonic Stress Field of the continental United States, *Mem. Geol.Soc. Am.,* 172: 523-539

Zoback, M.L., 1992, First and Second Order patterns of stress in the Lithosphere, The world stress map project, *J. Geophys., Res.* 97: 11.703-11.728.

Stress state in the Urals earth crust and its relationship with geological and tectonic evolution

Albert V. Zoubkov & Yakov I. Liepin
The Institute of Mining UD RAS, Ekaterienburg, Russia

ABSTRACT: Systematization of measurement results for original stresses in the rock masses at 22 Urals mines has provided the possibility for establishing some regularities in the distribution for elastic stress fields in the upper part of the Urals earth crust and for identification of its relationship with tectonic evolution and lithosphere structure in this region. Institute of Mining has carried out measurements at 17 from 22 above mentioned mines.

1 INTRODUCTION

An active human activity in the form of mining mineral deposits and construction of underground structures and communication lines is done in the upper part of the earth's crust. Reliable usage of these structures largely depend on the proper evaluation of the structure parameters and on the proper technical solutions based on the verified data concerning the stress state, mechanical properties of the parent rock masses surrounding the structures and their behavior in the existing stress fields.

The qualitative evaluation of the stress state in the earth's crust in the region considered is possible via study of tectonic processes beginning from global ones and terminating with regional ones. This approach allows to identity zones of tension and compression in the earth's crust and also determine approximately the orientation of principal stresses.

The relative magnitude and orientation of principal normal stresses may be judged by initial entrance of longitudinal and trans verse earthquake waves.

The results of in situ measurements of the rock mass stress state in the underground openings have particular importance. However it should be accounted that the values of original stresses and directions of their action in the rock mass depend essentially on the conditions of rock mass generation, its geological structure and tectonic fracture pattern.

There fore a reliable presentation of the stress state may be obtained only by complex usage of data concerning its present tectonic evolution and sufficiently large volume of results of in situ measurements of rock mass stress states in different areas of the region being considered.

2 RESULTS OF MEASUREMENTS

Such a condition is met by the Urals region where seven research institutes have carried out stress measurements for 22 ore deposits of North, Middle and South Urals over the 25-year period (see table). These measurements have been performed using following methods: full relief (F), part relief (P) and slot relief (S) methods, large base part relief method (LBR) and experimental analytical method (EA).

Gathered date present the original stresses in the virgin rock mass, that is they does not include the effects of mining openings and mined ont areas owing to introduction of applicable correction coefficients that have been found as a result of solution of three-dimensional geomechanical problems. The evaluation of measurements accuracy has been done with a confidence level of probability of 0.95.

From 43 measurement results obtained at various depths at 22 deposits 10 results have been processed with identification of directions of action and values for principal normal stresses in the horizontal plane where the measurements have been performed in mining openings driven in various directions.

In other cases the directions of horizontal stresses correspond to the orientation of two main types of mining openings at various mines driven along and across the strike of the deposit.

Table 1. Results of stress measurements

	City, deposit and institute that have carried out measurements	H, metres	Azimuth action $\sigma_x°$, degrees	Original stresses, MPa		
				horizontal		vertical,
				$\sigma_x°$	$\sigma_y°$	$\sigma_z°$
1	2	3	4	5	6	7
1	Severouralsk, III	800	90	-58,0	-38,0	-29,0
2	Krasnotouryinsk, Severopestchanskoye, I	Sf	6**	-9,6	-1,5	-
		300*	90	-10.3 ± 2.2	-7.9 ±2.7	-7.0
		380*	123± 9**	-13.0 ±2.4	-8.0 ±4.4	-11.3
		430*	90	-16.3	-12.5	-15.5
		500	90	-21.1 ± 2.1	-17.6 ± 8.3	-
3	Novopestchanskoye, I	370	146** ± 8	-14.0 ± 2.5	-6.4 ±2.7	-
4	Koushva, Valouyevskoye, I	125*	130	-5.6 ± 2.4	-2.9 ±4.4	-4.7 ± 2.2
		380	145	-26.1 ± 4.0	-21.1± 8.6	-22.2±3.2
5	Goroblagodatskoye, I	Sf	34**	-17.9	-5.3	-
		170*	188	-17.7 ± 3.4	-14.0±3.4	-
		260	188	-25.1	-18.7	-11.6
		600*	155**	-40.5	-21.3	-21.2
6	Nizhny Tagil, Lebyazhinskoye, I	300*	164	-15.5	-7.9	-6.9
		510	166** ±15	-22.3 ± 0.9	-19.3 ± 0.9	-21.1± 8.6
7	Vysokogorskoye, I	Sf	156**	-12.3	-6.7	-
		510	155	-41.0 ± 13.0	-37.0 ± 7.0	-32.0 ±5.2
		590	155	-43.6 ± 13.3	-39.4 ± 7.3	-34.2 ± 5.3
8	Yestyouninskoye, I	180	130	-25.4 ± 4.6	-24.2 ± 0.6	-20.9
		240	120	-37.0 ± 7.0	-28.5 ± 7.0	-34.3 ± 4.1
		360	124**± 7	-72.0 ± 8.9	-41.0 ± 3.4	-47.0± 2.1
		420	120	-140.0	-80.0	-53.0
9	Keezel, IV			-0.035H	-0.022H	-0.26H
10	Beryozovsky, VII	262	90	-17.9	-10.5	-10.5
		512	90	-25.3	-18.9 ± 3.4	-15.7 ± 2.5
11	Vishnevogorsk, III	320	40	-20.0	-13.0	-9.0
12	Satka, I	240	70	(10+0.029H)	(10+0.029H)	-0.029H
13	Bakal, Novobakalskoye, I	150	45	-14.0	-11.0	-4.0
14	Severo-Shikhanskoye, I	180	45	-15.0	-12.0	-4.4
15	Outchaly, Ouzelginskoye, VI	640*	0**	-24.0	-18.0	-18.0
16	Plast, Katchkarskoye, I	Sf	54	-34.0	-8.0	-
	Mine No.16, I, II	192	5	-13.7	-6.0	-3.7
	Mine "Centre", I, II	295	0	-31.3	-25.2	-9.5
	Froonzeh Mine, V	500	170	-47.0	-22.0	-15.0
	Mine "15th anniversary of October", VI	200-600	160	-0.058H	-0.033H	-0.03H
17	Mindyak, I	250*	125	-6.4	-6.2	-6.0
18	Roudny, Sokolovskoye, I	250	90	-10.0	-4.0	-7.0
19	Gai, VI	170	-	-(7.0 ÷ 10.0)	-(7.0 ÷ 10.0)	-6.0
		270	-	-12.0	-12.0	-11.5
		460	-	-(18.5÷22.0)	-(18.5 ÷ 22.0)	-18.0
20	Khromtau, Molodyozhnoye, I	530	140	-18.6	-18.0	-13.3
21	Almaz-Zhemtchouzhina, I	500	50	-20.9	-13.2	-13.2
22	Solikamsk	300	255	-15	-9	-11

* - results of new data processing by Institute of Mining UD RAS according to modern methodology based on original input data
**- Directions and values of principal stresses acting in the horizontal plane have been determined
Sf - The same as above but in the near surface rock mass based on rock deformations around subsidence area.

Research institutes: I - Institute of Mining, UD RAS; II - Institute of Geophysics, UD RAS;
III - UNIPROMED institute; IV - Urals Division of VNIMI; V - Polytechnical Institute, Perm city;
VI - Mining and Metallurgical Institute, Magnitogorsk; VII - IRGIREDMET Institute.

The length of these mining openings exceed 90% of total interval between mining openings in which measurements have been performed. It should be noted also that in the near surface layer of earth's crust up to the depth of 100-200 metres a relief of tectonic stresses onto weathered zones in the weak rock layers is observed. Therefore the stresses measured at these depths have maximum values in the direction parallel to the weathered layer and minimal ones in the normal direction to it. Furthermore in the area of each deposit the original stress state of the rock mass depend on the conditions of its formation, and on its geological and tectonic structure.

In view of above mentioned circumstances the evaluation of the stress state of the upper part of earth's crust in the Urals is recommended on the background of its tectonic evolution.

3 DISCUSSION OF RESULTS

The main features of its geological structure the Urals region has obtained in the Paleozoic period (Ivanov 1986). In the early stage of the Paleozoic period a break of Euro-Asian continent has occurred and the oceanic structure has formed that evaluated during a period of 20-30 million years. The width of the Silurian Urals ocean has been equal (based on paleo-magnetic data) to about 2000 kilometers. In the middle of the Silurian period the first island arcs have generated in the Tagil-Magnitogorsk download. The European continent has been driving to the East and in the same direction a zone of subduction has been lowering. In the beginning of the Carbon period a concentration of island are blocks and oceanic crust blocks has occurred as a result of collision with the periphery of the East European continent after which a period of quasiplatform development has come in the early Carbon period (Oushakov 1984).

Modern Urals mountains present the alpine intercontinental orogen that has generated as a result of renovation of the late paleozoic structure in the newest geological period (from the end of Paleogen). In terms of time this phenomena has coincided with the first signs of the collision between the Indostan peninsula and Eurasian Plate which has been dated as 45 million years ago (Stownili 1979).

The amplitude of newest upheavals of the axial part of North and South Urals is equal to 300-400 metres and may be up to 2000 metres and in the Middle Urals it equals to 200-250 metres. The amplitude of upheavals in the periphery of Russian Platform and West Siberian Plate adjacent to Urals does not exceed 150 metres (Sigov 1967)

Similar processes in the Urals have to be integrally related to gross stress-strain state of Eurasian Plate which has the following boundaries. In the North and in the West along the rift axis of the median oceanic ridges named Gackel, Mona and North Atlantic this Plate is directly bounded by North American Plate. This boundary is the zone of tension of the earth's crust. The south boundary of this Plate is presented by Azor-Gibraltar transform break, by the north edge of Pyrenian mountains, Alps, Carpathian, Caucasus and Copetdag. All these mountainy regions (except Crimean mountains and western part of the Main Caucasus Ridge) compose the Alps-Himalayas mountain belt of the lithosphere compression. The east boundary of the Euro-Asian Plate run along the west submountain regions of Pamir, Tyen-Shan, Altai, Sayan mountains and further to the east-along the north slope of the Stanovoy and Aldan ridges (along the rivers of Aldan and Lena). In its geodynamic nature the Predverkhoyansky downfold is the continental analogue for the deep-water channel (zone of compression).

Researchers analyzing relative linear velocities of lithosphere plate movement believe that the Euro-Asian Plate moves from the North-West to the South-East along the azimuth of 120-130° (Oushakov 1994). Specifically in the south-east a collision of Euro-Asian Plate with Indian and Pacific Plates occur whereby the greatest compression is noted along these plates.

Taking this fact into account one should expect in the Urals that maximum compressive stresses in the lithosphere of this region act along the azimuth of 120-130 °. The scheme of tectonic regioning in the Urals compiled by VNII Institute of Geology in 1972 and overlapped on the map of modern relief is presented in Figure 1. The newest north-west sectioning structures (tectonic zones) shown in this figure run at an angle of 10-30 ° to the direction of proposed maximum compression of lithosphere that ideally correspond to the planes of cleavage running at an angle α to the direction of largest compression (Vlokh 1987), where:

$$\frac{\arcsin B}{2} - \frac{\varphi}{2} < \alpha < 90° + \frac{\varphi}{2} - \frac{\arcsin B}{2},$$

$$B = \frac{2c + tg\varphi \cdot (\sigma_1 + \sigma_3)}{\sigma_1 - \sigma_3} \cdot \cos\varphi, \text{ when } B<1,$$

where c is cohesion of the rockmass, MPa; φ is angle of internal friction, degrees; σ_1 and σ_3 are correspondingly largest and smallest compressive stresses in the lithosphere, MPa. The average value of α is 20°.

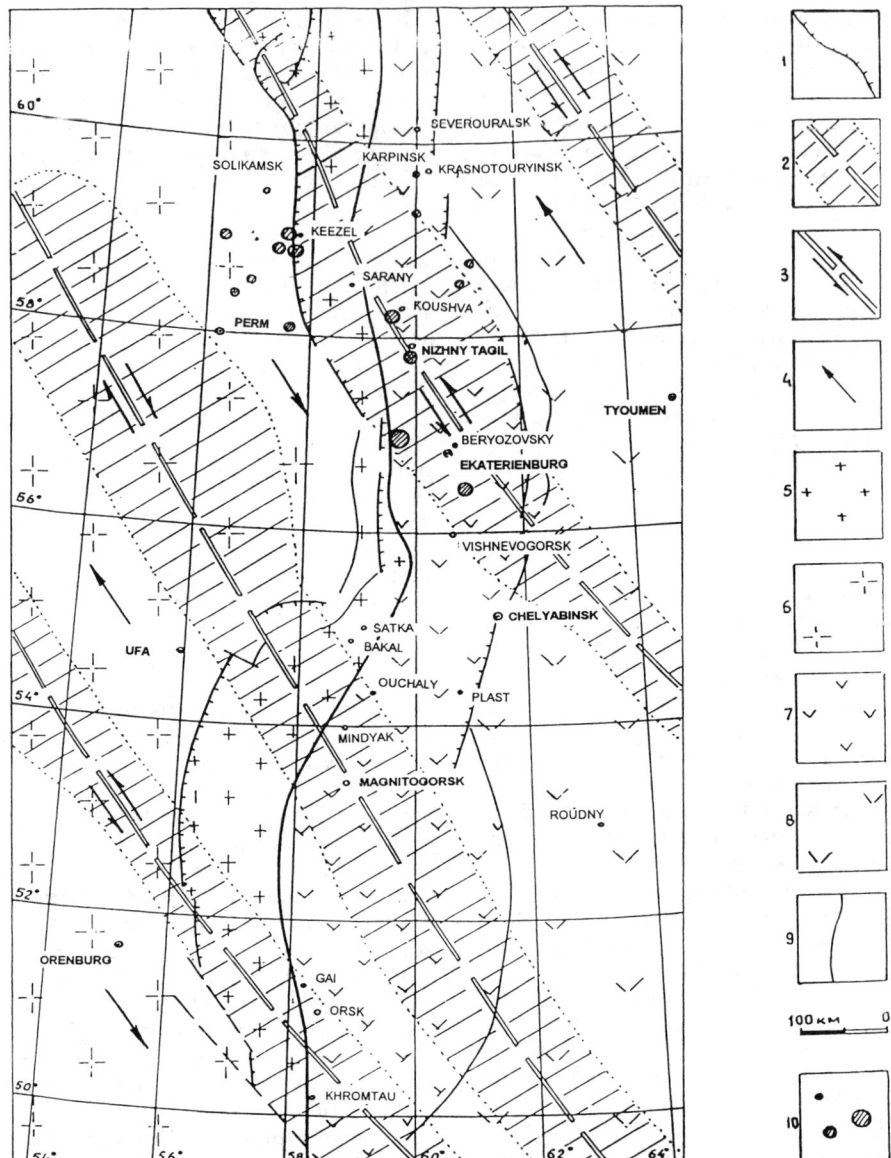

Figure 1. The scheme of newest tectonic structures in the Urals.
1- newest breaks, uplifts, uplifting shifts and uplifting overlap folds bounding the newest Urals orogen; 2- newest north-west sectioning structures deforming the newest Urals orogen manifested in the form of earth's crust upheavals running through Ekaterienburg (Timan-Kokchetav structure), through Magnitogorsk (Bashkiria-Oulutau), through Orsk (Karatau-Talas-Fergana); 3- proposed directions of relative displacement of earth's crust blocks along the sectioning northwest structures; 4- proposed directions of displacement of earth's crust blocks; 5- rocks of sedimentary covering and foundation of East-European Plat-form dislocated in the Urals gertsinian orogen; 6- rocks of the East European Platform not dislocated in the Urals gertsinian orogen; 7- rocks of the West Siberian Plate dislocated in the Urals gertsinian orogen; 8- rocks of the West Siberian Plate not dislocated in the Urals gertsinian orogen; 9- the Main Urals break-collision boundary between East European Platform and West Siberian Plate; 10 - epicenters of earthquakes with a magnitude of 3-6

In a line with the breaks shown in the figure turtner to the North two additional unnamed tectonic zones are located and further to the south the Mangyshlak-Gissar and Caucasus-Copetdag structures with north-west orientation are observed (Aleinikov 1993). In addition some tectonic zones with north-east strike can be traced out. The most large of them may be related to Arctic Urals being clearly demonstrated in the structures of Taimyr Peninsula. One may include in this group of zones the seismically active zone of Perm-Keezel-Severouralsk showing itself by specific features of structure of the foundation and covering of the Russian Platform in the form of wavy uplifts.

It is quite probable that the above mentioned tectonic zones are renovated more ancient tectonic breaks because in the Timan-Kokchetav zone some Baikal and even Carelian faults are identified, and in the Karatau-Talas zone one can identify the Gertsinian faults while in the Caucasus-Copetdag zone - the alpine ones. Is this case a deviation of tectonic zone (planes of cleavage) orientation from the direction of the highest compression amounting to 5-10 degrees is possible.

The most reliable results interns of values and directions of action for horizontal principal stresses have been obtained in the Tagil-Koushva and Krasnotouryinsk regions, that is in the area located to the north from the Timan-Kokchetav zone. The largest horizontal compressive stresses here act along the azimuth of 123-155° that is in accordance with direction of displacement of the Euro-Asian continent. Horizontal stresses in the perpendicular direction are 1.5-2 times lower in value and approach to loads from overburden rock weight when only gravitational stress component is acting. Measurements in Severouralsk and Beryozovsky indicate that the largest compression take place in the latitude direction and the least compression act in the meridianal direction. While these stress are not principal ones however the largest compression has orientation approaching to the direction of the Euro-Asian Plate movement.

In the zone between Timan-Kokchetav and Bashkiria-Oulutav structures at mines of the cities of Satka, Bakal, Ouchaly and Mindyak the measured normal stresses in two directions differ in value approximately 5-15% and this difference is in the range of measurement accuracy. Therefore one cannot say definitely about principal maximum horizontal compressive stress here (except Satka). However the equality of horizontal stresses in this region may be due to existence of very low angle of overlap folds with large horizontal displacement of overlapping wings in the zone of Ufa projection relieving the compression stresses in the south-east direction. In the region of Roudny city (Kazakhstan) the largest compression tend to be in the latitude direction that is in the direction more similar to the direction of Euro-Asian Plate movement.

In the zone of Karatau-Talas-Fergana structure the direction of the largest compression in the earth's crust cannot be judged based on results of measurements in the cities of Gai and Khromtau because equality of normal stresses is observed. The exception is the Almaz-Zhemchouzhina deposit located on the boundary of Kempirsai ultrabasic rock mass where maximum compression is in the normal direction to this boundary.

Reliable knowledge of stress vectors in the upper part of the earth's crust make it possible to update the general theory of geological and tectonic processes in the Urals and adjacent regions. And this task is achievable because there are no similar volumes of experimental data obtained on the limited area in all other regions except Sweden.

4 CONCLUSIONS

Stress measurements at 11 mines of the North and Middle Urals near cities of Severouralsk, Solikamsk, Krasnotourinsk, Karpinsk, Koushva, Keezel, Berezniki, Nizhny Tagil and Berezovsky show that the largest horizontal compressive stresses act along the azimuths having the range of 110-150°. This result is in good agreement with the direction of displacement of the Euro-Asian Plate and consequently with its dominant compression that takes place along the azimuth of 120-150° in the Urals region. The values of horizontal stresses in the normal direction are 1.5-2 times lower and approach to lithostatic pressure in value. Stress measurements at 14 mines of the South Urals and Bashkortostan near cities of Vishnevogorsk, Satka, Bakal, Outchaly, Plast, Mindyak, Gai, Roudny and Chromtau show that the largest horizontal compressive stress have random orientation. In some cases difference between values of maximum and minimum compression is negligible and consequently their orientation is indefinite. This can be explained by the tact that earthrelief-forming large - scale fractures along the west slope of the Urals in the region of Oufa console represent the low angle dipping overslides. Thus it may be suggested that in this area the West Siberian Plate have slided at low angle over the East European continent thereby providing the lower amount of mutual thrust and lower difference between minimum and maximum horizontal stresses and also the uncertainty in their orientation.

REFERENCES

Ivanov, S.N. et al, 1986. Formation of the earth's crust in the Urals. In Moscow: "Nauka" Publishing House.

Oushakov, C.A. et al,1984. The drift of continents and climates on the Earth. Moscow: "Mysl" Publishing House.

Stownili, R. 1979. Evolution of south continental periphery of the ancient Tetis. "Geology continental peripheries". Moscow: "Mir" Publishing House: 248-264.

Sigov, V.A. 1967. The map of newest tectonic structures in the Urals. "Tectonic movements and newest structures in the earth's crust". Moscow: "Nedra" Publishing House: 294-300

Vlokh, N.P. et al, 1987. Geomechanical analysis of tectonically faulted rock masses at Sokolovsky underground ore mine. Transactions of the VII- All-Union Conference on rock mechanics. Moscow: "Nauka" Publishing House: 149-153.

Aleinikov, A.L. et al, 1993. The Urals in the system of planetary lineations. Collection of scientific works. Ekaterienburg: "Nauka" Publishing House: 3-9

Intergranular cracking and relaxation of stress in deep crystalline rock as a result of physico-chemical influence of water

M.Z. Abdrakhimov
Joint-Stock Research Industrial Company GERS, Moscow, Russia

V.Yu. Traskin
Moscow Lomonosov University, Russia

ABSTRACT: A large number of data obtained at the Kola Superdeep well give evidence of rock volume discompaction in-situ below 7-8 km: low seismic velocities, high porosity and permeability, increasing drilling rate and hole cavity, core disking and etc. By these results it is possible to assume, that in-situ on the depth of 10-12 km, rocks in environment of water drilling liquid, can tend to discompaction. Our experimental study have demonstrated that the surface activity of water as the principal constituent part of the drilling fluid, combined with elevated temperatures and differential stresses, contributes to the development of intergranular microcracks under conditions for the lower part of Kola Superdeep Well.

1. INTRODUCTION

No attempt was made before to take into account the combined action of stress, high temperature and drilling fluid on partial disintegration and microcracking of core samples. For this purpose, we have used the ideas and experimental methods of the physico-chemical mechanics put forward by P.A.Rehbinder (Rehbinder P.A., Shchukin E.D., 1972) which proved to be successful in explaining many cases of premature failure of solids relating them to adsorption-induced strength decrease or stress corrosion (Atkinson B.K., 1978). This approach considers strength and fracture of solids as governed by physico-chemical (often only superficial) interactions between molecules when even small amounts of surface-active compounds (e.g. water) are able to lower considerably the surface free energy of the solid phase.

2. METHOD, TECHNIQUES AND MATERIAL STUDIED

We have employed a piston-cylinder testing apparatus allowing to perform triaxial tests of cylinder-shaped specimens (15 x 30 mm) in various liquid environments (water, drilling fluid, crude oil, acetone), within 300^0C temperature range and at confining pressures up to 300 MPa and axial loads until specimen failure. Before and after testing the petrophysical parameters (density, porosity, compressive and shear wave velocities) were measured and prints on photographic paper were made visualizing microcracks distribution (Abdrakhimov M.Z., V.Yu.Traskin... 1989)

3. RESULTS

The first set of experiments was aimed at determining fracture strength of amphibolite and gneiss specimens in the presence of liquids and in dry state. In the latter case the pressure liquid was prevented to contacted to contact the specimen by means of jacketing.

All the liquids investigated were found to lower rocks strength reducing it to 0,4-0,5 (amphibolite) or 0,65-0,7 (gneiss) of the initial value (Fig.1).

Water-acetone mixtures affect strength increasingly with the water content (Fig.2). This concentration dependence was used to estimate surface energy decrease and water adsorption. Data processing based on Griffith brittle fracture criterion and Gibbs adsorbtion equation gives the maximum adsorbed water amount of 1,5x10 moles/cm which

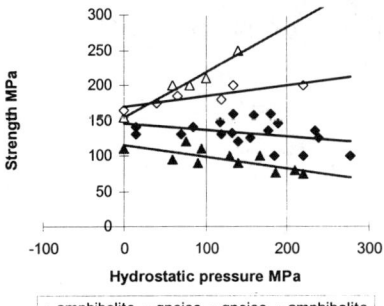

Fig.1. Compressive strength (Y) - hydrostatic pressure (X) trends of samples test of amphibolite (1-4) and gneiss (2-3) under constant temperature 200 C in dry condition (insulative envelope) (1-2) and in contact with water and bore mud (3-4)

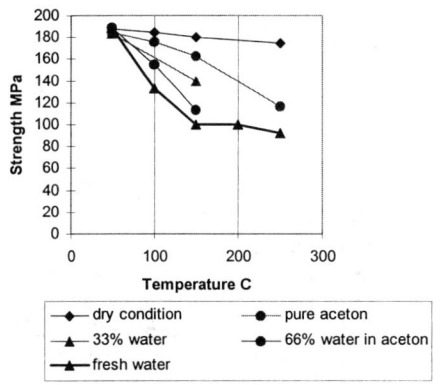

Fig. 2. Depedence of compressive amphibolite strength from temperature and composition of fluid

corresponds to area per water molecule of about 10 A, i.e. to monolayer adsorption (Pertsov N.V., 1985).

Print technique shows that in dry rocks the cracks are almost parallel to the compression axis and pass through the grains. In the presence of surface-active environments (water and moist fluids) the fracture path is essentially different: it follows a network of microcracks formed along grain boundaries.

It is well known that a typical feature of the Rehbinder effect on various types of solids is the preferential sensitiveness of polycrystals towards active environments as compared with monocrystals of the same nature (Rehbinder P.A., Shchukin E.D., 1972). Stresses necessary for grain boundaries disjunction decrease progressively if we increase the environment surface activity (by changing its chemical nature or by raising the temperature). The most active media can penetrate along grain boundaries with no external stresses at all, the grain boundary free energy being sufficient to produce the intergranular wetting. The relative free energy threshold beyond which the boundaries are permeable is known as Gibbs-Smith condition (Smith C.S., 1948): where is free interface energy, the subscripts GB and SL mean grain boundary and solid/liquid. The rock/water free energy estimates for the amphibolite tested in acetone-water mixtures indicate that above 100^0C the Gibbs-Smith condition should be valid.

To verify this supposition and to elucidate factors affecting the grain boundaries permeability, the next set of experimental was performed. amphibolite and gneiss specimens were exposed to water or drilling fluid at various temperatures, confining pressures and differential loads. Above 100^0C grain boundaries open, forming intergranular microcracks, after 3 hours exposure (Fig.3). The temperature and the axial load balance the affect. The most pronounced intergranular disintegration (manifesting itself in V and V decrease and in a sharp growth of the shear waves damping) occurs under combined action of high temperature, differential stresses and water. No one of these factors acting separately affects grain boundaries, neither does the combination of differential stresses and high temperature over the range investigated.

At the room temperature water does not penetrate along grain boundaries even in stressed rocks specimens (Traskin V.Yu., Pertsov N.V., 1987). The fracture occurs if the stresses are sufficiently high without formation of intergranular liquid films. It may be attributed to thermodynamical or kinetic factors related to the low stiffness of the testing machine. Supposedly, the grain boundaries in silicate rocks contacting with water are more sensitive to temperature increase than to mechanical loads.

It may be concluded that the specific features of the Kola well core in particular the frequent occurrence of intergranular microcracks increasing with depth from 9 to 12 km are consistent with the hypothesis about the Rehbinder effect as the mechanism of penetration of drilling fluid along grain boundaries into stressed rocks.

A special experiment was carried out with the goal to verify directly this hypothesis. A practically crack-free amphibolite specimen was sunk into the borehole to the depth of 9 km

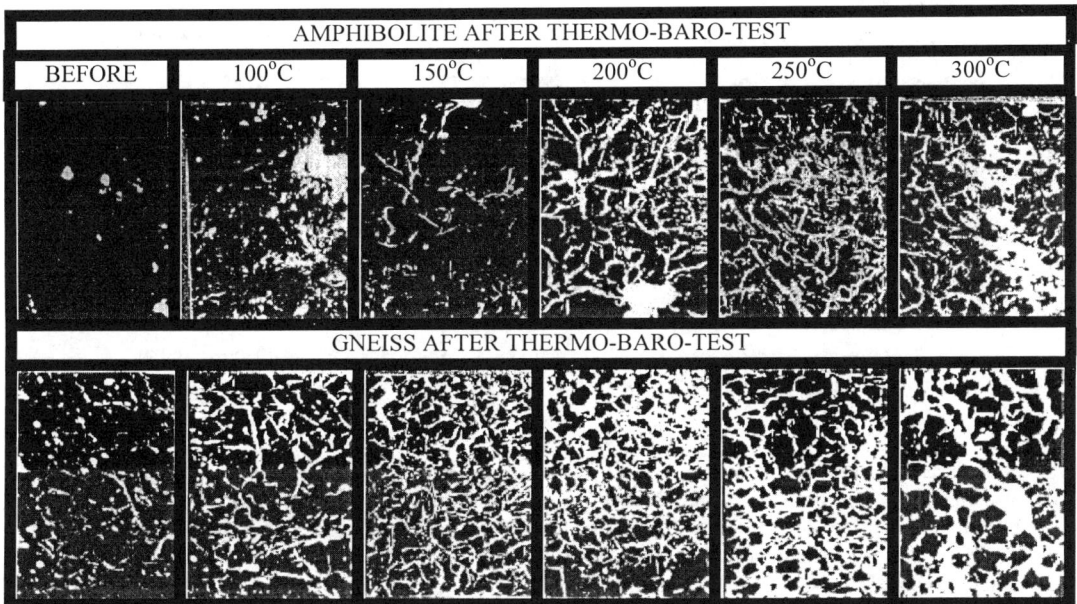

Fig. 3. Print images of open microcracks on surface of amphibolite and (1-6) and gneiss (7-12) (rocks - analogs of core SG-3) before (1, 7) and after tests during 3 hours in termo-baro-aparatus, under hydrostatic pressure of 100 MPa and temperature:100 (2, 8); 150 (3, 9); 200 (4,10); 250 (5, 11)°C

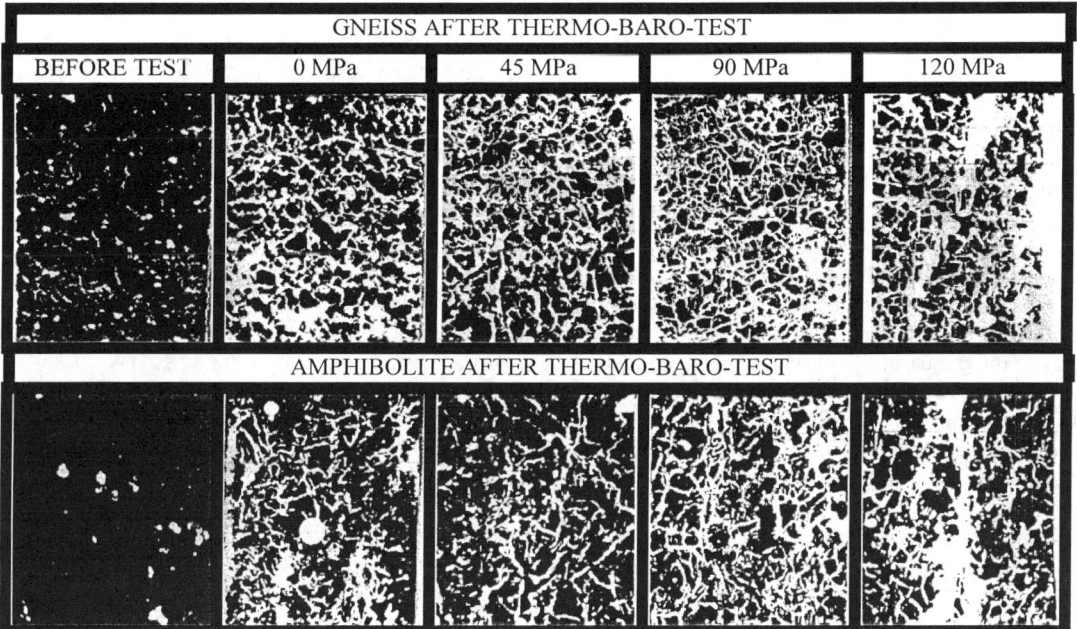

Fig. 4. Print images of open microcracks on surface of gneiss (rocks - analogs of core SG-3) before (1) and after tests during 3 hours in termo-baro-aparatus, under temperature 200°C, hydrostatic pressure 100 MPa and deviator pressures: 0 (2); 45 (3); 90 (4); 120 (5) MPa

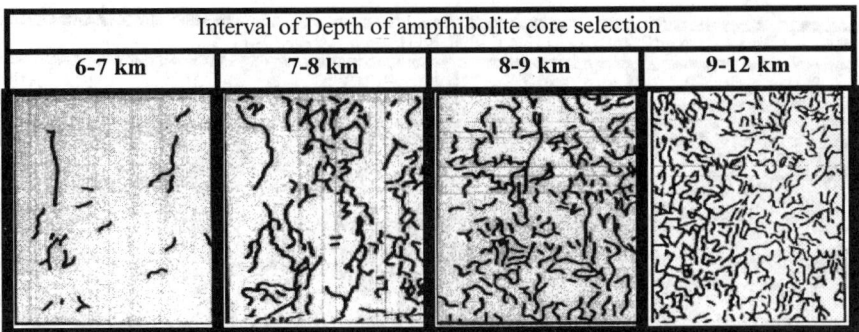

Fig. 5. Retouch print images of open microcracks on surface of amphibolite core collected from varies depths of Kola Super Deep Well.

(hydrostatic pressure 90 MPa, temperature 130^0C) and kept there in the drilling fluid during 24 hours. After that the specimen was found to become disintegrated along grain boundaries to the same extent as the samples tested under similar conditions in the laboratory pressure vessel. It should be emphasized that no additional axial stress was applied.

The study of the intergranular changes in the amphibolite over the depth range 6 to 12 km (temperature range 100 to 200^0C) has demonstrated that the number of open cracks streadily increases with depth, especially below 9 km (Fig.5). This observation is also consistent with the results of model experiments.

The time dependence of intergranular liquid penetration is known to follow a two-step law including linear and square terms. The data obtained previously for various kinds of materials enable us to estimate roughly the propagation velocity for the disintegrated zone front. It is expected to be about several meter/year. Comparison of core samples from neighboring boreholes drilled in 1980 and 1983 and separated by a score or two of meters reveals a marked difference in the occurrence of microcracks between the first (2,5 cracks/mm) and the second (4,2 cracks/mm) hole. This fact suggests that the rock massif around the more recent borehole had already been permeated with the drilling fluid from the first borehole before being drilled. A similar difference has often been observed between the amphibolites sampled in the beginning (3,5 cracks/mm) and in the end (1,7 cracks/mm) of each drilling run. Respective acoustic wave velocities are: $V =2,5$ $V =1,9$ and $V =3,4$ $V =2,7$ km/s.

The core samples taken from the lower part at the Kola well often display subhorizontal cracks with convexity turned upwards which are responsible for disk-shaped core fragments formation. We have succeeded in modeling this phenomenon in a laboratory experiment imitation borehole conditions at a depth of 6-7 km. A cylinder-shaped specimen with a "borehole" and a column (representing a core before its separation from the massif) was axially loaded at a temperature of 130^0C and confining pressure of 200 MPa in contact with drilling fluid or paraffin. It is shown that the drilling fluid felicitates the column rupture. The "core" analysis reveals the similarity between the shape of cracks in this case and in the real core.

4. CONCLUSIONS

This, our study demonstrated that the surface activity of water as the principal constituent part of the drilling fluid, combined with elevated temperatures and differential stresses, contributes to the development of intergranular micricracks under conditions characteristical for the lower part of Kola Superdeep Well.

REFERENCES

Abdrakhimov M.Z., V.Yu.Traskin and S.K.Belyaev. Method of revealing of microdefects in rocks. Bill of Invention. No.14, 1989 (in Russian)

Atkinson B.K., 1978. Subcritical crack growth in geological materials. J.Geoph. Res., vol. 89, N B6, June 10, p.4077-4114.

Pertsov N.V., 1985. Physico-chemical effect of liquid phases on rocks fracture. In: Physico-chemical mechanics of natural disperse systems. MGU, Moscow, p. 107-116. (in Russian).

Rehbinder P.A., Shchukin E.D., 1972. Surface effects in solid during their deformation and fracture. Progress in surface science. Pergamon Press, vol. 3, part 2.

Smith C.S., 1948. Grains, phases and interfaces: an interpretation of microstructure. Trans. AIME, vol. 175, p. 15-51.

Traskin V.Yu., Pertsov N.V., 1987. Physico-chemical mechanics of the intergranular wetting. In: Advances of colloid chemistry. FAN, Tashkent, p. 79-90 (in Russian).

Application of rock stress measurements in mining

Rock Stress, Sugawara & Obara (eds) © 1997 Balkema, Rotterdam, ISBN 90 5410 901 7

Determination of stress and strain fields around a horizontal fold and some applications in mining geomechanics: Correct and incorrect problems

V. Iv. Dimova
University of Mining and Geology, Sofia, Bulgaria

ABSTRACT: The problem of determining of the stressed and strained state in the rock mass around a horizontal fold is discussed. The problem is decomposed into two problems: a) a problem of determination of the stress and strain fields under the fold by a given fold shape, i.e. by given horizontal and vertical displacements of the points from the axis of a folded stripe whose thickness is neglected; b) a problem of determination of the filed of stresses and displacements between the horizontal fold and the Earth's surface by given horizontal and vertical displacements of the axis of the stripe whose thickness is neglected, and horizontal and vertical displacements of the points from the Earth's surface (land subsidence).

Assuming that the rock mass is linearly elastic and by making further suitable suppositions, the first problem is reduced to Dirichlet's problem for Laplace equation in a semiplane. The second problem is reduced to a biharmonic problem, which, when decomposed, leads to Dirichlet's problem for Laplace equation and to a problem of analytical continuation of a harmonic function which is improperly posed in J. Hadamard's sense problem of mathematical physics. It is solved by using A. Tikhonov's regularization method in the variant proposed by V.K. Ivanov.

The problems under discussion have both geodectonic and clearly mining interpretation: a) the first problem is the direct problem in the mining subsidence theory, i.e. for given subsidence of the immediate top, dictated by the order of mining, let us determine the land subsidence equation; b) the second problem is the problem of determining the stress and strain fields in the rock mass between a horizontal seam being mined and the Earth's surface by given land subsidence and immediate top equations. The knowledge of the solution to this problem is of particular importance for the future mining activity in the rock mass between the seam being mined and the Earth's surface.

1 INTRODUCTION

It is considered infinite, linear elastic and isotropic plain area, which represents a model of a rheological section of the Earth crust (Fig. 1).

At a given depth H, it can be observed the contour of a deformed stripe, whose thickness we neglect. In other words we monitor the fold L and the problem to be found the stress and strain distribution around the fold is posed (the 2D problem is examined).

The basic problem is decomposed to the following two problems:

1) determine the stress-strain field under the fold, for simplifying assumptions, which we will specify below.

2) determine the stress-strain field in-between the fold and the Earth surface, for assumptions, which we will specify below.

We will study the secondary stress-strain state, i.e. the state, which is caused by the fold existence. The prime stress-strain state (in a non-disturbed by the folded rock mass) in case of elastic mass, as it is known is determined by the formulas (Kleczek 1994) (2D problem is considered) (Fig. 1):

$$\bar{\sigma}_x = \frac{\nu}{1-\nu} \gamma_z$$

$$\bar{\sigma}_z = \gamma_z \qquad (1)$$

$$\bar{\tau}_{xz} = 0$$

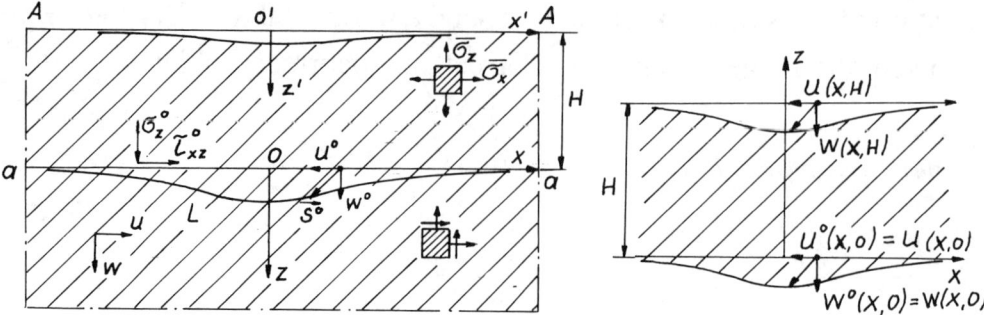

Fig. 1 Geological Earth's section

Fig. 2 Upper section of the rock mass

where z' is the bedding depth of the considered point, measured from the Earth surface, ν - Poisson coefficient, γ - volumetric weight of the mass.

We will be based on the basic static equations of the elasticity theory in displacements (Lame equations) (Timoshenko & Goodier 1951)

$$(\lambda+\mu)\frac{\partial\theta}{\partial x}+\mu\nabla^2 u+\rho X=0$$

$$(\lambda+\mu)\frac{\partial\theta}{\partial y}+\mu\nabla^2 v+\rho Y=0 \qquad (2)$$

$$(\lambda+\mu)\frac{\partial\theta}{\partial z}+\mu\nabla^2 w+\rho Z=0$$

$$\nabla^2(\ )=\frac{\partial^2(\ )}{\partial x^2}+\frac{\partial^2(\ )}{\partial y^2}+\frac{\partial^2(\ )}{\partial z^2}\ ,\ \theta=\frac{\partial u}{\partial x}+\frac{\partial v}{\partial y}+\frac{\partial w}{\partial x}$$

where λ, μ are Lame's elastic constants, X, Y, Z - intensity of the volumetric forces, ρ - density, θ - volumetric deformation.

2 STRESS-STRAIN STATE OF THE ROCK MASS UNDER THE FOLD

For achieving the aim, we accept the hypothesis, according to which the fold-forming is explained by deformation of the elastic plain alone the boundary a - a under the action of unknown loading $\left(\sigma_z^0 \text{ and } \tau_{xz}^0\right)$. This loading is however apparent, because it can be determined by the displacements on the line a - a. The location of the boundary a - a before the deformation, i.e. the axis of the band, whose thickness is neglected we accept, that can be identically determined for any particular case of fold forming analytically or experimentally.

The posed problem, is reduced to a problem in displacements for elastic semiplane. For solving it we accept such a distribution of u^0 and w^0 over the boundary a - a, which realize initially given form of the fold L (Fig. 1 - the coordinate system Oxy). Let us underline, that the last stage is not identical, because the preliminary given form of the boundary after the deformation can be realized by different assumptions about u^0 and w^0. Leaving this problem open, we proceed solving the posed problem.

We suppose, that
1) the media is incompressible, i.e. $\theta = 0$;
2) the mass is weightless (the weight is reflected in (1))., i.e. $X=Y=Z=0$.

For the assumptions made, from (2), for the plain case, we receive:

$$\nabla^2 u \equiv \frac{\partial^2 u}{\partial x^2}+\frac{\partial^2 u}{\partial z^2}=0$$

$$\nabla^2 w \equiv \frac{\partial^2 w}{\partial x^2}+\frac{\partial^2 w}{\partial z^2}=0 \qquad (3)$$

From (3) it follows, that the problems for determining $u(x,z)$ and $w(x,z)$, from mathematical point of view are identical, therefore we will consider only the problem for $w(x,z)$:

$$\frac{\partial^2 w}{\partial x^2}+\frac{\partial^2 w}{\partial z^2}=0$$

$$w(x,0)=w^0(x) \qquad (4)$$

Dirichlet's problem (4) has a solution from the type (Tikhonov & Samarskiy 1972):

$$w(x,z)=\frac{z}{\pi}\int_{-\infty}^{+\infty}\frac{w^0(\xi)}{(x-\xi)^2+z^2}d\xi \qquad (5)$$

By analogy, for $u(x,z)$ we receive:

$$u(x,z) = \frac{z}{\pi} \int_{-\infty}^{+\infty} \frac{u^0(\xi)}{(x-\xi)^2 + z^2} d\xi \qquad (6)$$

Thus the formulas (5) and (6) give the displacement field under the fold in the plain case $(v=0)$. In the considered case the stress field is determined on the base of (5) and (6), and according to the Hooke's Law (for known elastic constants):

$$\sigma_x = \frac{E}{(1+v)(1-2v)}\left[(1-v)\frac{\partial u}{\partial x} + v\frac{\partial w}{\partial z}\right]$$

$$\sigma_z = \frac{E}{(1+v)(1-2v)}\left[(1-v)\frac{\partial w}{\partial z} + v\frac{\partial u}{\partial x}\right] \qquad (7)$$

$$\sigma_z = \frac{Ev}{(1+v)(1-2v)}\left(\frac{\partial u}{\partial x} + \frac{\partial w}{\partial z}\right)$$

$$\tau_{xz} = \frac{E}{2(1+v)}\left(\frac{\partial u}{\partial z} + \frac{\partial w}{\partial x}\right)$$

where E is Young modulus of the rocks.

3 STRESS-STRAIN STATE OF THE ROCK MASS IN-BETWEEN THE FOLD AND THE EARTH SURFACE

Let us now only suppose, that the rock mass is weightless (X=Y=Y=0) and that the subsidence equation on the Earth surface, caused by the fold is given (measured), i.e. the functions $u(x,H)$, $w(x,H)$ are approximately given. Functions $u(x,0)$, $w(x,0)$ are also given (Fig. 2).

Under the suppositions made, system (2) (for the plane case - v=0) takes the form (Filonenko-Borodich 1959)

$$\nabla^4 u \equiv \frac{\partial^4 u}{\partial x^4} + 2\frac{\partial^4 u}{\partial x^2 \partial z^2} + \frac{\partial^4 u}{\partial z^4} = 0$$

$$\nabla^4 w \equiv \frac{\partial^4 w}{\partial x^4} + 2\frac{\partial^4 w}{\partial x^2 \partial z^2} + \frac{\partial^4 w}{\partial z^4} = 0 \qquad (8)$$

i.e. the horizontal and the vertical displacements holds the biharmonic equation.

For avoiding repetition, we will pose the second basic problem only for the vertical displacements (w). For determining the horizontal displacements (u), the analogic procedure is applied.

So, now the problem will be formulated as follows: in the semiplane $z > 0$ to be solved the biharmonic equation

$$\frac{\partial^4 w}{\partial x^4} + 2\frac{\partial^4 w}{\partial x^2 \partial z^2} + \frac{\partial^4 w}{\partial z^4} = 0 \qquad (9)$$

under the conditions:

$$w \to 0 \text{ when } z \to 0$$

$$w(x,0) = \varphi_1(x), \ w(x,H) = \varphi_2(x) \qquad (10)$$

where $\varphi_j (j=1,2)$ are given functions and

$$\varphi_j(x) = O(|x|^{-2-\varepsilon}), \quad \varepsilon > 0$$

The problem, posed in that way is incorrect in the sense of J. Hadamard (Tikhonov & Arsenin 1977) (Atahodjaev 1986). Hadamard's requirements for problems which have physical sense are: existence, uniqueness and stability of the solution. In the considered case, the third requirement is broken.

Since the following presentation is valid (Tikhonov 1972)

$$w(x,z) - w_1(x,z) + zw_2(x,z), \qquad (11)$$

where $w_1(x,z)$ and $w_2(x,z)$ are arbitrary harmonic functions, then for the conditions (10), we rich to the problems:

$$\nabla^2 w_1(x,z) = 0, \ z > 0$$

$$w_1(x,\infty) = 0, \ w_1(x,0) = \varphi_1(x) \qquad (12)$$

$$\nabla^2 w_2(x,z) = 0, \ z > 0$$

$$w_2(x,\infty) = 0, \ w_2(x,0) = \varphi_3(x) \qquad (13)$$

where

$$w'_{zz} = \nabla^2 w(x,z), \ \varphi_3(x) = \varphi_2(x) - w_1(x,H)$$

$$w_j(x) = O(|x|^{-2-\varepsilon}), \ j=1,2,3, \ \varepsilon > 0$$

Now it is clear, that the problem (13) is an incorrect problem for the harmonic continuation from $\{z > H\}$ into the stripe $0 < z < H$ (Atahodjaev 1986). When solving it we will apply the regularization method in a variant, proposed by Ivanov (Ivanov 1965) (Tikhonov & Arsenin 1977).

At first we will suppose, that the functions $\varphi_j(x)(j=1,3)$ are precisely given. We will seek a solution to the problem (12) (13) by applying Fourier's integral transformation by x. In this case

$$w_1(x,z) = \frac{1}{2\pi}\int_{-\infty}^{+\infty}\varphi_1(\omega)e^{-|\omega|z-i\omega x}d\omega \quad (14)$$

$$w_2(x,z) = \frac{1}{2\pi}\int_{-\infty}^{+\infty}\varphi_3(\omega)e^{-|\omega|z-i\omega x}d\omega \quad (15)$$

where

$$\varphi_j(\omega) = \int_{-\infty}^{+\infty}\omega_j(x)e^{i\omega x}dx \quad (j=1,3)$$

Let us immediately note, that formula (15) is unstable, which confirms one more time the incorrectness of the problem (13), hence alsoo the incorrectness of the problem (9) - (10).

After reguralizing (15) (Ivanov 1965), we receive

$$w_{2\alpha}(x,z) = \frac{1}{2\pi}\int_{-\infty}^{+\infty}R_\alpha(x-t,z)\varphi_3(t)dt \quad (16)$$

where

$$R_\alpha(x,z) = \frac{1}{2\pi}\int_{-\infty}^{+\infty}e^{-\alpha^2\omega^2-|\omega|(z-H)}\cos\omega x d\omega,$$

where α is a regularization parameter, which is determined according to the known methods (Tikhonov & Arsenin 1977).

Function $w_{2\alpha}$, determined by the equality (16) can be considered as an approximate solution to the problem (13), because (Atahodjaev 1986)

$$\lim_{\alpha \to 0} w_{2\alpha}(x,z) = w(x,z), \quad z \in [0,\infty] \quad (17)$$

uniformly in respect to x over $(-\infty,+\infty)$.

If instead of $\varphi_j(x)(j=1,3)$, their approximations $\varphi_{j\delta}(x)$ are given, and they are such that

$$|w_j(x) - w_{j\delta}(x)| \leq \delta, \quad (18)$$

acting by analogy we will receive the approximation

$$w_{2\alpha\delta}(x,z) = \frac{1}{2\pi}\int_{-\infty}^{+\infty}R_\alpha(x-t,z)\varphi_{3\delta}(t)dt \quad (19)$$

because (Atahodjaev 1986)

$$\lim_{\delta \to 0} w_{2\alpha\delta}(x,z) = w(x,z) \quad (20)$$

Having determined the displacements field, by differentiation and using Hooke's low, for given elastic constants, we can determine the strength fields.

4 SOME APPLICATIONS

Problem (4) and the analogical problem for the horizontal displacements $u(x,z)$ can be interpreted as a problem for determining as fare the displacement fields (i.e. the subsidence), as the stress fields above mined horizontal seam (for a coordinate system as in Fig. 2). In this case $u^0(x)$ and $w^0(x)$ are the displacements of the immediate roof. The real displacements of the points are determined as (Fig. 1):

$$\left|\vec{s}_0 = \sqrt{u^{0^2} + w^{0^2}}\right| \quad (21)$$

The displacements on arbitrary level z (the subsidence on the Earth surface is received for z=H), for a coordinate system directed as on Fig. 2, are determined from the formulas (5) and (6). The stress field above the seam is approximately determined from the formulas (7). This approximation come from the fact, that the boundary conditions on the Earth surface are not satisfied exactly (it is considered the area $D:\{-\infty < x < +\infty, z > 0\}$).

The second basic problem, treated in item 3 can be interpreted as a problem for determining the displacement and stress fields in the rock mass in-between the mined seam and the Earth surface (Fig.2) by measured displacements on the immediate roof and on the Earth surface both. This problem is incorrect in the sense of J. Hadamard and is solved by Tikhonov's regularization method (Tikhonov & Arsenin 1977) (Atahodjaev 1986).

5 CONCLUSIONS

The problem for determining the stress-strain state in the rock mass around horizontal fold was decomposed into two problems:

1) problem for determining the stress and displacement fields under the fold by given form (i.e. by given displacements) over the axis of the bended layer, whose thickness we neglect.

b) problem for determining the stress and displacement fields in-between a horizontal fold and the Earth surface by given displacements over the bended layer (whose thickness we neglect) and by given displacements of the points on the Earth surface.

Assuming that the rock mass is linearly elastic and after making some additional suppositions, the first problem is reduced to Dirichlet's problem for the Laplace's equation in a semiplane. The second problem is reduced to a problem for the biharmonic equation, which is incorrect in the sense of J. Hadamard. When solving it Tikhonov's regularization method, in variant, proposed by Ivanov is applied (Tikhonov & Arsenin 1977).

The problems considered have as fare as clear geotectonical, as mining interpretation:
- first problem leads to determining the Earth subsidence equation by given subsidence of the immediate roof.
- second problem is analogues to the problem for determining the stress and displacements fields in the rock mass in-between the undermined layer and the Earth surface by given equations of the Earth subsidence and the immediate roof subsidence.

The first problem leads to a correct, and the second to incorrect problem of the mathematical physics, which solution is achieved by Tikhonov's regularization method.

REFERENCES

Atahodjaev M.A. 1986 *Incorrect problems for the biharmonic equation*, FAN, Tashkent (in Russian).

Filonenko - Borodich M.M. 1959 *Theory of elasticity*, Fizmatiz, Moscow (in Russian).

Ivanov V.K. 1965 Caushy'e problem for Laplace'e equation in an infinite stripe, *ifferential equations*, Vol. I, No. 1 (in Russian).

Kleczek Z. 1994 *Mining geomechnaics*, SWT, Ktowice (in Polish).

Tikhonov A.N. & V.Y. Arsenin 1977. *Solution of ill-posed problems*. V.H. Whinston & Sons, Washington, D.C., USA.

Tikhonov A.N. & A.A. Samarskiy 1972 *Equation of mathematical physics*, Nauka, Moscow (in Russian).

Timoshenko S. & J.N. Goodier 1951 *Theory of elasticity*, McGraw-Hill, N.Y.

Evaluation of the effect of mine's rock bolts using a finite elements computer modeling

J.A. Ardito
Laboratorium of Rock Mechanics, The Pontifical Catholic University of Peru, Lima, Peru

G. De-La-Sota
Geomecánica Latina, Lima, Peru

ABSTRACT: This Study is a part of a larger project called "Rock bolting System in Mining Excavation" that aims to evaluate the different types of rock bolting used in mining. The first step was the evaluation of the Swellex bolt which is the most recent system of rock bolting.
The particular goal of this study is the evaluation of the effects of Swellex bolts in an arch of reiforced rock. The effect of the stress distribution of the variation of bolt length and of the mesh spacing is taken into account. The evaluation include comparison with field data gathered in a Chilean mine.
The simulation algorithm ALCODER (Computational Algorithm of Rock Excavations) using finite elements techniques has been used. It is a two-dimension algorithm which allows the modeling of the stress behavior of the rock mass in a mining excavation (arch type) before and after the placing of the bolts.
The results obtained with ALCODER reveal the interactive nature of the load-deformation phenomenon in rock mass and also in the support elements when the horizontal stresses are bigger than the vertical ones (big order cases). The variation of the bolt length and its spacing has noticeable effect on the rock mass stress distribution.

1 INTRODUCTION

1.1 General Aspects

In mining the complexity and geometric layout of excavations originate particular problems of stability. That is why the necessity of cheaper design of support systems arises. The temporal characteristic of excavations makes necessary to optimize the support system perfomances as well. In this context, Mining Engineering has developed able support systems to let release the stress of the geomechanical media by radial deformation in the openings, reaching the rock mass stress equilibrium in a low point of the rock mass - support interaction curve (fig. 1). It allows substantial resources economy. To save a substantial part of the resource originated by the search for more efficient support systems, the standard techniques have changed from external support (timber, steel and reinforced concrete support) to internal support (rock bolts, cables, etc.).

An important point to be mentioned and which found the interest of undertaking this study is the fact that the design and placing of the internal support are based on empirical models without considering the basic concepts of the rock-stress interaction (3,4) which are :
- The stress and strain of the excavation structure.
- The capability of the structure to resist the stress and strains.
- The stress field generated in the rock mass by support.

The analysis by numerical methods that may be processed in high speed computers has simplified the analysis of supported rock structures. It allows the study of problems like :
- The effect of rock bolts on the stress distribution of the rock mass.
- The reduction of the probable fault zones due to the placing of rock bolts or cables.
- The influence of the length of bolts and density of the rock bolts mesh.

The use of finite elements has allowed us to study the effect of a rock bolt (Swellex one), taking into account the bolt length and the density of the rock bolt mesh on the stress distribution of rock mass (3,4).

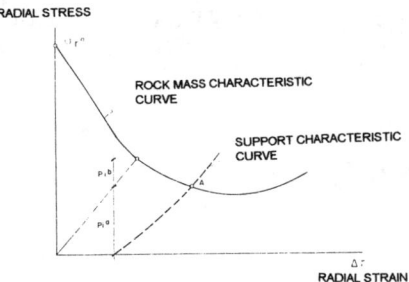

(Fig 1) Rock Mass - Support interaction curve.

2 METHODOLOGY FOR EVALUATING THE EFFECT OF BOLTS ON AN ARCH OF REINFORCED ROCK

2.1 Numerical Methods

With respect to the processing of rock masses four basic types of numerical methods are under consideration: Finite Elements Method (FEM), Finite Differences Method (FDM), Boundary Elements Method (BEM) and Discrete Elements Method (DEM). The Numerical Methods used in this study are based on the numerical resolution of differential equations that govern the mechanical behavior of the rock masses. Due to the complex behavior of the material, simplifications of their characteristics have been made. The solution of a problem is shown in a distribution form of main variables in the dominion considered, the variables are induced stress, strains and displacements (1).

2.2 Analysis Method Selection.

This research has used a simulation by finite element method in reason of its suitable capability of representing the main variables of rock. A useful and versatil tool for this research (5,6,7,8) has been used, practically the problem has been treated in two dimension using an Algorithm called ALCODER (6). This algorithm has been modified to represent the stress field generated by the use of rock bolts (5). The interpretation of the results permit us to:
- Identify the stress and strain conditions around the excavation.
- Know the effect of the rock bolt on the stress distribution of rock mass.
- Study the influence of rock bolt length and its mesh density on the rock mass stress.

2.3 Rock Mass Background.

The stability of a mining opening in a rock mass with high stress depends on the excavation and the magnitude and distribution of the stress around the opening.

2.3.1 Geometric Background.

The studied excavation geometry is a cross section of an arch type mining opening.

2.3.2 Geological Background.

The main rock of the mine used for the simulation is Andesite, where the 80% of the economical mineralization is presented.

2.3.3 Geomechanical Background.

The behavior of rock under stress conditions is based on the Mohr-Coulomb failure criterion and the stress-strain relationship by classical elasticity theory. The main geomechanical parameters are showed in table 1.

2.3.4 Tectonics in-situ Background.

The stress applied to the model are related to the place where is simulated the rock bolt effect on the mining opening. The values of σ_H and σ_V have been obtained in the literature (3). The values are showed in Table 2.

2.3.5 General Appraisal of Numerical Methods as Research Methods

In order to use a numerical code with confidence it

Table 1. Geomechanical Parameters

Young Mod. (Gpa)	Poisson Mod. (ν)	Cohesion (kg/cm²)	Friction Angle φ	Specific Weight (Tn/m³)
30	0,25	280	34°	2.81

Table 2. Stresses of Rock Mass

$\sigma_H = 2626\,Ton/m^2$	$\sigma_V = 1929\,Ton/m^2$

has to answer to some previous conditions. These requirements can be sorted in verification and validation.

- The verification process confirm that the mathematical calculus is made correctly.

- The validation process guarantees that the results obtained by the code are a sufficient and suitable representation of the real physical phenomena. The validation has to include comparison of simulation with *in situ* data. It is important to point that validation implies to study the simulation as a whole : equations, materials, boundary conditions, etc. (1)

2.4 Application of the ALCODER methodology

2.4.1 Mesh design

The simulation is made on a cross section of an arch type mining opening. The special rock bolt array around the opening requires a special mesh with regular or irregular quadrilateral elements in order to give a suitable geometric representation and rock bolt layout (see fig. 2 and 3).

The mesh finally used can be described as follows :

a) Bidimensional finite elements.

b) Smaller elements are concentrated around rock bolts, where a more precise simulation is critical.

c) 5228 Elements.

d) 5356 Nodes.

e) 1 Material (homogeneus rock).

f) Boundary conditions: The model is restricted in 254 nodes (the opening contour): 4 fixed nodes and 250 partially fixed.

2.4.2 IN PUT conditions

The compiled background with the mesh conditions are loaded to the simulation software by means of a file that is ordered as follows:

a) Number of elements - Number of nodes - Band width.

b) Number of nodes with boundary conditions - Number of rock types.

c) Rock type- Geomechanical parameters (Table 1).

d) Node coordinates.

e) Node - Boundary conditions.

f) Element - Four nodes - Rock type.

g) Elements and nodes excavated in the opening.

h) Stress system - Stress ratio.

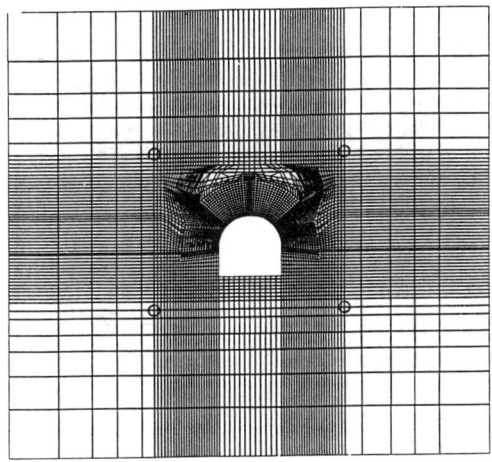

(fig. 2) Mesh of finite elements for five Rock Bolts Array
o: Refined Finite Elements Mesh

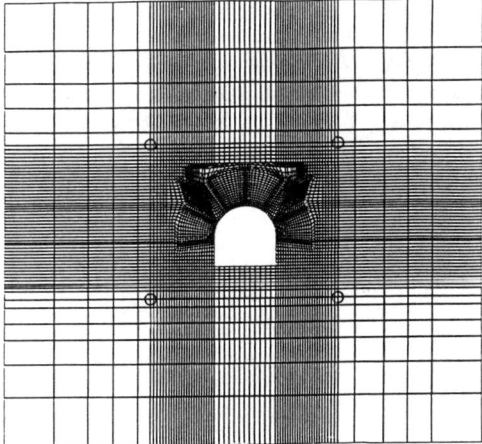

(fig. 3) Mesh of finite elements for seven Rock Bolts Array
o: Refined Finite Elements Mesh

In order to simulate the stress field generated on the rock mass, due to the rock bolt stress the in put conditions are loaded in the order as follows:

a) Excavated rock bolt holes, elements and nodes.

b) An additional in put file, called NOPPER allows the definition of the nodes that limit the bolt length and radial forces perpendicular to the positioning.

This file has the following characteristics:

- Total number of bolts and radial force.

- In clockwise direction, the bolt number and the bolt angle in the opening arch.

- Nodes that limits the bolt length

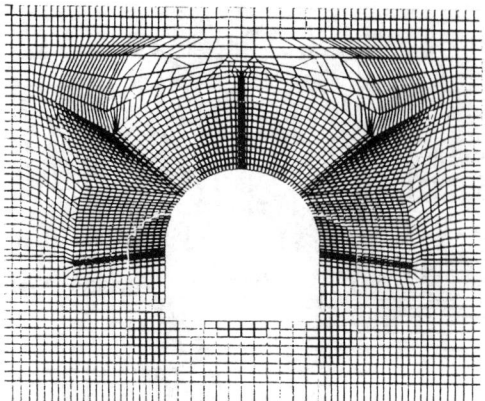

(fig 4) Stress Concentration for five rock bolts Array

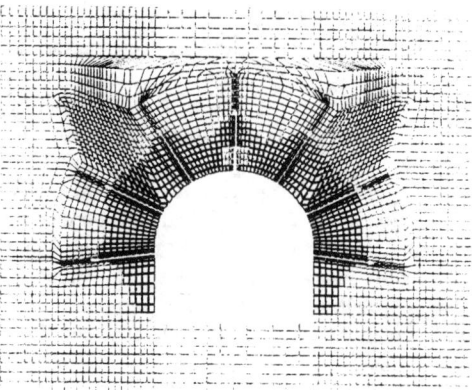

(fig 7) Effect of rock bolts on the Stress Concentration for 7 bolts array. Bolt length = 2.20 m. Space between bolts = 1.0 m. Percent of confinated elements = 14%

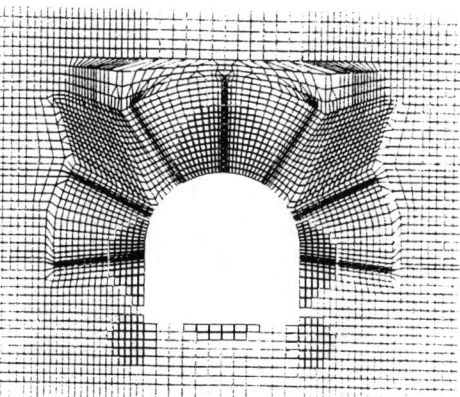

(fig 5) Stress Concentration for seven rock bolts Array

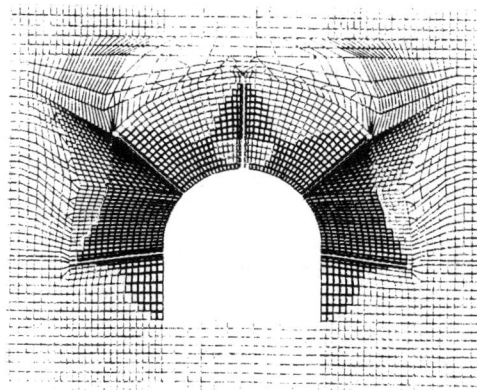

(fig 8) Effect of rock bolts on the Stress Concentration for 5 bolts array. Bolt length = 2.20 m. Space between bolts = 1.50 m. Percent of confinated elements = 22%

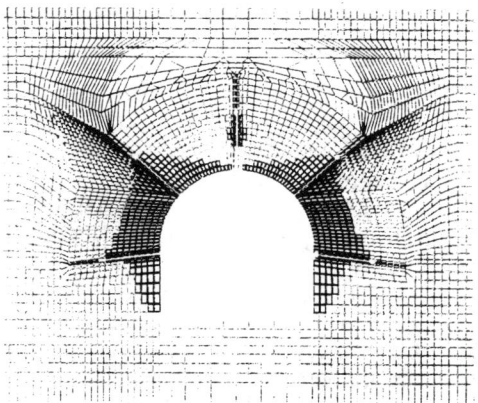

(fig 6) Effect of rock bolts on the Stress Concentration for 5 bolts array. Bolt length = 1.50 m. Space between bolts = 1.50 m. Percent of confinated elements = 12%

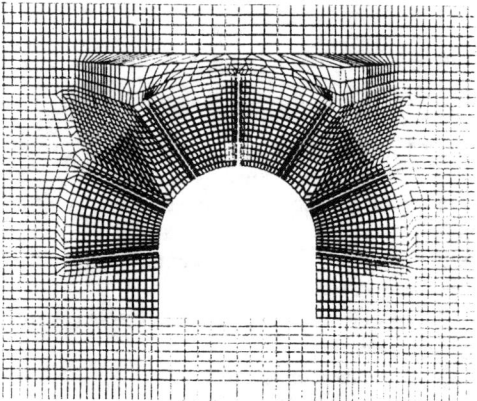

(fig 9) Effect of rock bolts on the Stress Concentration for 7 bolts array. Bolt length = 2.20 m. Space between bolts = 1.0 m. Percent of confinated elements = 25%

Table 3. Array of Bolts

Array	Number of Bolts	Length of Bolt	Figure
Array 1	5	1.50 m	figure 6
Array 2	7	1.50 m	figure 7
Array 3	5	2.20 m.	figure 8
Array 4	7	2.20 m	figure 9

The radial force has been calculated with rockbolt tests in order to obtain the elastic constant K of bolt (similar to a spring), then the radial force is:

$$F = K \times (\Delta\delta) \quad (1)$$

Where $(\Delta\delta)$ is the difference between the maximum diameter of Bolt when is expanded without confinement and the hole diameter (2).

3 PRESENTATION OF RESULTS

The work aims to simulate the rockbolt effect in the reinforcement arch of rock in four different arrays (see table 3).

3.1 Stress Concentration.

The stress concentration system is given by the mean of final stress versus the mean of initial stress in each element of the model:

$$C = \frac{(\sigma_x + \sigma_y)_{final}}{(\sigma_x + \sigma_y)_{initial}} \quad (2)$$

Where:
C is the Stress Concentration.
$(\sigma_x + \sigma_y)_{final}$ is the mean of final stress.
$(\sigma_x + \sigma_y)_{initial}$ is the mean of initial stress.

Due to the opening geometry and the layout of rock bolt arrays, C is the most representative ratio for the system as a whole (see fig. 4 and fig. 5).

Considering as a background the interaction between the rock mass and support, the most important remarks are:
- In graphical representation of stress concentration simulation (fig. 4 and 5) it is evident that the initial opening, immediately shows lost of rock confinement on the excavation walls and floor, there are low stress concentration (red color in fig. 4 and 5). On the other hand, the high stress concentration is set only on the ceiling and in the corners (blue color in fig. 4 and 5).
- When the opening is drilled it is clear in the rock-mass interaction curve (fig. 1) the drop to a determinated value of strain.

3.2 Rock Bolts effects

The alternatives investigated for the rock bolt simulation in the reinforced arch are showed in figures 6,7,8 and 9. In those figures, the increase of mean final stress ratio versus the original stress ratio is showed and its definition is the following:

$$INCREMENT = \frac{(R2 - R1) \times 100}{R1} \quad (3)$$

Where:
$R1$ is the mean of the final stresses and initial stresses in each element.
$R2$ is the mean of the final stresses with the radial force of rock bolt and the initial stresses in each element.

In general, it is evident that a distinct phenomenon is happening considering the stress state of the rock masses without rock bolts.

The stress increments supported by the elements are showed in the rock bolt effects (fig. 6,7,8 and 9). The important remarks are:
- It is clear that in the array of figure 9 the rock bolt effect generates an uniform increased bulb around the excavation. Due to the rock bolts separation this array influence the reduction of the potential fault zone.
- In figure 8, the increase of the rock bolt separation generates a less uniform stress bulb.
- When the rock bolts length decreases from 2.2 m. to 1.50 m. the reduction of the bulb stress is evident.
- Due to the stress concentration on the opening ceiling, parts of the rock bolt length (placed in the semicircle center of the excavation) do not exert any effect on the rock mass. This phenomenon is showed in all the arrays.

4 DISCUSIONS AND CONCLUSIONS

In this study the relationship between the main stress on a finite elements simulation model has been analysed.

The geometric configuration of the simulated opening modifies the original tectonic conditions, redistributing the *in situ* stress. As a result of this stress redistribution, there are sectors where there are compressed and relaxed rock.

In the rock mass - support interaction curve of the excavated opening (fig. 1), the constitutive rock must be suited to an equilibrium condition. This implies the deformation of rock toward the free face of the excavation.

The percentage of confined elements in function of the total number of model elements, indicates the influence of rock bolt density on the stress distribution on rock mass.

The most important difference is given by the size of the increment bulb of stress around the excavation in each array.

The array showed in fig. 9 is the best array for the mining opening studied.

Finally all this research will vary if there are another in put simulation conditions, but the procedures would be similar to the one used here.

5 BENEFITS AND LIMITATIONS

The use of a numerical model means obtaining an approximated solution of the real solution of the considered model. In our case the model represents the rock mass as a lineal and elastic continuum reinforced with rock bolts with lineal and elastic characteristics. For this reason the numerical method is approximation and its result must be interpretated with care. In this study it would be very difficult to have the certainty that the happening phenomena, when the simulations are made, correspond exactly to what might be happening in a heterogeneous rock mass. We may conclude that while there is no validation with field data, the model should not be considered as a kind of dimensioning a rock bolt array. We have to study more an adjustment of the model for each case. It could be by means of the observation and analysis of rock and support elements, whose results will show the dynamism of an opening mine in accordance with the exploitation method.

The ALCODER methodology has showed to be suitable to evaluate the stress behavior of a rock mass, before and after the placement of bolts, because this program has several interchangeable routines, by means of them was easy to effect all the simulation process of the reinforced mining opening with rock bolts.

REFERENCES

1. Alejano, L. and Ardito J.A., "Numerical Methods in Rock Mechanics", *Intercampus Research Peru-Spain,* University of Vigo, Spain, 1997
2. Atlas Copco MCT, "The Swellex Rockbolt System", *Information Bulletin*, 1990.
3. DeLaSota, G., "Application of Swellex in Bolivian and Peruvian Mines", *Internal Reports, Atlas Copco of Peru*, 1995.
4. DeLaSota, G., *Efecto del Perno Swellex en el arco de Roca Reforzada*. M Sc Thesis. University of Chile. 1995.
5. Krstulovic, L. and Cabello C., "Geomechanics for Rock Excavation Design", *Minerales*, Vol. 43, 1989.
6. Kenneth, H., *The Finite Element Method for Engineers*, New York, 1975.
7. Kulwahy, F., "Analysis of Underground Opening in Rock by Finite Elements Methods", *Final Technical Report*, Syracuse University, 1972.
8. Zienkiewicz, O., *The Finite Element Method*, 3rd Edition, Mc Graw Hill, 1977.

Influence of initial stress on rock slope stability

Katsuhiko Kaneko & Masaji Kato
Hokkaido University, Sapporo, Japan

Yoshifumi Noguchi & Naoaki Nakamura
Nittetsu Mining Co., Ltd, Tokyo, Japan

ABSTRACT : The influence of initial rock stress on the slope stability has been concretely discussed by the numerical analysis and field measurement. The numerical stress analysis indicates that both the stability factor at the failure initiation and the deformation behavior of rock slope are affected by not only the slope angle and the rock strength but also the initial stress state at the pre-excavation. The field displacement measurement has been performed in an open pit limestone mine, and the ratio of horizontal to vertical stresses at the pre-excavation in this field has been back analyzed. Furthermore, by comparing the values observed with those estimated by using the back analyzed result, it is confirmed that this slope is stable at present. From these results, it is concluded that the initial rock stress as well as the slope stability can be evaluated by the combination of the field displacement measurement and the numerical stress analysis.

1. INTRODUCTION

The stability assessment of rock slope is of fundamental importance for safety operation in open pit mines. For this purpose, various approaches to monitor the stability of rock slope have been carried out (Hoek and Bray, 1977; Kennedy et al., 1971).

In the stability monitoring of rock slope, it is mostly important to know whether rock slope is stable or not at present. For this purpose, a knowledge for the mechanical behavior of rock mass forming a slope is indispensable. Especially, if the deformation behavior of rock slope in the stable state can be predicted, the slope stability can be assessed by comparing the field observation result with predicted one. Furthermore, it is well known that the failure process of rock slope is progressive rather than instantaneous (Sugawara, et al. 1983 ; Kaneko, et al. 1997). This indicates that a knowledge on the failure process is also important. Especially, from the standpoint of stability monitoring, it requires to evaluate the condition of failure initiation.

In this paper, the influence of the initial rock stress as well as the slope geometry and mechanical properties of rock on the stability of homogeneous rock slope are analyzed and discussed. Firstly, the stress and displacement fields induced by bench cut excavation are analyzed by Boundary Element Method (Crouch and Starfield, 1983) and the influence of initial rock stress on the failure initiation is discussed. Secondarily, analyzing the result obtained by the field displacement measurement in a open pit mine, the initial stress state is estimated. Finally, a method to asses the slope stability by the combination of the field displacement measurement and the numerical stress analysis is proposed.

2. NUMERICAL ANALYSIS

The rock mass forming a slope is considered to behave as an elastic continuum when the slope is stable. Therefore, deformation behavior of rock slope in the stable state can be evaluated by the numerical stress analysis with the assumption that the rock mass is an elastic continuum.

A model for the computation is shown in Fig.1 and the stress and displacement field induced by bench cut excavation have been analyzed by Boundary Element Method (Kaneko et al. 1995). In this analysis, rock is treated as the homogeneous elastic material with Young's modulus, E and Poisson's ratio, v and the vertical and horizontal components of initial rock stresses at the pre-excavation are given by γz and $m\gamma z$, respectively, where γ, z and m are the unit weight of rock, the depth from the initial surface and the ratio of horizontal to vertical stresses. The slope height and the slope angle of the initial model are H and θ, respectively, and the stress and displacement fields induced by successive bench cut excavations have been analyzed. The height of each bench is $H/10$

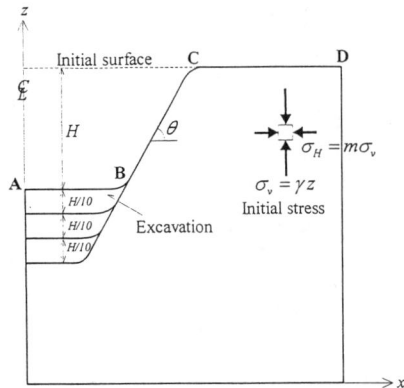

Fig. 1 A model for computation and definitions of slope geometry and initial rock stress, where m is the ratio of horizontal to vertical stresses, γ is the unit weight of rock and z is the depth from the initial surface.

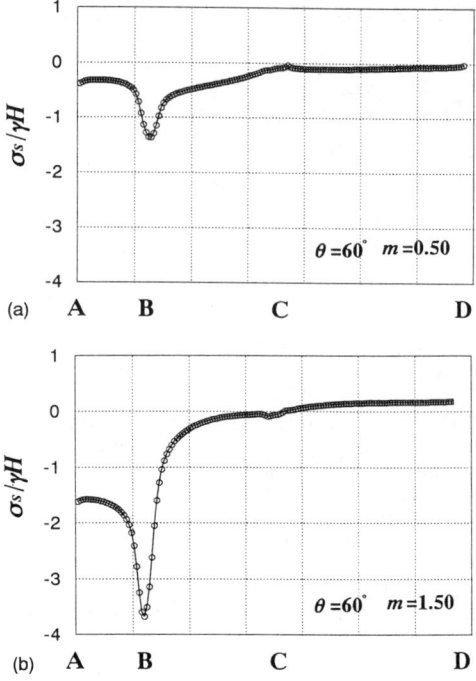

Fig. 2 Distribution of tangential stress σ_s along the rock surface. A, B, C and D are shown in Fig.1 and θ and m are slope angle and the ratio of horizontal to vertical stresses at the pre-excavation, respectively.

and three excavation steps have been calculated.

The distributions of stress parallel to the rock surface along the floor, slope and upper surface are shown in Fig.2, where (a) and (b) are those in the cases of $m=0.0$ and 1.0, respectively. From Fig.2, it is observed that the compressive stress concentrates at the toe of the slope and the concentration factor of the compressive stress increases with increasing the value of m. Furthermore, it is also found out that the stress at the upper surface changes from compression to tension with increasing the value of m. Theses results suggest that the failure initiates at the toe of the slope or the upper surface (Obara and Sugawara, 1991). The former is the compressive failure and occurs in the case that the value of m is relatively small. And the latter is the tensile failure and occurs in the case that the value of m is relatively high. To evaluate the potential of two types of the failure initiation mentioned above, we define the stress factor k_1 as the maximum value of compressive stress at the toe of the slope normalized by γH and k_2 as the maximum value of tensile stress at the upper surface normalized by γH. The relations between stress factors, k_1 and k_2, and the slope angle are shown in Fig.3, as a function of the ratio of horizontal to vertical stresses.

Using stress factors, k_1 and k_2, the criteria of failure initiation can be expressed as,

$$k_1 \gamma H = -Sc \quad (1),$$
$$k_2 \gamma H = St \quad (2).$$

Where Sc and St are the uniaxial compressive strength and the tensile strength of rock. The uniaxial compressive strength can be expressed by $Sc=2C\cos\phi/(1-\sin\phi)$, where C and ϕ are the cohesion and the internal friction angle, and the tensile strength can be written by $St=\zeta C$, where ζ is a constant. Substituting these relationships into eqs. (1) and (2), the stability factor, $\gamma H/C$, at the failure initiation is given by,

$$n_1 S = -2\cos\phi/\{k_1(1-\sin\phi)\} \quad (3),$$
$$n_2 S = \zeta/k_2 \quad (4),$$

where $n_1 S$ and $n_2 S$ correspond to the failure initiation at the toe and upper surface of the slope, respectively. Using eqs. (3) and (4), the critical slope height for the fracture initiation can be evaluated.

For an example of calculations, a contour map of the stability factor at the failure initiation in the case of $\phi=45$ degrees and $\zeta=0.2$ is shown in Fig.4. It is clear that the location of failure initiation changes from the toe of the slope to the upper surface with increasing the value of m and that the stability factor at the failure initiation decreases with

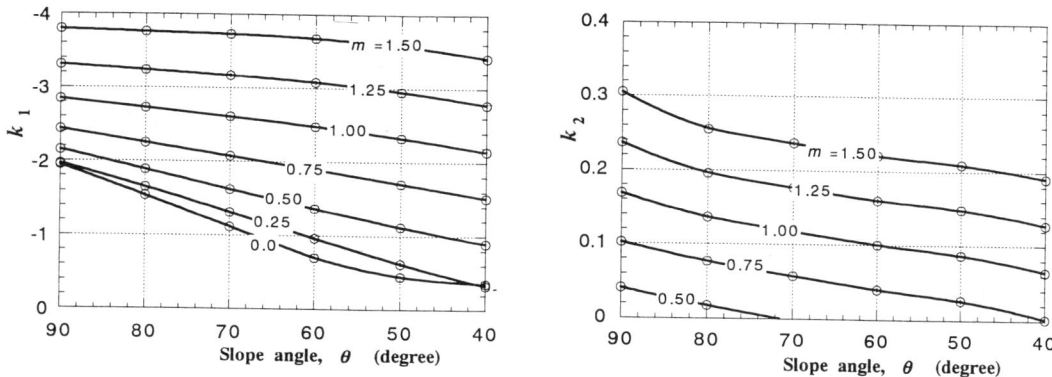

Fig. 3 Relation between the stress coefficient and slope angle θ, where m is the ratio of horizontal to vertical stresses at the pre-excavation.

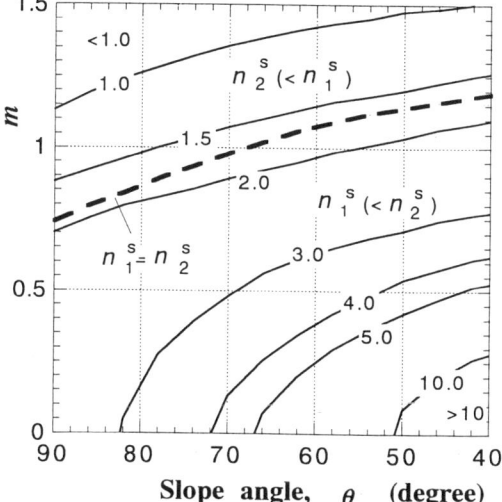

Fig. 4 Contour map of the stability factor at the failure initiation in the case that the internal friction angle is 45 degrees, where n_1^s and n_2^s are stability factors of the failure at slope toe and upper surface, respectively.

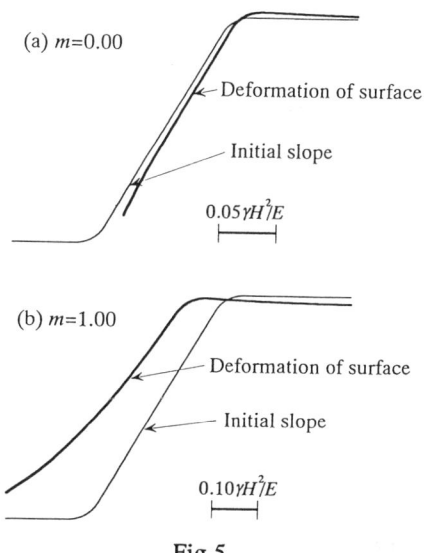

Fig. 5.

increasing the slope angle and the value of m. This result indicates that the slope stability is strongly affected by the initial stress state at the pre-excavation and that the evaluation of the initial rock stress is indispensable to assess the slope stability.

In order to estimate the value of m by the field displacement measurement, the deformation behavior of rock slope due to excavation has been analyzed. For an example of calculation results, the deformation of slope face and upper surface induced by the excavation of one bench is shown in Fig.5. It is clear that the deformation behavior of rock slope depends on the ratio of horizontal to vertical stresses. In the case of $m=0$, the slope surface moves to back of the surface and upper surface moves upward. This means that the rock mass forming the slope contracts in the horizontal direction and extends in the vertical direction. On the other hand, increasing the ratio m, the slope surface moves to front of the surface and upper surface moves downward. This means that the rock mass extends in the horizontal direction and contracts in the vertical direction. These results indicate that strain field in the rock mass is strongly affected by the initial stress state. It is pointed out that the value of m may be estimated by the field displacement measurement.

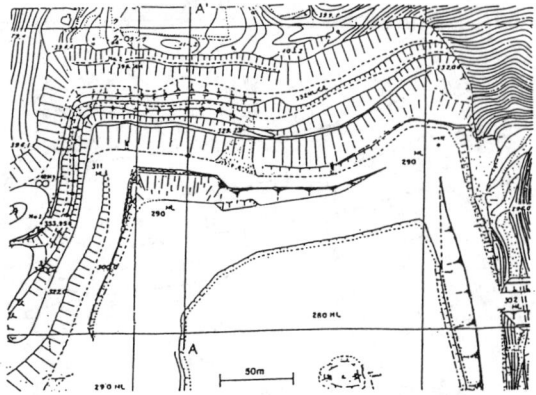
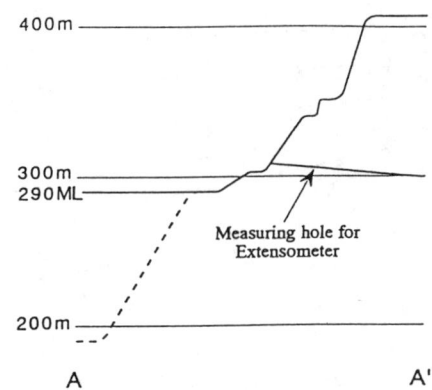

Fig. 6 Plan and section of the slope which is the object of the monitoring.

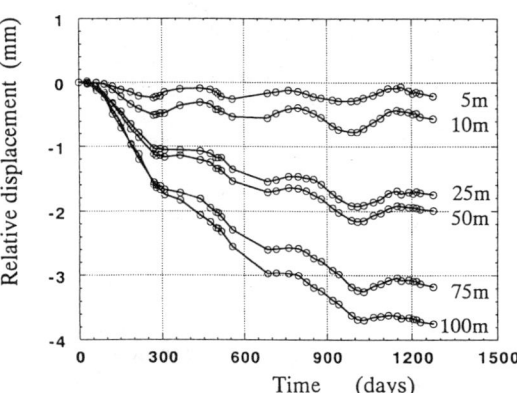
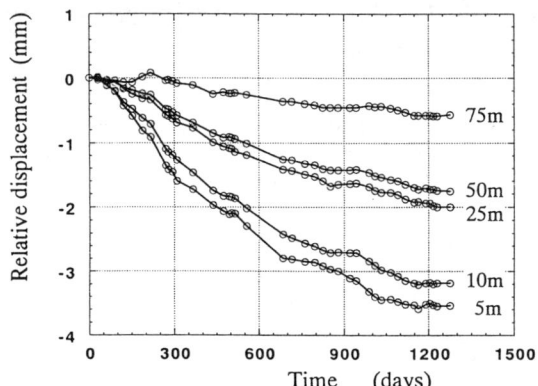

Fig. 7 Relative displacement observed by the extensometer. The reference point of the relative displacement is at the rock surface.

Fig. 8 Relative displacement observed by the extensometer. The reference point of the relative displacement is on the bottom of the measurement hole.

3. FIELD MEASUREMENT

The field measurement to assess the slope stability has been carried out in Ikura mine, a open pit limestone mine located in West Japan (Kaneko et al. 1996). A plan and a section of the present pit are shown in Fig.6. The broken line in the section is the final slope of the mine plan. A 6-channels extensometer was inserted and cemented in the horizontal bore-hole of 100m depth, as shown in Fig.6. The depth of anchor points are 5m, 10m, 25m, 50m, 75m and 100m from the slope surface and the relative displacement between the rock surface and each anchor point has been measured periodically. The slope height was 120m and the floor level was 280mL at the start of measurement.

Fig.7 shows the change of the relative displacement measured during about three years, where the reference point of the relative displacement is on the rock surface (the mouth of the hole) and extension is positive. During this period, two bench levels, 270mL and 260mL, were completely excavated. It is clear that the relative displacement decreases by the excavation. Furthermore, a periodic change with small amplitude can be found out in the relative displacement curve. This periodic change is interpreted to be thermal extension and contraction of rock due to temperature change, because the period is about one year. Therefore, the relative displacement curve in the case that the reference point is the bottom of the borehole is shown in Fig.8. From Fig.8, it is recognized that there is no periodic change due to the temperature effect in the region deeper than 10m. And it is confirmed that the relative displacement decreased by excavation. This means that the rock mass behind the slope surface contracted in the horizontal direction by the bench cut excavation. Considering the deformation characteristics shown in Fig.5, this observation result indicates that the ratio of horizontal to vertical stresses at the present field is relatively small.

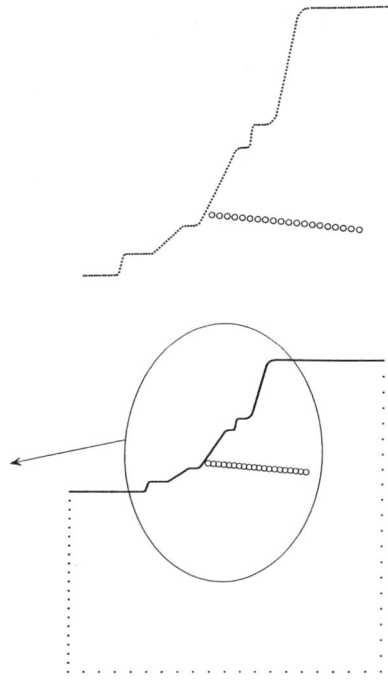

Fig. 9 Boundary element model for the back analysis where solid and open circles are nodes of boundary elements and the points for calculation of displacement, respectively.

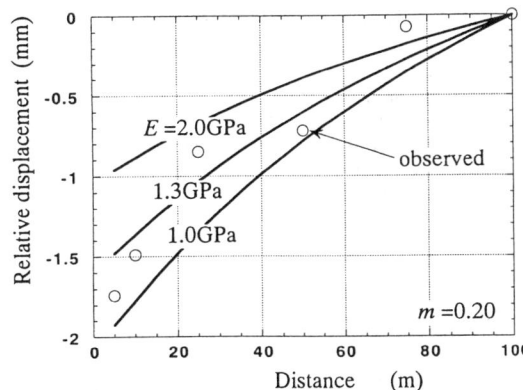

Fig. 10 Comparison of the relative displacement observed with that calculated by BEM, where E is Young's modulus of rock mass.

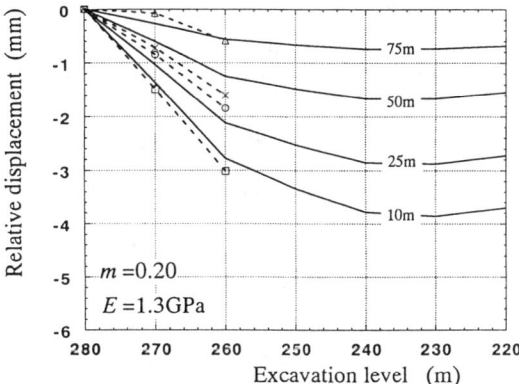

Fig. 11 Prediction of relative displacement due to excavation. Symbols indicate the values observed up to the present.

4. ESTIMATION OF INITIAL STRESS STATE

A back analysis to estimate the initial stress state and the deformability of rock was performed by using the result measured by the extensometer at the time 270mL bench was perfectly excavated.

Fig.9 shows a boundary element model for the back analysis. In this analysis, the rock mass is also treated as an elastic continuum and the displacement fields in the rock mass induced by 270mL excavation were calculated for cases that m=0.0 to 0.5. By comparing the relative displacements calculated along the measuring line corresponding to the extensometer and that measured by the extensometer, the value of m was estimated to be 0.2. In this analysis, Poisson's ratio of rock was assumed to be 0.25. Fig.10 shows the relationship between the relative displacement and the distance from the rock surface, where solid lines represent the relative displacements obtained by BEM with m=0.2 and open circles are those measured by extensometer. From Fig.10, Young's modulus of rock mass was estimated to be 1.3GPa.

In this pit, it is estimated that the failure will initiate at the toe of the slope if the rock slope has a potential of failure, because the ratio of horizontal to vertical stresses at the pre-excavation is relatively small. Therefore, the movement monitoring at the toe of the slope gives us an important information on the slope stability.

5. STABILITY ASSESSMENT OF SLOPE

In order to predict the slope movement, the relative displacements along the measuring line corresponding to the extensometer induced by successive bench cut excavations (from 260mL to 220m) were calculated by using the back analyzed result. Fig.11 shows the relation between the relative displacement predicted by BE-analysis and advance of excavation. In this pit, 260mL bench was perfectly excavated up to the present. Hence the relative displacement measured at the time 260mL bench was perfectly excavated is also plotted in Fig.11. It is clear that the observed values coincide fairly well with predicted ones. It is interpreted that the rock mass forming the slope has behaved as an elastic continuum, because the predicted values were obtained by assuming linear elasticity and continuum body. This means that there is no unfavorable and active discontinuities or failure does not mutter identified in the rock mass. From this result, it is confirmed that this slope is stable at present. It is concluded that the slope stability can be assessed by comparing the observed values with predicted ones. Furthermore, it is suggested that additional extensometers to monitor the movement at the toe of the slope will be required with advancing the excavation.

CONCLUSION

The influence of the initial rock stress on the slope stability has been concretely discussed by the numerical analysis and field measurement.

The numerical stress analysis indicates that both the stability factor at the failure initiation and the deformation behavior of rock slope are affected by not only the slope angle and the rock strength but also the initial rock stress at the pre-excavation. It is pointed out that the evaluation of the initial rock stress is fundamentally important to asses the slope stability.

The field displacement measurement by the use of multi-channels extensometer has been performed in a open pit limestone mine, and the ratio of horizontal to vertical stresses at the pre-excavation and the deformability of rock in this field have been back analyzed. Furthermore, by comparing the relative displacements observed by the extensometer with those estimated by using the back analyzed result, it is confirmed that the rock slope which is the object of monitoring is stable at present.

It is concluded that the initial rock stress as well as the slope stability can be evaluated by the combination of the field displacement measurement and the numerical stress analysis.

REFERENCES

Crouch, S.L. and Starfield, A.M. 1983. *Boundary Element Method in Solid Mechanics*, George Allen & Unwin.

Hoek, E. and Bray, J.W. 1997. *Rock Slope Engineering*, Institution of Mining and Metallurgy.

Kaneko, K., Noguchi, Y. Soga, K. and Hazuku, R. 1996. Stability Assessment of Rock Slope by the Displacement Measurement, *J. MMIJ*, **112**, 915-920.

Kaneko, K., Otani, J., Noguchi, Y. and Togashiki, N. 1997. Rock Fracture Mechanics Analysis of Slope Failure, *Proc. IS-Nagoya*, in press.

Kaneko, K., Noguchi, Y. Koga, M. and Hirayama, T. 1995. Effect of initial Rock Stress on Rock Slope Failure, *J. MMIJ*, **111**, 761-766.

Kennedy, B.A. and Niermeyer, K.E. 1970. Slope Monitoring System used in the Prediction of a Major slope Failure at the Chuquicamata Mine, *Planning Open Pit Mine*, 215-225.

Sugawara, K., Akimoto, M., Kaneko, K. and Okamura, H. 1983. Experimental Study on Rock Slope Stability by the Use of a Centrifuge, *Proc. Int. Cong. ISRM*, C1-4.

Obara, Y. and Sugawara, K. 1991. Elasto-plastic Analysis of Rock Slope by the Coupled Boundary Element-Characteristics Method, *J. MMIJ*, **107**, 455-460.

Physical changes due to reservoir compaction – A finite element solution

Y. B. Sukirman
Universiti Teknologi Malaysia, Johor Baharu, Malaysia

ABSTRACT: This paper presents a finite element method to study the physical changes due to the compacting of a saturated oil reservoir. The mathematical model was derived based on Biot's self consistent theory which describes a fully coupled governing equation system for a multiphase flow in a three dimensional reservoir system. It consists of the equilibrium and continuity equations for oil, gas and water-phases. An elastoplastic reservoir rock model based on the Mohr Coulomb yield criteria was used for simulating the deformation behaviour of of the reservoir. The compressibility factors are calculated based on the unknowns solved in each time step. Finally, the recent values of porosity and permeability are calculated for various type of reservoir rocks.

1 INTRODUCTION

In reservoir engineering practice, the reservoir rock deformation, also known as reservoir compaction, is normally neglected except in a few cases where unconsolidated formations can cause a considerable effect on reservoir performance. Although reservoir compaction and the associated subsidence are not commonly encountered their occurance may result in many problems. However, compaction due to effective compressibilty occurs in most undersaturated oil reservoir and this can act as a drive mechanism with a considerable effect on the ultimate recovery. Many papers in the literature have investigated the problem in various situation (Finol & Farouq 1975).

This paper deals with physical changes due to reservoir compaction processes for different type of reservoir rocks saturated with three immiscible and compressible flowing fluids. Initially, the reservoir and the overburden layers are in equilibrium hence the distribution of the effective stresses due to excess pore pressures are zero. As the withdrawal of fluids from the reservoir begins, the pore pressures start to decline in both systems, and therefore increase the overburden load at the top of the reservoir. If the reservoir system consists of unconsolidated sand, this load will reduce the thickness of the formation. The process is called reservoir compaction which in some cases result in a considerable amount of physical changes of reservoir rock (Lewis & Sukirman 1993). Merle et al (1975) have presented evidence that initially some aquifers and oil reservoirs behave as if the producing formation is relatively incompressible and becomes significantly more compressible after large pressure drops in the reservoir. At this stage, the formation rock may compact inelastically where further pressure decline can result in formation collapse, especially around the producing zones.

Lewis & Schrefler (1987) have investigated the effect of compaction on the physical properties of the reservoir formation. For example the influence of different values of Young modulus E, Poisson's ratio v, the degree of rock cohesion c, the friction angle ϕ and rock compressibility factors C_r on the degree of compaction has occured. In many cases, numerical solutions have been succesfully used to analyse the problems. However, very few cases have been reported in the literature which deal with the simulation of physical changes for three-phase fluids flowing in a compacting reservoir. In this paper, the developed fully coupled model was used to investigate the changes of porosity and permeability of a compacting saturated oil reservoir.

2 EQUILIBRIUM EQUATION

In order to describe the solid-phase behaviour, the equation of equilibrium, which takes into account the stress-strain relationship, must be considered. In the case of consolidation-fluid flow problems, the fundamental relationship is to define the interaction behaviour between the fluid and the soil skeleton. The well known Terzaghi 'effective stress principle' and its extension into more general three-dimensional consolidation relationships by Biot have been widely used in this class of problem. The derived relationships are the simultaneous partial differential equations with unknown parameters of the displacement of the skeleton and pore fluid pressures.

For a general non linear material, the effective stress relationship is expressed in a tangential form thus allowing for plasticity, creep and other factors influencing strains to be included (Lewis & Schrefler 1987). This can be written as follows

$$d\boldsymbol{\sigma}' = \mathbf{D}_T(d\boldsymbol{\varepsilon} - d\boldsymbol{\varepsilon}_c - d\boldsymbol{\varepsilon}_p - d\boldsymbol{\varepsilon}_o) \quad (1)$$

where $\mathbf{D}_T$ is the tangential elastic stiffness matrix, $d\boldsymbol{\varepsilon}$ represents the total strain of the skeleton, $d\boldsymbol{\varepsilon}_c$ is the creep strain and $d\boldsymbol{\varepsilon}_p$ represents the overall volumetric strain caused by uniform compression of the particles. Lewis & Schrefler (1987) defined the $\boldsymbol{\varepsilon}_o$ strains as all other type of strains not directly associated with stress changes (swelling, thermal, chemical etc) or referred as the 'autogeneous' strains.

The equilibrium equation relating the total stress $\boldsymbol{\sigma}$ to the body force $\mathbf{b}$ and the boundary traction $\hat{\mathbf{t}}$ specified at the boundary Γ of the domain Ω is formulated in terms of the unknown displacement vector $\mathbf{u}$. Based on the principle of virtual work, the equation can be written as follows

$$\int_\Omega \delta\boldsymbol{\varepsilon}^T d\boldsymbol{\sigma} d\Omega - \int_\Omega \delta\mathbf{u}^T d\mathbf{b} d\Omega - \int_\Gamma \delta\mathbf{u}^T d\hat{\mathbf{t}} d\Gamma = 0 \quad (2)$$

Incorporating the effective stress relationship into equation (2), the following expression is obtained,

$$\int_\Omega \delta\boldsymbol{\varepsilon}^T d\boldsymbol{\sigma}' d\Omega - \int_\Omega \delta\boldsymbol{\varepsilon}^T \mathbf{m} dP d\Omega - d\hat{\mathbf{f}} = 0 \quad (3)$$

where

$$d\hat{\mathbf{f}} = \int_\Omega \delta\mathbf{u}^T d\mathbf{b} d\Omega + \int_\Gamma d\hat{\mathbf{t}} d\Gamma \quad (4)$$

represents the change in external force due to boundary and body force loadings.

The final form of the equilibrium equation can be written as follows

$$\int_\Omega \delta\boldsymbol{\varepsilon}^T \mathbf{D}^T \frac{\partial \boldsymbol{\varepsilon}}{\partial t} d\Omega - \int_\Omega \delta\boldsymbol{\varepsilon}^T S_w'' \left(\mathbf{m} - \frac{\mathbf{D}_T \mathbf{m}}{3K_s}\right) \frac{\partial P_w}{\partial t} d\Omega$$

$$- \int_\Omega \delta\boldsymbol{\varepsilon}^T S_o'' \left(\mathbf{m} - \frac{\mathbf{D}_T \mathbf{m}}{3K_s}\right) \frac{\partial P_o}{\partial t} d\Omega - \int_\Omega \delta\boldsymbol{\varepsilon}^T S_g''$$

$$\left(\mathbf{m} - \frac{\mathbf{D}_T \mathbf{m}}{3K_s}\right) \frac{\partial P_g}{\partial t} d\Omega - \int_\Omega \delta\boldsymbol{\varepsilon}^T \mathbf{D}_T \mathbf{c} d\Omega -$$

$$\int_\Omega \delta\boldsymbol{\varepsilon}^T \mathbf{D}_T \frac{\partial \boldsymbol{\varepsilon}_o}{\partial t} d\Omega - \frac{\partial \hat{\mathbf{f}}}{\partial t} = 0 \quad (5)$$

Note that equation (5) can be used for simulating reservoir compaction problems in various conditions.

3 MULTIPHASE FLOW EQUATIONS

The multiphase flow model consists of the mathematical formulation of each flowing phase taking into account the effects of fluid and rock compressibility factors, capillary pressure, relative permeability contrasts and gas solubility in the liquid-phases. One of the main tasks of this paper is to develop three-phase fluid flow equations coupled with the deformation behaviour of the reservoir rocks. The following expression is obtained for a unit volume of fluid flowing at reservoir conditions,

$$(\text{Accumulation rate}) = \boldsymbol{\nabla} \cdot \left(\frac{\mathbf{k}\rho}{\mu} \boldsymbol{\nabla}(P + \rho g h)\right) \quad (6)$$

where P is the fluid pressure, ρ the density of fluid, $\mathbf{k}$ the absolute permeability matrix, μ is the dynamic viscosity, and h the height above an arbitrary datum (Sukirman 1993). The factors which contribute to the rate of fluid accumulation of each flowing phase are;
(a) rate of change of total strain

$$\frac{\partial \varepsilon_v}{\partial t} = \mathbf{m}^T \frac{\partial \boldsymbol{\varepsilon}}{\partial t} \quad (7a)$$

(b) rate of change of the solid particle volume due to pressure changes

$$\frac{(1-\phi)}{K_s} \frac{\partial \bar{P}}{\partial t} \quad (7b)$$

(c) rate of change of fluid volume (eg for the oil phase)

$$\phi S_o \frac{\partial}{\partial t}\left(\frac{1}{B_o}\right) \qquad (7c)$$

(d) rate of change of saturation (eg for the oil phase)

$$\frac{\phi}{B_o}\frac{\partial S_o}{\partial t} \qquad (7d)$$

(e) and finally the change of solid particle size due to effective stresses

$$-\frac{1}{3K_s}\mathbf{m}^T\frac{\partial \boldsymbol{\sigma}'}{\partial t} \qquad (7e)$$

The inclusion of each of the above terms in the continuity equations will define the simulation model used in this paper. The following continuity oil equation is finally obtained:

$$-\nabla^T \frac{kk_{ro}}{\mu_o B_o}\nabla P_o + \lambda_{oo}\frac{S_o}{B_o}\frac{\partial P_o}{\partial t} + \lambda_{wo}\frac{S_o}{B_o}\frac{\partial P_w}{\partial t} +$$
$$\lambda_{go}\frac{S_o}{B_o}\frac{\partial P_g}{\partial t}\frac{S_o}{B_o}\left(\mathbf{m}^T - \frac{\mathbf{m}^T\mathbf{D}_T\mathbf{m}}{3K_s}\right)\frac{\partial \varepsilon}{\partial t} + Q_o + \hat{F}_o = 0 \qquad (8)$$

where

$$C_{rm} = \left(\frac{1-\phi}{K_s} - \frac{\mathbf{m}^T\mathbf{D}_T\mathbf{m}}{3K_s^2}\right)$$
$$\hat{F}_o = \frac{S_o}{B_o}\frac{\mathbf{m}^T\mathbf{D}_T\mathbf{c}}{3K_s} - \nabla\left(\frac{kk_{ro}}{\mu_o B_o}\right)\nabla \rho_o gh$$
$$\lambda_{oo} = \frac{\phi}{S_o}\left(S_g' - S_w' + S_o B_o\left(\frac{1}{B_o}\right)' + \frac{S_o}{\phi}C_{rm}S_o''\right)$$
$$\lambda_{wo} = C_{rm}S_w'' + \frac{\phi}{S_o}S_w'$$
$$\lambda_{go} = C_{rm}S_g'' - \frac{\phi}{S_o}S_g' \qquad (9)$$

The derivations of the continuity equations for water and gas phases are essentially the same as that for the oil flow equation. The effect of the gravity term $\nabla \rho gh$ has been omitted throughout the study (Sukirman 1993). The total reservoir compressibility factor C_r can be defined as follows

$$C_r = \left[S_o\frac{\partial}{\partial P_o}\left(\frac{1}{B_o}\right) + S_w\frac{\partial}{\partial P_w}\left(\frac{1}{B_w}\right) + S_g\frac{\partial}{\partial P_g}\right.$$
$$\left.\times\left(\frac{1}{B_g}\right)\right] + \left(S_o C_{rm} + S_w C_{rm} + S_g C_{rm}\right)$$
$$\times\left(S_o' + S_w' + S_g'\right) + \left(\mathbf{m}^T - \frac{\mathbf{m}^T\mathbf{D}_T}{3K_s}\right) \qquad (10)$$

As the total fluid saturation values are equal to unity, similarly for $(S_o' + S_w' + S_g')$, therefore, equation (2.40) becomes

$$C_r = C_{rf} + C_{rm} + C_{rc} \qquad (11)$$

where

$$C_{rf} = S_o\frac{\partial}{\partial P_o}\left(\frac{1}{B_o}\right) + S_w\frac{\partial}{\partial P_w}\left(\frac{1}{B_w}\right) + S_g\frac{\partial}{\partial P_g}$$
$$\times\left(\frac{1}{B_g}\right) = S_o\left(\frac{1}{B_o}\right) + S_w\left(\frac{1}{B_w}\right) + S_g\left(\frac{1}{B_g}\right) \qquad (12)$$

represents the total fluid compressibility and

$$C_{rc} = \left(\mathbf{m}^T - \frac{\mathbf{m}^T\mathbf{D}_T}{3K_s}\right) \qquad (13)$$

is the total compressibility due to rock compaction as the result of pore pressure decrease during fluid withdrawal, whilst C_{rm} is the effective rock compressibility. The above equations indicate that the two rock compressibility components, C_{rm} and C_{rc}, depend on the type of rock i.e. these are determined by Young modulus E, Poisson's ratio v and solid bulk modulus K_s. Lewis and Schrefler (1987) and Finol et al (1975) have investigated the influences of these variables on the degree of reservoir compaction. In this paper the effects of the total compressibility factor C_r on the porosity and permeability changes were investigated in detail. The values of porosity and the absolute permeability were changed with time due to the occurance of reservoir compaction. Many authors agreed that these values are related to one another and therefore must be included when predicting the performance of a compacting reservoir (Finol & Farouk 1975). Aziz & Settari (1979) have defined porosity changes as a function of the reservoir pressure drop ΔP and the rock compressibility C_f, as follows;

$$\phi = \phi^o[1 + C_f\Delta P] \qquad (14)$$

where

ϕ^o – porosity at time zero
$\Delta P = \bar{P} - P^o$

$\bar{P}$ is the average reservoir pressure whilst P^o represents the initial pressure for the reservoir system. On differentiating equation (14) w.r.t time then

$$\frac{\partial \phi}{\partial t} = C_f\phi^o\frac{\partial \bar{P}}{\partial t} = \frac{\partial \phi}{\partial \bar{P}}\frac{\partial \bar{P}}{\partial t} \qquad (15)$$

where
$$\frac{\partial \phi}{\partial \bar{P}} = C_f \phi^o \qquad (16)$$

If the reservoir rock is assumed to be incompressible, i.e. $C_f \to 0$ then, the rate of change of porosity becomes zero or $\partial \phi / \partial t \to 0$ which means that the porosity is a constant value.

The changes of porosity with pressure can be approximated from equation (16) as follows

$$\phi^{m+1} = \phi^m [1 + c_p(P_o^{m+1} - P_o^m)] \qquad (17)$$

where
$$c_p = \frac{c_m + (1-\phi)c_r}{\phi} \qquad (18)$$

c_m is the uniaxial compaction coefficient
c_r is the rock matrix compressibility
c_k is a coefficient of permeability reduction
P_o is the pressure in the oil phase

and the superscripts $(m+1)$, (m) refer to new and old time step levels respectively. In practice, the uniaxial compaction coefficient c_m can be obtained from laboratory compressibility data by

$$c_m = \frac{1}{3}\frac{1+v}{1-v}(1-\beta)c_b \qquad (19)$$

where v is poisson's ratio
β is ratio of matrix/ bulk compressibility
c_b is the bulk compressibility

In cases where c_k is not known then, it can be assumed to be equal to the value of c_m.

Lewis and Schrefler (1987) defined the settlement/void ratio relationship for a one-dimensional consolidation model as follows

$$\delta = d \frac{e_1 - e_2}{1 + e_1} \qquad (20)$$

where δ is the average settlement of each element
d is the initial depth
e_1 is the initial void ratio
e_2 is the final void ratio.

In this paper, the variation of porosity with time was defined in a similar manner to the approach used by Aziz and Settari (1975). The rate of change of porosity can be written as

$$\frac{\partial \phi}{\partial t} = \left(\mathbf{m}^T - \frac{\mathbf{m}^T \mathbf{D_T}}{3K_s}\right)\frac{\partial \varepsilon}{\partial t} + \frac{\partial}{\partial t}\left(\frac{\mathbf{m}^T \mathbf{D_T c}}{3K_s}\right)$$

$$+ \left(\frac{1-\phi}{K_s} - \frac{1}{3K_s^2}\mathbf{m}^T \mathbf{D_T m}\right)\frac{\partial \bar{P}}{\partial t} \qquad (21)$$

Assuming the effect of creep strain is neglible. Therefore equation (21) can be simplified as follows

$$\frac{\partial \phi}{\partial t} = C_{rc}\frac{\partial \varepsilon}{\partial t} + C_{rm}\frac{\partial \bar{P}}{\partial t} \qquad (22)$$

The equation (22) calculates the porosity changes caused by the effective rock compressibility and the displacement of the solid skeleton. Finol & Farouk (1975) presented the variation of permeability with time as follows

$$k^{m+1} = k^m[1 + c_k(P_o^{m+1} - P_o^m)] \qquad (23)$$

where
k^{m+1} – is the permeability at time level (m+1)
k^m – is the permeability at time level m

In this paper, the time derivative of permeability can be defined in similar manner as for the porosity changes in equations (23). Lewis & Schrefler (1987) reported that the variable permeability scheme is of practical use only if the expected consolidation is important.

4 NUMERICAL SOLUTIONS

The finite Element method was developed simultaneously with the increasing use of high speed electronic digital computers and with the growing emphasis on numerical methods for petroleum engineering analysis. In this paper, the finite element method, which is Galerkin-based, was used to discretize the developed governing equation which describes three-phase fluid flow coupled with the equilibrium equations in a three dimensional model.

Since the accuracy of the final solution is the main concern for every numerical method, the continuity of the unknowns between elements must be maintained. For this purpose, the finite element method requires a sufficient number of nodes on the element boundary in order to satisfy the shape function $\mathbf{N}$ being used. An eight-noded brick element was used in the present three-dimensional model.

Applying the finite element discretization method to the governing equations will result as follows
For the equilibrium equation

$$\mathbf{K}\frac{d\bar{\mathbf{u}}}{dt} + \mathbf{L}_w\frac{d\bar{\mathbf{P}}_w}{dt} + \mathbf{L}_o\frac{d\bar{\mathbf{P}}_o}{dt} + \mathbf{L}_g\frac{d\bar{\mathbf{P}}_g}{dt} - \mathbf{C} - \frac{d\mathbf{f}}{dt} = 0 \quad (24)$$

where

$$\mathbf{K} = -\int_\Omega \mathbf{B}^T \mathbf{D}_T \mathbf{B} d\Omega$$

$$\mathbf{L}_w = \int_\Omega \mathbf{B}^T S_w'' \left(\mathbf{m} - \frac{\mathbf{D}_T \mathbf{m}}{3K_s}\right) \bar{\mathbf{N}} d\Omega$$

$$\mathbf{L}_o = \int_\Omega \mathbf{B}^T S_o'' \left(\mathbf{m} - \frac{\mathbf{D}_T \mathbf{m}}{3K_s}\right) \bar{\mathbf{N}} d\Omega$$

$$\mathbf{L}_g = \int_\Omega \mathbf{B}^T S_g'' \left(\mathbf{m} - \frac{\mathbf{D}_T \mathbf{m}}{3K_s}\right) \bar{\mathbf{N}} d\Omega$$

$$\mathbf{C} = -\int_\Omega \mathbf{B}^T \mathbf{D}_T \mathbf{c} d\Omega$$

$$d\mathbf{f} = -\int_\Omega \mathbf{N}^T d\mathbf{b} d\Omega - \int_\Gamma \mathbf{N}^T d\hat{\mathbf{t}} d\Gamma - \int_\Omega \mathbf{B}^T d\varepsilon_o d\Omega \quad (25)$$

and for the oil-phase, equation (8) will take the form

$$\mathbf{H}_p \bar{\mathbf{P}}_o + \mathbf{H}_w \frac{d\bar{\mathbf{P}}_w}{dt} + \mathbf{H}_o \frac{d\bar{\mathbf{P}}_o}{dt} + \mathbf{H}_g \frac{d\bar{\mathbf{P}}_g}{dt} + \mathbf{H}_u \frac{d\bar{\mathbf{u}}}{dt} + \bar{\mathbf{F}}_o = 0 \quad (26)$$

where

$$\mathbf{H}_p = \int_\Omega (\boldsymbol{\nabla}\bar{\mathbf{N}})^T \frac{k k_{ro}}{\mu_o B_o} \boldsymbol{\nabla}\bar{\mathbf{N}} d\Omega$$

$$\mathbf{H}_o = \int_\Omega \bar{\mathbf{N}}^T \lambda_{oo} \frac{S_o}{B_o} \bar{\mathbf{N}} d\Omega$$

$$\mathbf{H}_w = \int_\Omega \bar{\mathbf{N}}^T \lambda_{wo} \frac{S_o}{B_o} \bar{\mathbf{N}} d\Omega \quad (27)$$

$$\mathbf{H}_g = \int_\Omega \bar{\mathbf{N}} \lambda_{go} \frac{S_o}{B_o} \bar{\mathbf{N}} d\Omega$$

$$\mathbf{H}_u = \int_\Omega \bar{\mathbf{N}}^T \frac{S_o}{B_o} \left(\mathbf{m}^T - \frac{\mathbf{m}^T \mathbf{D}_T \mathbf{m}}{3K_s}\right) \mathbf{B} d\Omega$$

$$\bar{\mathbf{F}}_o = \int_\Gamma \bar{\mathbf{N}}^T q_o d\Gamma + Q_o$$

The finite element discretization for water and gas-phases are essentially the same as that for oil flow equation. These equations represent a set of ordinary differential equation in time In this paper, the time discretization method used is based on a Kantorovich (Lewis & Schrefler 1987) scheme which may be regarded as a one-dimensional finite element scheme. The time integration takes the same form as used for the spatial integration which gives the following form

$$\begin{bmatrix} \mathbf{K} & \mathbf{L}_w & \mathbf{L}_o & \mathbf{L}_g \\ \mathbf{W}_u & \mathbf{W}_w' & \mathbf{W}_o & \mathbf{W}_g \\ \mathbf{H}_u & \mathbf{H}_w & \mathbf{H}_o' & \mathbf{H}_g \\ \mathbf{G}_u & \mathbf{G}_w & \mathbf{G}_o & \mathbf{G}_g' \end{bmatrix}_{k,\alpha} \begin{Bmatrix} \bar{\mathbf{u}} \\ \bar{\mathbf{P}}_w \\ \bar{\mathbf{P}}_o \\ \bar{\mathbf{P}}_g \end{Bmatrix}_{n+1} =$$

$$\begin{bmatrix} \mathbf{K} & \mathbf{L}_w & \mathbf{L}_o & \mathbf{L}_g \\ \mathbf{W}_u & \mathbf{W}_w'' & \mathbf{W}_o & \mathbf{W}_g \\ \mathbf{H}_u & \mathbf{H}_w & \mathbf{H}_o'' & \mathbf{H}_g \\ \mathbf{G}_u & \mathbf{G}_w & \mathbf{G}_o & \mathbf{G}_g'' \end{bmatrix}_{k,\alpha} \begin{Bmatrix} \bar{\mathbf{u}} \\ \bar{\mathbf{P}}_w \\ \bar{\mathbf{P}}_o \\ \bar{\mathbf{P}}_g \end{Bmatrix}_n + \begin{Bmatrix} \bar{\mathbf{F}}_u \\ \bar{\mathbf{F}}_w \\ \bar{\mathbf{F}}_o \\ \bar{\mathbf{F}}_g \end{Bmatrix} \Delta \quad (28)$$

where

$$\mathbf{W}_w' = (\mathbf{W}_w + \mathbf{W}_p \alpha \Delta t)$$

$$\mathbf{W}_w'' = (\mathbf{W}_w + \mathbf{W}_p (1-\alpha) \Delta t)$$

$$\mathbf{H}_o' = (\mathbf{H}_o + \mathbf{H}_p \alpha \Delta t)$$

$$\mathbf{H}_o'' = (\mathbf{H}_o + \mathbf{H}_p (1-\alpha) \Delta t) \quad (29)$$

$$\mathbf{G}_g' = (\mathbf{G}_g + \mathbf{G}_p \alpha \Delta t)$$

$$\mathbf{G}_g'' = (\mathbf{G}_g + \mathbf{G}_p (1-\alpha) \Delta t)$$

Equations (29) are applied at all nodes within the domain and those on the boundary where the unknowns are not prescribed. These equations represent a fully coupled, and highly non linear system, for three-phase flow in a deforming porous media. Since all the coefficients are dependent on the unknowns, iterative procedures are performed within each time step to obtain the final solution.

A material balance error check per unit time was performed by calculating the algebraic sum of the residuals of each phase in every gridblock. In this paper, an implicit pressure-explicit saturation solution scheme (IMPES) has been applied to solve the unknowns.

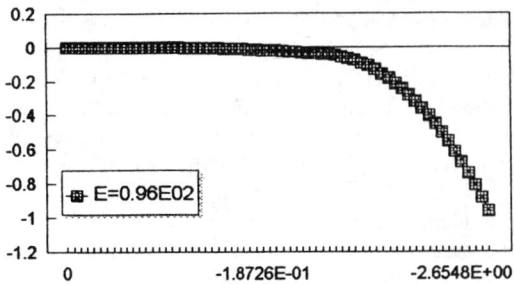

Figure 1 Changes in Res. Vol. (%) Vs Por. (%)

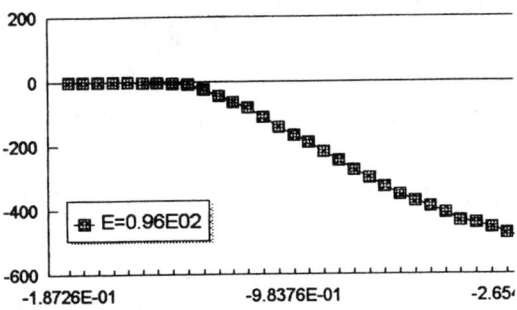

Figure 2 Reservoir Press. Drops Vs Porosity (%)

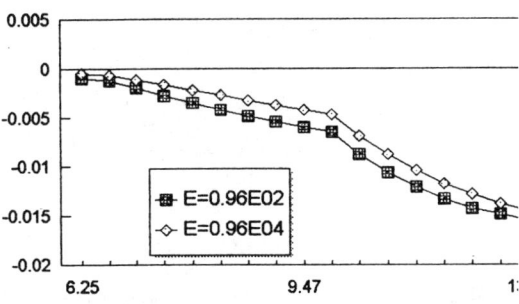

Figure 3 Permeability Changes Vs Prod. Time, yr

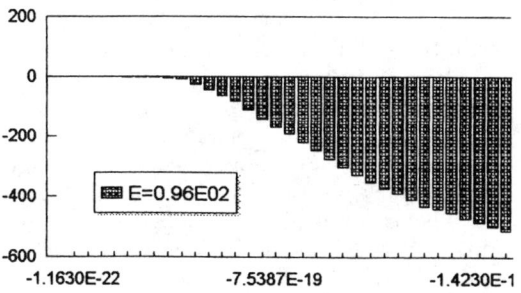

Figure 4 Reservoir Press. Drops Vs Perm. Change

5 EXAMPLES

The developed finite element model was employed to analyse the physical changes due to the reservoir compaction. In this paper, for a hypothetical saturated reservoil model was used (Sukirman 1993). The simulations results for the reservoir compaction and the consequent changes in porosity and permeability values with production time are shown Figures 1 to 4. It can be seen that the changes in porosity and permeability values are minimum for higher value E and vice versa. This is an expected results because a higher value of E implies a more rigid formation rock and therefore tending to incompressible behaviour. The results obtained show the reduction of porosity and permeability values with production time.

6 REFERENCES

Finol A. and Farouq Ali S.M. 1975, 'Numerical Simulation of Oil Production with simultaneous Ground Subsidence', *SPEJ* (1975), **15**, 411-24

Lewis R.W. and Schrefler B.A.1989 *'Finite Element Method in the Deformation and Consolidation of Porous Media'*, John Wiley, Chichester, 1987 *Transport in Porous Media*, **4**: 319-334, (1987

Merle H.A *et al.*1975; 'The Bachaquero Study - Composite Analysis of the Behaviour of a compaction Drive/Solution Gas Drive Reservoir,' *JPT* 1107-14, SPE 5529

Sukirman Y.B.; 1993. Petroleum Reservoir Simulation Coupling Flow and Subsidence,' PhD Thesis, University of Wales Swansea, UK

Insitu stress measurement and its application in mining – Case studies of Indian mines

Pradeep Sharma
Regional Engineering College, Rourkela, India

ABSTRACT: Insitu stress field measurements have significant application in design of stoping parameters and stress analysis to evaluate new designs. The stope geometry and layout, sequence of mining, mining method, controlled blasting and ground control methods are influenced by the magnitude and orientation of the principal stresses and the resulting induced stress field. With increasing depth of operations especially in metalliferous mines stress induced structural failures are frequent. This paper reviews the insitu stress field measurements with case studies of some deep metalliferous mines in India and correlates it to the geo-mining conditions, optimisation of stoping operations and stope design parameters. Measurements of insitu stress field in mines has lead to better understanding of the geo-mining environment and also to improved mining methods with greater safety, conservation and productivity.

1 INTRODUCTION

1.1 *Review of common insitu stress measurement methods*

All insitu stress measurement techniques disturb the rock to create a response that is measured and analysed making use of a theoretical model to estimate the insitu stress tensor. Some common principles utilized are complete strain relief as in USBM over coring guage (Merril and Peterson 1961), CSIRO strain Gauge(Worotnicki and Walton 1976); partial strain relief as in Flat Jack Method (Rocha et al 1966); rock flow or fracture as in Hydraulic fracturing method, Double fracture method (Serata etal 1992) and some other methods utilizing correlation between rock properties and stress such as resistivity, rock noise (Kaiser effect), wave velocity etc.

1.2 *Comparative advantages and limitations*

Over coring methods using triaxial strain cells glued to the pilot hole walls have advantage over USBM gauge that record changes in pilot hole diameter that they provide complete stress tensor from one bore hole while the latter requires three orthoganal boreholes for complete stress tensor making it more time consuming and expensive. Martin and Christiansson (1991) state that USBM gage gave consistently higher magnitude of principal stresses by about 3 % to 15 % than the CSIR cell and that mean stress tensor for the USBM results fall within the 90 % confidence limits for the CSIR results. Flat Jack method introduced by Tincelin in France in 1952 offers and inexpensive method for determining one stress component of the stress tensor if one has access to a rock face for example wall of an underground gallery. The procedure consists of null displacements caused by cutting a tabular slot in rock wall. The limitation is that measured stress lies in the region of disturbance of the gallery. Hence its applicability is possible when the following conditions are satisfied that is a relatively undisturbed surface of the opening, an opening geometry for which closed form solutions exist, relating the far field stresses and the boundary stresses and a rock mass which behaves elastically. With hydraulic fracturing it is possible to estimate the stresses in rock at considerable depth using boreholes where water is pumped into a section of the borehole isolated by packers until a tensile fracture is induced in the rock. Stress determination requires measurement of following pressure data; breakdown pressure during fracture induction, the refracture pressure for fracture reopening and the shut-in pressure to keep the induced fracture open against the acting normal stress. The assumptions are that borehole axis is parallel to the direction of one of the principal stress component; the pressurisation occurs sufficiently fast to avoid fracture fluid permeating into the rock so that pore pressure within the rock matrix is not altered; fracture occurs at the point of least tangential compression stress on the bore hole wall and the fracture propagates perpendicular to the direction of the least principal stress; the shut-in pressure is equal to the stress component perpendicular to the fracture plane. The difference between the initial breakdown pressure and the fracture reopening pressure is taken to be the hydraulic fracture tensile strength (Bredehoeft technique) assuming that stress state around the bore hole during pressurization is the same with or without the fracture(provided all stresses are compressive) and in the case when fracture exists the tensile strength of the rock is assumed to be zero. Ratigan (1992) proposed fracture reopening pressure based on Linear Elastic Fracture Mechanics where it is shown that fracture reopening pressure is a function of fracture geometry, pumping rate and fracturing fluid and insitu stress field. The Double fracture method developed by Serata et al (1992) differs from hydraulic fracturing in that the loading fluid is prevented from penetrating into the induced fracture. Here the instrument stressmeter determines in situ material properties in addition to measuring stresses. The advantage of this method is that it can be applied to elastic as well as non elastic and less than ideal grounds where it consolidates the ground during a loading/unloading cycle. The first fracture is initiated similar to that in hydraulic fracturing however the length is minuscule compared to latter due to difference in method of loading. It is this limited length of first fracture plane that allows the second fracture to occur perpendicular to the first. From the two pressure-diametral deformation curves obtained across the two fracture planes, the elasticity breakdown points for respective fracture and the loading pressure at reopening of each fracture determines the state of stress.

2 CASE STUDIES

Case studies of Kolar Gold Field and Singhbhum Copper Belt both important and famous mining areas in India are reviewed with respect to insitu stress determination and its significance and impact on mining.

2.1 *Kolar gold field*

One of the earliest studies in insitu stress field determination was conducted in the deep mines of Kolar Gold field, India under the Indo-German Collaboration project between National Geophysical Research Institute, Hyderabad,India and the Institut Fur Geophysi, Ruhr Universitat Bochum, Federal Republic of Germany during 1980-83, (Gowd 1983).

2.1.1 *Location and geology*

K.G.F. has been a major gold production centre in India and has some of the deepest mines in the world namely Champion Reef mine, Nundydurg mine and Mysore mine. The gold field is located in Kolar Schist belt, a 100 Km long N-S trending Precambrian Greenstone belt. The three prominent lodes are Champion Lode, Oriental lode and Mc-Taggart Lode. Lodes trend N-S and dip towards west. Rock formations show moderate dip near to surface which at depth of around 1500 m becomes nearly vertical. Diagonal faults trending NW-SE have dislocated the rock formation. The major faults being Balaghat North fault which defines the northern limit of the ore bodies in Nundydroog area, The Mysore North fault in Champion Reef- Mysore mine area and The Gifford's system of faults in Champion Reef mine area. The mineralisation in K.G.F. is hydrothermal fissure vein type and native gold is major mineral.

2.1.2 *Insitu stress field in kolar gold field and its impact on mining*

Measurement using hydraulic fracturing technique were carried out in short (25 m) boreholes of 48 mm diameter at five sites located at 20th level and 40th level in Nandydroog mine and at 40th level, 74th level and 100th level in Champion Reef mine. Based on a total of 75 tests data, identification and distribution of regional stress field and stress field affected by mine opening were determined.

Major and minor horizontal stresses (S_H and S_h) increase with depth (h) as per the following equations (Gowd, Rummel 1983).

S_H (bars) = 255 + 100 h (Km)

S_h (bars) = 135 + 52 h (Km)

It is apparent that the major and minor principal

stresses are rather high in the order of 250 and 125 bars respectively. The data for principal stress direction show enough scatter. The major principal horizontal stress and minor principal stress are approximately oriented in the North-South and East-West direction respectively. From focal mechanism solutions based on studies of earthquakes in peninsular India it is also obtained that direction of maximum and minimum compression are nearly North-South and East-West direction respectively (Chandra 1977). This stress pattern is due to the continental collision caused by the northward movement of India. The stress pattern and the geology of gold bearing quartz veins which strike in North South direction and are nearly vertical suggest that intrusion of quartz veins in the schist rock in K.G.F. area might have been a natural hydraulic fracturing process.

The regional vertical stress in K.G.F. area is only 35 % - 70 % of the over burden pressure. The rock in the vicinity of the mine opening has been destressed in the vertical direction and state of equilibrium achieved by transfer of overburden stress to far field through formation of pressure arches. The interaction between the mine opening and regional stress field have resulted high stress concentration in the vertical as well as the East-West direction in the abutment of the North South openings. The sidewalls are highly destressed within 5 - 10 m from the mine openings. The above study reveals that for stress concentration factors of the order of 10 - 15, 7 - 11 and 5 - 8 are a prerequisite for causing rock bursts at one, two and three kilometer depth respectively in the K.G.F. mines as shown in Table 1.

Due to depth of working and associated geological structures rockburst have frequently occurred and some major rockburst tremors in the range of 4.5 to 5.0 on Richter Scale. Monitoring of seismic activity occurring around mine workings with geophone network was started in 1978. Co ordinates of the computed foci using the regional P wave velocities have agreed to within $\pm$ 25 m of the location of damage. Micro seismic monitoring in collaboration with Bhaba Atomic Research Centre, Bombay is also being done to forecast the occurrences. PC 386 based microseismic monitoring system installed at Northern folds area of Champion Reef mine provides real time data analysis capability for short range rockburst prediction which can then help prevent occurrence of the rockburst by applying destressing technique (Raju 1991).

Statistical analysis of rock bursts reveal that only a small percentage of recorded bursts were traceable underground, frequency of reported bursts is minimum on Sundays and maximum on Fridays; there is a significant peak in occurrence during the time of stope blasting or afterwards; there appears a specific relationship between rainfall and rockburst; frequency and severity of events are not directly related to depth. The important factors being physical properties of rock, stress, size and shape of excavation and inhomogeneity of the rock such as faults, pegmatites, dykes and calcite stringers all involving plane of weakness either in themselves or at the contact (Krishnamurthy 1990).

Due to the problem of rockbursts a system of mining is essential which would permit a considerable increased rate of advance to be achieved and maintained; limit the area to be exposed after each machine cycle to the minimum and adopt a quick support system; the support system which will sufficiently yield and will relax to the general strata movement of the rock mass but which is sufficiently strong to support the immediate walls or skins of the stoping area or drive and deliberately assist the main body of the rock mass to attain static and dynamic equilibrium quickly. The Stope Drive system of extraction with concrete fill as the medium of support has been developed and practiced in deep levels.

2.2 *Case study of singhbhum copper belt*

Insitu stress field determination in various mines of this thrust belt have been conducted by various institutions and organisations including CMRI (Singh 1989), HCL (Robertson Research 1989).

Table 1. Stress concentration factor required for causing rock burst in K.G.F. mines (Gowd 1983).

Depth Km	Principal Stress S_h bar	S_H or S_{V*} bar	Triaxial Strength, C_m bar	C_m/S_H or C_m/S_{V*}
1	200	355$^+$	3500-5000	10 -15
2	250	366^{++}	4000-6000	7 -11
3	300	849^{++}	4500-6500	5.5-7.7

* S_H (+); S_V (++)

2.21 Location and geology.

Singhbhum Copper belt is primarily a zone of over thrust and shearing. The formations within the area are predominantly metamorphosed sediments and metavolcanics both of precambrian age. The rocks within the shear zone are highly sheared and mylonitised equivalents of quartz chlorite biotite schist and quartzite. Mosabani Mine is the second most deepest mine in India with a vertical depth of 1.23 Km and a strike length of 4.6 Km. The lodes dip at an average of 30 degrees toward NE and with an average strike of N 10 degrees W. Mosabani mine is presently being phased out and other mines namely Surda, Pathargora, Rakha etc are being expanded. Surda is the second largest in terms of production having been developed over a strike length of 2.2 Km and a depth of 474 m. In central portion of the mine lodes have merged to form a wide ore body upto 20 m at places which leads to bulk mining.

2.22 Insitu stress field in Singhbhum Copper Belt and its impact on mining.

Insitu test have been conducted in Surda by the USBM over coring method. The major principal stress is horizontal and parallel to the strike. Intermediate principal stress dips 20° opposite to dip[direction of lode (nearly vertical) and the minor principal stress dips 70° in the same direction as the lode as shown in figure 1.

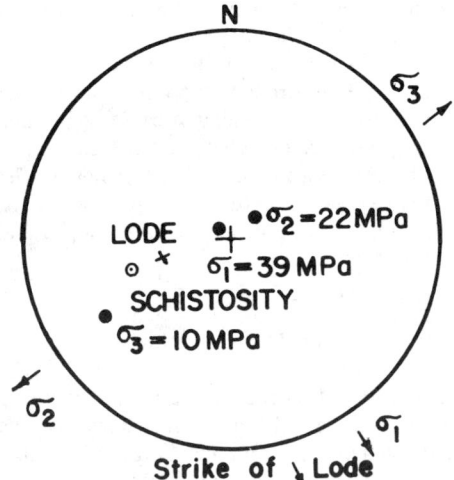

Figure 1. Orientation of major principal stresses in Surda Mine (Robertson Research 1989)

Insitu stress determination using USBM borehole deformation gauge was also done in 6L/865m SE in Rakha mines in a 7 m long cross-cut from the above hangwall drive. The values for the insitu stresses were found to be abnormally high as given in Table 2 (Singh 1989).

The orebody geometry constraints the selection of high productivity mining methods. Room and Pillar Stoping is applied when true lode width is less than 4 m with room span of 15 m and at deeper levels between 10 -12 m. Horizontal Cut and Fill stoping is applied in stopes with a true lode width of 4 -6 m and HCF Post Pillar stoping where the true width of orebody is more than 7 m with spacing of pillars 13 m along strike and 9 m across. A post pillar is a column of ore 4 m x 4 m dimension, open on four sides and designed to fail below the fill line. A distinct feature of the post pillar is that it deforms progressively with advance of mining upwards. Large size pillars on the other hand with higher safety factor tend to store high energy concentration and may cause deteriorating ground conditions in the stope back.

In general the orientation of the stopes is favorable with respect to the principal stress direction, for example the long axis along the lode is parallel to the major principal stress and in section with the intermediate stress normal to the lode. Ground conditions at Surda mine are relatively better compared to Pathargora and Rakha which show evidence of higher tectonic stresses. At deeper levels of Mosabani mine footwall drives show signs of shear failure along lode side wall edge especially where the location is beneath the sill pillar and under high abutment stress. In level drives also shear failures along the corner of hangwall side walls are seen (shear kink band) due to high stresses. Stress induced failures of post pillars was occurring even at first cut needing reinforcement. Deterioration of ground conditions are also related to mining practices. Regulations require that mining of lodes should progress from footwall to hangwall and depending on the parting this leads to considerably greater disturbances to the hangwall; leaving of poor mineralization along the hangwall contact in Cut and Fill stopes later tends to open and rockbolts are usually insufficiently long to pin the walls; during HCF stoping where the orebody pinches there is a tendency to back strip the footwall side to meet the production requirement thereby excavating an overhang ledge which at times results in falls; adequate and early installation of supports is essential and usually the time between initial raise development and completion of mining is far to

Table 2. Results of insitu stress measurements at Rakha Mine 6L, 865 m SE (Singh 1989)

Hole No.	Bearing	Inclination	Depth of overcore (m)	U1	U2	U3	Modulus of Elasticity (MPa)	Poissons ratio
RM_3	N40° E	94°	3.34	-1400	-1043	-1290	2.47×10^5	0.2
RM_4	N50° W	94°	5.49	-782	-444	-821	2.47×10^5	0.2
RM_5	vertical	vertical	3.5	-185	+233	-1075	1.24×10^5	0.2

Average ground stress components

$\sigma x = -36 \pm 28$ MPa
$\sigma y = -22 \pm 20$ MPa
$\sigma z = -62 \pm 43$ MPa
$\tau xy = -7 \pm 12$ MPa
$\tau yz = +2 \pm 34$ MPa
$\tau zx = -5 \pm 34$ MPa

Principal stresses and directions

Stress	Bearing	Inclination
$S1 = -63 \pm 42$ MPa	S86.3° E	169.7°
$S2 = -26 \pm 31$ MPa	S23.2° E	85.3°
$S3 = -53 \pm 33$ MPa	N66.0° E	80.9°

Vertical up = 0°
Horizontal = 90°

great. At depths time dependent deformation plays a prominent role even for spans of 2.5 m. Due to inadequate filling in top levels severe ground control problems were faced in North Badia zone between 22nd level and 23rd level of Mosabani mine caused by severe stress concentration in the unmined area forming the abutment zone. Leaving a pillar along the strike to create a rigid barrier between zone of high concentration and the working involved a loss of 17 % ore reserves on 23rd level. Despite increased depth of working no incidence of rock burst as well as possibility exists. This is due to the fact that unlike K.G.F. here the rocks are comparatively weak and structurally inhomogeneous with a high energy dissipation function due to structural inhomogeneities such as foliation planes, joints etc and a low capacity to store strain energy. The performance of the stopes has generally been good with the exceptions of blockfalls which are structurally controlled.

3. CONCLUSION

Insitu stress determination have significant application in deep metalliferous mines. Studies in India in K.G.F. and Singhbhum Copper Belt have resulted in better understanding of the geo-mining environment and to improved mining methods with greater safety, conservation and productivity.

REFERENCES

Chandra, U., 1977, Earthquakes of peninsular India - A seismotectonic study., Bull. Seis. Soc. Amer. 67(4), 1367-1413.

Goodman, R.E., 1989, Introduction to Rock Mechanics, John Wiley and Sons, New York.

Gowd, T.N., Rao, M.V.M.S., Krishnamurthy, P., Rummel, F. and Alheid, H.J., 1981(83), Proc. Indo-German Workshop on Rock Mechanics, NGRI, Hyderabad, India.

Gowd, T.N. Rummel F., 1983, Insitu stress measurements by hydraulic fracturing in the underground mines of Kolar Gold Fields, India, CSIR Project Report.

Jeremic, M.L., 1987, Ground Mechanics in Hard Rock Mining, A A Balkema.

Krishnamurthy, R. and Shringarputale, S.B., 1990, Rockburst hazards in Kolar Gold fields, Proc. of 2nd symp. on rockburst and seismicity in mines, A A Balkema publishers, 411-420.

Martin, C.D. and Christiansson, R.C., 1991, Overcoring in highly stressed granite: comparison of USBM and modified CSIR devices, Rock Mechanics and Rock Enginering, Vol 24, No. 4, 207-235.

Merril, R.H. and Peterson J.R., 1961, Deformation of a borehole in rock, U.S.B. Mines R.I. 5881

Ratigan, J.L., 1992, The use of fracture reopening pressure in hydraulic fracturing stress measurements, Rock Mechanics and Rock Enginering, Vol 25, No. 4, 225-236.

Raju, R.M., Jha, P.C., Shringarputale, S.B., Srinivasan, C. and Sivakumar, C., 1991, Combating the problem of rockbursts at KGF-contribution of National Institute of Rock Mechanics, Jl. of Mines, Metals and Fuels, Vol XXXIX, Nos 11 & 12, 370-376.

Robertson Research Australia,1989, IDSCB Rock Mechanics study for underground mining, HCL Report No. Z45/1-AN

Rocha, M., Baptista Lopes, J. and Dasilva, J.,1966, A new technique for applying the method of flatjack in the determination of stresses inside rockmasses, Proc. 1st Conf. ISRM(Lisbon),Vol 2, 57-65.

Sereta, S., Sakuma S., Kikuchi, S. and Mizuta Y., 1992, Double fracture method of insitu stress measurement in brittle rock, Rock Mechanics and Rock Enginering, Vol 25, No. 2, 89-108.

Singh, B., 1989, Ground Control and Rock Mechanics studies for evolving new mining methods to promote productivity, safety, and conservation in non coal mines, R & D Report, CMRI, India.

Worotnicki, G. and Walton R.J., Triaxial hollow inclusion guages for determination of rock stresses insitu, Proc. Symp. on investigation of stress in rock, Sydney, Supplement 1-8, ISRM and Inst. of Engineers of Australia.

Characteristics of in-situ stress state and control methods of ground pressure in Jinchuan nickel mine

T. Liu & C. Zhou
Jinchuan Non-ferrous Metal Corporation, Jinchang, People's Republic of China

ABSTRACT: This paper introduces *in-situ* stress measurement results and distribution characteristics of *in-situ* stress state in Jinchuan Nickel Mine. Some successful methods for maintaining stability of underground openings and mining areas in poor rock formations under high stress condition in Jinchuan mine are also provided.

1 BRIEF INTRODUCTION TO THE MINE GEOLOGY

Jinchuan nickel mine is located in the middle of Hexi Corridor in Gansu Province, northwest of China. It is about 400km to the west of Lanzhou City. The nickel orebody zone is 6.5km long, tens to above 500 meters wide and more than 1,000 meters deep. The ore bearing parent rock is ultrabsic rock. The NEE oriented heterotropic fault separated the whole parent rock mass into four independent mine areas : No. 3, No. 1, No. 2, and No. 4 form west to east. At present, the annul ore output in mine area No. 1 is one million tons and in mine area No. 2 is two million tons. The mine areas No. 3 and No. 4 have not been excavated yet. The reserve of mine area No. 2 covers 75% of the total reserve with an average grade of two percent.

The mine region underwent many tectonic movements and the intrusive actions of magmatic rock. So there are many faults and joints and the rock mass is badly broken which caused the rock conditions very poor and complicated. Both the contact zone between the ore bodies and surrounding rock and the contact zone between poor orebody and rich orebody are soft and fractured. The stability of these zones is very poor.

2 IN-SITU STRESS STATE IN JINCHUAN MINE

Since 1973, *in-situ* stress measurement has been carried out by means of optic elastic strainometer, resistance strainometer, piezomagnetic stressometer and triaxial hollow inclusion strain cell in different levels and rock masses(Liao and Shi, 1983). The

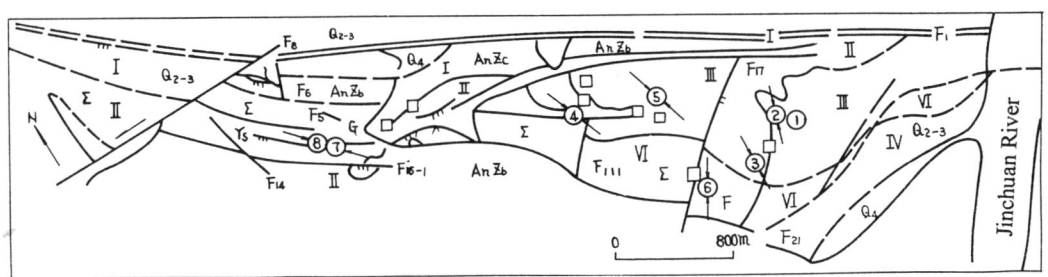

□- shaft   ① - stress measuring point   I - migmatite zone   II - schist and gneiss zone   III- marble zone
IV - streak-homogeneous migmatite zone   V -granite zone   VI -ore bearing ultrabasic zone

Figure 1. Planar distribution of *in-situ* stress measuring points in Jinchuan mine

Table 1. Results of *in-situ* stress measurement in Jinchuan mine

Measuring points	Rock type	Depth (m)	σ₁ value (MPa)	σ₁ bearing (degree)	σ₁ dip (degree)	σ₂ value (MPa)	σ₂ bearing (degree)	σ₂ dip (degree)	σ₃ value (MPa)	σ₃ bearing (degree)	σ₃ dip (degree)
1	marble	20	2.4						2.3		
2	marble	44	4.2	20					3.5		
3	marble	120	16.8	352	57	12.1	215	16	5.8	117	28
4	rich ore	240	34.4	338	39	21.1	48		2.6	139	51
5	marble	375	19.8	3					10.8		
6	marble	460	50.0	347	6	33.4	76	6	28.2	117	81
7	granite	480	24.5	335					15.4		
8	very rich ore	480	32.0	32	6	21.4	137	67	20.6	300	22

Planar distribution of the measuring points is shown in Figure 1. The results of *in-situ* stress measurement are shown in Table 1.

3 CHARACTERISTICS OF *IN-SITU* STRESS STATE IN JINCHUAN MINE

1. The major principal stress is horizontal and is oriented in NE-SW direction. Observation has showed that *in-situ* stress in Jinchuan mine is in the state of energy accumulation. The rate of strain concentration is between 10^{-7} and 10^{-6}.

2. The major horizontal principal stress in the surface is about 3MPa. The magnitude of *in-situ* stress is increased with depth and the major horizontal principal stress in depth of 200-500m is 30-50MPa as shown in Figure 2. In the Figure, between two solid lines is the region of maximum horizontal stress and between two dashed lines is the region of minimum horizontal stress. It is also showed that the difference between two horizontal principal stresses has the trend of increasing with depth, which has bad effect on the stability of the mine in deep level.

3. The ratio of average horizontal stress to vertical stress ($k = \sigma_{h.av}/\sigma_v$) changes with depth as shown in Figure 3. In a certain range of depth (smaller than 1,000m), the value of k is between 1.4 to 2.5, which means the horizontal stress is predominant. The value of k in Jinchuan mine is higher than the averaged value of k in the world.

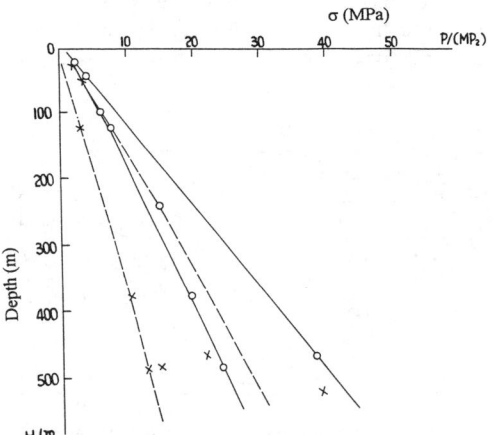

Figure 2. The major horizontal principal stress increased with depth

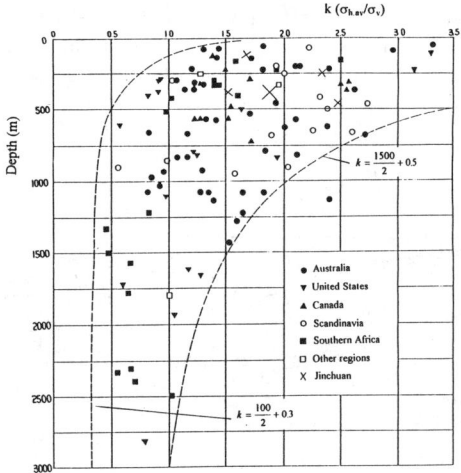

Figure 3. Ratio of average horizontal stress to vertical stress with depth below surface (after Hoek and Brown, 1980)

4 DEFORMATION AND CREEP CHARACTERISTICS OF THE ROCK SURROUNDING UNDERGROUND OPENINGS IN BAD ROCK FORMATIONS UNDER HIGH STRESS CONDITION

Both convergence meters and multipoint extensometers were used to monitor displacement of rock surrounding underground openings. Monitoring results showed that the displacement of the surrounding rock was quite large and presented remarkable creep characteristics in bad rock formation.

One of the typical surrounding rocks in bad rock formations is iherzolite, in which about 50 percent of openings were excavated. In iherzolite stratum deformation took place immediately after beginning of excavation of the openings. The deformation could be divided into three stages: fast deformation, slow deformation and stable deformation, i.e. the deformation gradually became stabilized. The three stages totally took about 250-300 days. The first stage took 30 days and 50 to 80 percent of total deformation was completed in this stage. The second stage took 100-120 days and 90 percent of total deformation was completed after this stage. Through test of iherzolite rock blocks sized $\phi 40mm \times 90mm$, it was obtained that Young's modulus of the rock blocks was 84GPa and uniaxial compressive strength was 191MPa. However, field test on a rock mass sample sized $650mm \times 650mm \times 1300mm$, which contained more than 10 joints, showed that the Young's modulus was only 7.8Gpa and uniaxial compressive strength was only 8MPa. Developed joints and fractures in the rock masses and high virgin stress are the main reasons to cause remarkable creep behaviour of the rock mass in Jinchuan mine.

5 CONTROL OF GROUND PRESSURE DURING MINING EXCAVATION

Ore body No.1 of mine area No.2 in Jinchuan is lenticular and has a very large scale and thickness. In its centre is sponge-shaped rich ore. Its hanging wall and bottom wall are disseminated poor orebody. Discending cut-fill stopping method was adopted in the design on the principle of "rich ore first, poor ore later". In order to maintain stability of the mine, following measures were taken.

5.1 Optimum layout of development openings and stopping areas

It has been found that the stress orientation has much influence on stability of underground openings and stopping areas. If the opening's strike was identical with the major principle stress orientation, the stress surrounding the opening was low and well-distributed. When the angle between the opening's strike and the major principal stress orientation increased, the stress concentration surrounding the opening subsequently increased and uneven stress state occurred. So, orientation of the major principle stress should be considered when to design the layout of development openings. It is better to make strike of the openings as close to the orientation of major principal stress as possible. Of course, production benefit and other geological conditions should also be considered. It is one of the effective step to reduce deformation and damage of the openings. The deformation and damage in stope were also related to orientation of the principal stress. When the stope was put along with strike of the ore body and its axis was vertical to orientation of the major principal stress, the side walls of the stope were easy to deform and became unstable. On the contrary, when axis of the stope was vertical to the orebody's strike, the side walls were quite stable. In addition, the cross-section shape of the opening was also related to the stress state. If the ratio of width to height of the opening was equal to the ratio of horizontal to vertical stresses in the cross section of the opening, the opening would be stable. For example, many transport roadways were in poor rock formations and parallel to the strike of the orebody and vertical to the orientation of major principal stress, which caused big difficulty to maintain their stability. In order to solve this problem, the oval-like cross section of the roadways and totally-enclosed support with bottom arch were adopted. Thus, the long-term stability of the roadways has been achieved successfully(Yu et al., 1985). Based on the same principle, we changed the shape of cross-section of the stope from square of 4m × 4m to hexagon whose hanging and bottom width was 3m, middle width 5m and height 4m, as shown in

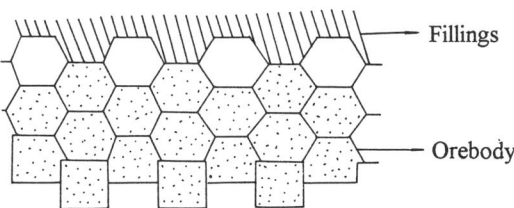

Figuer 4. Square stope changed to hexagonal stope.

Figure 4. FEM analysis showed that the stress concentration factor in surrounding rock decreased from 6.8 to 3.4, the maximum principal stress decreased from 91.65Mpa to 46.26MPa.

5.2 *Continuous mining of large area with no pillars*

The original design divided the mining operation into two steps. The first step stopped the panel (mine room) and the second step stopped the pillars between panels. However, after the first step, high stress concentration in pillars made them damaged seriously and could not stope them. So, the mining method was changed to continuous cut-fill method of large area with no pillars. This method can transfer the stress to the hanging wall, bottom wall and the surrounding rock. Using this method, the orebody No.1 has been safely and effectively stopped for 10 years. The stopped mine area have attained 56000m^2. This method will be continuously used to stope a mine area of 100000m^2 without pollars.

5.3 *Two-step support method*

In order to suit the deformation characteristics of surrounding rock under high stress after excavation in poor rock formations, Jinchuan nickel mine widely adopted the two-step support method which called "first yield and then resist". The first-step support with shotcrete of thickness less than 5cm and injekto rock bolting should be carried out immediately after excavation. Stress release and creep deformation of surrounding rock were permitted. When the surrounding rock became stable basically, i.e. 30-50 days after the first step support, the second step support was carried out with 10-15cm thick shotcrete and metal net. This method effectively increased the stiffness and integrity of the support structure and achieved long-term stability of the openings.

5.4 *High quality of cement filling*

Cement filling can effectively improve the stable state of surrounding rock. It could reduce the peak stress magnitude 5-25 percent in surrounding rock. The underhand stope roof might become stable if the filling thickness was above 15m. Through long-term of study, the supporting mechanism of fillings has been found as follows(Yu et al., 1983):
  1. To absorb and transfer stress. When the mined-out area was filled, part of stress was transferred into the filling and redistribution of stress will make the surrounding rock stable.
  2. Contacting support effect. The filling contacted surrounding rock and provided side pressure. So it increased the resisting ability of underground structure and limited the deformation, displacement and damage of the surrounding rock.
  3. To separate stress concentration areas. The filling stiffness was small but its deforming capacity was large. So it could play a role to separate stress concentration areas.

According to the stress separating theory, the lower the stiffness of the filling, the greater the effect of stress separating. But, the higher the filling stiffness, the greater the effect of contacting support. So, the coordination of the two kinds of effect should be considered carefully. The elastic modulus of filling currently used accounts for 1-2% of that of the surrounding rock. Paste filling will be adopted soon, its elastic modulus will be increased to 3-4% of that of the surrounding rock. It will be hopeful to improve stress distribution in stope and increase the stability of large scale mining area without pillars.

REFERENCES

Hoek, E. and Brown, E.T., 1980, Underground Excavations in Rock, IMM, London.

Liao, C. and Shi, Z., 1983, In-situ stress measurement and their application to engineering design in the Jinchuan Mine, Proc. Fifth ISRM Congr., Melbourne, PP. D. 87-89

Yu, X. et al., 1983, Analyses of stability of Underground Excavations(in Chinese), Coal Industry Publishing House, Beijing.

Yu, X., Cai, M. and Chi, F. 1985, The philosophy and measures of maintaining stability of underground openings in poor rock formations in Jinchuan Mine District, Proc, Int. Symp. On Mining Science and Technology, China Institute of Mines, Xuzhou, China, Paper No. Cd6

Some experiences on rock stress measurements and its application in mining

Fernando Fujimura
Mining Engineering Department, Polytechnic School, University of São Paulo, Brazil

Antonio Carlos Campos Fernandes
CPTI Technology and Development, Brazil

Carlos Manoel Nieble
Geodinâmica International Consulting and Design Company, Brazil

ABSTRACT: Considerable progress has been made over the last decade in the development of new equipment and methodology for measuring the natural field stress, due its importance to underground excavations. There are many papers dealing on rock field stress phenomena, but measurements of stress variations in rock structures related to excavation plan, pillar extraction, excavation sequences and mining methods are comparatively in lack. These aspects are very important in mining, since its frequently represent a way to solve complex balance problem between economical and safety operations. This paper presents some experiences that have been done in two Brazilian underground zinc mines to analyze the stope enlargement and effects of pillar extraction located between two chambers, using a new stress meter manufactured by São Paulo Research Institute of Technology.

1 INTRODUCTION

Rock masses and ore bodies inevitably contain physical discontinuities owing to the presence of joints, fractures, voids, fault zones and so on, which become the rock medium completely hetcrogcneous.

Even in fairly good little jointed rock mass it's very difficulty to characterize all properties influencing stability of underground excavation.

The stability analysis of mine structures frequently brings enormous problems to the designer hoping to get quantitative rather than qualitative information on strcss distribution around the mine excavations.

As well known, the excavations resulting from ore extraction may be very complex in size and shape of pillars, rooms, chambers, stopes, shafts, etc., and almost all structures are tri-dimensional

Therefore, monitoring stress variation in mine structures is a challenge task, since near of excavation surfaces high stress concentration occurs and can reach several times those of natural stress field.

In mines, stress analysis is a problem also related to the ore bodies that requires techniques of mining methods for achieving a feasible balance between economical and safety operations. The dimensions of ore bodies with economic significance frequently exceeds hundred meters and excavation of individual stope can attain dimensions not less than those of ore bodies.

The main feature of mining stresses is its dynamic and changeable character that represents a reaction to the particular mining method.

Additionally, the nature of loads on underground openings is quite different from other types of structures.

The classic way of loads in conventional structures the geometry and its mechanical strength of each parts take an important role in defining the loads imposed on them.

On the contrary, for an underground opening, the rock medium presents a pre-mining stress and the final loads depend on the initial state of stress and stresses induced by excavations.

Induced stresses are closely related to the pre-mining state of stress, and so it has been matter of field researches for decades by many investigators, among them: Obert and Stephenson (1965), Fairhust (1968), Hyett; Dyke and Hudson (1986), and more recently by Sugawara and Obara (1993).

As well noticed by Cornet (1993), while a lot of efforts has been done for determining the natural field stress or induced stress, comparatively few works have been carried out toward monitoring the variation of stress with the time.

It's true specially for human activities in mining works, where the ore extraction ratio is a crucial factor to define the economical feasibility and safety mining operations.

2 VARIABLE STRESS METER (V.S.M.)

According to Franklin & Dusseault (1989), three types of monitoring devices are used in stress variation: borehole diameter variation meter, soft inclusion and rigid inclusion. Almost all operate based on principle that stress changes around a borehole result in deformation measurable by a sensor. The main advantage for rigid inclusion is claimed on it sensitivity that is much less dependent on the rock modulus, if the device stiffness is 2 to 5 times that of the surrounding rock.

For over 30 years past very valuable information has been collected in the field, however the high costs of devices, qualified technicians and instruments that need remain embedded and working correctly for a long period, have discouraged its more frequently application.

Recently a very cheap instrument for monitoring borehore diameter change and consequently stress variation in rock with reliable resolution was developed by São Paulo Institute of Technology - Brazil, which is described below.

2.1 Apparatus descriptions

The VSM was designed to be installed in 3" (76mm) borehore and can be installed in holes longer than 20 m length. For a complete evaluation of stress variation on the borehole plane it's needed at least three VSM installed in the same hole. The instrument is composed by 5 pieces: two brackets, a conical hollow cylinder, sensor gage and conductor cable, as shown in the figure 1.

The VSM is relatively simple to be assembled because it consists basically in a small circular steel plate with a hole in the center with two strain gages, connected to conductor wire and inserted into hollow conical cylinder. The deformation in borehole diameter is followed by this plate that implies in proportional changing in the measurement of electric sensor gages glued at the circular hole (figure 2).

This arrangement is very useful to measure stress changes in the structures under increasing or decreasing loads promoted by excavations.

The theoretical basis of stress concentration on homogeneous and elastic plate with single hole was presented by Timoshenko & Goodier (1951) and demonstrated the stress concentration around the hole. Therefore, the strain gauges glued at points of stress concentration the sensor sensitivity results rather amplified.

2.2 Installation procedures

Two brackets are used to insert the VSM into the borehole and compress the conical hollow cylinder by action of small hydraulic jack connected to this with two rivets. Two conical surfaces diametrically opposed allow the brackets slide over these surfaces and the VSM can set very tightly inside hole.

The stiffness of the VSM apparatus makes it a semi-rigid to rigid inclusion for the great majority of rocks. The hydraulic jack with guide positioner set the VSM in the required depth and position into the borehole. The operator acts a manual hydraulic pump and presses the ring of brackets, forcing to slide over conical frame until rupture of rivets.

2.3 Calibration curves

Each sensor is individually calibrated, performing at least 3 crescent cycles of five stages of loading and unloading. Maximum loads are limited to 3,92 kN, for assuring the elastic linear properties of sensor, provided by a couple of load distribution pads with

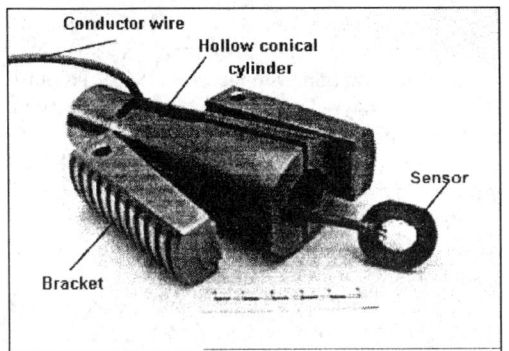

Figure 1 - View of Variable Stress Meter (VSM)

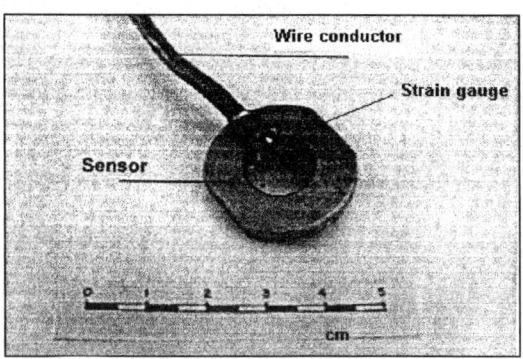

Figure 2 - Detailed view of sensor gauge

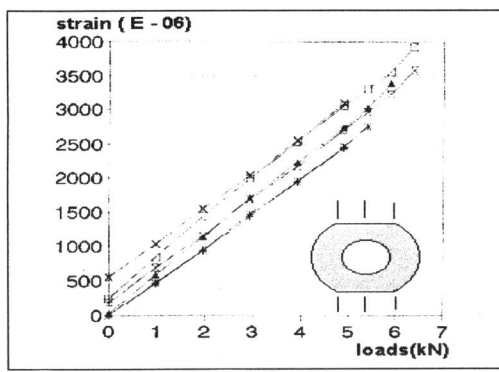

Figure 3 - Calibration curves of sensor

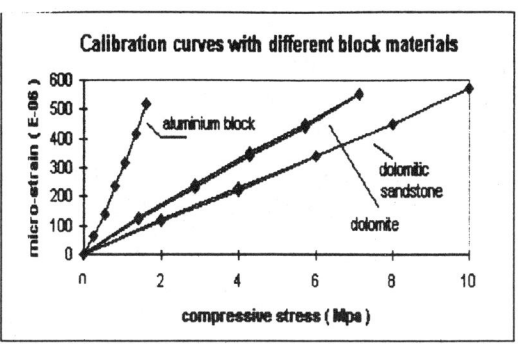

Figura 5 - Calibration curves of VSM meter

smooth and plane surfaces. At each load increments the sensor variation is recorded to find gauging constant by linear regression. Basically, all sensors have had similar behavior.

Figure 3 presents the calibration curves of one of them submitted to six cycles of eight stages of loading and unloading, where the sensor shows a fairly good linearity until 5,0 kN, in spite of its residual deformations.

Considering that each VSM has different gauging constant and depends on its mechanical and assembling characteristics, the VSM is also calibrated with rock block of rectangular base not shorter than 200 millimeter and 500 mm of height, cut by a diamond saw disk. The rock sample should be the same type of that where the VSM will be installed. The block is pre-loaded with 2% of uniaxial compressive strength before inclusion of VSM to avoid block rupture during its inclusion. After this uniaxial loading is started, in successive increments, until 80% of full capacity of VSM. (figure 4)

The figure 5 is an example of calibration curves obtained in dolomite and dolomitic sandstone blocks collected at Morro Agudo Mine. In the same figure the curve obtained in aluminum block (E = 70.000 Mpa) is also shown.

Each tested material presents a straight lines with different angular coefficients that represent inverse relationship of different elasticity modulus of each blocks. More detailed design and instrument assembling were presented by Fujimura; Hennies & Fernandes (1995).

3 FIELD APPLICATIONS

Two Brazilian zinc mines, both located at Minas Gerais State, were selected to apply the VSM apparatus to monitor the mining operation and rock behavior under stress variation. For this, the studies were carried out through the stope enlargement and pillar recovery between two chambers to verify the feasibility of mining works with spans much larger than those practiced actually.

The main characteristics of each mine are presented at Table 1, below:

Table 1 Characteristics of Brazilian Zinc Mines

Discrptions	*Morro Agudo Mine*	*Morro da Mina Mine*
Mining Method	room and pillar	sublevel stoping shinkage stop.
Rock Type	dolomite	dolomitic sandstone
Bieniawski Rock Mass Classification	I very good rock	III fair with big blocks
VSM application	pillar extraction	stope enlargement

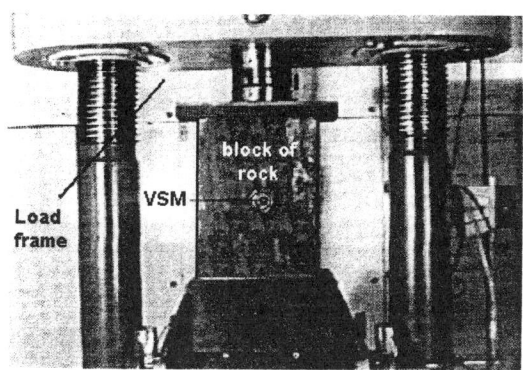

Figure 4 - VSM calibration with block of rock

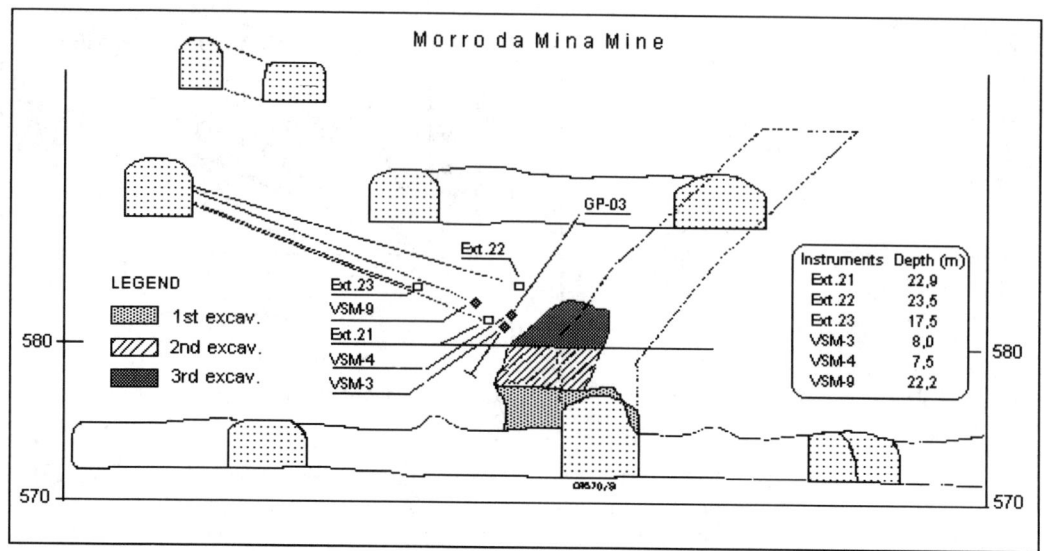

Figure 6 - Longitudinal section of Morro da Mina Mine with instruments

3.1 Morro Agudo Mine

The main goal of WSM application in this mine was to analyze the chamber stability under the effect of pillar recovery between two chambers. The local was carefully selected, since the pillar extraction could results in high concentration stress and promote failure of remained pillars or roofs. In this case, the risk of compromising other mining areas or future mine planning would be very serious.

The experimental mining was developed by gradual extraction of the rib pillars between two chambers that resulted in one big chamber of almost 1,100 m^2 of free area, with more than 36 m span.

3.2 - Morro da Mina Mine

The Morro da Mina Mine is a high zinc content deposit distributed in several bodies of irregular shape and size. The VSM application, in this case, was installed in order to verify the geomechanical behavior of rock masses under stress variation to define the mining method that could be safely applied. For this purpose an experimental mining by sublevel stoping and shrinkage stoping was developed. The evaluation of rock masses behavior was obtained in three selected areas monitored by VSM meters and single extensometers.

The longitudinal section of one of these areas is presented at figure 6. The extensometers were installed in three sub horizontal NX borehole, perforated from upper gallery and inclined conveniently to monitor stope wall movements toward its perpendicular direction.

Two VSM meters were installed in sub vertical hole, properly inclined to monitor the stress relief in conjunction of wall movements recorded by the extensometers. One 3rd VSM was installed in sub horizontal hole and intend to record stress variation in perpendicular direction. All instruments apparently worked well, despite of presence of water filling up the holes and heavy water inflows. The water tightness was assured by coat of paint, specially to protect the sensor gauge.

4 RESULTS

4.1 Morro Agudo Mine records

The VSM meters and extensometer, respectively in pillars and roof of chamber, after approximately 1000 hours (41 days) installed, start to shows anomalous performance and despite of efforts to restore the equipment the problem was not solved and all records were unconsidered for analysis. The bad function of devices was attributed to the sulfuric gas derived from zinc ore (zinc sulfide) and irregularities of borehole wall perforated by percussive rotary drilling.

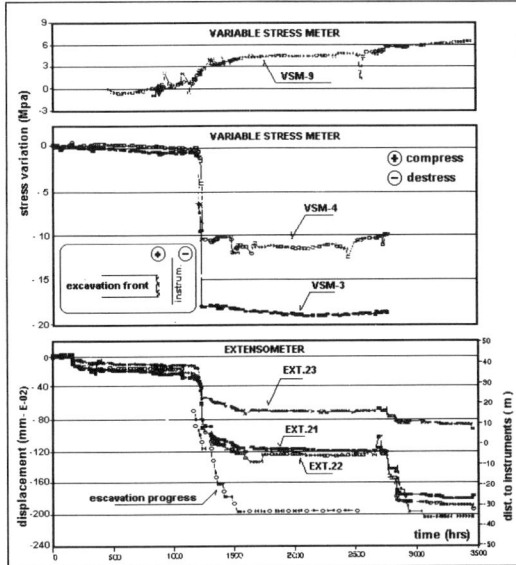

Figure 7 - Instrumentation records

4.2 Morro da Mina Mine records

The diagrams are presented at figure 7. The record variations were plotted in function of excavation rate of the sublevel stoping . One second axis is also provided for indicating the distance of excavation from instrumentation plane in the same time basis.

The overall behavior of extensometers is very similar, showing relief displacements about 2 mm, except the Ext.23 (0,8 mm) located farther from the stope wall than the other two extensometers. This fact is an evidence of bulk stress distribution phenomena on surrounding of underground openings.

When the excavation passed through the instrumentation plane all instruments showed sudden drops in its records, including VSM-4 and VSM-3 meters that represented the stress relief in perpendicular direction to the stope wall.

On the contrary, the VSM-9 after slight stress relief showed a constant increase of compression stresses, with some increase acceleration when the excavation front passed through the instrument.

5 CONCLUSIONS

The VSM meter is not a "stress meter" as it sensitivity is dependent to some extent on the properties of the rock in which it's set. The accuracy of instrument can't be assured without a calibration on the rock block. The VSM was primary idealized for measuring stress changes and worked well with relatively degree of reproducibility and low costs when compared with similar equipment. Instead of bad results of Morro Agudo Mine the practical application has shown that the VSM can help the mining engineer to improve safety in mining operations.

6 ACKNOWLEDGEMENTS

The authors wish to thanks the Companhia Mineira de Metais - CMM for permission to publish the research data.

7 REFERENCES

Cornet, F. H. 1993. Stresses in rock and rock masses. In: Comprehensive Rock Engineering, Principles, Practice and Projects. Chapter 12, John A. Hudson Editor, Vol. 3, pp.297-327, Pergamon Press, New York.

Fairhust, C. 1968. Methods of determining in-situ rock stress at great depth. Technical Report n° 1-68, Missouri River Division, Corps of Engineers, Omaha, NE.

Franklin, J. A.; Dussealt, M. B. 1989. Methods of Stress Measurement. In: Rock Engineering, Chapter 5- Stress, pp. 144-159, McGraw-Hill, New York

Fujimura, F.; Hennies, W. T.; Fernandes, A. C. 1995. Variable stress meter for monitoring rock mass structures. In: Mine Planning and Equipment Selection, 4, pp.881-885, Raj k. Singhal Editor, A. A. Balkema, Rotterdam.

Hyett, A.J.; Dyke, C.G.& Hudson, J. A. A.1986. A critical examination of basic concepts associated with the existence and measurements of the in situ stress. In: *Rock Stress and Rock Stress Measurements*. O. Stephansson Editor, pp.387-396, Centek, Luleá, Sweden.

Obert, L.; Stephenson, D. E.1965. Stress conditions under which core discing occurs. *Trans. Soc. Min. Eng.* AIME 232, 227-234.

Sugawara, K.; Obara, 1993 Y. Measuring rock stress: Case examples of rock engineering in Japan. In: Comprehensive Rock Engineering, Chapter 21, John A. Hudson Editor, Vol.3, pp. 533 - 552, Pergamon Press, New York.

Timoshenko, S. & Goodier , J. N. 1951. Theory of Elasticity, Chapters 1, 2 and 8, McGraw-Hill Book Co., New York.

Evaluation of rock stress in the mines of Kolar Gold Fields – A seismological approach

C. Srinivasan, P.C. Jha & N.M. Raju
National Institute of Rock Mechanics, Champion Reefs, Kolar Gold Fields, Karnataka, India

ABSTRACT: Mine induced seismicity is a common phenomenon in the mines of Kolar Gold Fields (KGF) in southern India. Seismicity induced by mining is usually defined as the appearance of seismic events caused by rock failure as a result of changes in the stress field in the rock mass near mining excavations. In order to analyse the behaviour of mine induced stress as regards its genesis and migration over the years with the progress of mining operations, the recorded seismic data from the deep mines of Champion reef mine in KGF consisting of hypocentral location and energy released by each event has been analysed and found that delineation of high stress zones and systematic movement of the seismic or stress front leading to prediction of rockbursts are possible with considerable success.

1. INTRODUCTION

Lithostatic stresses and their redistribution around mine excavations are the dominant driving force in the generation of most mine tremors and rockbursts. Seismicity induced by mining is usually the seismic events caused by rock failures as a result of changes in stress field in the rock mass near mining excavations (Cook, 1976). The total state of stress around a mine excavations is the sum of ambient stresses in the rock mass and the stresses induced by mining. The ambient stress state tends to be little static corresponding to the weight of overburden whereas stresses induced by mining are dynamic in nature, being dependent mostly on the rate of mining activity. Comprehensive studies of seismicity in deep mines have been carried out in South Africa to confirm these observations. The gold bearing reef of the Witwatersrand mine are mined by stoping at depths down to 4Kms. below the surface (Cook, 1976). A close relationship of seismicity to mining is observed at this mine and also in the Orange Free State district, with some events located above and below the mining horizons at depths from 400 to 2300m.

Seismic events and rockbursts are observed in metalliferous, potash and coal mines in Canada (Hasegawa et.al. 1989). There has been a growing rockburst problem in Northern Ontario hard rock mines operating at depths down to 2Kms. In the US, the best documented cases of mine seismicity occur in the silver, lead and zinc mining districts of Coeurd'Alene in Northern Idaho and the coal mining areas of the eastern Wasalch Plateau and Brook cliffs in Central Utah. Both cases occur within the western US, where several tectonic regimes exist (Zoback and Zoback, 1989) in large part because of the proximity to a major plate boundary along the Pacific coast and the high level of associated tectonics. The response of solid bodies to externally imposed stress was studied by several scientists all over the world during the last couple of centuries (Robertson, 1964). The behaviour of rock when the stress distribution is altered due to mining is studied with a view to improving the safety of personnel and equipment in mining regions (Hardy and Leighton, 1980).

One of the oldest mining areas in the world is the Kolar Gold Fields (KGF), where the mining activity reached a depth of 3.2 Kms. In the last 100 years of the mining history of KGF, there are virtually no places left where the incidence of rockbursting has not been reported. A regional seismic network was established in the mining region in 1978 and it is continuously operated for round the clock monitoring of the rockburst activities. Analysis of seismic data collected from this network helped in a better understanding of the rockburst mechanism and in choosing a safe course of mining (Subbaramu et.al 1989). The microseismic monitoring and the data analysis has revealed a distinct pattern of higher rate of microseismic activity prior to the rockburst (Srinivasan, 1992).

The in-situ stress measurements have been relied upon by rock mechanics engineer to set stress data for designing & stability evaluation of civil engineering structures such as dams, tunnels, underground power houses and mining excavations. Stress measurements are possible in deep bore holes using hydraulic fracture methods. It requires the measurement of fluid pressure data during inducing and propagating hydraulic fractures. Similar stress measurements were carried out for mines mainly at shallow depths or in close distance from mine openings. Stress measuring techniques developed in the past were stress or strain relief methods. They are extensively discussed by Fairhurst (1968), McGarr and Gay (1978). Due to various reasons such as the existence of joints, time-dependent deformations or discing, most of the techniques have serious drawbacks and the stress values derived from such measurements may often be questionable (Jaeger and Cook, 1968).

A second source of information on the active tectonic stress field at greater depths are earthquake focal mechanism solutions (Stauder, 1962), and they yield, though with some error, the directions of the active principal stresses. The major advantage of the seismological approach is that the field data is already available where seismic monitoring station is established. Almost all mining districts of the world, where mining has gone to a deeper level in hard rocks are reported to have been plagued by this hazard of rockbursts. So far only the seismological investigation has proved helpful in a clear understanding the phenomenon of origin of rockbursts on a regional scale. This paper attempts to investigate and evaluate rock stress, delineate high stress zones and movement of seismic stress front leading to prediction of rockbursts utilising the recorded seismic data from one of the deepest mines of India, i.e. the Champion Reef mines of KGF.

2. SOURCE PARAMETERS

Source parameters are usually determined by carrying out spectral analysis of seismic waveform data. From the stress drop calculated from this method, the stress accumulated and released due to a rockburst can be calculated. The relationships between seismic moment (Mo), zero frequency intercept, hypocentral distance, propagation velocity etc., are described by Keils-Borok (1960), as

$$M_0 = \frac{4 \Pi \rho \alpha^3 R |\Omega_0|}{F} \quad (1)$$

where $|\Omega_0|$ is the zero frequency intercept of the P-wave.
ρ – density of the source material,
α – P-wave velocity,
R – hypocentral distance,
F – radiation pattern of the P-wave

In situations where the focal mechanism is not known, a mean value of F = 0.39 is chosen for P-waves of the mine tremors in gold mines (Spottiswoode et.al. 1975).

Estimates of source radius (r_0) of the mine seismicity is normally obtained by assuming Brunes (1970) model.

$$r_0 = \frac{K_p \alpha}{2 \pi f_c} \quad (2)$$

Where K_p is equal to 2.34 and f_c is the corner frequency. The corner frequency f_c can be obtained from the spectrum. Substituting the above mentioned parameters the static stress drop ($\Delta\sigma$) can be calculated as follows:

$$\Delta\sigma = \frac{7M_0}{16r_0^3} \quad (3)$$

The corner frequency obtained from these two signals vary from 120 to 180 Hz as obtained from the case studies (Srinivasan et.al. 1997). By substituting these corner frequencies in the equation (2) for two cases, the source parameters namely seismic moment, seismic energy and stress drop computed for the Champion reef mines of KGF have been tabulated in Table 1.

Source parameter	Event 1	Event 2
Origin time	12/12/1990 11:03:38	13/12/1990 08:34:20
Seismic moment M, N.m	2.1288×10^2	3.1921×10^2
Seismic energy E, J	5.1668×10^3	1.1625×10^4
Stress drop Pa	1.59×10^2	8.082×10^2
Displacement m	0.000568	0.001919
Source radius r, m	18	12

The most vital link added by the seismic monitoring for better understanding of rockbursts is the determination of the energy release. The energy released in a rockburst sequence is characteristic of the state of stress prevailing in that region before the rockburst. Based on this concept, a method has been adopted in analysing the stress regime of Champion reef mine (Jha et.al 1990 and Jha 1991). A brief description is provided to understand the methodology.

3. EVALUATION OF STRESS REGIME

The recorded rockburst data from Champion Reef mine for the years 1985-1989 are considered for the data analysis here. The log data consists of hypocentral location of each events in terms of mining coordinates along with maximum amplitude, energy released in each event and duration of ground vibration as recorded by the seismic network. The underlying principle of this approach is that the square root of seismic energy released can be taken during an event is proportional to the state of strain in the rockmass prior to the occurrence of that seismic event (Benioff, 1951). Keeping in view, the proportionality of the stress and strain within elastic limits, the square root of energy released as a measure of the stress build-up prior to the occurrence of that event.

A mathematical formulation of Benioff's method in calculating the quantity proportional to the stress prior to seismic event is given below. Suppose the elastic strain accumulated prior to a seismic event was is uniformly distributed in a volume V of the rock, then the elastic energy stored is expressed by

$$E = \mu V \varepsilon^2 / 2 \qquad (4)$$

Where E = elastic energy,
μ = shear modulus,
ε = strain prior to the seismic event and
V = volume of rock.
If σ = stress prior to the seismic event, then from equation (4)

$$E = \kappa 0.5 \mu V \sigma^2 \qquad (5)$$

Since σ is proportional to ε within elastic limits (Hookes Law) and κ is the constant of proportionality. A fraction of this energy released as seismic wave, if the said fraction be η, and seismic energy released be J, then

$$J = \eta E \qquad (6)$$

Substituting (5) in (6) we get

$$J = (\eta \kappa 0.5 \, \mu V) \, \sigma^2$$
$$\sigma = (2/ \mu \kappa \, \eta \, V) \, J^{0..5}$$
$$\sigma \propto K \, J^{0.5} \qquad (7)$$

where K = ± (2 / $\mu\kappa \, \eta \, V$) is a constant for a particular rock type in a particular seismic zone. Equation (7) shows that stress build-up prior to a seismic event release is proportional to square root of seismic energy J (released due to that event). This method provides significant information of an impending seismic event in a particular seismic zone based upon past strain accumulation rate projected to expected time slot.

Based upon this approach, square root of seismic energy released for each rockburst event is computed and taken as the representative stress build up in the region prior to the event. A typical plot of the stress section of the Champion Reef mine for July-December 1985 is shown in Figure 1.

The important point to note in this figure is the concentration of stress contours in certain packets. It is worthwhile mentioning that, though rockbursts occur randomly at all the places, but the anomalous stress concentration is located in certain regions in both mining and old mine working areas. Such areas are known as high stress zone. Thus this approach has helped to delineate high stress zone in the burst prone area. Continuous mining through one particular shaft leads to continuous loading whereby the resulting stress build up reaches to a brink of instability. Any further mining in that region acts as a triggering agent leading to a chain of severe and damaging rockburst, thereby bringing the production to a standstill. Therefore A prior knowledge of high stress zone help the mine management in planning their mining operation in such a way, that the adverse build up of stress may get properly diffused and spread over the region, so that severity of burst can be minimised.

4. PREDICTION OF ROCKBURST

In order to determine the spatio-temporal location of future rockburst activity, the principle of seismic migration is used (Mogi, 1968). In order to obtain the migration pattern and rate of migration, stress maps of an annual time window is made use of. The maximum value stress contour in each zone is traced out separately within the boundary of that zone for the 5 year period. Later the centers of these maxima are joined to obtain the migration axis. Figure 2 shows a typical migration pattern of the stress front for the zone III of the Champion Reef mine.

Once a clear migration pattern and the rate of migration are obtained, the axis of migration is suitably interpolated in its own direction to an extent equal to the average annual rate, so as to project the center of activity of impending rockbursts in the following year. The coordinates of projected location gives the locale of the future seat of rockburst activity and size of the projected maxima determines the area under its influence in which the majority of rockbursts during the projected period should take place.

While moving to the step of quantification of rockbursts, use is made of the quantitative parameters of each seismic zone, i.e. total stress value, peak stress value, number of damaging bursts and number total bursts. Three sets of graphs are then drawn for each active seismic zone by using the following parameters.

1. Total stress value VS. number of damaging bursts;
2. Peak stress value VS number of damaging bursts; and

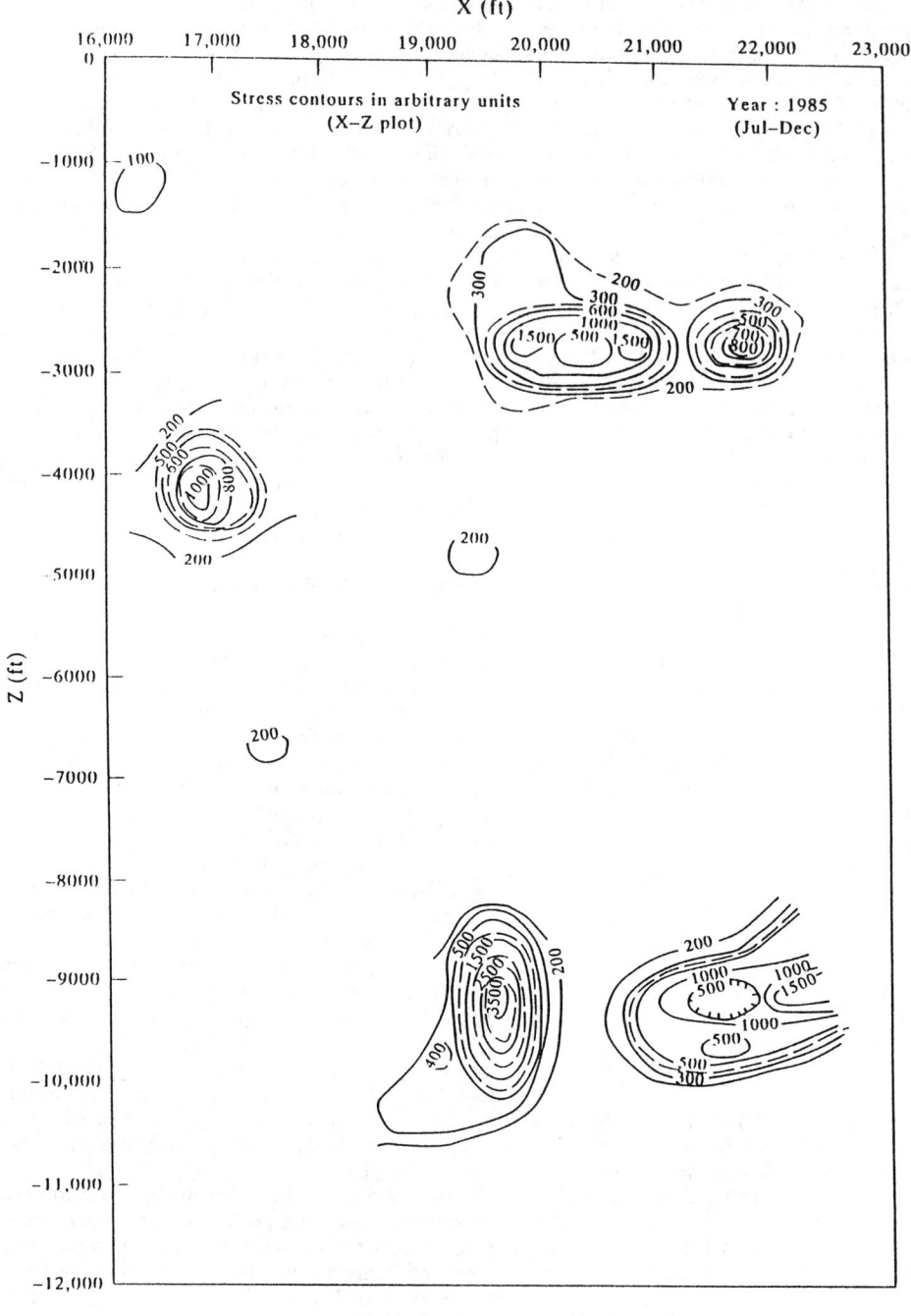

Figure 1. Longitudinal section of the stress build-up pattern in the Champion Reef mine, KGF during July-December 1985.

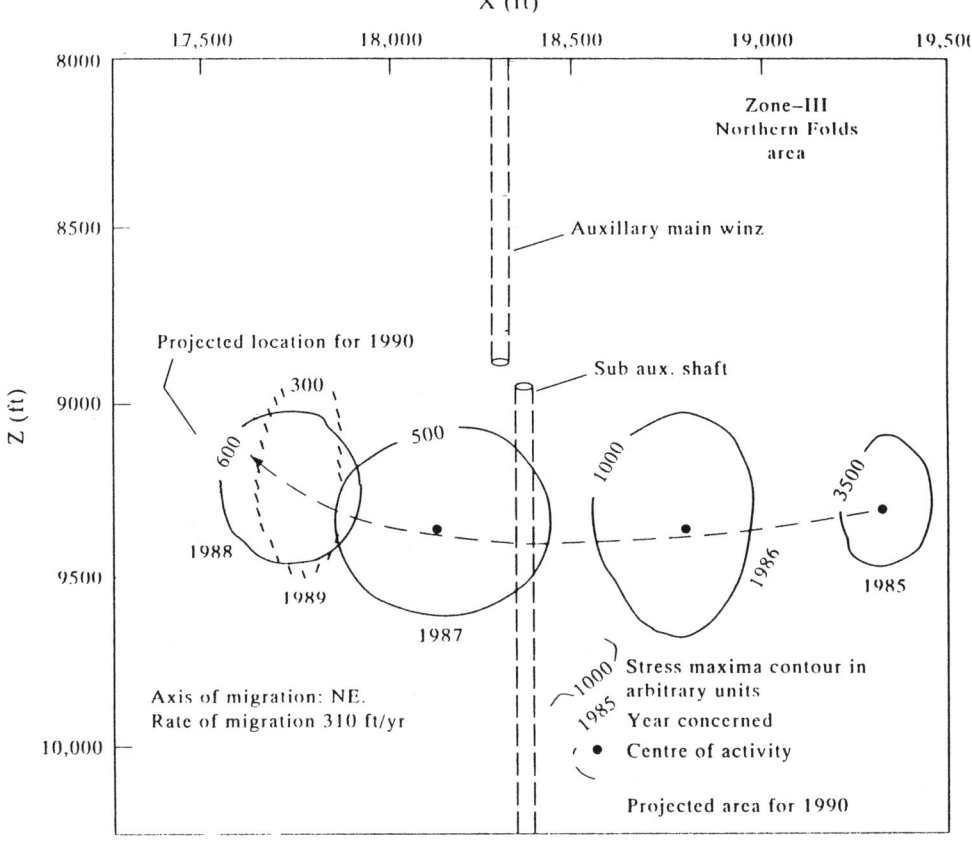

Figure 2. Migration of the stress front in the zone III of the Champion Reef mine, KGF during 1985-1989.

3. Number of damaging bursts VS number of total bursts.

A set of nomograms are prepared using the above parameters and used for estimating the number and size of expected rockbursts in future. Using this approach the predicted number and size of rockbursts are duly listed on half-yearly basis for each of the seismic zones in Table-2.

It is observed from the table-2 that there is a good agreement between the figures predicted and the actually recorded ones. No restriction is made in this approach as regards the mine and the type of data. Hence this can be used for any seismological data set with the above objective.

Table-2 Summary of predicted rockbursts for 1991

Zones	Period	Predicted rockbursts		Recorded rockbursts	
		Damaging	Total	Damaging	Total
I	Jan-Jun	Not expected		00	02
	Jul-Dec	Not expected		00	03
II	Jan-Jun	05	12	02	07
	Jul-Dec	04	11	03	15
III	Jan-Jun	06	10	04	12
	Jul-Dec	06	15	03	19
IV	Jan-Jun	Not expected		00	01
	Jul-Dec	Not expected		00	02
V	Jan-Jun	Few bursts		02	05
	Jul-Dec	Not expected		Nil	

CONCLUSION

The seismic investigation carried out in the Kolar Gold Fields provided a extensive database for understanding the phenomenon of rockburst. With the seismological approach, the data collected from the seismic network has been made use to obtain stress drop value and evaluate the state of rock stress through the energy of individual event. This approach has been extended to delineate high stress zone, monitor the migration of peak stresses as the mining progressed and for the prediction of rockburst with considerable success.

ACKNOWLEDGEMENTS

The authors are thankful to the management of M/S. Bharat Gold Mines Ltd. for providing all the support in collecting the seismological data of rockbursts. We also thank all the staff of Seismology section for their continued assistance.

REFERENCES

Cook, N.G.W. 1976. Seismicity associated with mining, Engineering geology 10,99-122.

Hasegawa, H.S., Wetmiller, R.J., and D.J. Gengzwill 1989. Induced seismicity in mines in Canada - an overview, Pure Applied Geophysics 129, 423-453.

Zoback, M.L. and M.D. Zoback 1989. Tectonics stress field of the conterminous United States. In L.C. Pakiser and W.D. Mooney (eds.), Geophysical Framework of the Continental United States, Geol.Soc.Am.memoir 172, p. 523-539.

Robertson, E.C. 1964. Visco elasticity of rocks. Proc.Inter-national conference on state of stress in earth's crust, Santa Monica California, Elsevier, N.Y. (Ed). W.R. Judd., pp. 181-224.

Hardy, H.R.and F.W.Leighton 1980. Proc.Second Conference on acoustic AE/MS activity on geological structures and materials. Pennsylvania State University. Trans Tech Publications.

Subbaramu K.R., Rao B.S.S, Krishnamurthy R. and C.Srinivasan 1989. Seismic Investigation of Rockbursts in the Kolar Gold Fields, Proc.of the 4th conference on acoustic emission/microseismic activity in geological structures and materials, Pennsylvania State University, Trans. Tech. Publication, Germany, Pp. 265-274.

Srinivasan C. 1992. Seismic and Microseismic precursory signals for monitoring and prediction of rockburst in Kolar Gold Fields, Ph.D thesis, Karanataka Regional Engineering college, Mangalore University, (unpublished)

Srinivasan C, Nair G.J and N.M.Raju 1992. Precursor analysis of microseismic events prior to seismic events in Kolar Gold Fields - A case study. Proc.of the 5th conference on acoustic emission/microseismic activity in geological structures and materials, Pennsylvania State University, Trans. Tech. Publication, Germany. Pp. 372-381

Fairhurst, C. 1968. Methods of determining in-situ rock stress at great depth. Tech. Rep. No. 1-68, U.S. Arms Corps Eng., Missouri River Div., Ohmaha.

McGarr, A. and N.C.Gay 1978. State of stress in the Earth's crust. Ann.Rev.Earth Sci., 6 405-436.

Jaeger, C.B. and N.G.W.Cook 1969. Fundamentals of Rock Mechanics. P. Methuen, London.

Stauder, W.S.J. 1962. The focal mechanism of earthquakes, Advances in Geophys., 9, 1-76.

Keilis-brook,V.I. 1960. Investigation of the mechanism of Earthquakes, Eng. Trans. Sov. Res. Geophys. Ser.,4 (English translation), Am.Geophys. Union .Consultants Bureau, New York, Pp.201.

Spottiswoode,S.M., and A. McGarr 1975. Source Parameters of tremors in a deep-level gold mine. Bull.Seism.Soc.Am.,64,Pp. 1295-1317.

Brune J.N. 1970. Tectonic stress and the spectra of seismic shear waves. J.Geophys. Res.75, Pp. 4997 - 5009.

Srinivasan C., M.V.M.S.Rao M.V.M.S., Shivakumar K. and K. Kusunose 1997. Stability Evaluation of Deep Underground Caverns - Field and laboratory Investigations using microseismic and acoustic emission monitoring techniques. Interim Report #3 (Oct94-Oct96) India-Japan S & T collaboration project.

Jha P.C. and Y.A. Willy 1990. Analysis of the stress regime of the Champion Reef mine with reference to rockbursts. NIRM Internal Report. Pp. 1-75.

Jha P.C. and R.K.S. Chouhan 1994. Long Range Rockburst Prediction: A Seismological Approach. Int.J.Rock Mech. Min.Sci. & Geomech.Abstr. Vol.31, No.1,Pp. 71-77.

Benioff H. 1951.Earthquake and rock creep. Bull. Seis. Soc.Am. 41, 31-62.

Mogi K. 1968. Migration of seismic activity, Bull.Earthquake Res. Inst. Univ. Tokyo 46, 175-203.

Possibility of estimating in-situ stress of virgin coal field using acoustic emission technique

M. Seto
National Institute for Resources and Environment, Tsukuba, Japan

V. S. Vutukuri
The University of New South Wales, Sydney, N.S.W., Australia

D. K. Nag
Monash University, Churchill, Australia

ABSTRACT: In this study a thorough laboratory investigation has been conducted to investigate the Kaiser effect in coal and to explore the possibility of its application in the estimation of stress in a virgin coal field. AE signals were measured by two piezoelectric transducers in different frequency ranges, 50-200 kHz and 200-1200 kHz. Coal specimen exhibited an obvious Kaiser effect both in lower frequency and higher frequency AEs. The time interval, up to 20 days, did not strongly influence the Kaiser effect of coal. The previous stress was more pronounced in lower amplitude range than in the higher one. The vertical in situ stress determined from cored coal and rock specimens coincided well with the overburden pressure estimated from the depth.

1. INTRODUCTION

A knowledge of the magnitude and directions of the in situ and induced stresses in a rock mass is an essential concern in underground excavation design. Reliable evaluation of in situ stress is an important step in the analysis and design of any underground excavations, particularly for excavating the stability of underground structures to prevent failure or collapse of underground openings.

A number of approaches have been developed to determine in situ stress, but none of them are universally applicable and all suffer from deficiencies and limitations. Particularly, coal seam has such a fragile and fractured property in nature that most of the established techniques have not been successfully applied to determine in situ stress of coal seams. One of the promising techniques relies on the Kaiser effect, obtained from measurements of AE in stressed rock. This phenomena, termed the "Kaiser effect", suggests that previously applied maximum stress might be detected by stressing a rock specimen to the point where there is a substantial increase in AE activity. This technique has been developed and tried by various researchers in the past (Kanagawa et al., 1976; Kurita and Fujii, 1979; Heughton and Crawford, 1987; Seto et al., 1989, 1992, 1996; Holocomb, 1993) with the aim of providing a practical technique for retrieving the Kaiser effect. That is a recollection of the maximum previous stress to which a rock had been subjected in its in situ environment. The technique is functionally workable technology, and is anticipated that the rapid and economical determination of the in situ rock stress is possible. Few research works, however, have been done with the Kaiser effect in coal. In this study a series of laboratory experiments was conducted to understand the Kaiser effect in coal and tried to explore the possibility of its application in the estimation of stresses in coal seams. In addition, the AE technique was applied to estimate in situ vertical stresses from cored rock and coal specimens taken from a deep vertical borehole.

2. EXPERIMENTAL PROCEDURE

2.1 *Coal specimen*

In test specimen preparation, all cutting, sanding and grinding were done in dry condition to prevent the adding of moisture to specimens. Cubic specimens were prepared and were 110 mm in height and approximately 105 mm × 105 mm in cross-section. Parallelism between the top and bottom faces of each cube, to within 1/50 mm, was accomplished. Cored rock and coal specimens, which were taken from the depth up to 356 m, 8 to 45 days before the test, had a dimension of 61 mm in diameter and 144.5 mm in height. Besides, rock cores from another borehole of 400 m depth, which was drilled 2 years before the test, were tested in order to evaluate the time dependency of stress recollection.

2.2 *Testing procedure*

In the experiments, the previous stress was memorized in a coal specimen by cyclic uniaxial loading up to a certain stress level (nearly 5 MPa) under a constant displacement rate of 100 μm/min by means of a servo-controlled testing machine, Schenck TREBEL. After the previous loading, specimens had been kept in room temperature until reloadings for 1 day, 2 days, 6 days and 20 days. In reloading of the specimen, each loading-unloading cycle was repeated four times while AE signals were measured.

The AE instrument, MISTRAS-2001 system, is a computerised AE system that performs AE signal measurements and stores, displays and analyses the resulting data. AE signals were amplified by a pre-amplifier (Gain: 40 dB, frequency filter: 50 - 1200 kHz) and a post-amplifier inside the system (Gain: 20 dB). The threshold could be set in the screen set-up menu of the test running code. Each AE signal was described in terms of its counts, energy, amplitude, rise time and duration in the record. Two different types of piezoelectric transducer (PAC nano-30 (sensor-1) and NF AE-901S (sensor-2)) were employed. The resonant frequencies of sensor-1 and sensor-2 are 500 kHz and 120 kHz, respectively. Lower frequency emissions were monitored by sensor-2 through a lower frequency band from 50 to 200 kHz, and higher frequency emissions were monitored by sensor-1 through a higher frequency window from 200 to 1200 kHz. Two of these transducers were attached to a specimen and cemented with electron wax. In the present experiment, the two transducers were placed adjacent to each other to minimize the difference in propagation path from emission sources between the two transducers.

3. RESULTS AND DISCUSSIONS

3.1 *Kaiser effect of coal*

Fig. 1 shows a typical example that indicates the existence of Kaiser effect in a coal specimen. Data for a specimen tested just after the previous cyclic loading are shown. An arrow indicates the previous maximum stress. The take-off point of AE activity coincides with the maximum previous stress. The previous stress level of 5.7 MPa was within elastic stage. In all experiments, conducted within the short delay time, the existence of Kaiser effect in coal specimens could be clearly observed and the assigned stress from the take-off point of AE signature was within 7 %.

3.2 *Effect of delay time on Kaiser effect*

The question is how long the stress memory can be retained in coal specimen. Since a coal specimen has more complicated fracture system than a rock does, the recovery process of the hysterisis due to delay time is important for the application of the Kaiser effect to the stress estimation.

In the previous section, time interval between preloading and reloading was quite short. Further experiments were conducted with time interval of 1, 2, 6 and 20 days. The previous stress level was chosen within the elastic stage. Fig. 2 shows the AE signatures in the first reloading at 20 days after the previous loading in the amplitude range from 40 to 100 dB. Previous stress is indicated by an arrow. In both AE signatures of AE(H) and AE(L), the Kaiser effect can be clearly observed. The previous stress (5.24 MPa) could be estimated with reasonable accuracy of 4.7 %.

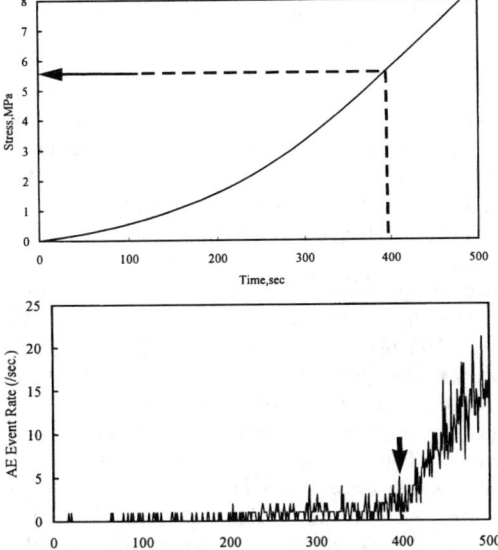

Fig. 1 A typical example of Kaiser effect of coal

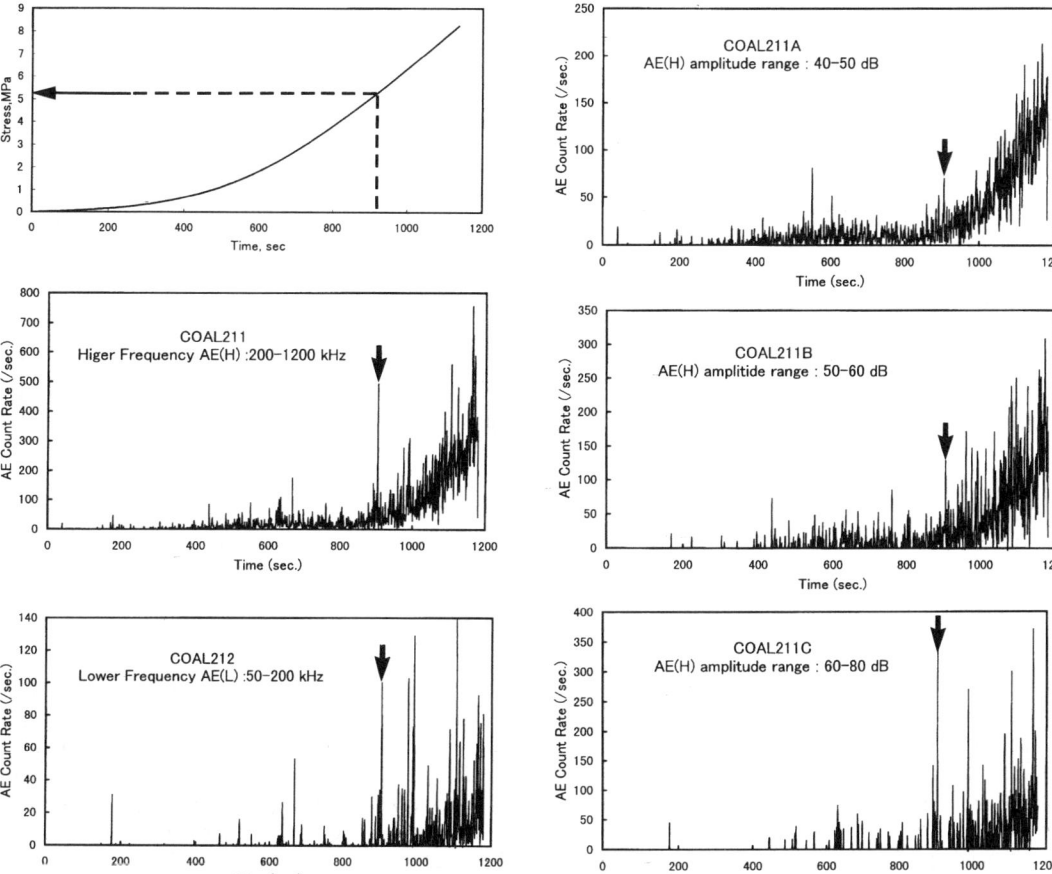

Fig.2 AE(H) and AE(L) behavior of coal (20days)

Fig.3 AE behavior in different amplitude ranges

Fig. 3 shows the AE signatures of AE(H) in the first reloading separately in the amplitude ranges of 40 - 50 dB, 50 - 60 dB and 60 - 80 dB. AE increase at the previous stress can be more easily identified in the highest amplitude range than in the two lower ranges. The higher AE amplitude is shifted to, the clearer AE increase at the previous stress level becomes.

As the delay time was increased, the Kaiser effect in coal was obscured by lower amplitude emissions produced below the previous stress level. Thus, in case of long delay time, the Kaiser effect in coal can be clearly identified by the AE signature of higher amplitude emissions.

Fig. 4 shows the AE signatures of AE(L) and AE(H) in the second reloading. Although the emissions below the previous stress level was significantly reduced in the second reloading, the AE take-off point can be recognized at the previous stress level in both AE(L) and AE(H) signatures. From these experiments, it is confirmed that no recovery of Kaiser effect in coal is observed up to 20 days interval under room temperature condition.

Delay time effect on the stress memory is interpreted as follows: In the elastic stage, stress memory would be retained through the microcrack system which is grown to an equilibrium configuration corresponding to the previous stress (Seto et al., 1995). After unloading, tensile cracks would be closed and shear cracks would be opened and slid with friction along the crack surface. This is the healing process of the crack configuration corresponding to the previous stress. In the healing process, other microcracks would be generated and

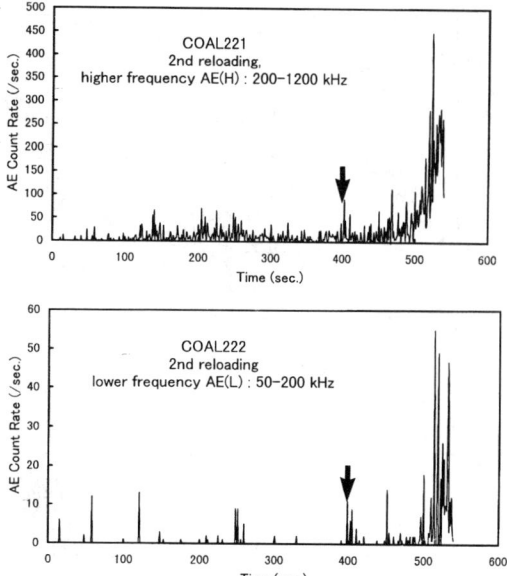
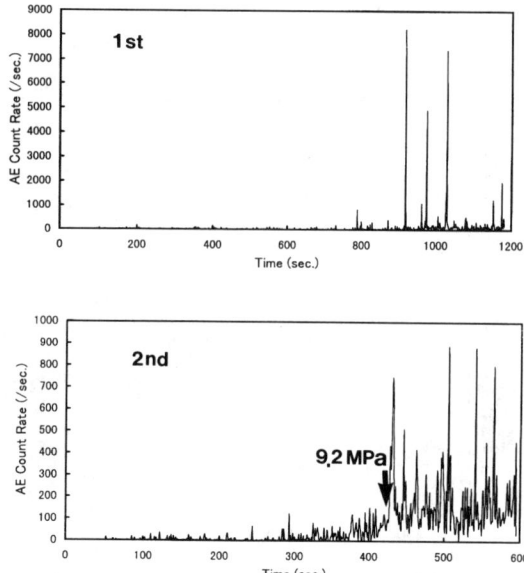

Fig.4 AE(L) and AE(H) in the second reloading

Fig.5 AE behavior of cored coal specimen

the existing cracks would be rearranged. The new formation and rearrangement of microcracks is responsible for the noise emissions produced below the previous stress level in the first reloading. Since the first reloading let the newly formed and rearranged cracks grow to an equilibrium state corresponding to the applied stress of cyclic reloadings, the noise emissions due to the cracks produced in the healing process would be significantly reduced in the subsequent reloading. In the subsequent reloadings, the growth of cracks, whcih have been produced in the preloading, is only responsible for acoustic emission. The AE increase, consequently, at the previous stress was more pronounced in the second reloading than in the first reloading.

3.3 *Estimation of in situ stress from cored rock and coal specimens*

Cored coal and rock specimens were taken from the exploratory borehole of 400 m depth drilled in Newcastle, NSW, Australia area. The estimation of in situ stress was conducted under uniaxial compression condition 8 to 45 days after the drilling. The specimens were loaded repeatedly four times at a constant displacement rate of 100 μm/min.

Fig. 5 shows the AE signatures of cored coal specimen from the first and second loading up to 15.7 MPa. In the second loading the emissions below the stress level was significantly reduced, and AE take-off point can be identified more easily than in the first loading. The estimated stress from the AE signatures was 9.2 MPa, which was very close to the overburden pressure (8.5 MPa) estimated from the depth of 356 m. Fig. 6 shows AE signatures in the first and second loading of a rock core taken depth of 301.6 m 43 days before the test. Although the AE take-off point is not clear in the first loading, the stress can be estimated from the AE signature in the second loading. The estimated stress was 7.4 MPa. Fig. 7 represents the relation between the depth and estimated stresses. The broken line represents the overburden pressure. Since the borehole was vertically drilled from the flat surface, it could be expected that the estimated stresses were consistent with the overburden pressure. As it can be seen from the figure, the estimated stresses significantly vary with the depth and well agree with the overburden pressure with reasonable accuracy.

Fig. 8 shows the relation between the estimated vertical stresses and the depth. The cored rocks were taken from a vertical borehole drilled 2 years before the test. The estimated stresses are higher than the overburden pressure, but they are still within 10 %. There were several cases where the AE take-off point was not clear in the first loading but could be identified in the second loading.

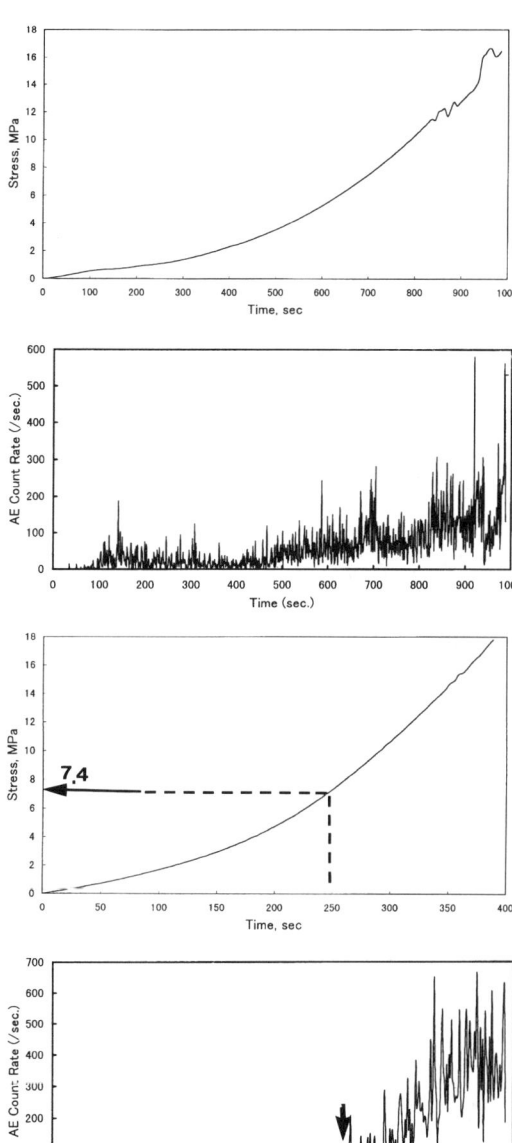

Fig.6 AE behavior of a rock core specimen

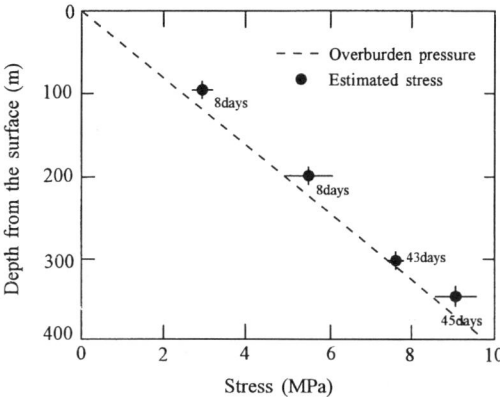

Fig. 7 Variation of estimated stresses with depth

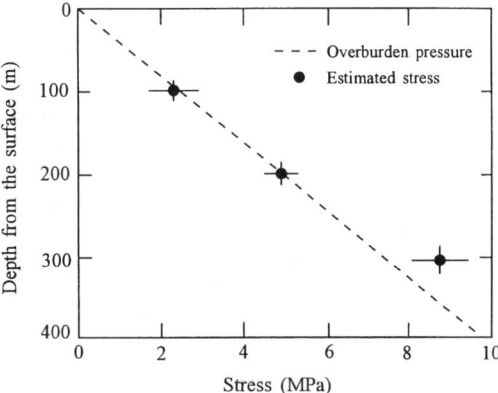

Fig.8 Variation of estimated stresses with depth

4. CONCLUSIONS

The Kaiser effect in coal has been investigated to explore the applicability of AE technique to in situ stress measurement in virgin coal field. The conclusions obtained here are as follows:
(1) Coal specimen exhibits an obvious Kaiser effect. The time interval, in the tested range up to 20 days, did not strongly influence the Kaiser effect of coal.
(2) The previous stress in coal can be estimated more accurately in higher amplitude range than in lower one.
(3) There was significant correlation between overburden pressure (estimated from the depth) and the Kaiser effect of cored coal specimen taken from underground 45 days before the test. It was confirmed that maximum previous stress memory can be retained in coal for periods of up to at least 45 days. Besides, the vertical stress could be estimated with reasonable accuracy from AE technique using rock cores taken 2 years before the test.

REFERENCES

Houghton, D.R. and A.M. Crawford (1987). Kaiser effect gauging: The influence of confining stress on its response, *Proc. 6th ISRM Congress,* Montreal, Canada, Vol.2, pp.981-985

Holocomb, D.J. (1993). Observations of the Kaiser effect under multiaxial stress state: Implications for its use in determining in situ stress, *Geophys. Res. Lett.,* 20, pp.2119-2122

Kanagawa, T., Hayashi, M. and H. Nakasa (1976). Estimation of spatial geostress components in rock samples using the Kaiser effect of acoustic emission, *Rep. No. 375017,* Central Res. Inst. of Electrical Power Industry, Abiko, Japan

Kurita, K. and N. Fujii (1979). Stress memory of crystalline rock in acoustic emission, *Geophys. Res. Lett.,* 6, pp.9-12

Seto, M., Utagawa, M. and K. Katsuyama (1989). Estimation of rock pressure using the acoustic emission (in Japanese), *Proc. 7th National Conf. on Acoustic Emission,* The Jap. Soc. for NDI, Shizuoka, Japan, pp.54-59

Seto, M., Utagawa, M. and K. Katsuyama (1992). The estimation of pre-stress from AE in cyclic loading of pre-stressed rock, *Proc. 11th Int. Symp. on Acoustic Emission,* The Jap. Soc. for NDI, Fukuoka, Japan, pp.159-166

Seto, M., Utagawa, M. and K. Katsuyama (1995). The relation between the variation of AE hypocenters and the Kaiser effect of Shirahama sandstone, *Proc. 8th Int. Cong. on Rock Mechanics,* Vol.1, Tokyo, Japan, pp.201-205

Seto, M., Nag, D.K. and V.S. Vutukuri (1996). Experimental verification of the Kaiser effect in rock under different environment conditions, *Proc. for Eurock'96* , Vol.1, Torino , Italy, pp.395-402.

A review of recent in-situ stress measurements in United Kingdom Coal Measures strata

P.B. Cartwright
Rock Mechanics Technology Ltd, Burton on Trent, UK

ABSTRACT: The in-situ stress regime is recognised by United Kingdom coal mine operators as a significant design parameter related to efficient mine design. The results obtained from recent overcore stress measurements undertaken in Coal Measures strata are analysed and presented. A relationship has been deduced which relates the maximum horizontal stress to the depth and to the elastic properties of the rock. This relationship is considered more suitable for estimating the maximum horizontal stress magnitude in Coal Measures strata than existing methods based solely on the depth of cover. This study also indicates that all in-situ stress determinations in sedimentary strata should be quoted with the elastic properties of the test horizons.

1. INTRODUCTION

It is now recognised that the stability of underground excavations in Coal Measures strata is significantly influenced by the in-situ stress regime. In recent years a large number of in-situ stress measurements have been undertaken in Coal Measures strata within the United Kingdom. This occurred as a response to a change in support strategy within the coal mining industry from standing steel framework support to rockbolt support. An understanding of the in-situ stress field is now considered by the coal producers of the United Kingdom to be a parameter directly relevant to mine design (Altounyan et al., 1997).

Assessing the in-situ stress regime at a particular site without a stress measurement can be difficult and often many assumptions are made. Whilst stress directions and the magnitude of the vertical stress can be estimated from data banks, such as that held by the World Stress Map Project, and the depth of cover, estimation of the magnitude of the horizontal stresses presents significant problems. In the past, it has often been the case that a relationship between the horizontal stress and the depth below the surface has been sought. The normal practice has been to relate either the ratio k (k = $\sigma_{H,h}/\sigma_V$ or σ_{Hav}/σ_V) to depth or the maximum or minimum horizontal stress to depth by some linear function, Hoek & Brown (1980), Rummel et al. (1986), Pine et al. (1990), Stephansson (1993) and Sugawara (1993). Relationships of this form have often resulted in a general trend with depth but with considerable scatter especially at shallow depths. Only in rock types which have fairly consistent elastic properties does a reasonable depth-horizontal stress relationship exist. In rock formations which are interbedded and hence have potentially variable elastic properties, such as sedimentary basins, horizontal stress relationships based on depth are far less precise, Bigby et al. (1992). In Coal Measures strata horizontal stress profiles based on depth have indicated a poor relationship and it has been necessary to undertake stress measurements to describe the state of stress. A relationship which would take account of the variable elastic properties of interbedded Coal Measures strata and give a reasonable estimate of the maximum horizontal stress magnitude would therefore be advantageous in the initial design stages.

2. IN-SITU STRESS MEASUREMENTS IN COAL MEASURES STRATA USING CSIRO HI CELLS

Over the past six years a series of underground stress measurements have been undertaken in UK coal mines by overcoring CSIRO Hollow Inclusion (HI) cells. The programme provided design data for mine layout and tunnel support. Despite the weak rock which generally surrounds most productive British coal seams over 80 successful overcores have been completed at 22 mine sites. Of these, 26 stress measurements at 16 mine sites represent what is considered to be virgin or near virgin conditions.

The location of the stress measurement sites ranged from the Longannet Complex, near Alloa in Scotland to Lyn Mine in South Wales, some 600 km apart. The deepest site was at Hem Heath Colliery at 1060 m and the shallowest was at Lyn Mine at a depth of 90 m. Details of the measurement sites are summarised in Table 1.

In undertaking the measurements a conscious effort was made to measure the stress at a point in excess of twice the average roadway width from the edge of the opening. This was assumed sufficient to reduce the influence of the opening on the stress to a satisfactory level.

In all cases, the tests were undertaken at a distance greater than 1.5 times the roadway width from the edge of the excavation with the exception of Lyn Mine in South Wales, which occurred at approximately one roadway width. The depth of cover at this site was only 90 m and the visible deformation was minimal suggesting that the extent of influence of the opening on the stress may be less than would otherwise be the case. Although the test was closer to the mine opening than desired it provided the only data at this shallow depth and has been included in the data set for analysis.

The measurement procedure generally conformed to ISRM suggestions and the HI cell manufacturer's handbook (ISRM, 1987; Mindata, 1986). Data reduction and analysis was performed using in-house software based upon the Duncan, Fama and Pender isotropic solution (Duncan et al., 1980).

In any stress measurement there are several sources of both random and systematic errors, only a few of which are quantifiable. Useful discussions of the problems and errors in in-situ stress measurements using HI cells can be found in papers by Pine, Tunbridge and Kwakwa (1983) and Price Jones and Simms (1984).

3. ANALYSIS OF HI OVERCORE STRESS MEASUREMENT RESULTS

The results of the stress determinations are presented in terms of the magnitude, bearing and dip of the principal stresses in Table 1. These measurements confirm that an anisotropic stress regime prevails in the UK Coal Measures.

If the principal stresses are resolved to give the stresses in the horizontal plane, the orientation of the maximum horizontal stress can be plotted on a rosette. The resulting plot is shown in Figure 1. The length of

TABLE 1 - DATA ON VIRGIN STRESS MEASUREMENTS IN UNITED KINGDOM

Colliery	Depth (m)	Tunnel Size (m)	Test borehole Bearing (deg)	Test borehole Dip (deg)	Depth into Rib (m)	Sigma 1 (MPa)	Bearing (deg)	Dip (deg)	Sigma 2 (MPa)	Bearing (deg)	Dip (deg)	Sigma 3 (MPa)	Bearing (deg)	Dip (deg)	Rock Type	Elastic Modulus (GPa)	Poisson's Ratio	Measure of Elastic Property
N Selby	987	4.9x3.7 arched	4	-18	7.7	25.7	18	69	18.8	162	17	12.1	256	12	Sandy Siltstone	21	0.44	Biaxial
Wistow	440	4.5x3.0 rect	100	-45	7.5	17.3	267	-28	15.7	140	-49	7.9	13	-28	Siltstone	22.2	0.4	Biaxial
Bolsover	660	4.9x3.7 arched	154	-28	10.05	19.8	309	0	18.9	300	88	12.1	39	0	Siltstone	25.4	0.4	Biaxial
	660				11.06	21.5	308	9	18.3	119	81	10.8	38	-1	Siltstone	30	0.35	Assumed
Coventry	825	4.9x3.7 arched	3	-26	7.92	27.8	325	-18	24.5	206	-56	15.4	65	-28	Silty Sandstone	30	0.44	Biaxial
Lea Hall	810	4.9x3.7 arched	326	-39	7.65	20.6	58	-71	14.1	182	-11	6.5	275	-15	Sandstone	15.4	0.36	Biaxial
	810				8.25	19.5	78	-78	11.9	193	-5	6.4	284	-11	Muddy Silts	16	0.4	Assumed
Asfordby	495	5.0x3.0 rect	12	-33	7.37	44.5	321	-12	12.8	263	69	5.2	47	18	Sandstone	56	0.2	Biaxial
	495				7.86	43.7	324	-14	13.5	159	-75	4.3	55	-4	Sandstone	53	0.3	Biaxial
Welbeck	800	4.9x3.7 arched	135	-8	8.18	24.3	85	63	11.7	181	3	8.3	273	26	Siltstone	18.3	0.22	Biaxial
	800				8.92	22.4	5	-68	12.2	186	-22	7.9	276	1	Siltstone	18.6	0.15	Biaxial
	800				9.52	26.1	72	75	12.4	211	12	8.3	303	10	Siltstone	17.5	0.31	Biaxial
Prince of Wales	450	4.5x2.7 arched	236	-15	10.96	12.3	335	48	11.4	158	42	6.3	67	1	Silty Muds	16.1	0.34	Biaxial
Thoresby	780	4.9x3.0 arched	154	-33	9.05	22.1	335	87	16.8	120	2	12.1	30	-2	Interbedded Sand/silts	21.5	0.4	Biaxial
	780				10.7	21.4	297	73	16.1	111	17	10.9	21	-2		25.4	0.24	Biaxial
Longannet Aberdona	430	4.9x3.7 arched	272	-31.5	9.1	11.1	76	-73	9.7	174	-2	4.1	85	16	Mudstone	12	0.3	Biaxial
	430				10.3	11.6	351	-47	10.3	155	-41	6.7	72	8	Mudstone	12	0.3	Assumed
Longannet Solsgirth	292	4.5x2.8 rect	92	-30	9	8.8	338	14	7.8	213	67	6.9	73	18	Mudstone	12.8	0.39	Biaxial
	292				10.1	9	7	37	7.7	138	41	3.4	74	-27	Mudstone	21	0.22	Assumed
Harworth	960	4.5x2.8 rect	191	-42	9.8	29.2	7	-65	23.7	145	-19	11.7	61	15	siltstone	25.5	0.4	Biaxial
Maltby	974	4.9x3.0 rect	257	-7	9.48	25	346	75	16.2	182	14	6.8	271	-4	Siltstone/ sandstone	28.2	0.26	Biaxial
	974				>9.60	25.6	85	-77	17.29	163	3	6.46	72	13	sandstone	29.4	0.26	Biaxial
Hem Heath	1060	4.8x3.6 rect	n/a	n/a	10.7	29.8	320	-64	23.8	356	22	20.2	260	14	Siltstone/ sandstone	32.7	0.34	Biaxial
Littleton	560	5.0x3.0 rect	n/a	n/a	7.4	15.6	135	83	10.3	327	7	6.9	236	1	Sandstone	13.9	0.36	Biaxial
Lyn Mine	90	7.0x1.2 rect	210	-25	6.33	9.39	327	1	2.8	238	-41	1.98	56	-49	Sandstone	17.3	0.32	Biaxial
Pentra/ clwydau	400	4.8x3.6	325	-36	10.7	15.2	285	63	8.8	252	-23	7.3	348	-13	Siltstone	17.6	0.39	Lab tests

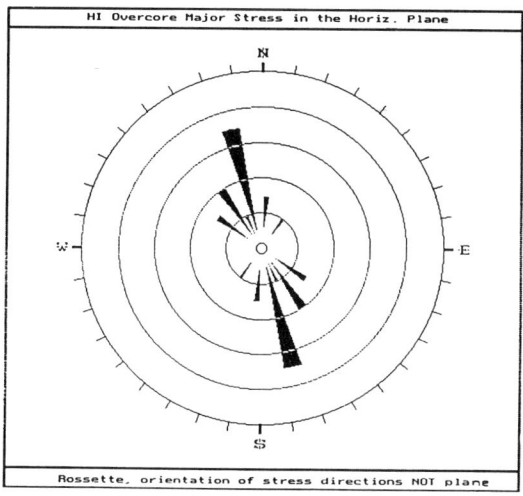

Figure 1 - Rosette indicating orientation of the major stress in the horizontal plane

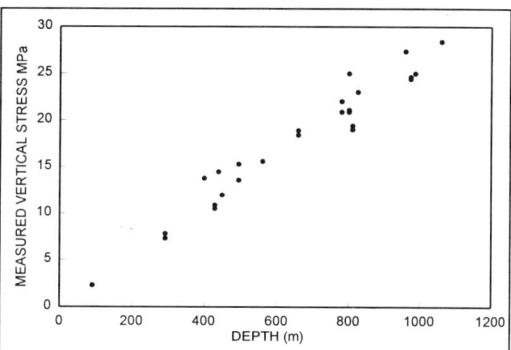

Figure 2 - Graph of vertical stress against depth.

a sector on the rosette indicates an increasing frequency of the maximum horizontal stress orientation in that direction. The most frequent orientation of the maximum stress resolved into the horizontal plane is between 340 and 350 degrees.

Comparison of the in-situ stress orientation in the United Kingdom with those of other parts of western Europe suggests that the NW-SE maximum horizontal stress direction is dominant over much of this area and originates from plate tectonic forces associated with the northerly to north westerly collision of the African and Eurasian plates and the south easterly push of the North Atlantic spreading ridge (Evans, 1987).

Based on the measured data, an analysis has been conducted on the magnitude of the stress components. In all cases the stresses have been resolved into the vertical and maximum and minimum horizontal normal components for ease of analysis.

The relationship between the measured vertical stress and depth below the surface is shown in Figure 2. This confirms the accepted theory that vertical stress is related to depth. Where γ is the unit weight (MN/m^3) of the overburden and z is the depth (m).

$$\sigma_v = \gamma.z \quad \text{(MPa)} \qquad (1)$$

A regression indicates that the gradient of the line is 0.025 MN/m^3 (the unit weight) with an R^2 correlation coefficient of 0.95. If the line is forced through the origin the value of the unit weight increases slightly to 0.027 MN/m^3 with an R^2 = 0.94. The results of the regression analysis are consistent with that expected from theory and other published data.

The relationship between the horizontal stress and depth is shown in Figure 3. It can be seen that a strong correlation with depth does not occur with either horizontal stress component. In both cases there is a general increase in the horizontal stress with depth, but there is considerable spread. Two tests indicate exceptionally high values of maximum horizontal stress. These were both undertaken at Asfordby Mine in a thin very stiff (53 - 56 GPa) sandstone bed.

The ratio of maximum to minimum horizontal stress has been plotted with respect to depth in Figure 4. With the exception of three tests, the ratio is fairly consistent with depth. If these three tests are not included in a statistical analysis the mean H_{max}/h_{min} ratio is 1.68 with a sample standard deviation of 0.35. It is not clear why the three anomalous ratios are much higher than the other test values and further investigation is required.

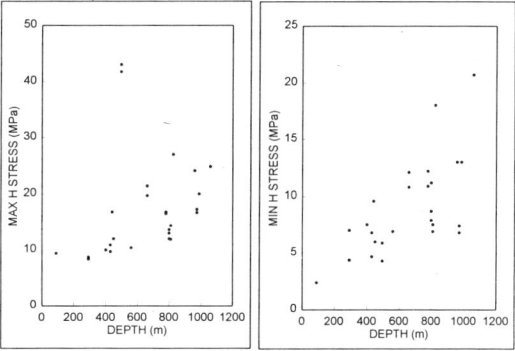

Figure 3 - Graphs of measured maximum and minimum horizontal stress against depth.

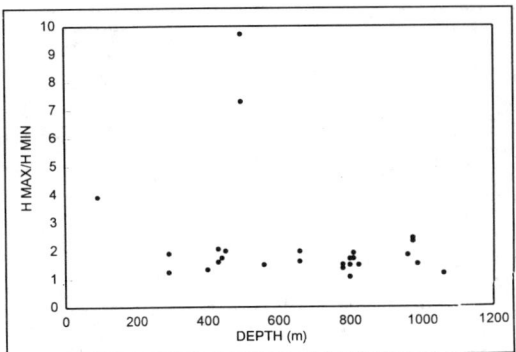

Figure 4 - Ratio of maximum to minimum horizontal stress against depth.

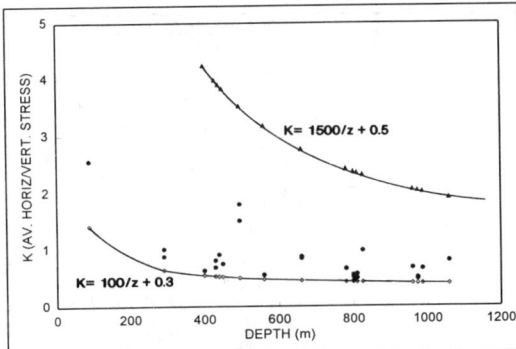

Figure 6 - Graph of k ($k = \sigma_{Hav.}/\sigma_V$) against depth.

Variations in the in-situ stress observed from earlier underground overcoring work have been shown to be related to formation stiffness (Bigby et al., 1992). Since this initial work further stress measurements have been undertaken which confirm the relationship between horizontal stress and rock stiffness. The graph of maximum horizontal stress against elastic modulus (E) which is shown in Figure 5 indicates a strong correlation between these quantities.

For the maximum horizontal stress a regression analysis gives :

$$\sigma_H = 0.782E - 0.98 \quad (MPa) \qquad (2)$$

$R^2 = 0.898$ and the standard error in the y estimate = 2.95 MPa.

A graph of k ($k = \sigma_{Hav.}/\sigma_V$) against the depth is shown in Figure 6. The results from the overcore stress measurements are consistent with those presented by Hoek and Brown (1980) and reside towards the lower bound for k as defined by Hoek and Brown and shown in Figure 6.

In summary, the above stress measurement results indicate that:

a. an anisotropic stress regime prevails within the UK Coal Measures.
b. the vertical stress is related to depth of burial with a mean unit weight of the overburden of approximately 0.027 MN/m^3.
c. there is a strong correlation between the maximum horizontal stress and the elastic modulus.
d. there is a general increase in the horizontal stress with depth of burial.

4. ESTIMATE OF MAXIMUM HORIZONTAL STRESS MAGNITUDE

The above analysis indicates that the maximum horizontal stress component is related to both the depth below the surface and the formation stiffness. In the following analysis a relationship has been investigated based upon two components. One is due to the depth of burial and the other which is termed the "tectonic component".

With regard to the depth of burial, using an elastic analysis, the induced horizontal stress of confined sedimentary strata is related to the vertical stress ($\sigma_v = \sigma_z = \gamma.z$) and the Poisson's ratio (v) by the formula:

$$\sigma_x = \sigma_y = \gamma.z.(v/1-v) \qquad (3)$$

This implies a constant induced stress in the horizontal plane at a given depth, irrespective of direction.

With regard to the tectonic component, a correlation

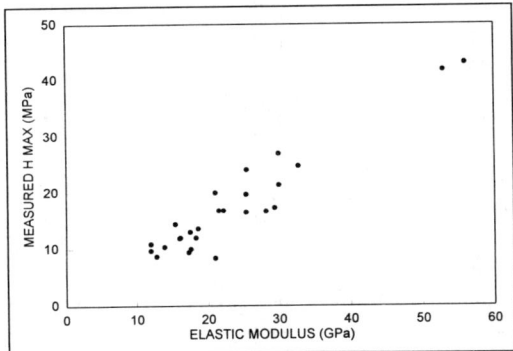

Figure 5 - Graph of maximum horizontal stress against elastic modulus.

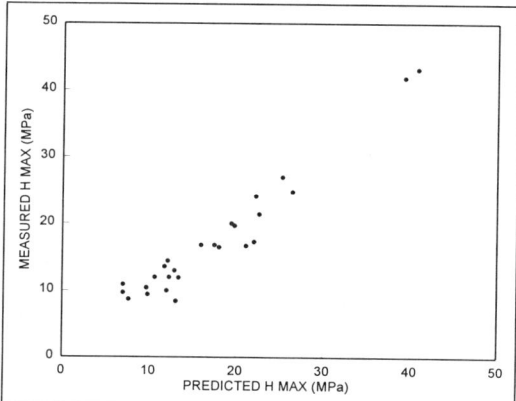

Figure 7 - Graph of measured against predicted maximum horizontal stress.

Table 2 Multiple Correlation Results for Maximum Horizontal Stress.

mines analysed	a_1	a_2	a_3	R^2	std. err. in σ_H est. MPa
all UK	0.0092	0.779	-3.998	0.936	2.39
all UK	0.0049	0.688	0	0.912	2.72
English	0.0090	0.803	-4.566	0.947	2.17
English	0.0038	0.716	0	0.93	2.45

has already been found linking the maximum horizontal stress to the elastic modulus of the rock. The tectonic component of the maximum horizontal stress is considered to be the product of the elastic modulus of the rock formation and a coefficient which can be thought of as a "tectonic strain". In the initial analysis a constant is also included in the tectonic component since a constant was evident in the relationship between maximum horizontal stress and elastic modulus. The approach brings together the above components in the following form:

$$\sigma_H = a_1 \cdot z \cdot (v/1-v) + a_2 \cdot E + a_3 \quad \text{(MPa)} \qquad (4)$$

where a_1 is a coefficient which includes the unit weight of the rock and therefore has units of MN/m^3, a_2 is a measure of tectonic strain and a_3 is a constant with the units of stress (MPa).

A multiple correlation analysis has been undertaken using the stress measurement data to generate values for the coefficients a_1, a_2, and the constant a_3 which allow a "best fit" estimation of the dependant variable σ_H. Using all the data in Table 1:

$$\sigma_H = 0.0092 \cdot z \cdot (v/1-v) + 0.779 \cdot E - 3.998 \qquad (5)$$

The statistics generated in the regression analysis give $R^2 = 0.94$ and the standard error in the y estimate $(\sigma_H) = 2.39$ MPa. This equation has been used to calculate a predicted value for the maximum horizontal stress for each site from the depth and the elastic properties of the test horizon. A graph of measured against predicted maximum horizontal stress is shown in Figure 7.

The above graph and statistics indicate that a good correlation exists between the measured and predicted stress magnitudes.

Additional multiple correlation analyses have been conducted without the constant a_3 and using only data for English mines which, due to their relative geographical proximity, are more likely to be part of the same regional stress environment. The results are summarised in Table 2.

The regression data indicates that the fit of the model improves when only English Mines are considered and although improved correlation does occur when the constant a_3 is included in the analysis, the effect of removing the constant (i.e. $a_3 = 0$) from the model is not significant.

A similar analysis was been conducted for the minimum horizontal stress using a model of similar form. The degree of correlation of this model with measured data was not as good as that obtained with the maximum horizontal stress model.

A sensitivity analysis indicates that the model is most sensitive to changes in the elastic modulus of the rock, with the depth and Poisson's ratio having only a marginal overall effect. This would indicate that the tectonic component is the major driving force in the development of the horizontal in-situ stress field.

5. CONCLUSIONS

Based on recent virgin in-situ stress measurement results obtained by overcoring in the United Kingdom Coal Measures, it is possible to make the following conclusions:
a. The results confirm that an anisotropic stress regime prevails in the UK Coal Measures.
b. The trend of the maximum horizontal stress component is NNW - SSE with anomalies related to structural features.
c. With the exception of three anomalous values, the

ratio of maximum to minimum horizontal stress remains fairly consistent with depth giving a mean ratio of 1.68. The reasons for the exceptional values are unclear and further investigation is required.

d. The vertical stress is related to the depth of burial and the unit weight of the overburden. From this data the unit weight of the overburden has been found to be 0.027 MN/m^3.

e. The relationship of k (k = σ_{Hav}/σ_V) with depth for the measured in-situ stress data is consistent with that found by Hoek and Brown (1980). In addition, a strong relationship has been confirmed between maximum horizontal stress and the elastic modulus of the rock.

f. A formula has been developed to estimate the maximum horizontal stress that occurs within the Coal Measures strata of the United Kingdom. The relationship relates the maximum horizontal stress to the depth, the elastic modulus and Poisson's ratio of the rock formation.

g. In sedimentary strata the magnitude of the horizontal stress should always be quoted with the elastic properties of the test horizon and the method of elastic property determination.

ACKNOWLEDGEMENTS

The author is grateful for the assistance provided by both his colleagues at Rock Mechanics Technology Ltd. and the advice of Professor R.J. Pine formerly of the Camborne School of Mines (now Golder Associates). The investigative work reported was funded by the mine operators and the European Coal and Steel Community.

REFERENCES

Altounyan P.F.R., Hindmarsh W.E., Leeming J. and Freeman P. 1997, Rapid gate road development for high production longwalls in deep mines. KOMAG Conference, Katowice, Poland.

Bigby D.N., Cassie J.W. and Ledger A.R. 1992 Absolute stress and stress change measurement in British Coal Measures. Eurock 1992, 390-395.

Evans C.J. 1987 Crustal Stress in the United Kingdom. Investigation of the Geothermal Potential of the UK, British Geological Survey.

Hoek E. and Brown E.T. 1980, Underground Excavations in Rock. Institute of Mining and Metallurgy, London.

ISRM. Suggested methods for rock stress determination. Int. J. Rock Mech. 1987, vol 24, 1, 53-73.

Mindata Ltd. CSIRO HI Stress Gauge, Field Manual, 1986.

Pine R.J., Jupe A. and Tunbridge L.W. 1990, An evaluation of in-situ stress measurements affecting different volumes of rock in Carmenellis granite. Scale Effects in Rock Masses, Pinto da Cunha (ed.), Balkema, Rotterdam, 269-277.

Pine R.J., Tunbridge L.W. and Kwakwa K. 1983, In-situ stress measurement in the Carmenellis granite. I - Overcoring tests at South Crofty Mine at a depth of 790 m. Int. J. Rock Mech. Min. Sci. and Geomech. Abstr. 20, 51-62.

Price Jones A. and Simms G.P. 1984, Measurement of in-situ rock stresses for a hydroelectric scheme in Peru. Proc. Design and Performance of Underground Excavation. pp191-198. ISRM/BGS, Cambridge, London.

Rummel F., Mohring-Erdman G. and Baumgartner J. 1986, Stress constraints and hydrofracturing stress data for the continental crust. Pageoph, Vol 124, Nos 4/5.

Stephansson O. 1993, Rock stress in the Fennoscandian Shield, Comprehensive Rock Engineering, Volume 3, Chapter 17, Pergamon Press.

Sugawara K. and Obara Y. 1993, Measuring rock stress: Case examples of rock engineering in Japan. Comprehensive Rock Engineering, Volume 3, Chapter 21, Pergamon Press.

Stability of interpanel-pillar due to longwall mining

K. Matsui, H. Shimada & M. Ichinose
Department of Mining Engineering, Kyushu University, Fukuoka, Japan

ABSTRACT : The Department of Mining Engineering, Kyushu University, in cooperation with Miike Colliery and the Coal Mining Research Center, Japan (CMRCJ), conducted research into an optimum design of interpanel-pillar in retreat longwall mining.

Field measurements of the deformation of the gateroads and of stress distribution in the pillar show that the designed layout of the longwall panel and interpanel-pillar and the supporting system are proper from the viewpoint of gateroad maintenance and spontaneous combustion in the pillar.

1 INTRODUCTION

Retreat longwall method with re-use of gateroad has been traditionally employed in Japan, mainly because of the advantage of higher recovery. But a new mining system or an interpanel-pillar system has been introduced to maximize the production efficiency. In this mining system, optimum design of interpanel-pillar is of critical importance for achieving safety, economy and efficiency of longwall mining. An optimum pillar must be designed so that it is able to maintain the gateroads until the passage of the second-panel longwall face and collapse soon thereafter. Improper designed pillars left in place are not only a waste of precious coal resources, but also create some problems such as excessive roadway closure and spontaneous combustion.

The purpose of this study is to assess the stability of the interpanel-pillar under the influence of longwall mining by means of continuous pillar load measurements using hydraulic borehole pressure cell and roadway closure measurements, on-site observations and gas injection technique.

2 SITE INVESTIGATION

2.1 Site Description

Figure 1 shows the study site located in the Second Upper seam in the West-80 area at Miike Colliery. There are no panels in the other two seams below the investigated area. In this area, the Second Upper seam is at a depth of about 430 m below sea level and the seam thickness varies between 4.0 m and 4.3 m. The seam is overlain and underlain by sandstone, but is locally underlain by shale. Mechanical properties of these rocks and coal deteriorate greatly

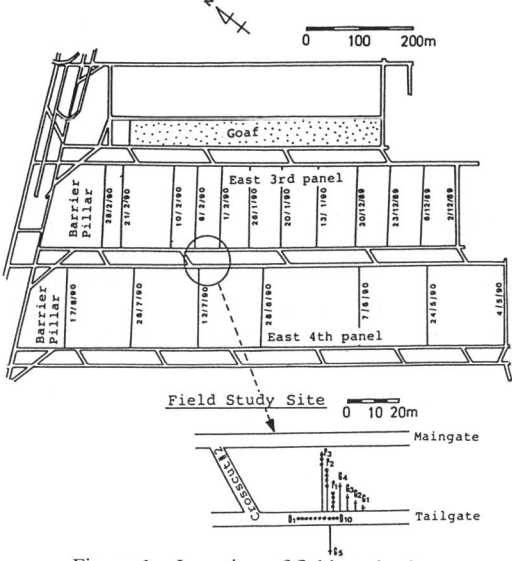

Figure 1 Location of field study site.

in the presence of water and shale exhibits a slaking phenomenon when it comes in contact with water.

The study site was selected in the tailgate of the East 4th panel. This gateroad was developed utilizing 25-m-wide diamond-shaped pillars, and was affected by the extraction of both panels (East 3rd and East 4th). Both faces were 150 m wide. The retreat distance of the East 3rd and the East 4th panels were approximately 680 m and 840 m, respectively. These faces are called the Miike High Power Plant (MHP) face, a new longwall mining system, using the larger powered, more efficient and mechanized mining equipment (Furukawa, 1989). The extracted height was about 2.8 m, leaving floor coal 1.5 m thick unworked. The rate of face advance was approximately 10 m/day in both cases.

The gateroads were driven by a roadheader of the MRH S-65 from Mitsui Miike Machinery Co., Ltd., and supported by a three-piece set of a trapezoidal shape with a 4.2 m steel beam and two 3.0 m wooden props at 1.0 m centers as shown in Figure 2. The supports were tied and lagged with wood. In the tailgate, strata bolting was used. Resin-grouted steel bolts and wooden dowels were not installed immediately after the excavation by the MRH S-65, but at about 50 m ahead of the active longwall face. Under poor strata conditions, supplemental wooden props along pillar were also erected ahead of the active face.

2.2 Instrumentation

Eight boreholes with 80 mm in diameter were drilled horizontally in the pillar and the tailgate rib of the next panel (East 4th) at the study site, as shown in Figure 1.

Three holes P1 to P3 were used to measure vertical load in the pillar by means of 11 borehole pressure cells developed by the CMRCJ. These pressure cell were arrayed to determine a profile of vertical load distribution across the instrumented pillar. Cell pressures were transmitted continuously through a phone line to a computer at a surface station and were also available at the site by reading a Bourdon pressure gauge.

Five boreholes G1 to G5 were used to measure permeabilities of the coal seam by means of nitrogen gas injection technique (Barron, 1978), as shown in Figure 3. This technique consists of two types of packers, movable type packer and fixed type packer.

A distribution of fractures along borehole was also observed using a borehole-scope.

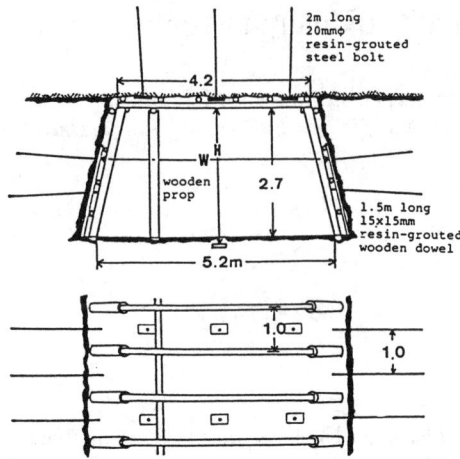

Figure 2   Support system in tailgate.

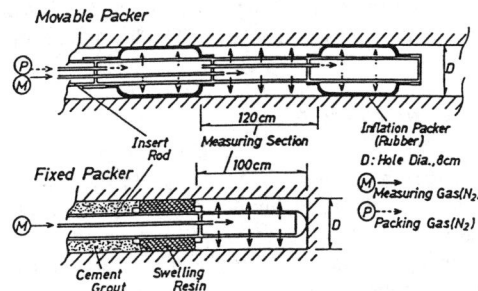

Figure 3   Apparatus of gas injection technique.

Supplemental information was obtained from the measurements of vertical and side closure at the ten station D1 to D10, as shown in Figure 1. Roadway deformation was determined by the variation of height between the marks at the roof and the floor, H, and of width between the marks on the heads of wooden dowels at the sides, W, as shown in Figure 2.

Monitoring of these variables was conducted during the extraction of both adjacent panels (East 3rd and 4th).

2.3 Results and Discussion

A borehole-scope investigation shows that several large open cracks and borehole wall collapses were clearly observed within 1.5 m from the mouth of the each hole. This implies that failure zone was created around the roadway during and after the roadway development. This was also confirmed by nitrogen gas injection technique using movable type packers.

Figure 4 shows the profiles of vertical load distribution across the instrumented pillar corresponding to several face positions, which clearly exhibits the high magnitude asymmetric loading across the pillar. As the face approaches the study site, the greatest loading takes place within 3 m of the pillar edge near the active panel. After the passage of the face, the greatest loading transfers to the center of the pillar, indicating that coal fracture yielding occurs within about 7 m of the face-side pillar edge and a pillar core is formed in the center of the pillar.

Figure 5 presents the changes in permeability in the pillar during extraction of the East 3rd panel. As mentioned above about pillar loading, the changes in permeability in the coal near the tailgate (G1) shows a higher value than those at the pillar center, representing the fracture formation in the proximity of tailgate during and after development. As the face pulls even with the site, the permeability decreases remarkably because of the installation of fully resin-grouted dowels into the pillar rib, as shown in Figure 2. However, as the face advances beyond the site, the value becomes greater, indicating the occurrence of fracturing by the side abutment loading. The permeability from G2 also increases after the passage of the face. On the other hand, the permeability in the pillar core shows a low value even after the extraction of the East 3rd panel, indicating that no fracture yielding occurs in the pillar core.

Figure 6 presents the profiles of vertical load distribution across the pillar at several face positions of the next East 4th panel. As the next panel face approaches, the maximum pressure of the cell in the pillar center decreases, indicating that coal yielding occurs in the pillar core. Afterwards the pressures of cells nearer the 4th panel begin to increase. However, as the face approaches within 30 m of the study site, the cell pressures decrease and reach the residual strength level of the pillar. This indicates that the fractured yield zone is created across the entire pillar. Figures 7 and 8 are observed patterns of the vertical closure in the tailgate of the East 4th panel during the extraction of the East 3rd and 4th panels. The gateroad begins to deform at 20-40 m ahead of the faceline. After the passage of the face, the deformations increase rapidly, and tend to reach the constant levels within 200 m behind the faceline. The vertical and side closures exhibit a similar trend, but the former is less than the latter, because the roof rock is relatively strong and almost intact. With the

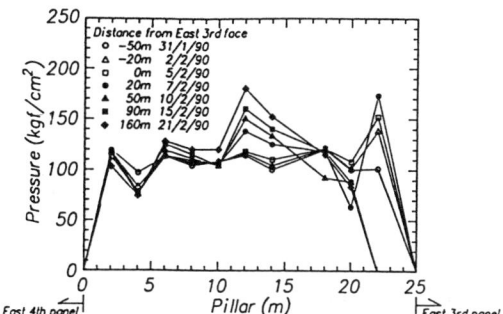

Figure 4 Vertival pressure profile across the instrumented pillar.

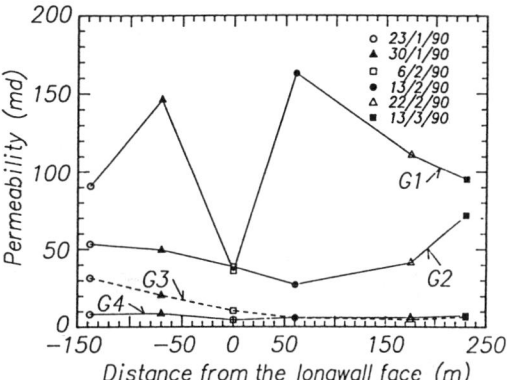

Figure 5 Changes in permeability during the extraction in the East 3rd panel.

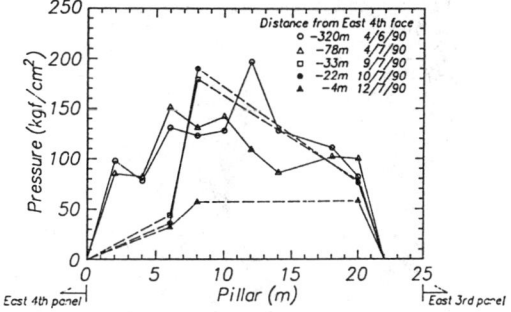

Figure 6 Vertical pressure profile across the instrumented pillar.

approach of the next East 4th face, the gateroad begins to deform rapidly at 40-50 m ahead of the faceline and reaches the peak value at the faceline. Although the study site was located under relatively good strata conditions, pillar and rib spallings were

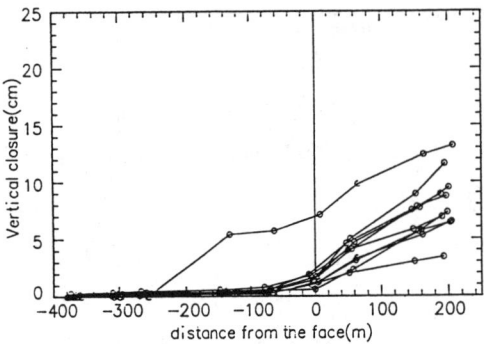

Figure 7 Roadway closures in the tailgate during the extraction of the East 3rd panel.

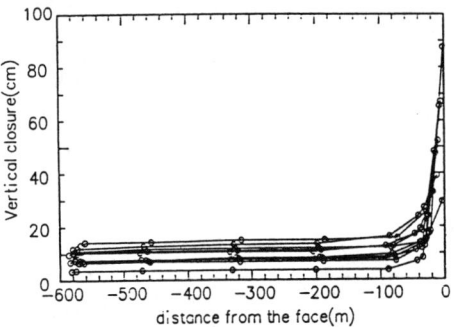

Figure 8 Roadway closures in the tailgate during the extraction of the East 4th panel.

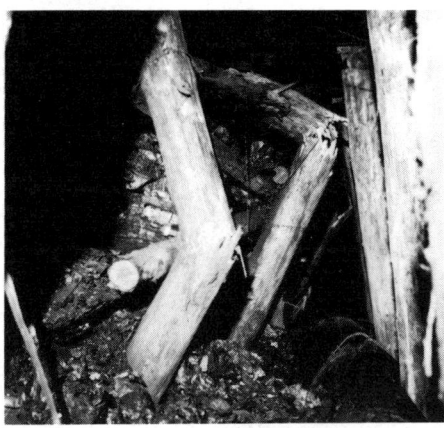

Figure 9 Spalling of pillar and failure of wooden props after the passage of the East 3rd face.

observed and some installed dowels were failed when the face approaches within 30 m. This behavior is anticipated from the results of pressure monitoring in the pillar. However, thanks to the strata bolting, the supports were kept stable without failure and excessive distortion. In order to improve the situation further, longer dowels should be installed into both sides. Under poor strata conditions, however, excessive spalling of pillar and rib and floor heaving occurred and wooden props along the pillar were almost broken even after the passage of the first East 3rd face, as shown in Figure 9. However, it should be noted that under poor strata conditions, roof bolting contributes to the stability of roof without excessive bending or distortion of the roof beam of the support.

3 CONCLUSION

Field measurements and observation for assessment of stability of interpanel-pillar of longwall mining for roadway maintenance and spontaneous combustion were performed.

Results show that the stability of the pillar is sufficient to maintain the gateroad and prevent air leakage through the pillar under good strata conditions, although under poor strata conditions, excessive deformation was observed. In order to establish the optimum pillar design method, more research should be carried out.

ACKNOWLEDGMENTS

During the preparation of this paper, Miike Colliery, the largest coal mine in Japan, closed down because of adverse market conditions.

The authors would like to thank the many mining engineers and workers at Miike Colliery for their help and cooperation in this research project.

Any opinions stated in this paper are those of the authors themselves and not necessarily those of the colliery, or the CMRCJ.

REFERENCES

Barron, K. 1978. An Air Injection Technique for Investigating the Integrity of Pillars and Ribs in Coal Mines, Int. Journal of Rock Mechanics & Mining Sciences & Geomechanics Abstracts, Vol. 15, 69-76.

Furukawa, H. 1989. Development of High Productivity Plant (called MHP), Journal of Mining and Material Processing Institute of Japan, Vol. 105, No. 11, 808-811, (in Japanese).

Experimental study on the relation between in-situ stress and permeability of coal

T.Yamaguchi, Y.Oikawa, T.Narita & H.Kobayashi
Department of Geo Engineering, National Institute for Resources and Environment, Tsukuba, Japan

X.M.Zhang
New Energy and Industrial Technology Development Organization, Japan

ABSTRACT: *In-situ* permeability of coalbed plays an important role in mining of CBM(Coalbed Methane). As permeability of coal is greatly affected by *in-situ* stress, the differential strain curve analysis was applied to coal specimen to estimate the stress state. A permeability of coal specimen as a function of confining pressure was also measured. From these experiments, it is shown that *in-situ* permeability of coal can be estimated from a mechanical behavior or coal.

1 INRODUCTION

In a coal mine, CBM (coalbed methane or coalseam gas) had been studied from the point of view of preventing disasters like gas explosion. Recently, CBM have been utilized as one of the clean natural energy resources. Especially in United States, a total amount of annual product of CBM was 156 billion cubic-meter and it occupied about 3 % of total natural gas product in 1992 and has been still increasing. In Japan, CBM has not been produced commercially, so far. But a total reserve of CBM is estimated about 2,500 billion cubic-meter and regarded as one of the promising domestic energy.

In developing CBM, like other natural gas, wells are drilling from ground surface to penetrate coal seams. Thus the in-situ permeability of coal seams determines productivity of a CBM mining system. Because a methane gas mainly flows through cracks within a coal, and cracks are closed by *in-situ* stress, estimation of *in-situ* stress state is very important. In this paper, *in-situ* stress state was estimated by laboratory tests at first. Then the permeability of coal specimen was measured as a function of confining pressure. Finally, permeability of coal is related to the strain behavior observed at DSCA experiment.

2 EXPERIMENTAL PROCEDURE

2.1 *Differential strain curve analysis (DSCA)*

A coal specimen used for DSCA were taken from the Kushiro coal mine in Hokkaido, Japan. An overburden of a face, from where a coal block was taken, was about 700-m. In coal specimen preparation, all cutting and grinding was done in dry condition. Five cubic specimen which has a side length of 50 mm were made from one coal block. Twenty-four foil strain gauges were attached to each cubic coal specimen with epoxy resin adhesive. Before attaching strain gauges onto the coal specimen, the same epoxy resin adhesive were used to fill up hollows on a specimen surface. Each coal specimen was sealed by a silicone sealant. Figure 1 shows an arrangement of strain gauges on a development surface of a cubic coal specimen. In this figure, Z direction consists with vertical direction. Because the coal block was not oriented as to magnetic direction, there is no information about relationship between magnetic direction and X or Y direction of strain gauges. But of all five cubic coal specimen, the direction of X coinsides with each other.

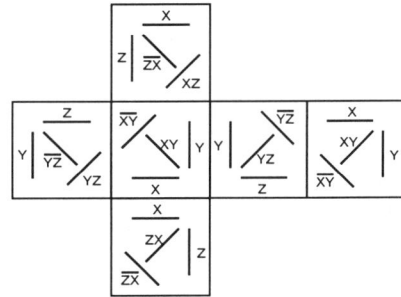

Figure 1. Development surface of a cubic coal specimen.

2.2 Transient pressure build-up analysis (TPBA)

Air permeability of coal specimen was measured by TPBA. Two cylindrical specimen were made from coal blocks. This coal blocks were taken from the same coal mine mentioned above, but an overburden of the face was about 560m. A dimension of the cylindrical specimen is 50mm in diameter, and 100mm in height. In this experiment, the specimen was prepared that the air is flowing along the X-Y plane shown in Figure 1. Figure 2 shows a schematic view of TPBA. The coal specimen is set into the confining pressure vessel. At first, a confining pressure in the vessel is kept at atmospheric pressure. Then by closing valve 5 and opening valve 7, the gas pressure vessel is evacuated by the vacuum pump. Immediately after the valve 5 is open, the air flows through coal specimen, the pressure in the gas vessel is continuously increasing to atomosperic pressure. By monitoring and analyzing the transient pressure in the gas vessel, permeability is calculated. After increasing the confining pressure to higher value and kept constant at that value, the same procedure is repeated to obtain another permeability under higher confining pressure. Usually, for the purpose of measuring permeability, differential pressure between both sides of a specimen is kept constant, and flow rate of gas is measured. Comparing with this conventional method, TPBA has an advantage that the apparatus is simpler. On the other hand, TPBA has a disadvantage that it takes long time before the pressure of gas vessel converges to atomosperic pressure under high confining pressure.

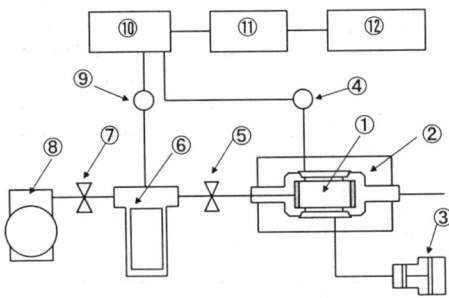

Figure 2. Schematic view of TPBA apparatus
(1.Coal sample, 2.Confining pressure vessel, 3.Servo-controlled intensifier, 4.Pressure transducer, 5.Valve, 6.Gas pressure vessel, 7.Valve, 8.Vacuum pump, 9.Pressure transducer, 10.Signal conditioner, 11.A-D converter, 12.Data logger)

3 RESULTS

3.1 DSCA

In DSCA experiment, a confining pressure was applied up to 20 MPa. Figure 3 shows typical strain curves as a function of the confining pressure observed during experiment. These strain curves are classified into three types as is shown in Figure 3. Type A is most commonly observed during experiments. 91 strain gauges out of 120 show this tendency. In Figure 3, β indicates an intrinsic compressibility. ε^* indicates a difference between straight line on a intrinsic strain part and observed strain. Here, ε_0^* is defined as zero-confining pressure intercept along the straight line. P^* indicates a confining pressure at which all cracks are completely closed. Type B, which was observed 16 cases out of 120, shows straight part at low confining pressure (from 2MPa to 5MPa in Figure 3). Then the inclination of strain curve is increasing. In this case, it is difficult to define β. Type C, which was observed 13 cases, has apparently obvious tendency. Although a straight part is observed, ε_0^* is a negative value.

Excluding the strain curves which fell into categories of type B or C, direction of principal stress were estimated by DSCA for each five coal specimen. The detailed procedure of DSCA is shown by Oikawa (1993), although Oikawa applied DSCA not for coal specimen but crystalline rock. In Figure 4, estimated direction of principle stress are shown. Except for coal specimen no.3, which includes many type B or C strain curves, directions of maximum stress indicated by solid circles are almost vertical. Although, there is no distinct tendency for directions of intermediate(solid triangles) and minimum (solid squares) principle stress, it seems that intermediate principle stress directions are 45 degrees rotated unclockwisely from X-direction, and minimum principle stress directions are 45 degrees rotated unclockwisely from Y-direction. The DSCA also gives a ratio of

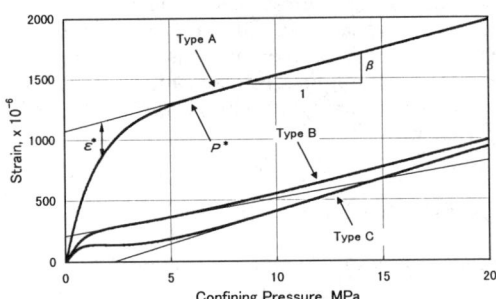

Figure 3. Typical strain curve observed in DSCA.

maximum, intermediate and minimum principle stress magnitude. Excluding coal specimen no.3, which showed different tendency of principle stress compared to other specimen, these ratios are summarized in Table 1. The average of these ratio is 1.00:0.65:0.26. The overburden was about 700m. If the specific gravity of the overburden was assumed to be 2.0, then the magnitudes of *in-situ* maximum, intermediate and minimum are 14.0, 9.1 and 3.6 MPa, respectively.

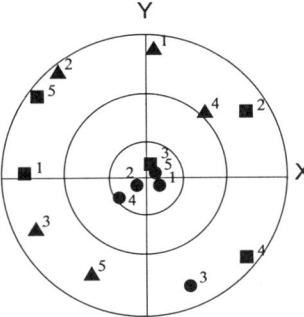

Figure 4. Estimated principle stress directions on lower hemisphere. Circle is maximum, triangle is intermediate and square is minimum stress direction.

Table 1. Estimated ratios of principal stress magnitude

Sample ID	Ratio of principal stress magnitude Max. : Int. : Min.
D1	1.00 : 0.74 : 0.45
D2	1.00 : 0.36 : 0.12
D4	1.00 : 0.80 : 0.16
D5	1.00 : 0.68 : 0.31

3.2 TPBA

In Figure 5, bold lines are experimental results of pressure build-up curves under confining pressure of 0 MPa(atmospheric pressure) to 5.9 MPa. Thin lines in Figure 5 are numerical results calculated by a differential element method to fit experimental result under each confining pressure. As is seen from this figure, there are good agreement between measured and calculated results. Thus a permeability under each confining pressure can be estimated from this analysis.

Figure 6 shows relation between confining pressure and permeability for specimen T1 and T2. In this figure, confining pressure is expressed by a gauge pressure. Following relationship between confining pressure P and permeability k is obtained empirically. In this equation, confining pressure, P is normalized by atmospheric pressure P_0. Thus, a permeability k_0 is a permeability of a specimen under atmospheric pressure P_0. In equation (3.1), coefficients a and b in equation (3.1) for both T1 and T2 coal specimen are 0.6 and 0.5, respectively.

$$k = \frac{k_0}{\exp a \left(P / P_0 \right)^b} \tag{3.1}$$

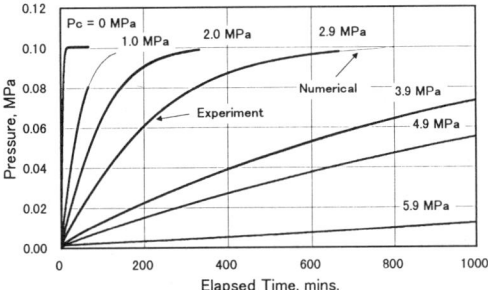

Figure 5. Observed pressure build-up curves.

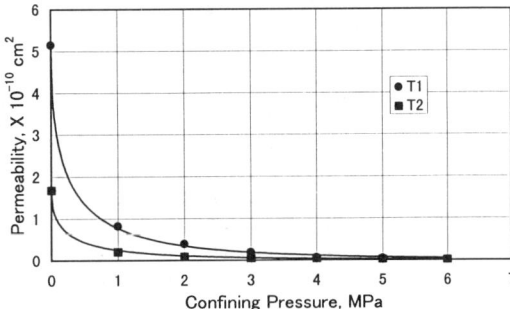

Figure 6. Confining pressure vs. permeability.

4 DISCUSSION

A permeability of coal specimen is strongly affected by confining pressure as is shown in Figure 6. Because a gas flows through cracks or pore within coal, a permeability should be related to deformability of coal. In both DSCA and TPBA experiments, coal specimen were made from intact coal blocks and did not include any visible open cracks on a surface of specimen. It is more likely that visible open cracks plays a main role on *in-situ* permeability. A following discussion is limited to only an intact part of a coal.

A coal generally has a plane anisotropy in deformablity. To confirm a plane anisotropic behavior, strain curves and ε^*, defined in Figure 1, are plotted in Figures 7 and 8.

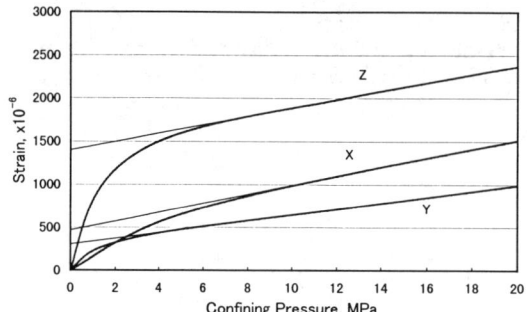

Figure 7. Strain curves for X, Y and Z direction

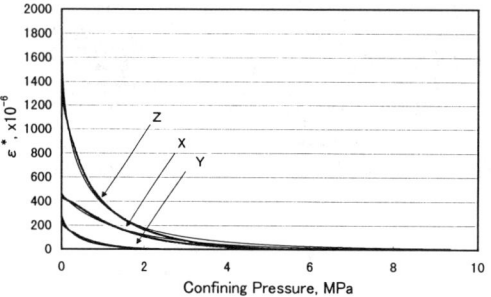

Figure 8. Confining pressure vs. ε^*.

In Figure 8, ε^* for X, Y and Z directions are plotted as a function of confining pressure. Apparently, ε^* along Z-direction, which is parallel to vertical direction, has a largest value compared to another direction. Empirical equation (4.1) is fitted to ε^* curves which have direction along X, Y or Z.

$$\varepsilon^* = \frac{\varepsilon_0^*}{\exp c \left(P/P_0 \right)^d} \quad (4.1)$$

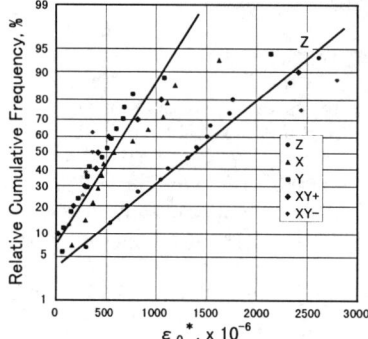

Figure 9. Distribution of ε_0^* along Z direction, and directions within X-Y plane.

It is shown from Figure 9 that the average of ε_0^* along Z-direction is about 1400×10^{-6}, which is almost twice as large as another direction.

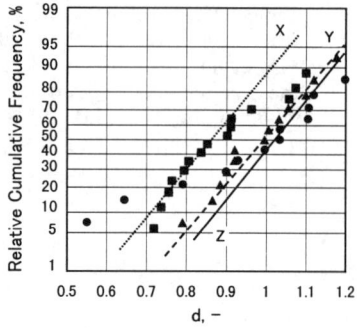

Figure 10. Distribution of d in equation (4.1).

A coefficient d in equation(4.1) was calculated and a distribution are plotted in Figure 10. The average of coefficient d is almost 1. A coefficient c fall into a range 0.01~0.40. An average of intrinsic compressibility β was about 60 MPa^{-1} and there is no distinct difference in direction.

From equations (3.1) and (4.1), a following equation is derived.

$$\ln \frac{k_0}{k} = \alpha \left[\ln \frac{\varepsilon_0^*}{\varepsilon^*} \right]^\gamma \quad (4.2)$$

Coefficients α and γ are calculated from a, b, c and d in equations (3.1) and (4.1). Using equation (4.2), permeability can be estimated from ε^*.

5 CONCLUSIONS

1. The differential strain curve analysis (DSCA) was applied to coal specimen. *In-situ* stress state were estimated.
2. Permeability of coal specimen was measured by the transient pressure build-up analysis (TPBA). The relation between confining pressure and permeability can be expressed by an empirical equation (3.1).
3. In DSCA experiment, coal specimen shows a strong plane anisotropic behavior. This behavior can be expressed by equation (4.1).
4. Equation (4.2) is proposed to estimate a coal permeability from ε^*, defined in Figure 3.

REFERENCES

Oikawa, Y et al. 1993.Differential strain curve analysis to estimate the stress state of the Hijioiri hot dry rock field, *Int.J. Rock Mech. Min. Sci. & Geomech. Abstr*, 30:1023-1026.

Application of rock stress measurements in civil engineering

Significance of in-situ stress measurement in the practice regarding engineering projects

Li Fangquan
Institute of Crustal Dynamics, SSB, Beijing, People's Republic of China

ABSTRACT: In-situ stress state has been shown to be important for engineering constructions. As for large and medium-size works, it is imperative to have in-situ stress measurement as a key procedure, so that we can use the favorable and avoid the unfavorable aspects of the stress state to achieve reasonable designs.
    The relationship between the in-situ stress measurement and engineering as well as the applications of the stress data to various fields of engineering are discussed in the present paper.

1 INTRODUCTION

In the analysis of stability of construction of rock engineering, and taking power source and mineral source, the in-situ stress state in the crust of the earth has to be known. For rock mechanics and engineering, the in-situ stress measurement appears to be more important. Because the basic task of rock mechanics is to research the mechanical behavior of rock and rock mass under static and dynamic load, which deals with the stress measurement and deformation. By the above reasons, in the designing of engineering, the magnitude, the direction and the distribution of in-situ stress is the one of the important data, which can not be lack of. Some scientists consider: once we can not determine the in-situ stress in the earth crust and rock around tunnels, the rock engineering is a kind of techniques only. If rock mechanics were developed to be a kind of science which was used in the engineering practically, the proper method of measurement of in-situ stress would have to be figured out(Stagg and Zienkiewicz 1978). For important engineering, the measurement of in-situ stress, studying the stress state of rock mass, is to recognize the mechanical nature of rock, clearly failure mechanism of round rock mass fully, make engineering designing more reasonably, safely and economically.

2 THE RELATIONSHIP BETWEEN TUNNEL AND STABILITY OF ROUND ROCK MASS

In the region of high stress and deep rock mass, because of existing high magnitude of stress, which makes the wall of tunnel and under-ground house fall apart, deformation of tunnel, even failure and burst of rock. The direction and shape of the intersection of tunnel are selected reasonably, which reduce the tensile stress of boundary of tunnel to be least, and reduce the concentration of the compressive stress least, so that the engineering can keep to be stable. The stability of the round rock mass of under-ground house is determined by the ratio and absolute magnitude of two stresses, σ_H is the horizontal stress and the σ_v is the vertical stress, the direction of them is perpendicular to the axis of tunnel. For the circular-shape of intersection of under-ground house, when the absolute magnitude of the in-situ stress is not too big, and $\sigma_H/\sigma_v=1$, the distribution of perimeter stress of opening is uniform, the stability of the round rock mass is the best. When $\sigma_H/\sigma_v<1/3$, the tensile stress will be on the roof of the under-ground house, the compressive stress is on the side wall, magnitude of which is bigger than $2.67\sigma_v$. When $\sigma_H/\sigma_v>3$, the tensile stress is on the side wall, the compressive stress is on the roof, the magnitude of which is bigger than $8\sigma_v$(Yamaguch and Nishimatsu 1982).
    Because of those above, when the horizontal stress is bigger than the vertical stress, the long axis of the under-ground house will be put on to the direction of the maximum horizontal principal stress; and when the vertical stress is bigger than the horizontal stress, the long axis will be on the direction of the minimum horizontal principal stress. For example, in a tunnel of a mine where is in Jing Chuan in our country, the depth of the mine is 450 meters below the ground, the intersection of the tunnel is like the shape of the horse hoof, which was lined by precast concrete, $\sigma_H/\sigma_v=2$, there were some serious longitudinal tensile fracturings in the central

part of the tunnel, the roof was compressed into a peach-shape. In Russia, in a mine named Laswumchor where was located in Kola peninsula Shibin land mass, when the principal and assistant tunnels were dug, the rock burst once appeared. By observation, the rock burst occurred on the roof of the tunnel which was made of ijolite-urtite rock with brittle elasticity; and the serious rock burst occurred in the tunnel, the orientation of which was in the direction of south-north, in the tunnel, the orientation of which was in the direction of west-east, there was almost no rock burst to occur. In mine body, even though there were some rock bursts to occur, but the intensities of which were weaker. The occurring regulation of rock burst in the region indicated, that exception of nature difference of rock, it was controlled by the field of in-situ stress of the earth crust. Measuring the in-situ stress in the region, there was high horizontal stress there, and the direction of the maximum horizontal principal stress was almost in the east-west(Peiwei et al. 1978).

The compressive strength of rock is much bigger than it's tensile strength. Even though the compressive stress is so large, but there is no problem to be worried. And the tensile strength of rock is usually less than 10MPa, so existing tensile stress, the tensile strength of round rock is over easy, which makes the tunnel to be failure. By said above, it is very important that the shape of the tunnel is selected reasonably, therefore make the tensile stress of round rock to be least.

3 THE STABILITY AND THE BEARING LOAD CAPABILITY OF ROUND ROCK IN THE TUNNEL WITH HIGH PRESSURE

In the designing of tunnel with high pressure, from coordinating condition of deformation of lining and rock mass, how many inner hydraulic pressure loading on the rock mass can be calculated. But is the rock mass able to bear this part of inner hydraulic pressure? There is a problem of the bearing capacity of round rock. Therefore exception of researching nature of deformation of rock mass, and the bearing capacity of round rock has to be researched. In the condition of the tunnel with high pressure, the high deformation in the radius direction can make steel pipe yield and failure the construction of liner. So if the stress and strength of the round rock were analyzed, the capability of bearing load of the round rock could be determined reasonably.

For the rock mass with fractures, the limited inner hydraulic pressure that the surrounding rock mass can bear is given below:

$$P_i = 1/2[(P+Q)+2(P-Q)\cos2\theta](1-\sin\Phi)+C\cos\Phi$$

In the formula P, Q are the major and minor horizontal principal stresses in the surrounding rock; P_i is the inner hydraulic pressure of the tunnel; θ is an angle between P_i and Q; Φ is the internal friction angle; C is the cohesion of rock mass.

From formula being known, the limited inner hydraulic pressure that the surrounding rock can bear is consisted of two parts, one is the nature stress and the another is the internal viscous stress. So, when the values of C and Φ are known, the essential is determined by the in-situ stress. In designing, the in-situ stress is able to make the value of permissible bearing stress of the rock mass go to be high, and make the rock mass bear much more inner hydraulic pressure. This is why in many engineerings, when the inner hydraulic pressure is high, the thickness of the overburden of the rock mass is not too big, and the liner is more thinner, but the stability is still good.

In Yun Nan province of our country, in a hydropower station, the steel pipe which bore high pressure was buried in basalt of Permian Period, the overburden is only 32 meters, once the stability of surrounding rock mass was worried about in the effect of the inner hydraulic pressure. But however by the measurement of the in-situ stress, it discovered that in that region the horizontal stress was much more larger than the vertical stress, the designing plan which let the nature stress of the round rock mass bear a part of the inner hydraulic pressure was adopted. After the hydropower station was constructed, and operated, the stability of the round rock mass was good. By the data of practical measurement of the deformation of the tunnel and the steel, the round rock mass was bore by some inner hydraulic pressure the magnitude of which was 11.5 to 12 MPa which was about 83% to 86% of the designing inner hydraulic pressure(Jin and Wu 1976).

Because of the test of hydraulic fracturing and the measurement of the in-situ stress, there is a full basis of the designing of the tunnel with high pressure, so the requirement of the quality of the steel was reduced, the thickness of the steel plat was reduced to be thinner, let the technology more simple, speed up the engineering, and save a lot of investment. Therefore in the designing of the tunnel with high pressure and the steel pipe with high pressure that buried underground, considering the strength and the distribution of the stress of the round rock mass which is a great practical meaning for the economic and reliable designing of liner.

4 THE RELATIONSHIP BETWEEN THE IN-SITU STRESS AND THE STABILITY OF THE SIDE SLOPE

The re-distribution stress field of the rock mass of the side slope is the comprehensive result of the effect of the nature stress field of the rock mass and the local stress field which is from the unloading effect. So the state of the stress in the rock mass influences the stability of the rock mass of the side slope. The degree of the influence of the state of the nature stress on the stability of the side slope relies on the relationship between the direction of the surface of slope and the direction of the nature stress, and also relies on the ratio of the horizontal stress and the vertical stress, that is σ_H/σ_v. When the vertical stress is the least principal stress, and one of the two horizontal principal stresses is perpendicular or parallel to the orientation of the side slope strike separately, the more the ratio of the horizontal principal stress and the vertical stress, (σ_H/σ_v) the direction of which is perpendicular to the orientation of the side slope, is large, and the more the shear stress (σ_τ) which is parallel to the orientation of the side slope is large, the more the side slope is not stable(Li and Pan 1970).

Research indicated that the largest magnitude of the shear stress in the side slope is usually distributes at the foot of the side slope and near the region of the side slope surface, and the magnitude of the largest shear stress often increases when the ratio of the original horizontal principal stress to the original vertical principal stress and the angle of the slope increase. Under the effect of the gravity, hydraulic pressure, vibration and the other external forces, the angle of unstable nature slope and the man-made slope of the angle of which is too large when it is designed, is able to slide and failure often, which can make the people injure and lose their properties. On the other hand, if the unstable of the slope is considered too seriously, the angle of the man-made slope is designed to be too gentle, or some unnecessary measures are adopted, which makes the term of the construction postpone, waste the money and the manpower. Therefore, measuring the in-situ stress, studying the characteristic of the redistribution stress field of the rock mass of the slope, testing in advance, designing and controlling the stability of the slope, has a great important meaning.

5 MEASUREMENT OF THE IN-SITU STRESS AND THE STABILITY OF BASEMENT OF DAM

When the concrete dam is constructed on the rock mass, because the unloading effect while digging is going on, which makes the basement pit rise and rebound, at the same time makes the rock mass of the wall of the pit displaced towards to the inside of the pit in the radial direction. This deformation of the rock mass under the least principal stress in the vertical direction, the stress in the horizontal direction is larger; when there is a horizontal weak plane in the rock mass, the situation said above, is more remarkable. At the same time, which is able to make the rock mass of the pit wall dislocate along the weak plane in the near horizontal direction. This deformation and dislocation of the rock mass might make the quality of the engineering worse, and influence the stability of the construction.

By the measuring data, the value rebound rising of the pit bottom, and the distance of dislocation along the near horizontal weak plane of the rock mass of the pit wall, is usually from millimeters to centimeters, the largest is to tens centimeters, sometimes to several meters. For example, in a hydropower station of our country, during construction of the basement pit for the generator, the rock mass near the bottom of the pits on the upper reaches pit walls of generator pits number one and two, in the mud-changing plane of number 212 layer the appear tilt of which is from 1.0° to 3.0°, dislocated reverse ,the largest dislocation distance was to 8 centimeters.

From said above, it can be seen that the nature stress state of the rock mass influences very much to the displacement of the basement pit and sliding dislocation of the rock mass of the pit wall along the horizontal weak plane.

The rebound rising, displacement and dislocation of the rock mass of the basement pit, which makes the permeability of the basement rock mass increase, and make it's mechanical nature worse. The another, because the displacement and the dislocation of the basement pit is a course which needs some time, if the course effects until the touch part of the construction with the rock mass has been done, the continuous displacement and the dislocation of the rock mass will make the construction be effected by the extra stress even make the construction displacement and fracturing(Li 1985).

6 THE MEASUREMENT OF THE IN-SITU STRESS AND PROCESS OF THE NUCLEAR WASTE

In the wake of development in the nuclear industry, how to process the radiant nuclear waste, more and more attention is paid to by the people. One effective method of the processing the nuclear waste liquid is the use of the hydrofracturing that compresses mixture of cement paste and the nuclear waste into the rock mass which is located down below the ground for hundreds meters by high pressure and solidify, the purpose of which is seal up for safekeeping for ever, reduce the pollution to the least limit for the relationship between organisms and their environment. Using this method of processing the nuclear waste, the problem to which the people pay attention is if the tensile fracture which perpendicular to the surface of the earth and the steep tilt tensile fracture can be made while the paste is injected in the rock mass; because, this kind of fracture is able to make the nuclear waste liquid flow out and to destroy the safekeeping effect of the overburden, and connect with the ground water, which pollutes the environment seriously. Therefore, the orientation of the fracture by the hydrofracturing should be near the horizontal direction, and the layer with the mixture of the cement paste with the nuclear waste should be near to the horizontal direction too, this is the basic require when the process of the hydrofracturing is used.

Obviously, making the near horizontal fracturing is related to geology, the original stress field of the rock mass and the variation of the stress field when the paste is injected into. So measuring the in-situ stress, knowing the character of the original stress field and the variation of the stress field is undoubtedly very important for the processing the nuclear waste safely.

By the theory studying and a lot of hydrofracturing tests in the laboratory and practice in the field, in agreement the orientation of the fracturing by the hydrofracturing is dominated by the state of the stress of the point fractured. If there is no other disturbing the direction fractured by the hydrofracturing is always perpendicular to the direction of the least principal stress. This means that the fracturing orientation is controlled by the state of the in-situ stress.

The fracturing orientation is influenced by the in-situ stress, which can be varied by the other factors, the important one is the unisotrope of the strength of rock. For example, shale, the strength being perpendicular to the layer plane is smaller, and the strength being parallel to the layer plane is larger, so it is easy fractured along the direction of the layer plane. For the rock formation the layer plane of which is near horizontal, if the difference of the in-situ stress is smaller than the difference of the tensile strength, even though the vertical portion of the in-situ stress is larger than the horizontal portion, it is possible to make a horizontal fracturing. At a one fields of the processing nuclear waste, the data of the measuring the in-situ stress in two boreholes indicated: the stress state of the processing field was $\sigma_H > \sigma_h > \sigma_v$, from the shallow to the deep, and the more the deep, the more the difference of the horizontal principal stress with the vertical principal stress was large, which was good for making and extending of the horizontal fracturing when the hydrofracturing was going. Afterwards, according to the injecting test, it was discovered that the boundary of the paste piece and the tilt angle were more stable; The tilt angle of the paste piece was 7° to 25°, the fracturing was basically thought to be near horizontal(Li et al. 1993).

7 THE RELATIONSHIP BETWEEN MEASUREMENT OF THE IN-SITU STRESS AND THE REGION STABILITY

At any region, the property and the intensity of the present tectonic movement is determined by the stress state of that region and the mechanical property of the rock mass. By the view of the geo-engineering, earthquake is the most important kind of the present tectonic movement.

In some regions the reservoirs were built, which changed the original stress state, and coursed reservoir induced earthquake. Studying indicated that the burst of the reservoir earthquake was mainly related to the seismic geologic condition where the earthquake burst, especially to the state of the in-situ stress at that region. The storing water of the reservoir makes the pore pressure raise, which reduces the effective normal stress of the faults under the reservoir and the nearby regions, so makes the shear stress increase of the peripheral faults of the reservoir, which let the fault tend to slide. However, because storing water in the reservoir makes the shear stress and shear strength decrease, the sum of decreasing value of the shear stress and the shear strength is only several MPa, so the occurrence of the induced earthquake of reservoir is dominated by the geological condition of the region where the earthquake occurs, especially by the state of the in-situ stress.

M. D. Zoback and S. Hickman have studied the induced earthquake which occurred in Monticello, South Carolina. At that region where the hypocenter of the induced earthquake was located two holes the depth of which was 1.1 kilometers were bored, the in-situ stress, the pore pressure, the permeability, and the distribution of the fault fracturing and joints were measured. According to the measured data, the original plane of the fault which had borne rather large shear stress near the surface of the earth, because the pore pressure increased to be enough, was triggered the reverse faulting and the earthquake occurred. The result of the measured data indicated: a. for the reverse fault movement, the depth near to the critical difference stress was less than 200 to 300 meters; b. at the deep region, the increasing pore pressure was related to the condition of the water storing of the reservoir; c. the direction of the original fault plane was the same as the direction of the earthquake hypocenter plane which was gotten from the resolution of the combined earthquake hypocenter. d. the diffusing rate of the hydropressure in-situ was consistent with the extent of the active region of earthquake and with the expecting time of liquid transiting to the active region of earthquake. Therefore it was thought that the action of the earthquake in Monticeilo reservoir would be constrained in very small area in the future, and the magnitude of the earthquake would be constrained too. Afterwards, the fact indicated that the conclusion said above was correct(Zoback 1982).

When there is fault near to the nuclear power station, the data of the state of the in-situ stress is extremely needed while the action of the fault is considered.

8 THE RELATIONSHIP BETWEEN THE MEASUREMENT OF THE IN-SITU STRESS AND EXPLOITATION OF SOURCE OF POWER

At the present, in The United States of America, Germany, France and Japan, the measurement of the in-situ stress is combined with the exploitation of the source of power and resources. Especially, there is a close relationship between the measurement of the in-situ stress by hydrofracturing and the exploitation of petroleum, nature gas and geothermal energy which is gotten from the hot dry rock mass. Because, in the exploitation of petroleum and nature gas, the fracturing face is needed to be as transiting pass so that they are assembled in one place and extracted, and in the exploitation of the geothermal energy by dry hot rock mass the thermal-interchange face must be constructed, in this way the geothermal energy can be extracted. In all of these the hydrofracturing has to be done. And the fracturing face by the hydrofracturing is related to the state of the stress in the crust of the earth. The original crack system was as a result of the effect of the stress in the crust of the earth usually, so that the research of the stress in the crust of the earth is more important.

9 CONCLUSION

The measurement of the in-situ stress has great practical meaning for the engineering construction. In order to use the favorable part of the stress state of the rock mass, and overcome it's unfavorable part, it is needed reasonably to arrange the axis of the under-ground house, the axis of the dam, and the orientation of the man-made side slope, to calculate accurately the redistribution of the stress in the rock mass and the deformation of the rock mass, select correctly the engineering measures for the stability of the rock mass, so that make the engineering designing more reasonable and safe. For the big and middle engineering project, the measurement of the in-situ stress should be arranged to be as a task which is necessary to be done.

In recent years, the measurement of the stress has been developed greatly, and is used widely. Many geologists, rock mechanists and engineers pay more attention to the measurement of the in-situ stress. The measurement of the in-situ stress has very wide future not in studying basic geological theory but also in the practical usage of the engineering construction.

REFERENCE

Jin, H. P and M. J. Wu 1976. Significance of In-situ Stress Measurement for the Design of High Pressure Tunnel Project, *Collected Papers and Notes on Geomechanics*, No. 3, (in Chinese), Science Press.

Li, F. Q. 1985. The Measurement of Rock Stress In-situ, *Chinese Journal of Rock Mechanics and Engineering*, Vol. 4, No. 1(in Chinese).

Li, F. Q. et al. 1993, Application of In-situ Stress Measurement to the Assessment of A Site for Nuclear Waste Disposal, *Chinese Journal of Rock Mechanics and Engineering*, Vol.12, No.1(in Chinese).

Li, T. H and B. T. Pan 1970, *Rock Mass Mechanics*, Geological Publishing House, (in Chinese).

Peiwei, A. B et al. 1978. *Crustal Stress State*, Seismological Press(in Chinese, translated from Russian): 27-31.

Stagg, K, G, and O, C, Zienkiewicz 1978. *Rock Mechanics in Engineering Practice*(John Wiley and Sons), Geological Publishing House(in Chinese, translated from English).

Yamaguch, U. and Y. Nishimatsu 1982. *Fundamentals of Rock Mechanics*, Metallurgical Industry Press(in Chinese, translated from Japanese).

Zoback, M. D. and S, Hickman 1982. In Situ Study of The Physical Mechanisms Controlling Induced Seismicity at Monticello Reservoir, South Carolina, *J. Geophys., Res.*, 87: 6959-6974.

Rock stress measurement for design of underground powerhouse and considerations

Y. Ishiguro, H. Nishimura & K. Nishino
Chubu Electric Power Co., Inc., Nagoya, Japan

K. Sugawara
Department of Civil Engineering and Architecture, Kumamoto University, Japan

ABSTRACT: This paper reports the initial rock stress measurements performed at two adjacent underground powerhouses, Sites I and II, by means of three types of stress relieving method, the borehole deformation method, the modified doorstopper method, and the conical-ended borehole technique, as well as the hydraulic fracturing method, and presents some considerations concerning the results obtained. The results of measurement of initial rock stress at Sites I and II agree that the maximum principal stress is compression and that its orientation is generally horizontal in the East-West direction, but a rather large difference was found concerning the magnitude of stress. The cause of this is thought to be a difference in rock bearing stress due to changes in the rock mass stiffness.

1 INTRODUCTION

Various methods and techniques have been proposed to measure the initial rock stresses, and improvements have been made in several techniques with resulting improvement in their reliability and economy. The borehole deformation method based on the stress relief principle has been used extensively in the past at underground powerhouse sites in Japan, and judging from the results of construction up to the present, measurement of initial rock stress by this method is believed to be highly reliable. Several other methods have also been performed recently at underground powerhouse sites.

This paper reports the results of measurement of initial rock stress performed at underground caverns of two adjacent pumped storage power plants, sites I and II, by means of three types of stress relieving method, the borehole deformation method, the modified doorstopper method, and the conical-ended borehole technique, as well as the hydraulic fracturing method, and presents some considerations concerning a point of agreement and differences in measured results at the two sites.

2 OUTLINE OF MEASUREMENTS

2.1 Outline of measurement sites

The sites I and II are located in the central part of Japan. The power station at Site I commenced the operation two years ago, and the measurements of initial rock stress for design were performed 15 years ago. Site II is located at a point of approximately 4.5km in horizontal distance in the northeast direction from Site I. This power plant is presently in the pre-construction stage and the measurements of initial rock stress for design were performed one year ago.

The geological map of the area is shown in Figure 1. And the east-west sections through the sites are shown in Figure 2.

The topographical conditions surrounding the two sites are generally the same, but the geology at Site I consists of rhyolite of the Cretaceous period of the Mesozoic era, while that at Site II is granite of the same period. The elevation at which measurements were performed is 460m at Site I and 478m at Site II. The depth is 340m at Site I and 550m at Site II. A comparison of the Young's modulus of rocks is shown in Table 1.

Almost equivalent values are shown for the Young's modulus found from uniaxial compression tests of rock cores. However, from the average joint

Table 1. Comparison of the geological conditions and the Young's modulus of rocks at Sites I and II.

Condition & properties	Site I	Site II
Rock type	Rhyolite	Granite
Depth (m)	340	550
Joint spacing (cm)	50	200
RQD (%)	69	90
The Young's modulus of core under uniaxial compression (GPa)	39	38
The Young's modulus of rock mass by in-situ jack test (GPa)	13	23

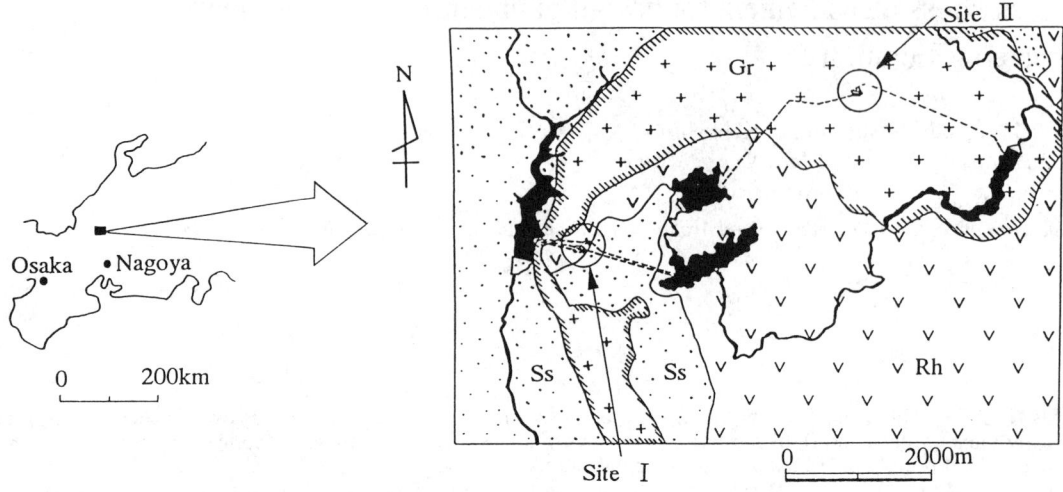

Figure 1. Geological map of the sites. (Gr: granite; Rh: rhyolite; Ss: sandstone)

spacing in test adits and the RQD values at the vicinity of initial rock stress measurement points, it is expected that the rock mass at Site II has a greater stiffness. The Young's modulus of the rock mass obtained from in-situ jack tests at Site II is on the order of approximately 1.8 times of that at Site I. Such a difference in rock mass stiffness and the deformability of rock mass are considered to play an important role in determining the magnitude and orientations of in-situ stresses at the two sites, as discussed later.

2.2 *Outline of measurement methods*

At Site I, the borehole deformation method and the modified doorstopper method have been applied to evaluate the three-dimensional state of in-situ stress. The location and arrangement of the boreholes and measurement points are shown in Figure 3.

The stress measurements by means of the borehole deformation method were performed using the five-element borehole deformation gauge (Ishida et al. 1982). A gauge incorporating a total of five strain gauge elements, four radial elements and one axial element, is embedded in a 56mm diameter borehole using cement paste, and then, after a curing period of about one week, large diameter (218mm) overcoring is performed and the change in strain accompanying stress relief in the rock surrounding the embedded gauge due to this overcoring is measured. By performing a large-scale triaxial laboratory test on the rock core including the gauge which was removed by the overcoring, strain sensitivity coefficients are experimentally determined and the initial rock stress is computed by the elasticity theory.

The stress measurement by means of the modified

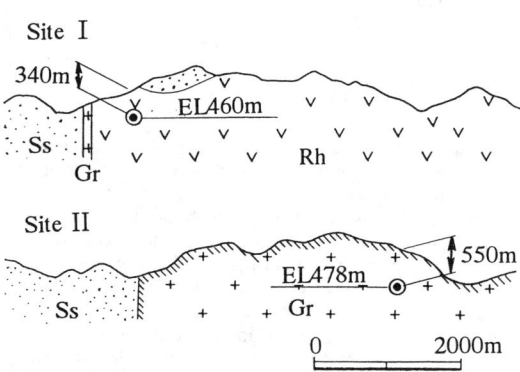

Figure 2. East-west sections through the sites.

doorstopper method was conducted using the eight-element strain cell (Kameoka et al. 1978). The strain cell is affixed by adhesive to the flat finished end of a 76mm diameter borehole, and then, after a curing period of several hours, large diameter (218mm) overcoring is performed and the changes in strain due to this overcoring are measured. By a uniaxial compression test on the recovered core, the Young's modulus and the Poisson's ratio are determined, and the initial rock stress is computed assuming that the rock is an isotropic homogeneous elastic body.

At Site II, the borehole deformation method and the conical-ended borehole technique have been applied as well as the hydraulic fracturing method. The location and arrangement of the boreholes and measurement points are shown in Figure 4.

The stress measurement by means of the borehole deformation method was carried out using the eight-

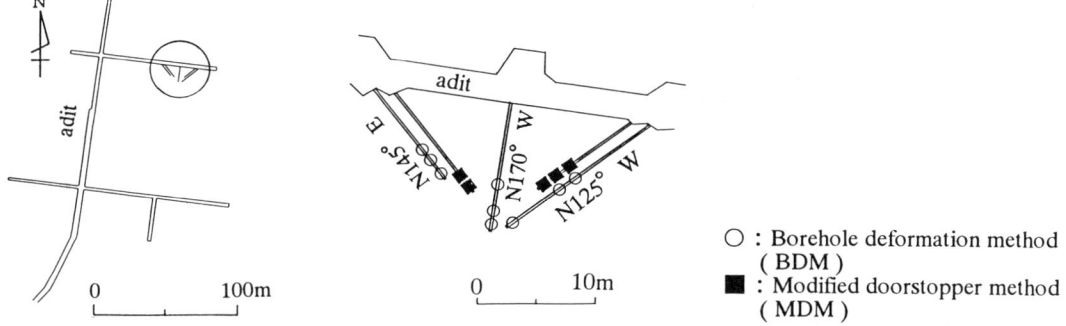

Figure 3. The location and arrangement of the boreholes and measurement points at Site I.

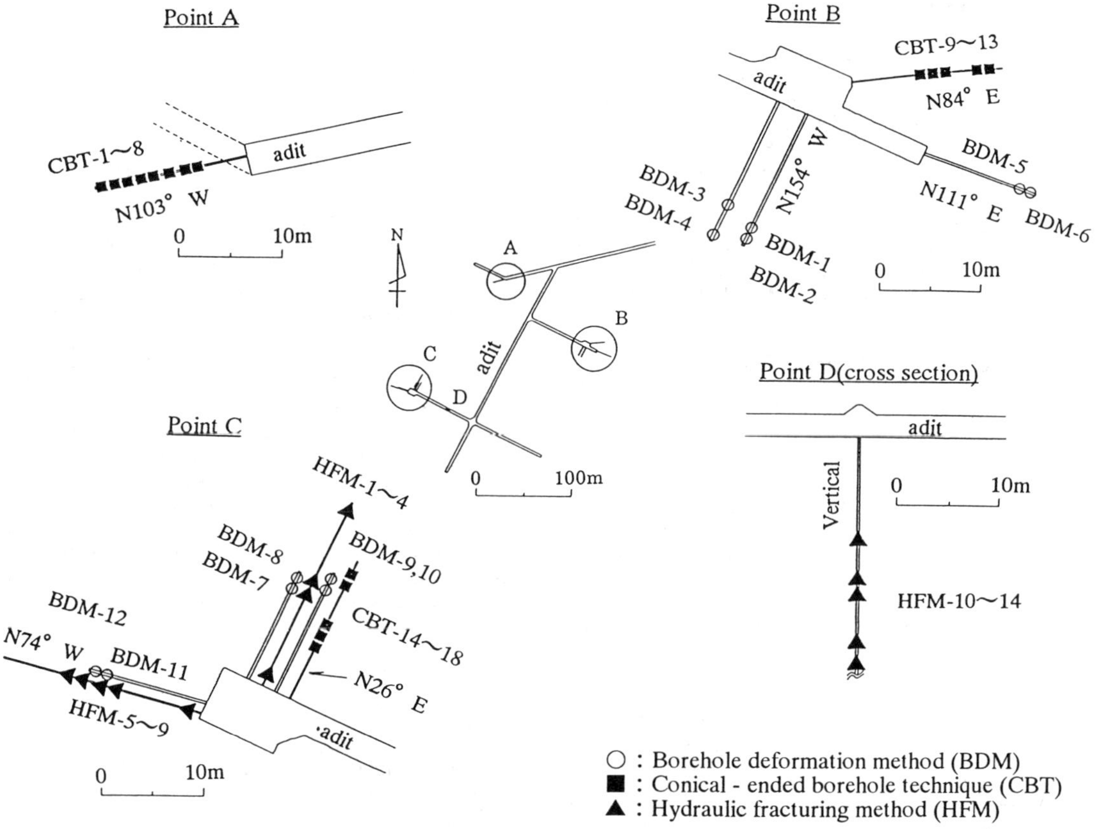

Figure 4. The location and arrangement of the boreholes and measurement points at Site II.

element borehole deformation gauge (Kanagawa et al. 1986). This is a gauge incorporating a total of eight strain gauge elements, four elements in borehole radial directions and four elements in directions diagonal to the borehole axis. In principle, the three dimensional stress state can be determined from the measurement in a single borehole. The overcoring procedure of this method is the same as that of the borehole deformation method using the five-element borehole deformation gauge described previously.

The measurement by means of the conical-ended borehole technique was conducted using the sixteen-element conical strain cell (Sakaguchi et al. 1994). This is a gauge incorporating on a conical surface eight cross gauges to measure strain in the longitudinal and latitudinal directions. The strain cell is affixed by adhesive to the conical finished end of a 76mm diameter borehole, and then overcoring of the same diameter is performed and the changes in strain accompanying stress relief are measured. Initial rock stress is computed in the same way as in the case of the modified doorstopper method, assuming that the rock is an isotropic homogeneous elastic body. In the same way as with the borehole deformation method, the three dimensional stress state is determined by the measurement in a single borehole.

Stress measurement by means of the hydraulic fracturing method was performed utilizing 66mm diameter boreholes. Using a borehole scanner, a section of borehole is selected, where there are no natural joints. Water pressure is applied until a fracture develops and then the pressure is relieved. Subsequently, water pressure is applied until the fracture re-opens and secondary breakdown. After that, water injection is ceased, and when the water pressure becomes nearly constant the water is drained. This operation is repeated three to six times. To find the three dimensional state of stress, measurements were performed in boreholes laid out in three directions generally corresponding to the principal directions of stress evaluated by the stress relieving method.

3 MEASUREMENT RESULTS

3.1 *Measurement results at Site I*

The measurement results at Site I, by means of the borehole deformation method and the modified doorstopper method, are shown in Table 2 and Figure 5. Compressive rock stress is shown as positive. In the case of the borehole deformation method, the principal stresses σ_1, σ_2 and σ_3 are computed by weighting all of the measurement data and applying the method of least squares, and are the results obtained from the data from 7 points which were considered to be

Table 2. Initial rock stresses observed at Site I.

Stress	BDM	MDM
σ_1 (MPa)	9.0	15.9
azimuth	N100° E	N104° E
dip	6°	4°
σ_2 (MPa)	6.2	11.3
azimuth	N195° E	N204° E
dip	37°	73°
σ_3 (MPa)	4.6	3.1
azimuth	N3° E	N13° E
dip	52°	17°
σ_{AVE} (MPa)	6.6	10.1
σ_V (MPa)	5.2	10.6

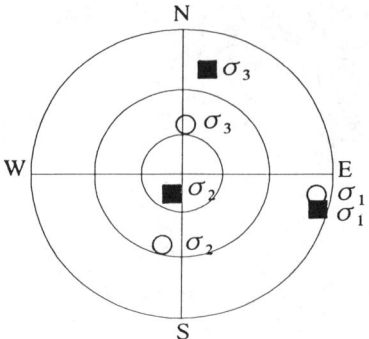

○ : Borehole deformation method (BDM)
■ : Modified doorstopper method (MDM)

Figure 5. Orientation of principal stress at Site I.
(Stereographic lower hemisphere projection)

significant among the data of 9 points. The principal stresses by the modified doorstopper method are the results obtained from all of the data of 5 points.

Comparing the results obtained by the borehole deformation method and the modified doorstopper method, both methods showed the orientation of the maximum principal stress to be horizontal in the east-west direction, agreeing extremely well. Regarding the magnitude of stress, it can be noted that the modified doorstopper method gave greater values. The value of average principal stress σ_{AVE} from the modified doorstopper method was 10.1MPa as opposed to 6.6MPa from the borehole deformation method. Regarding the vertical stress σ_V, because the depth of overburden at this site is 340m, the vertical stress obtained by the borehole deformation method is smaller than the overburden pressure, and the vertical stress obtained by the modified doorstopper method is larger than the overburden pressure.

3.2 *Measurement results at Site II*

The measurement results at Site II, by means of the borehole deformation method, the conical-ended borehole technique and the hydraulic fracturing method, are shown in Table 3 and Figure 6. The principal stresses of the borehole deformation method are computed by weighting all of the measurement data and applying the method of least squares. Because data of 8 elements is measured at each measurement point, data was obtained on 96 elements at 12 measurement points, and the results shown were obtained from the data of 61 elements which were considered to be significant among 10 measurement points. The principal stresses by the conical-ended borehole technique are obtained from the data of 17 measurement

Table 3. Initial rock stresses observed at Site II.

Stress	BDM	CBT	HFM
σ_1 (MPa)	21.9	28.1	26.9
azimuth	N102° E	N89° E	N286° E
dip	17°	25°	5°
σ_2 (MPa)	11.2	11.4	14.2
azimuth	N193° E	N353° E	N184° E
dip	3°	13°	18°
σ_3 (MPa)	6.1	7.5	8.5
azimuth	N293° E	N239° E	N21° E
dip	73°	62°	71°
σ_{AVE} (MPa)	13.1	15.7	16.5
σ_V (MPa)	7.4	11.3	9.2

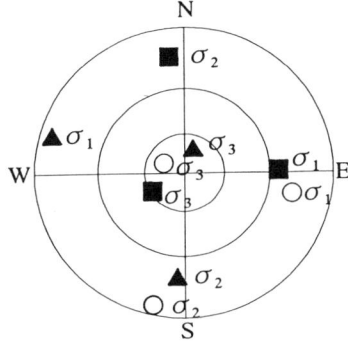

○ : Borehole deformation method (BDM)
■ : Conical - ended borehole technique (CBT)
▲ : Hydraulic fracturing method (HFM)

Figure 6. Orientation of principal stress at Site II. (Stereographic lower hemisphere projection)

points which were considered to be significant among 18 measurement points.

Comparing the results obtained by the borehole deformation method and the conical-ended borehole technique, both methods showed the orientation of the maximum principal stress to be horizontal in the east-west direction, agreeing extremely well. Regarding the magnitude of stress, a result in which the value from the conical-ended borehole technique is approximately 1.3 times of the value from the borehole deformation method. The average principal stress σ_{AVE} from the conical-ended borehole technique was 15.7MPa as opposed to 13.1MPa from the borehole deformation method. Regarding the vertical stress σ_V, because the depth of overburden at this site is 550m, both methods gave smaller values than the overburden pressure, respectively.

With the stress relieving method used here, it is theoretically possible to find by either technique the three-dimensional stress state from the data of a single borehole. In case of the borehole deformation method, significant data is required from at least three of the four elements in each of the radial and diagonal directions. From the results of the present measurements, it was possible to find the three-dimensional stress condition independently at five measurement points. The results of finding three-dimensional stress at each point are shown in Figures 7(a) and 7(c).

Although a certain amount of scattering is to be found, there is a good agreement regarding both the magnitude and the orientation of principal stress. Similar results of the conical-ended borehole technique obtained at 17 measurement points are shown in Figures 7(b) and 7(c). The Young's modulus evaluated from uniaxial compression tests is also given in Figure 7(b). There is a good agreement regarding the orientation, but regarding the magnitude of stress, the amount of scattering is somewhat greater than that of the borehole deformation method. At the points where the value of the Young's modulus is large, the value of rock stress computed also tends to be large.

The results of measurement by the hydraulic fracturing method, shown in Table 4, are the results obtained from the data of 6 measurement points which were considered to be significant among the data of 14 measurement points. Longitudinal fractures were observed at these 6 measurement points. An example of the time-pressure curve obtained from the measurements is shown in Figure 8. The shut-in pressure Ps, after Gronseth et al. 1982, was found from the point where the time-pressure curve diverges from the initial tangent line after ceasing water injection following fracture re-opening. The vertical stress evaluated from the results of measurement in horizontal borehole was ranging from 7.2 to 10.9MPa. Because these are values which were measured directly without using strain gauges and the elasticity theory as in the stress relieving methods, it is thought that the vertical stress acting in the rock mass is being found with a fairly good accuracy. The estimation of the three-dimensional stress state has been carried out by applying the scheme presented by Mizuta et al.(1987). The results are shown in Table 3. The principal stresses obtained by the hydraulic fracturing method differs from the values obtained by the stress relieving methods, by a margin on the order of only 5MPa, an extremely good agreement.

4 DISCUSSION

From the in-situ measurement of initial rock stress at Sites I and II, it has been made clear that the orientation of the maximum principal stress is horizontal in about the east-west direction. However, there is a clear difference in the magnitude of stress. The maximum principal stress at Site I was ranging from 9.0 to 15.9 MPa, while that at Site II was 21.9 to 28.1 MPa, a result which shows the maximum principal stress at Site II to be about 2.4 to 1.8 times of that at Site I.

Figure 9 shows the results of measurement of hori-

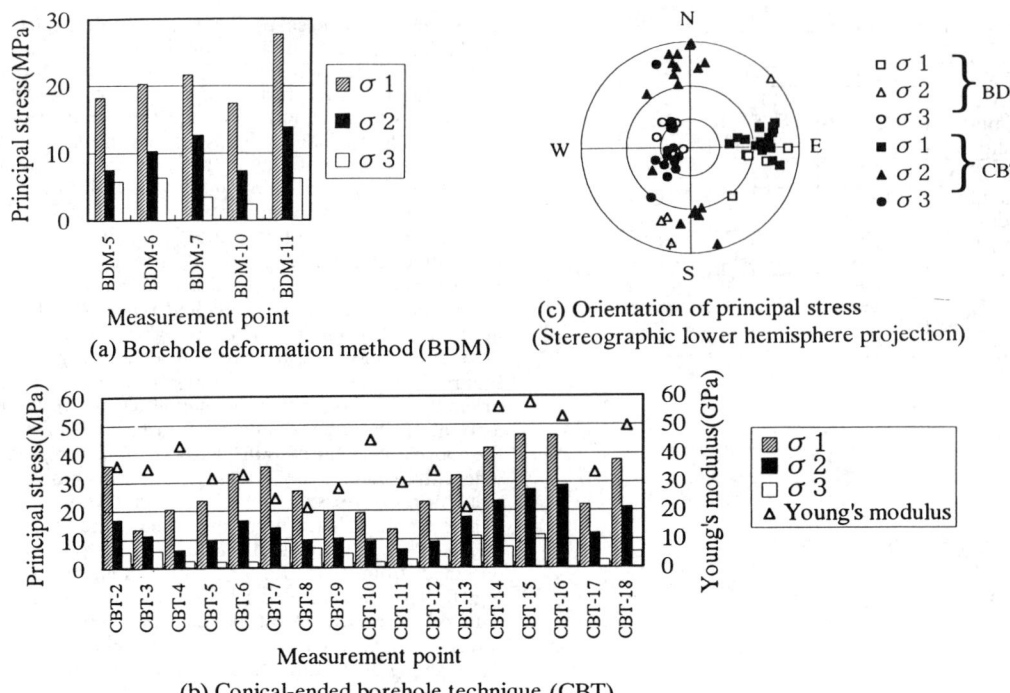

Figure 7. Three - dimensional principal stress obtained from each measurement points at Site II.

Table 4. Results of measurements by the hydraulic fracturing method.

Point No.	HFM-3	HFM-4	HFM-7	HFM-9	HFM-11	HFM-14
Direction of borehole	North-South (N26° E)		East-West (N74° W)		Vertical	
Re-opening pressure Pr (MPa)	11.9	12.0	8.4	7.7	16.9	20.1
Shut-in pressure Ps (MPa)	10.6	10.7	7.4	7.0	16.0	16.4
Vertical stress σ_v (MPa)	10.9	10.9	7.9	7.2	-	-

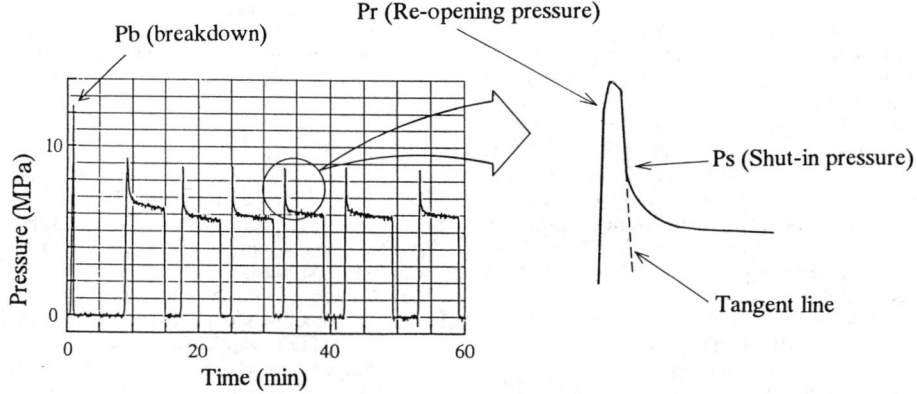

Figure 8. Example of time-pressure curve.

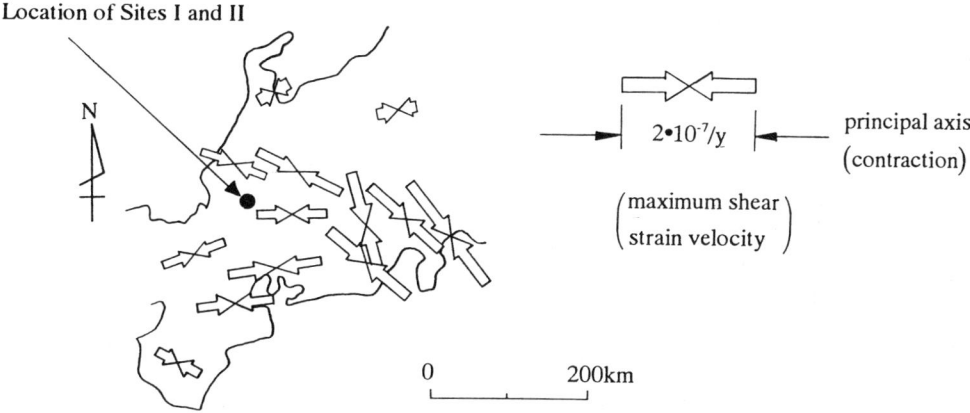

Figure 9. Horizontal tectonic strain by first order triangulation over the past 60 years.

zontal tectonic strain by first order triangulation over the past 60 years (Nakane 1973). Compressive strains in about the east-west direction have been measured at the vicinity of Sites I and II, and this is considered to be due to the action of tectonic compression in the east-west direction accompanying activity of the Pacific Plate. The orientation of rock stress obtained as a result of the measurements agrees well with this tectonic movement.

Possible causes of the differences in magnitude of rock stress between the two sites include overburden depth, rock type, rock mass stiffness and local disturbance of stress due to geological heterogeneity and discontinuities such as faults. Regarding the rock mass stiffness, as mentioned previously, the Young's modulus obtained by in-situ jack tests in Site II is much greater than that of Site I. This tendency agrees well with that of magnitude of initial rock stress. On the other hand, the sites are surrounded by the Median Tectonic Line and the Itoigawa-Shizuoka Tectonic Line, and the Neodani Fault and several other faults are found in the vicinity. Consequently, it is possible to think that the geological structure is relatively complex, causing a disturbance in the distribution of strain. However, a large-scale, continuous fault which would cause a difference in rock stress is not to be found in the near vicinity of these sites.

As described above, the orientations of initial rock stress observed in the Sites I and II correspond with the geodesic compressive strain in the east-west direction accompanying the action of the Pacific Plate against the Japanese Islands, and the cause of the difference in magnitude can be concluded to be the result of a difference in rock bearing stress due to changes in rock mass stiffness.

5 CONCLUSIONS

Measurements of initial rock stress have been performed for the design of underground caverns at two adjacent pumped storage type power plants. The knowledge obtained from the measurements is as follows:

1. Comparing the borehole deformation method and the modified doorstopper method at Site I, the orientations of initial rock stress obtained by the two methods agree well, but the absolute values of initial rock stress obtained by the modified doorstopper method tend to be greater.

2. Comparing the borehole deformation method and the conical-ended borehole technique at Site II, the orientation of initial rock stress obtained by the two methods agree well, but the absolute values of initial rock stress obtained by the conical-ended borehole technique tend to be greater.

3. The results of measurement by the hydraulic fracturing method at Site II agree extremely well with the stress measurement results by means of the stress relieving methods.

4. The initial rock stresses at Sites I and II are concluded to be caused by the compressive strain in the east-west direction accompanying the action of the Pacific Plate against the Japanese Islands, and the orientations of initial rock stress at both sites agree well with this tectonic movement.

5. The absolute values of the maximum principal stress at Site II are clarified to be approximately twice of Site I, and the cause of this has been considered to be chiefly a difference in rock bearing stress due to changes in rock mass stiffness.

ACKNOWLEDGMENTS

Initial rock stress measurements were performed with

the help of the Central Research Institute of the Electric Power Industry. The authors would like to express their sincere thanks to persons concerned for their invaluable suggestions.

REFERENCES

Ishida, T., T. Kanagawa and S. Hibino 1982. In-situ Initial Stress Measurements in the Underground Power Station and Some Studies on the Results. Central Research Institute of Electric Power Industry, Japan. Rept . No.382025.

Gronseth J.M. & P.R. Kry 1982. Instantaneous shut-in pressure and its relationship to the minimum in-situ stress, Workshop on Hydraulic Fracturing Stress Measurements, U.S. Geol. Surv. Open File Report, 82-1075, pp.147-166.

Kameoka, Y. 1978. Study on rock stress measurement with stress relief on the bottom of the borehole. Ph.D.Thesis, Kyoto University.

Kanagawa, T., S. Hibino and T. Ishida 1986. In-situ Stress Measurements by Over-coring Method - Development of 8-elements Gauge for 3-dimensional Estimation. Central Research Institute of Electric Power Industry, Japan. Rept. No.385033.

Mizuta, Y., O. Sano, S. Ogino and H. Kato 1987. Three dimensional stress determination by hydraulic fracturing for underground excavation design. International Journal of Rock Mechanics and Mining Science, 24, 1, 15-29.

Nakane K. 1973. Horizontal tectonic strain in Japan (2). J. geod. Soc. Japan, 19, 200-208.

Sakaguchi, K., T. Takehara, Y. Obara, T. Nakayama and K. Sugawara 1994. Rock Stress Measurement by means of the Compact Overcoring Method. MMIJ, 110, 4, 331-336.

Rock Stress, Sugawara & Obara (eds) © 1997 Balkema, Rotterdam, ISBN 90 5410 901 7

Two-dimensional elastic analysis for a circular tunnel lining in the pre-deformed ground due to initial stresses – An approach to quantitative evaluation of the load bearing capacity of the surrounding rock mass

Hideo Kiyama, Hisashi Fujimura, Tsuyoshi Nishimura & Yasuo Ikezoe
Department of Civil Engineering, Tottori University, Japan

ABSTRACT: The behavior of a tunnel lining is a typical ground-lining interaction problem which depends on the relative stiffnesses of the lining and the ground as well as the initial stress conditions. In this paper a strict solution of the relative stiffness is derived for both full-slip and no-slip conditions at the ground-lining interface; moreover, the solution is modified for the interaction to be not affected directly by the ground movements due to the initial stresses before tunneling. The analytical results of stress-displacement behaviors of the tunnel lining, the surrounding ground and the total are quantitatively evaluated by using a common index, "support-stiffness", which must be useful for practical implications and the further development of tunnel support design.

1 INTRODUCTION

The NATM is characterized by a concept that the ground surrounding an underground opening becomes the main load bearing component. By excavating a tunnel opening the surrounding ground surely displays to support the opening. However, no quantitative expression of this bearing capacity has ever been recognized.

A support load of the surrounding ground and a support load of the lining are always coupled in a lined tunnel, and they share the total support load of the tunnel in different ratios depending on their relative stiffnesses. It is clear that the total support load is equal to the initial load supported by the ground mass removed from the opening (constant in a given tunnel opening). Thus the tunnel deformation, e.g. a radial convergence of the opening, depends mostly on the total stiffness of the lining and the surrounding ground.

The authors proposed[1] support-stiffnesses, $\bar{K}_L$, $\bar{K}_E$ and $\bar{K}_T$, which are defined as the relative stiffness of each support to the initial stiffness of the rock mass removed from the opening, K_0^* : $\bar{K}_L$ is a support-stiffness of lining, $\bar{K}_E$ a support-stiffness of surrounding ground, and $\bar{K}_T$ the total support-stiffness of tunnel.

In order to give a quantitative evaluation of each support-stiffness, a strict solution of a two-dimensional elastic circular lined tunnel is derived for both full-slip and no-slip conditions at the ground-lining interface. The solution is the assumption of surface overpressure loading condition. This "external loading" condition implies that the tunnel opening has been excavated and supported before the load corresponding to the initial stresses is applied (in the cases of buried culverts, ordinary tunnel model experiments, etc.).

The solution is modified for the actual "excavation unloading" condition, where the tunnel opening is excavated and lined after the load corresponding to the initial stresses has been applied.

The stresses and displacements in the lining and the surrounding ground were discussed for both loading conditions, and from the circumferential stress-displacement relationships of the lining we determined the support-stiffnesses, $\bar{K}_L$, $\bar{K}_E$ and $\bar{K}_T$, which enable us to give a quantitative expression of the support capacity of the surrounding ground.

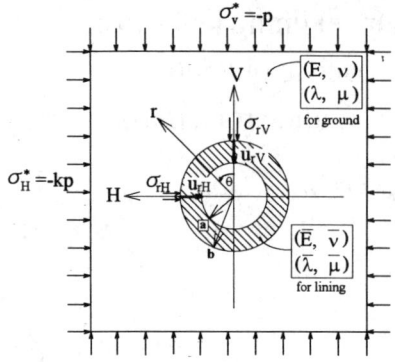

Figure 1. Analytical model of a circular lined tunnel in plane strain

2 ELASTIC ANALYSIS FOR A CIRCULAR LINING IN PLANE STRAIN ; THE "EXTERNAL LOADING" SOLUTION

For the purpose the simplified analytical solutions derived by Muir Wood[2] and Einstein et.al.[3] are well known, but such an orthodox analytical solution as described in this paper has never been recognized.

Figure 1 shows an analytical model of a circular tunnel lining. a and b are the inner and outer radii of the lining, λ, μ are Lamé constants for the ground, and $\bar{\lambda}$, $\bar{\mu}$ are for the lining. Those elastic constants are suitably alternated with Young's modulus and Poisson's ratio: E, ν for the ground and $\bar{E}$, $\bar{\nu}$ for the lining. Initial stresses in the ground are assumed $\sigma_V^* = -p$ and $\sigma_H^* = -kp$ where k is called as a lateral stress ratio.

The Airy's stress function, Eq. 1, is adapted for both ground and lining

$$\phi = \frac{\lambda + \mu}{2} C_0 r^2 - 2\mu E_0 \log r + \left\{ \frac{\lambda + \mu}{6} A_2 r^4 \right.$$
$$\left. - \frac{\lambda + \mu}{2} C_2 - \mu E_2' r^2 + \mu E_2 r^{-2} \right\} \cos 2\theta \quad (1)$$

where the arbitrary constants C_0, E_0, $\cdots$, E_2' are used for the ground and $\bar{C}_0$, $\bar{E}_0$, $\cdots$, $\bar{E}_2'$ are for the lining. The corresponding stress and displacement components are
in the surrounding ground ($\infty > r \geq b$),

$$\sigma_r = (\lambda + \mu)C_0 - 2\mu E_0 r^{-2}$$
$$+ \left\{ 2(\lambda + \mu)C_2 r^{-2} + 2\mu E_2' - 6\mu E_2 r^{-4} \right\} \cos 2\theta \quad (2a)$$

$$\sigma_\theta = (\lambda + \mu)C_0 + 2\mu E_0 r^{-2}$$
$$+ \left\{ -2\mu E_2' + 6\mu E_2 r^{-4} \right\} \cos 2\theta \quad (2b)$$

$$\tau_{r\theta} = \left\{ (\lambda + \mu)C_2 r^{-2} - 2\mu E_2' - 6\mu E_2 r^{-4} \right\} \sin 2\theta \quad (2c)$$

$$u_r = \frac{C_0}{2} r + E_0 r^{-1}$$
$$+ \left\{ -\frac{\lambda + 2\mu}{2\mu} C_2 r^{-1} + E_2' r + E_2 r^{-3} \right\} \cos 2\theta \quad (2d)$$

$$u_\theta = \left\{ \frac{C_2}{2} r^{-1} - E_2' r + E_2 r^{-3} \right\} \sin 2\theta \quad (2e)$$

in the lining ($b \geq r \geq a$)

$$\bar{\sigma}_r = (\bar{\lambda} + \bar{\mu})\bar{C}_0 - 2\bar{\mu}\bar{E}_0 r^{-2}$$
$$+ \left\{ 2(\bar{\lambda} + \bar{\mu})\bar{C}_2 r^{-2} + 2\bar{\mu}\bar{E}_2' - 6\bar{\mu}\bar{E}_2 r^{-4} \right\} \cos 2\theta \quad (3a)$$

$$\bar{\sigma}_\theta = (\bar{\lambda} + \bar{\mu})\bar{C}_0 + 2\bar{\mu}\bar{E}_0 r^{-2}$$
$$+ \left\{ 2(\bar{\lambda} + \bar{\mu})\bar{A}_2 r^2 - 2\bar{\mu}\bar{E}_2' + 6\bar{\mu}\bar{E}_2 r^{-4} \right\} \cos 2\theta \quad (3b)$$

$$\bar{\tau}_{r\theta} = \left\{ (\bar{\lambda} + \bar{\mu})\bar{A}_2 r^2 + (\bar{\lambda} + \bar{\mu})\bar{C}_2 r^{-2} \right.$$
$$\left. - 2\bar{\mu}\bar{E}_2' - 6\bar{\mu}\bar{E}_2 r^{-4} \right\} \sin 2\theta \quad (3c)$$

$$\bar{u}_r = \frac{\bar{C}_0}{2} r + \bar{E}_0 r^{-1} + \left\{ -\frac{\bar{\lambda}}{6\bar{\mu}} \bar{A}_2 r^3 \right.$$
$$\left. - \frac{\bar{\lambda} + 2\bar{\mu}}{2\bar{\mu}} \bar{C}_2 r^{-1} + \bar{E}_2' r + \bar{E}_2 r^{-3} \right\} \cos 2\theta \quad (3d)$$

$$\bar{u}_\theta = \left\{ \frac{2\bar{\lambda} + 3\bar{\mu}}{6\bar{\mu}} \bar{A}_2 r^3 + \frac{\bar{C}_2}{2} r^{-1} - \bar{E}_2' r + \bar{E}_2 r^{-3} \right\} \sin \theta \quad (3e)$$

In this case the tunnel opening is excavated and lined, and then it is subjected to the load corresponding to the initial stresses, $-p$ and $-kp$.

The boundary conditions are

at $r = \infty$ $\quad (\sigma_r)_{r=\infty} = -p\left\{ \frac{1+k}{2} + \frac{1-k}{2} \cos 2\theta \right\} \quad (4)$

$\quad (\tau_{r\theta})_{r=\infty} = p\frac{1-k}{2} \sin 2\theta \quad (5)$

at $r = a$ $\quad (\bar{\sigma}_r)_{r=a} = 0 \quad (6) \quad (\bar{\tau}_{r\theta})_{r=a} = 0 \quad (7)$

at $r = b$ (at the ground-lining interface)

$(\sigma_r)_{r=b} = (\bar{\sigma}_r)_{r=b} \quad (8) \quad (u_r)_{r=b} = (\bar{u}_r)_{r=b} \quad (9)$

ⓐ for the Full-slip(no shear stress transmission)

$(\tau_{r\theta})_{r=b} = (\bar{\tau}_{r\theta})_{r=b} = 0 \quad (10)$

ⓑ for the No-slip(no relative shear displacement)

$(\tau_{r\theta})_{r=b} = (\bar{\tau}_{r\theta})_{r=b} \quad (11) \quad (u_\theta)_{r=b} = (\bar{u}_\theta)_{r=b} \quad (12)$

From these boundary conditions the eleven constants in Eqs.2 and 3 are determined as follows :
the five constants are independent of the interface conditions,

$$C_0 = -p\frac{1+k}{2(\lambda + \mu)} \quad (13) \qquad E_2' = -p\frac{1-k}{4\mu} \quad (14)$$

$$\frac{\bar{E}_0}{b^2} = \left\{ \frac{\lambda + 2\mu}{2\mu} C_0 \right\} \left(\frac{a}{b}\right)^2 \Bigg/ \left[\left(\frac{a}{b}\right)^2 + \frac{\bar{\mu}}{\bar{\lambda} + \bar{\mu}} + \frac{\bar{\mu}}{\mu}\left(1 - \left(\frac{a}{b}\right)^2\right) \right] \quad (15)$$

$$\bar{C}_0 = \frac{2\bar{\mu}}{\bar{\lambda} + \bar{\mu}} \frac{\bar{E}_0}{b^2} \Bigg/ \left(\frac{a}{b}\right)^2 \quad (16)$$

$$\frac{E_0}{b^2} = \frac{\lambda+\mu}{2\mu}C_0 - \frac{\bar{\mu}}{\mu}\left(1-\left(\frac{a}{b}\right)^2\right)\frac{\bar{E}_0}{b^2}\bigg/\left(\frac{a}{b}\right)^2 \quad (17)$$

a matrix expression, $\{x\}$, of the other six constants depending on the interface conditions,

$$\{x\} = \begin{Bmatrix} C_2/b^2 & E_2/b^4 & \bar{A}_2 b^2 & \bar{E}_2 & \bar{C}_2/b^2 & \bar{E}_2/b^4 \end{Bmatrix}^T \quad (18)$$

is determined by

$$[A]\{x\} = \{B\} \quad (19)$$

ⓐ Full-slip

$$[A] = \begin{bmatrix} -2(\lambda+\mu) & 6\mu & 0 & 2\bar{\mu} & 2(\bar{\lambda}+\bar{\mu}) & -6\bar{\mu} \\ -(\lambda+\mu) & 6\mu & 0 & 0 & 0 & 0 \\ 0 & 0 & (\bar{\lambda}+\bar{\mu}) & -2\bar{\mu} & (\bar{\lambda}+\bar{\mu}) & -6\bar{\mu} \\ \frac{\lambda+2\mu}{2\mu} & 1 & \frac{\bar{\lambda}}{6\bar{\mu}} & -1 & \frac{\bar{\lambda}+2\bar{\mu}}{2\bar{\mu}} & -1 \\ 0 & 0 & 0 & 2\bar{\mu}\left(\frac{a}{b}\right)^4 & 2(\bar{\lambda}+\bar{\mu})\left(\frac{a}{b}\right)^2 & -6\bar{\mu} \\ 0 & 0 & (\bar{\lambda}+\bar{\mu})\left(\frac{a}{b}\right)^6 & -2\bar{\mu}\left(\frac{a}{b}\right)^4 & (\bar{\lambda}+\bar{\mu})\left(\frac{a}{b}\right)^2 & -6\bar{\mu} \end{bmatrix} \quad (20)$$

$$\{B\} = \begin{Bmatrix} 2\mu E_2' & -2\mu E_2' & 0 & -E_2' & 0 & 0 \end{Bmatrix}^T \quad (21)$$

ⓑ No-slip

$$[A] = \begin{bmatrix} -2(\lambda+\mu) & 6\mu & 0 & 2\bar{\mu} & 2(\bar{\lambda}+\bar{\mu}) & -6\bar{\mu} \\ -(\lambda+\mu) & 6\mu & (\bar{\lambda}+\bar{\mu}) & -2\bar{\mu} & (\bar{\lambda}+\bar{\mu}) & -6\bar{\mu} \\ \frac{\lambda+2\mu}{2\mu} & 1 & \frac{\bar{\lambda}}{6\bar{\mu}} & -1 & \frac{\bar{\lambda}+2\bar{\mu}}{2\bar{\mu}} & -1 \\ -\frac{1}{2} & -1 & -\frac{2\bar{\lambda}+3\bar{\mu}}{6\bar{\mu}} & -1 & \frac{1}{2} & 1 \\ 0 & 0 & 0 & 2\bar{\mu}\left(\frac{a}{b}\right)^4 & 2(\bar{\lambda}+\bar{\mu})\left(\frac{a}{b}\right)^2 & -6\bar{\mu} \\ 0 & 0 & (\bar{\lambda}+\bar{\mu})\left(\frac{a}{b}\right)^6 & -2\bar{\mu}\left(\frac{a}{b}\right)^4 & (\bar{\lambda}+\bar{\mu})\left(\frac{a}{b}\right)^2 & -6\bar{\mu} \end{bmatrix} \quad (22)$$

$$\{B\} = \begin{Bmatrix} 2\mu E_2' & -2\mu E_2' & -E_2' & -E_2' & 0 & 0 \end{Bmatrix}^T \quad (23)$$

3 MODIFIED SOLUTION WITH SUBTRACTION OF THE GROUND DEFORMATIONS DUE TO INITIAL STRESSES BEFORE TUNNELING ; THE "EXCAVATION UNLOADING " SOLUTION

The solution above implies that the lining associates with the initial ground deformation. As analysed by Einstein et al.[3], an actual tunnel opening is excavated and lined after the initial ground deformation has been completed. The lining begins to support a load corresponding to the incremental displacement due to the "excavation unloading" condition.

An idealized image of this in elastic analysis is that the ground mass in the opening which is loaded and deformed by the initial stresses is replaced instantaneously with a lining of zero stress and zero deformation. The surrounding ground instantly loses the initial equilibrium of stresses and begins to exchange stress and deformation with the lining through the interface until reaching a new equilibrium in both support components.

The modifications of the "external loading" solution to the "excavation unloading" solution are as follows: the initial displacements in the ground due to the initial stresses are

at $r=b$
$$u_r^* = \ell^* + m^*\cos\theta \quad (24)$$
$$u_\theta^* = -m^*\sin\theta \quad (25)$$

where
$$\left.\begin{aligned} \ell^* &= -(1+\nu)(1-2\nu)(1+k)pb/2E \\ m^* &= -(1+\nu)(1-k)pb/2E \end{aligned}\right\} \quad (26)$$

The incremental displacements of the lining at $r=b$ can be obtained from the displacements under the external loading condition, the left of Eqs. 9 and 12, minus these initial displacements. As a result, there need three modifications in the external loading solution described in 2.

(M1) the term in the bracket $\{\}$ of the numerator in Eq. 15 is changed

from $\left\{\dfrac{\lambda+2\mu}{2\mu}C_0\right\}$ to $\left\{\dfrac{\lambda+2\mu}{2\mu}C_0 - \dfrac{\ell^*}{b}\right\} \quad (27)$

(M2) the matrix $\{B\}$ in Eq. 21 for ⓐ full-slip is replaced by

$$\{B\} = \begin{Bmatrix} 2\mu E_2' & -2\mu E_2' & 0 & \left(-E_2' + \dfrac{m^*}{b}\right) & 0 & 0 \end{Bmatrix}^T \quad (28)$$

(M3) the matrix $\{B\}$ in Eq. 23 for ⓑ no-slip is replaced by

$$\{B\} = \begin{Bmatrix} 2\mu E_2' & -2\mu E_2' & \left(-E_2' + \dfrac{m^*}{b}\right) & \left(-E_2' + \dfrac{m^*}{b}\right) & 0 & 0 \end{Bmatrix}^T \quad (29)$$

The other expressions in Eq. 2-Eq. 23 for the "external loading" condition hold good here also.

4 RESULTS OF ANALYSIS

4.1 *Circumferential stresses and displacements of lining*

To compare the "external loading" solution, F, N, and the "excavation unloading" solution, $F(C)$, $N(C)$, stresses and displacements at a circumference of lining in both solutions are for example shown in Figure 2, where $a/b=0.95$, $k = \sigma_H^*/\sigma_V^* =0.5$, $\nu=0.4$ and $\bar{\nu}=0.2$, $\bar{E}/E =10$ and 100, and conditions of the ground-lining interface are full-slip, F, $F(C)$, and no-slip, N, $N(C)$.

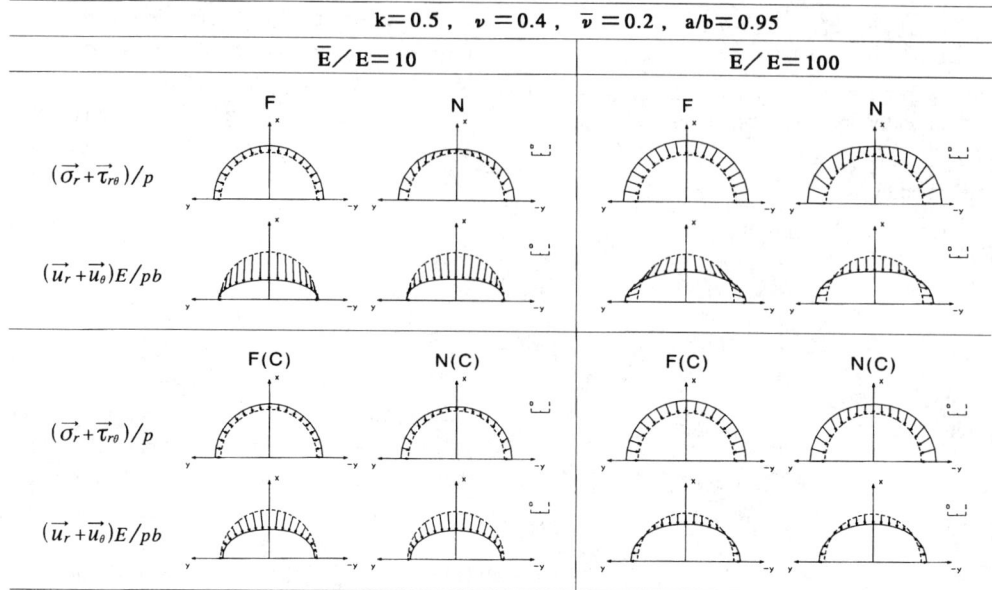

Figure 2. Circumferential stress and displacement vectors of lining : F and N indicate full-slip and no-slip at the ground lining interface for the "external loading" condition, as well as $F(C)$ and $N(C)$ for the "excavation unloading" condition.

In the figures circumferential stresses and displacements at $r=b$ are expressed by the resultant vectors, $(\vec{\sigma}_r + \vec{\tau}_{r\theta})(1/p)$ and $(\vec{u}_r + \vec{u}_\theta)(E/pb)$. All the stresses in F, N, $F(C)$ and $N(C)$ are total stresses, and the displacements in F, N are total displacements, whereas the displacements in $F(C)$, $N(C)$ are incremental displacements from the initial ground displacements (= total displacements for the lining).

Here the results are briefly summarized as follows:
① Circumferential stress distributions and lining deformations are quite different between the interface conditions of full-slip and no-slip(between F and N, and between $F(C)$ and $N(C)$).
② Circumferential stresses and displacements of the external loading solution, F, N, are larger than those of the excavation unloading solution, $F(C)$, $N(C)$.
③ Stress distributions of $F(C)$ and $N(C)$ are more smooth and possible than those of F and N, especially $N(C)$ than N.
④ In any case circumferential stresses of the lining show a strong tendency to become more uniform in spite of the lateral stress ratio, k, even though under uniaxial stress state, $k=0$. It must be the most important characteristics of lining and also very desirable for the lining.

4.2 Support-stiffnesses of lining and ground and the total support-stiffness of tunnel

The support-stiffnesses, $\overline{K}_L$, $\overline{K}_E$ and $\overline{K}_T$ are determined from a representative stress σ_0 and a representative displacement u_0 of such circumferential stresses and displacements as shown in Figure 2. To express suitably the representative stress and displacement, two typical points at the ground-lining interface are selected: one is a crown ($r=b$, $\theta = 0$) and the other is a center of side wall ($r=b$, $\theta = \pi/2$).

The stress and displacement at $r=b$, $\theta = 0$ are σ_{rV} and u_{rV} after excavation and lining as well as σ_{rV}^*, and u_{rV}^* for the initial ground; those at $r=b$, $\theta = \pi/2$ are σ_{rH} and u_{rH} as well as σ_{rH}^* and u_{rH}^*, correspondingly. Hence, σ_0 and u_0 after excavation and lining as well as σ_0^* and u_0^* for the initial ground are defined as follows:

$$\left. \begin{array}{l} \sigma_0^* = \left(\sigma_{rV}^* + \sigma_{rH}^*\right)/2, \quad \sigma_0 = \left(\sigma_{rV} + \sigma_{rH}\right)/2 \\ u_0^* = \left(u_{rV}^* + u_{rH}^*\right)/2, \quad u_0 = \left(u_{rV} + u_{rH}\right)/2 \end{array} \right\} \quad (30)$$

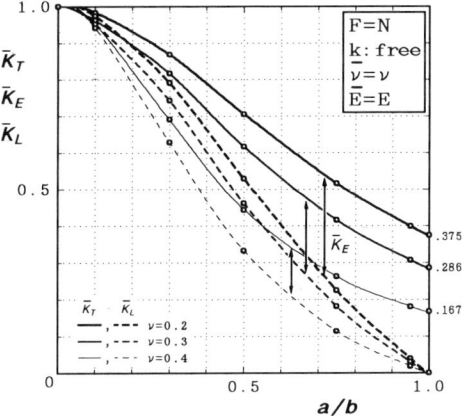 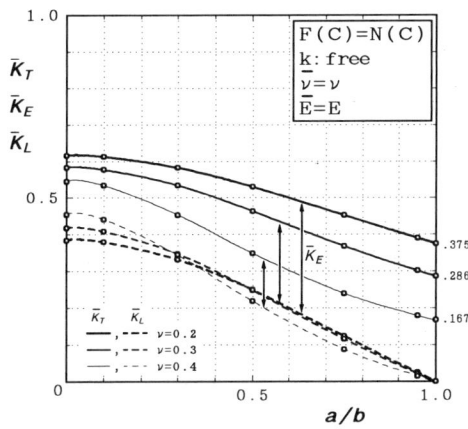

(a) External loading solution (b) Excavation unloading solution

Figure 3. Relationships between support-stiffnesses, $\bar{K}_L, \bar{K}_E, \bar{K}_T$, and specific lining thickness a/b for different values of Poisson's ratio ν

The elastic theory of elasticity indicates that those representative stress and displacement are mean values of the circumferential stresses and displacements in any case, moreover that σ_0 and u_0 become independent of the interface conditions, full-slip and no-slip.

From the expressions of the initial stress, $\sigma_r^* = -p\{1+k+(1-k)\cos 2\theta\}/2$, and the displacements in Eqs. 24-26, σ_0^* and u_0^* can be given by

$$\left.\begin{array}{l}\sigma_0^* = -(1+k)p/2 \\ u_0^* = \ell^* = -(1+\nu)(1-2\nu)(1+k)pb/2E\end{array}\right\} \quad (31)$$

Using the analytical results of σ_0 and u_0 as well as σ_0^* and u_0^*, the support-stiffnesses, $\bar{K}_L, \bar{K}_E$, and $\bar{K}_T$ can be calculated by the following equations,

$$\bar{K}_T = u_0^*/u_0 \quad (32)$$
$$\bar{K}_L = (u_0^*/u_0)\sigma_0/\sigma_0^* \quad (33)$$
$$\bar{K}_E = \bar{K}_T - \bar{K}_L = (u_0^*/u_0)(\sigma_0 - \sigma_0^*)/\sigma_0^* \quad (34)$$

in which u_0 is the total displacement of ground and $u_0 - u_0^*$ is the incremental displacement of ground or the circumferential displacement of lining under the excavation unloading condition, $F(C)$ and $N(C)$.

Fortunately as the representative stress and displacement are the mean stress and displacement, the lateral stress ratio, k, vanishes in the terms of σ_0/σ_0^* and u_0/u_0^* in the above equations.

Therefore the following figures of the support-stiffnesses, $\bar{K}_L, \bar{K}_E$, and $\bar{K}_T$ are established for an arbitrary lateral stress ratio, k, and for both full-slip and no-slip conditions at the ground-lining interface.

First, as a basic example of the external loading solution, $F=N$, relationships between each support-stiffness and a/b in the case of $\bar{E}/E=1$, $\bar{\nu}=\nu$ are shown in Figure 3(a). In this case, a smaller concentric opening of radius a ($0 \leq a \leq b$) in side the projected opening of radius b is excavated in the ground of E, ν, and the unexcavating ground ring between the radius a and b is regarded as a lining of $\bar{E}/E$, $\bar{\nu} = \nu$, and a/b.

There are shown in the figure three solid lines of $\bar{K}_T$ as well as three broken lines of $\bar{K}_L$ corresponding to different ν of the ground, $\nu=0.2$, 0.3, and 0.4. The support-stiffness of surrounding ground, $\bar{K}_E$ ($=\bar{K}_T - \bar{K}_L$), appears as the difference of ordinate between the corresponding two lines of $\bar{K}_T$ and $\bar{K}_L$.

On one extreme of the initial ground ($a/b=0$), the result of $\bar{K}_T = \bar{K}_L = 1$ and $\bar{K}_E = 0$ means that the initial ground core in the projected opening, as a lining, bears all the support-load belong to the opening. In this case the absolute stiffness of the lining is the same one of the initial ground core; so the support-stiffness of lining, $\bar{K}_L$ (= the total support-stiffness of tunnel, $\bar{K}_T$) is regarded as 1.0, as a relative stiffness to the value of the initial ground core, K_0^*. On the other extreme of the unlined opening ($a/b=1$), the result of $\bar{K}_L = 0$ and $\bar{K}_T = \bar{K}_E < 1$ shows that the surrounding ground bears all the support-load, that

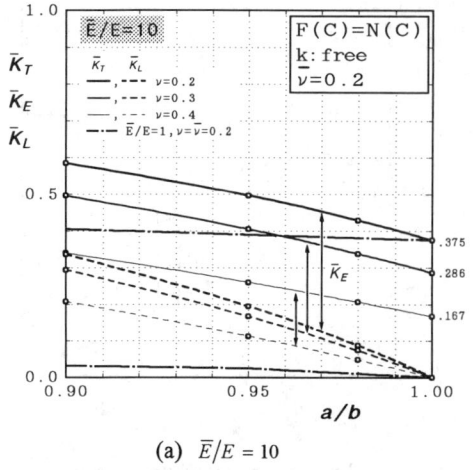
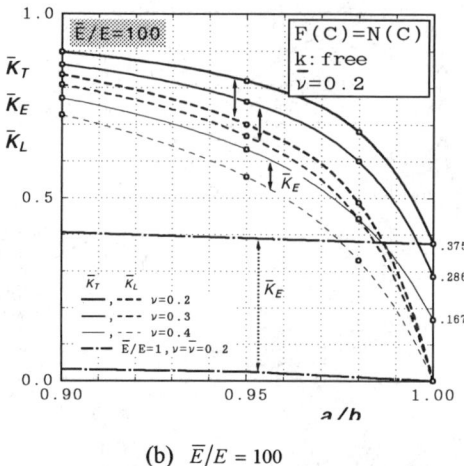

(a) $\bar{E}/E = 10$ (b) $\bar{E}/E = 100$

Figure 4. More practical examples of the support-stiffnesses of excavation unloading solution, $F(C)=N(C)$ ($\bar{\nu} = 0.2, a/b = 0.9 - 1.0$)

the representative displacement u_0 becomes much larger than u_0^* of the initial ground, and that $\bar{K}_E(=\bar{K}_T)$, depending on ν alone, becomes much lower than 1.0.

Next, Figure 3(b) shows the result corresponding to the "excavation unloading" solution, $F(C)=N(C)$. Comparing with Figure 3(a), the support-stiffnesses $\bar{K}_L$ and then $\bar{K}_T$ become much lower at the full range of a/b except $a/b=1$ than those of the "external loading" solution, and both results only coincide at $a/b=1$ (the same unlined condition).

Finally, Figures 4(a) and (b) indicate more practical examples of the support-stiffnesses, $\bar{K}_L$, $\bar{K}_E$, and $\bar{K}_T$, of the "excavation unloading" solution, $F(C)=N(C)$, for the practical range of lining thickness, $a/b=0.9-1.0$. The Poisson's ratio of lining is $\nu=0.2$, and the relative Young's modulus are $\bar{E}/E=10$ in Figure 4(a) and 100 in Figure 4(b).

From the results, we may summarize important characteristics of the support-stiffness as follows:
① The lower the Poisson's ratio of the surrounding ground, ν, is, the higher become all the support-stiffnesses.
② Increasing the relative Young's modulus of the lining, $\bar{E}/E$, increases the support-stiffness of lining and then the total support-stiffness of tunnel.

It should be recognized that one cannot estimate the support-stiffnesses of lining, surrounding ground, and the total without accurate knowledge of E and ν of a given ground.
③ For low $\bar{E}/E$ (=1-10), the support-stiffness of surrounding ground, $\bar{K}_E$, is higher than $\bar{K}_L$ of lining, and it keeps through $a/b=1-0.9$ almost constant near the value of the unlined condition, $a/b=1$.
④ For high $\bar{E}/E$ (=100), the support-stiffness of lining, $\bar{K}_L$, constitutes about 90% of the total support-stiffness of tunnel, $\bar{K}_T$, at $a/b=0.90$-0.96 where $\bar{K}_T$ reaches 80-90% of the stiffness of the initial ground core.

As a conclusion we may estimate the total support-stiffness of tunnel, $\bar{K}_T$, is 0.2-0.35 for ordinary tunnelling, consisting of $\bar{K}_L=0.05$-0.20 and $\bar{K}_E=0.13$-0.17; since $\bar{\nu}=0.2$, $\bar{E}/E=1$-10, $a/b=0.9$-1.0 for the practical lining of shotcrete and/or field concrete and $\nu=0.4$ as weakening the surrounding ground.

REFERENCES

1) Kiyama, H., Fujimura, H., Nishimura, T., & Ikezoe Y. : Theoretical Construction of bearing characteristic curve in tunnelling (in Japanese), *Journal of the Society of Material Science, Japan*, Vol. 41, No. 463, pp.417-423, 1992.
2) Muir Wood, A. M. : The circular tunnel in elastic ground, *Géotechnique* 25, No.1, pp.115-127, 1975.
3) Einstein, H. H. & Schwartz C. W. : Simplified analysis for tunnel supports, *Journal of the Geotechnical Engineering Division, ASCE*, Vol.105, No.GT4, pp.499-518, 1979.

Induced stress measurements in damaged region around a tunnel

A. Hirata
Department of Civil Engineering, Kumamoto Institute of Technology, Japan

M. Yamamoto
Asahi Chemical Industry Co., Ltd, Japan

T. Inaba
Nishimatsu Construction Co., Ltd, Japan

Y. Obara
Kumamoto University, Japan

ABSTRACT: This paper presents the results of induced stress measurement in damaged regions around a test tunnel excavated by smooth blasting. The blasting design was for a test tunnel excavation 8 m^2 in cross section, with an advance per round of 2.5 m. Five rounds were performed by two types of detonators, each with a large-hole cut and perimeter holes in a 0.4 m spacing. One is electronic detonators (EDs) which were used in the holes on the perimeter of the right half, the other is conventional pyrotechnical long period delay detonators of 0.25 deci second interval (PDs) which were used in the holes on the perimeter of the left half. In order to compare the delay accuracy of two detonators, a series of stress measurement was performed from the tunnel wall. It was made clear that EDs had little influence on remaining rock and surface, and PDs generated a damaged region. The damaged region generated by PDs was within 1 m from the tunnel surface and vertical stress hardly acted on the damaged region.

1 INTRODUCTION

Tunnel blasting causes several undesirable effects such as overbreak and underbreak at the perimeter, and damage of the remaining rock around a tunnel. Control blasting has been employed for the prevention of these undesirable effects. Smooth blasting, one of control blasting, is the standard method for underground rock excavation, to reduce overbreak and remaining rock damage and obtain a smooth remaining rock surface. These are important for structural integrity of an excavated tunnel or underground chamber, and also for economy in the use of rockbolts, shotcretes, and other structural supports.

Many studies have elucidated the effects of explosive type and charge volume, decoupling indexes, hole spacing and drilling precision, burden, and tamping length on smooth blasting. And quasi static gas pressure contributes very much to the completion of a smooth wall in the smooth blasting operation (Ito et al., 1970). Notched blast hole technique (Nakagawa et al., 1986) and ligamented split tube charge holder (Fourney et al., 1978) have been suggested as countermeasures to achieve an optimum smooth blasting. These techniques allow the fracture plane to smoothly grow with an arbitrary direction. It has been reported on the basis of a detailed analysis of an actual tunneling survey that the improvement of drilling precision can save 7 - 10 % of the total expense (Furukawa et al., 1987). The influence of detonator delay accuracy on the achievement of smooth blasting remained unclear, because of the inaccuracy of the delay times provided by conventional pyrotechnical delay detonators.

Microseismic activity induced by blasting excavation in tunneling was monitored in a highly stressed area (Hirata et al., 1991). The epicenters localized in the vicinity around the tunnel. The damaged region plays an important role for stability of an underground structure. The estimation of stress field in the damaged region is essential. But, stress measurement in the region damaged by blasting has not been previously carried out. Therefore, we had no knowledge in enough detail about the induced stress field around rock cavity.

The electronic delay detonator was developed in order to improve initiation time accuracy. It consists of an integrated circuit that controls delay time, an instantaneous electric detonator, and an electric capacitor. The electric capacitor supplies electric energy to drive the IC and initiate the electric detonator. All of them are incorporated in a plastic cartridge measuring approx. 110 mm in overall length and 10 mm in maximum diameter. EDs are connected to the connecting wire in series, and electric energy is supplied to the ED's capacitor through the legwires. When electric energy from the blasting machine brings the capacitor to a designed charge level, the counter reset circuit activates the counter circuit. When the counter reaches the time entered in the detonation time preset circuit, the switching circuit releases the remaining capacitor charge into the instantaneous electric detonator. The coefficient of variation of ED's delay time is 0.37 % at 1 second in nominal time, and that of PD is 4.45 % (Sakamoto et al., 1989). The delay time of ED has smaller variations than that of PD.

The blasting experiments were conducted in a deep mine. We adopted smooth blasting method in tunneling for reduction of overbreak, remaining rock damage and stress concentration on rock surface. Two types of detonators were used in smooth blasting. One is the conventional deci second detonator of 0.25 second interval, that is not good on delay accuracy. The other is the electronic delay detonator, that is highly accurate. The EDs were used in holes on the perimeter of the right half, and the PDs in all the other holes. Induced stress in the remaining rock around a test tunnel was measured by the compact overcoring method (Sugawara et al., 1992, Obara et al., 1995).

2 OVERVIEW OF TEST

2.1 Site of test blasting

The test site shown in Figure 1 is 550 m above sea level, and is consisted of very hard and uniform granodiorite. The overburden at the test site is about 340 m. The compression wave velocity in the test site is over 6.0 km/s. The uniaxial compression strength and the tensile strength are 300 MPa and 12 MPa, respectively. The geological discontinuity is shown as contours on the map of pole concentrations determined from the pole plot in lower hemisphere stereographic projection in Figure 2. Two major types of the discontinuities exist. First major discontinuities have a strike in an east-west direction, and the angle of inclination is broadly vertical. The discontinuity group intersects the test tunnel axis at an angle of 30 degrees. Second major discontinuities intersect the tunnel axis at right angles, and the dip angle is about 40 degrees toward a south-east direction. The geological discontinuities stay in closer touch, and so underground water hardly soaks from a rock surface and the discontinuities. The key block around the test tunnel is composed of these major geological discontinuities and tunnel walls.

The co-ordinates are defined in such ways that axis y is horizontal along the test tunnel axis toward the face, that axis x is horizontally perpendicular to axis y, and that axis z is upward. The test tunnel is 3.8 m in width, 3 m in height, and 8 m² in cross section, and the advance per round is 2.5 m. Five rounds were performed, each with a large-hole cut and perimeter holes in a 0.4 m spacing charged with a 20 mm diameter water gel explosive to obtain low charge concentration. After excavation of the tunnel, The smoothness of the walls and the damaged region of the remaining rock around the tunnel are observed by in-situ seismic prospecting, and stress measurements.

2.2 Overbreak and surface smoothness

In general, overbreak and surface smoothness are largely influenced by drilling accuracy. The position of each perimeter hole and the excavation cross section after each shot were measured. The three-dimensional position of the perimeter hole was determined by reading the scale on a measuring rod inserted in the hole by laser surveying at two points. The excavated cross section was determined every 0.5 m in the direction of advance by laser survey for cross-section dimensions and configurations.

The area of the excavation cross section and its quantity in each advance were evaluated. Excavation accuracy is expressed as the ratio the excavation quantity calculated from this area to the area of a cross section bounded by straight lines connecting the perimeter hole positions. The ratio is named a cross

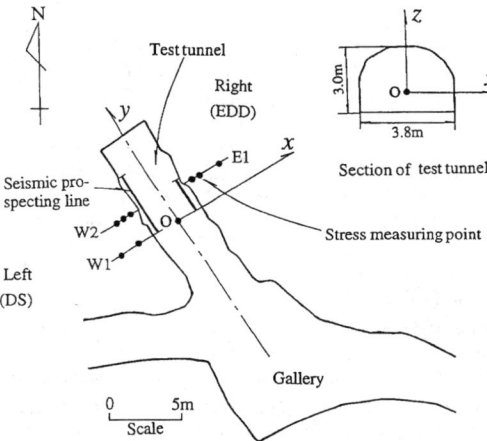

Figure 1. Map of the test site and the co-ordinates. Stress measurements were performed at the points of solid circles in borehole, E1, W1 and W2.

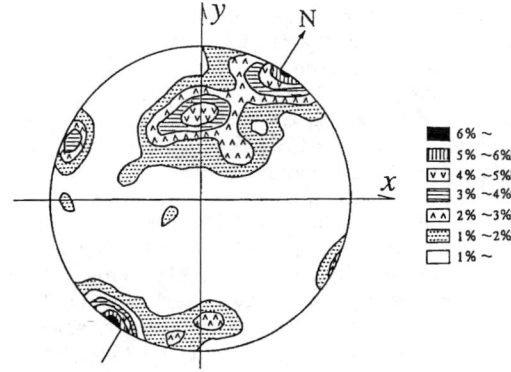

Figure 2. Contours of pole concentrations determined from the pole plot as lower hemisphere stereographic projection. Two major types of discontinuities exist in the test region. Tunnel direction y rotates 30 degrees in an west direction to the north.

section ratio. Figure 3 shows the cross section ratio for the ED and PD bounded halves, at various points of advance. The cross section ratio larger than 1.0 represents overbreak, and that smaller than 1.0 represents underbreak. The range of cross section ratios obtained for the ED and PD initiations are 0.92 to 1.07 and 0.83 to 1.16, respectively. The average and standard deviation of the cross section ratio for the ED and PD are 1.01, 0.03 and 1.06, 0.05, respectively. Overbreak and underbreak in case of the ED is lower than that of PD.

2.3 Laboratory test using core samples

The core samples were obtained from three boreholes. One is samples to a depth of 3 m on the ED side and two are samples to a depth of 3 m on the PD side, as shown in Figure 1. Boreholes and core samples are named as E1 on the ED side, and W1, W2 on the PD side.

In the core samples taken from the ED side, cracks obviously caused by the blasting exist up to a depth of only about 10 cm, with no observable cracks in any deeper region. In each of the core samples taken from the PD side, cracks obviously caused by the blasting exist to a depth of 20 cm, and many cracks probably attributable to the blasting were observed at depths of 0.5 to 1.0 m.

Young's modulus E, Poisson's ratio ν and compression wave velocity V_p of core samples were measured. These results are shown as a series of measurements running along the boreholes in Figure 4 and Figure 5. Compression wave velocity is measured in the borehole direction. Young's modulus and Poisson's ratio are 60 GPa and 0.21 on the average respectively on both sides, and the compression wave velocity is 6 km/s on both sides. There is no significant difference between the ED side and the PD side. It has become evident that the measurements by core samples do not lead to the difference between the both sides, because the damage by blasting hardly find in the core samples.

2.4 Damage determined by in situ seismic prospecting

In situ seismic wave prospecting was conducted in the test tunnel in order to determine the seismic wave velocity and the extent of remaining rock damage. Figure 6 shows plan view in which measurements were conducted. The vibration sensors and striking points were arranged on the right and left walls of the region excavated by the third and fourth rounds, as shown by open circle and arrow in Figure 6.

The incident wave transmits to the points in remaining rock at which the sensors are fixed. Damage in remaining rock generally consists of cracks generated by blasting. The seismic wave velocity in damaged regions is therefore lower than in non-damaged regions, decreasing in proportion to the size and number of the cracks within rock. The shortest interval between sensors was 10 cm. The waveforms

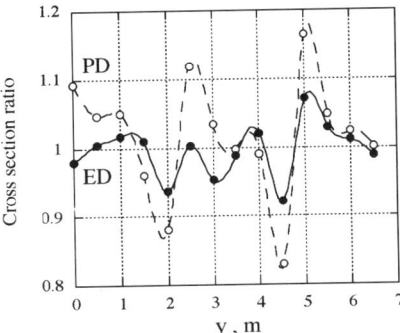

Figure 3. Advance distance and the cross section ratio. Solid circles are the measurement on the ED side, and open circles are that on the PD side.

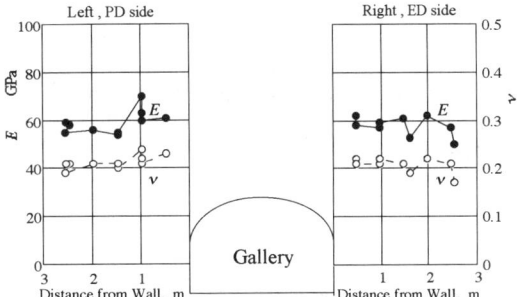

Figure 4. Distribution of Young's modulus and Poisson's ratio observed by the core samples.

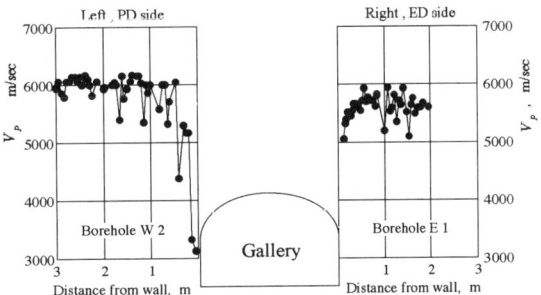

Figure 5. Distribution of the P wave velocity observed by the core samples.

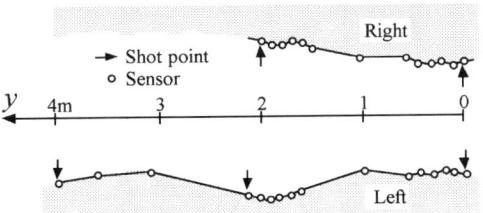

Figure 6. Arrangement of shot point (arrow) and sensors (open circle).

were recorded to obtain travel time to the sensors at a sampling frequency of 20 MHz.

Figure 7 shows that travel time curves along measurement lines on both the ED and the PD side. The travel time to 2 m from the striking point was approx. 800 micro seconds on the PD side and approx. 400 micro seconds on the ED side. This means that the damage caused by the PD-initiated blasting was substantially larger.

The seismic wave velocity distribution and the depth of damaged layers in remaining rock were determined by the seismic refraction method. As the results in Figure 8 show, the surface layer with a seismic wave velocity of between 1.0 km/s and 2.0 km/s, which indicates serious damage, was 20 cm in depth on the PD side, and 10 cm on the ED side. Next to this surface layer on the ED side was a layer with a seismic wave velocity of about 6.0 km/s, exactly the same value as that obtained by the measurement of boring cores. This indicates that the blastings initiated by the ED caused no damage to the bedrock at a depth exceeding 10 cm. On the PD side, however, a layer with a seismic wave velocity of approx. 4.5 km/s extended to a depth of 1 m, suggesting significant damage in the rock to that depth.

In all cases, the regions containing many cracks obviously caused by blasting are coincident with the regions which showed a seismic wave velocity of 1.0 km/s to 2.0 km/s in the in situ seismic prospecting. The regions, in the PD-side cores, containing cracks probably attributable to the blastings corresponded largely to the region showing a seismic wave velocity of about 4.5 km/s on the PD side, although they were also found at a greater depth. Overall, the boring core observations were in close agreement with the results of the in situ seismic prospecting, and therefore confirm their validity.

3 STRESS DISTRIBUTION AROUND TUNNEL

The compact overcoring technique developed by Sugawara et al., in which the borehole bottom has the geometry of conical surface, was adopted to stress measurement of remaining rock around the tunnel. The technique enables the three dimensional stress tensors to be determined from a measurement in a single borehole. The strains on the conical bottom of a borehole, which are eight longitudinal and latitudinal strains, are measured with the stress relief technique using the overcoring operation. They are measured by means of a conical strain cell made from epoxy resin with eight cross gauges.

Stress measurements were carried out in three boreholes, E1, W1 and W2. Solid circles in Figure 1 are the points of stress measurement, and the induced stresses were determined at eight points in total. Stress components determined in a series of measurements are shown as a function of distance from the tunnel

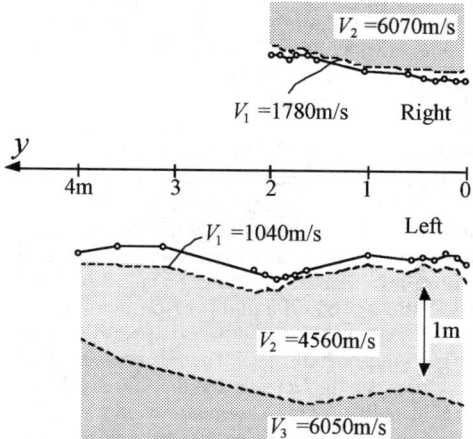

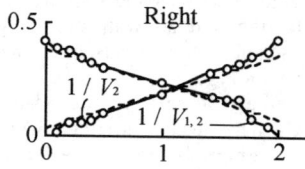

Figure 8. The P wave velocity and the damaged depth in remained rock by seismic prospecting. The damaged region of 1 m in depth exists on left side, in which P wave velocity is 4560 m/s, but that damaged region hardly exists on right side.

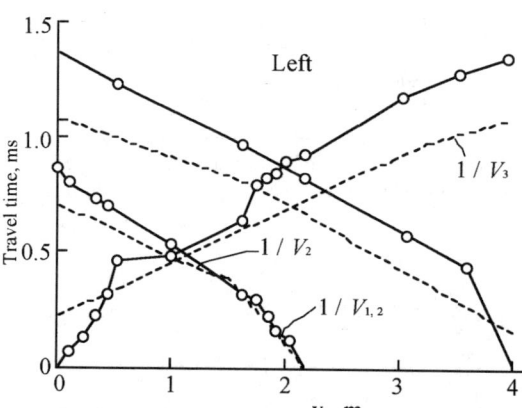

Figure 7. Travel time curve along measurement lines on the ED (right) side and the PD (left) side by in-situ seismic wave prospecting. Compression wave transmits in the damaged rock, and the first arrival reaches at most fast pass to each sensor. Open circle represents the travel time of vibration induced by hitting to each sensor from shot point. Broken line represents reciprocal of P wave velocity in each region.

wall in Figure 9. Open circles are the measurements of ED side, and closed circles are those of PD side, respectively. Long dashed lines and short dashed lines estimate the stress distribution on the ED side and PD side basing on the measurement, respectively. In this paper, minus in magnitude of stress shows a compression.

σ_x on either the ED side or the PD side shows equally zero to 0.5 m from the tunnel wall, and increases in magnitude of -7 MPa on the ED side and -5 MPa on the PD side to 1 m from 0.5 m in depth. Both of σ_x on the right and the left side equally converge to -5 MPa to the back of 1 m in depth. These characteristic curves along the boreholes of σ_x are quite similar, one to the other. σ_y on either side is nearly zero at the tunnel surface, and reaches a maximum of -17 MPa on the ED side and -10 MPa on the PD side at 1 m in depth, respectively. σ_y decrease by degrees and converges to

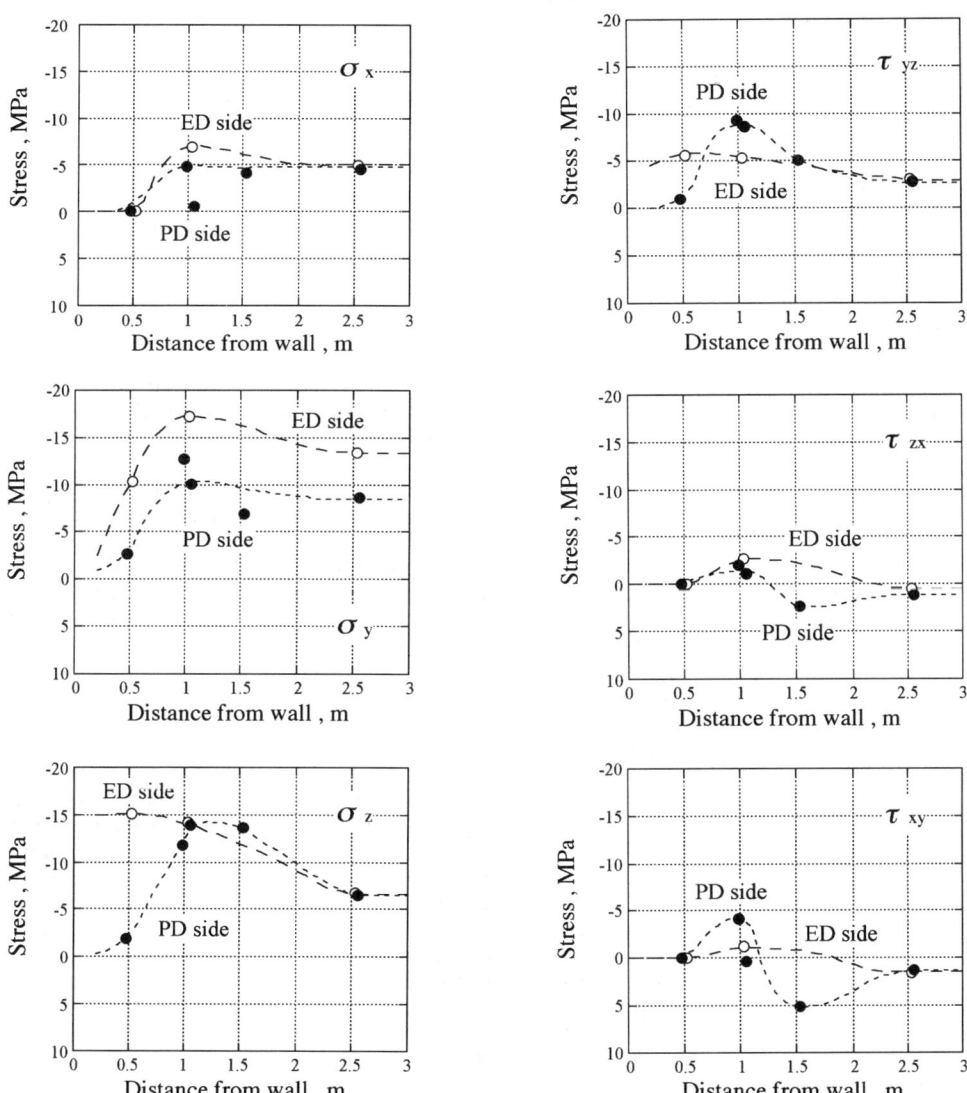

Figure 9. Comparison of the stress distribution as a function of the distance from gallery wall. Open circle is the measurement of the ED side, and closed circle shows that of the PD side. Long dashed line and short dashed line represent the estimation of the stress distribution on the ED side and the PD side, respectively. Minus in magnitude of stress shows a compression. The difference between vertical stresses on the PD side and the ED side is clear within 1 m from the tunnel wall.

-13 MPa on the right side and -8 MPa on the left side, respectively. It is considered that the damaged region on the PD side changes the maximum magnitude of -17 MPa on the right side into the maximum magnitude of -10 MPa on the left side. σ_z on the ED side shows the magnitude of -15 MPa to 0.5 m from rock surface, and decreases by degrees to the magnitude of -7 MPa at the back of 2.5 m in depth. On the other hand, σ_z on the PD side shows nearly zero at the surface, and the peak of σ_z is -14 MPa in range of 1 m from 1.5 m in depth. And σ_z at the back of 2.5 m in depth coincides with σ_z on the ED side. Vertical stress is not transferred in the damaged region on the left side.

τ_{yz}, that is shear stress in plane in parallel with the tunnel side wall, is greater than τ_{zx} and τ_{xy}. τ_{yz} on the ED side is -5 MPa at 0.5 m in depth, and -3 MPa at 2.5 m in depth. The characteristic curve of τ_{yz} on the PD side is generally similar to that of the ED side with the exception of the magnitude of zero to 0.5 m in depth from the surface. τ_{zx} and τ_{xy} on both sides are zero in the vicinity of the surface since the surface is free, show no-zero at 1 m from 1.5 m in depth, and converge to zero at the back. We consider that the discontinuity of type of N60° E45° SE causes the steep change of τ_{xy} in range of 1 m to 1.5 m in depth on the left side. The influence of the discontinuity gives the great change to the magnitude of τ_{xy} at 1.5 m in depth. The magnitude of τ_{xy} at 1.5 m in depth should be eliminated in the distribution of the shear stress τ_{xy} on the PD side.

It is concluded at a rough guess that one of principal stresses is in a direction of axis x, and the others are included on y-z plane. Maximum principal stress in compression acts on the tunnel face from above, since maximum normal stress in compression is σ_y, and τ_{yz} is negative. The measurements on the ED side and the PD side are similar to each other at 2.5 m in depth. This leads to the conclusion that the excavation of test tunnel affects within 2.5 m from the rock surface. Initial stress before excavation is obtained by averaging of the data on the ED and the PD side measured at 2.5 m in depth.

4 CONCLUSION

The present study was conducted to investigate the effect of high accuracy of delay time on surface smoothness and remaining rock damage, in comparison with that of less accurate-delay times. The test tunnel was excavated with blast initiation by periphery EDs on one side and by PDs on the other. The resultant surface smoothness and remaining rock damage were determined by cross sectional area measurement, in situ seismic prospecting, core sample test, and stress measurement in remaining rock.

It was recognized that the smooth blasting using EDs could decrease the damaged region in remaining rock and create the smooth surface, and PDs generated a damaged region.

Stress components in the damaged region were determined as a function of distance from the tunnel wall on both side. The maximum magnitude of σ_y on the PD side was -17 MPa, and that on the ED was -10 MPa. σ_z on the ED side indicated the magnitude of -15 MPa to 0.5 m from the tunnel wall, and decreased by degrees to the magnitude of -7 MPa at the back of 2.5 m in depth. σ_z on the PD side was nearly zero at the surface, and the peak of σ_z was -14 MPa in range of 1 m from 1.5 m in depth. σ_z on the PD side coincided with σ_z on the ED side at the back of 2.5 m in depth. Vertical stress hardly acted in the damaged region on the left side. The severe damaged region generated by PDs was within 1 m from the tunnel surface.

The stress measurements on the ED side and the PD side were similar to each other at 2.5 m in depth from the tunnel wall. It is concluded that the influence of the test tunnel excavation is within 2.5 m from the tunnel wall. Virgin stress state before excavation is obtained by averaging of the measurements at 2.5 m in depth on the ED and the PD side.

REFERENCES

Fourney, W. L., J. W. Dally and D.C. Holloway 1978. Controlled blasting with ligamented charge holders. *Int. J. Rock Mech. Min. Sci. Geomech. Abstr.* 15:121-129.

Furukawa, K., K. Yoshimi, H. Setoguchi and K. Nakagawa 1987. Optimum design of smooth blasting in tunneling hard rock. *Proceedings of Japan Society of Civil Engineers* 379:107-115.

Hirata, A., K. Ishiyama, N. Taga and Y. Kameoka 1991. AE monitoring and rock stress measurement in rockburst site. *Proceedings of International Congress on ISRM*: 505-508.

Ito, I. and K. Sassa 1970. Mechanism of rock breakage by the pressure of explosion gas. *Proceedings of the 3rd Japan Symposium on Rock Mechanics*:173-178.

Nakagawa, K., Y. Nishida, Y. Ono and J. Kawakami 1986. Blast crack control and smooth blasting using notched blast hole technique. *Proceedings of Japan Society of Civil Engineers* 373:52-61.

Obara, Y., K. Sugawara and K. Sakaguchi 1995. Rock stress measurements by the conical-ended borehole technique using the compact overcoring. *Proceedings of International Congress on ISRM*: 145-148.

Sakamoto, M., M. Yamamoto, K. Aikou, E. Suzuki, H. Fukui, and K. Ichikawa 1989. A study on high accuracy delay detonator. *Proceedings of 15th Annual Conference on Explosives and Blasting Techniques*: 185-200.

Sugawara, K., K. Sakaguchi, Y. Obara, T. Nakayama and H. K. Jang 1992. Rock stress measurement and numerical approach for cavern designing. *Journal of Korean Rock Mechanics Society* 2-1:164-176.

In site measurement of geostresses in a tunnel of Nanning-Kunming railway

Fang Zhaoru & Bai Shiwei
Institute of Rock and Soil Mechanics, Wuhan, The Chinese Academy of Sciences, People's Republic of China

ABSTRACT: In site measuring results of geostresses of a soft and fractured rockmass obtained using hollow inclusion borehole stainmeters are described in detail through a practical engineering case of a tunnel of Nanning-Kunming Railway. Based upon the testing results and the geomechanical environments, the basic reasons causing large deformations in the rockmass surrounding the tunnel are analysed, which provides scientific basis for the supporting design of the tunnel.

1 INTRODUCTION

Measurements of rockmass stresses are an important aspect of the study on rockmass' in site mechanical behavior. Our institute has been for years dedicating to the study on this topic closely in combination with engineering practice. The geostress measuring performed in a tunnel of Nanning-Kunming Railway using self-developed hollow inclusion borehole strainmeters is a successful practical case of in site rockmass stress study.

Of the total length of 4900m of the tunnel, about 1085m passes through coal measure seams belonging to Longtan series of Neogene series of Dyas with an extremely complicated geological environments. During excavation, gas inrushes once occured for many times in succesion, large quantity of outgush of underground water took place, the surrounding rockmass swelled and some segments of the tunnel seriously deformed. The maximum deformation is high up to over one meter, resulting in serious bending and twist of steel arch frames, considerable fracture of concrete lining and even cave-in in many places. To ascertain the reason causing the large deformation and to ensure smooth proceeding of the engineering works, we carried out various field tests including in site measuring of geostresses in the large-deformation sections to seek effective supporting measure. According to the measuring results about the magnitude and the acting orientation of the geostress, the constructing unit took effective supporting measure in time, thus ensuring the completion of the tunnel on scheldule.

2 GENERALIZATION OF ENGINEERING GEOLOGY AROUND THE TUNNEL

The tunnel passes through a mountain range with a relative elevation difference of about 380m, and the range feature is governed by the geological structure to form a pedion mountain. The northwest slope is a structure one, its gentle surface has a dip of 25°~30°, approximately the same as that of the rock stratum; the southeast terrace slope is a denudated one with a local steep landform and developed cleuches on the two sides of the subdivide.

The tunnel is located in the east wing of the discoid sycline belonging to unicline structure. The strike of the rock stratum is N20°~30°E/NW$\angle$25°~30°. The tunnel passes through the basalt stratum groups of Dalong, Changxing and Longtan of the Emei Mountain (Pliosene series of Dyas) and the stratum groups of Feixianguan and Yongning (Eogene series of Triassic system). The stratification is developed. Owing to the effects of structural movements, joint cracks are quite developed and flexible folds have formed locally between beddings. There are two orthogonal faults, F_1 and F_2, in the region where the tunnel axis penetrates through. Fault F_1, at an angle of 80° with the tunnel near IDK-597 ± 340, is large in scale with a 15~20m wide fractured zone.

A length of about 1085m of the tunnel is in the coal seams with 15 beds. Every bed contains gas and of these beds, three have a gas pressure over 1MPa.

The outcrop of the rockmass exposed by the excavation shows that large deformations mainly

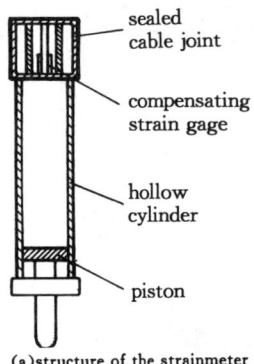 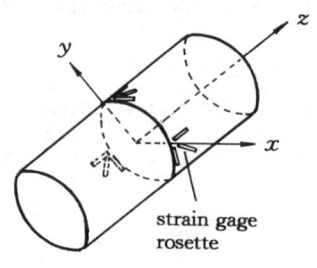 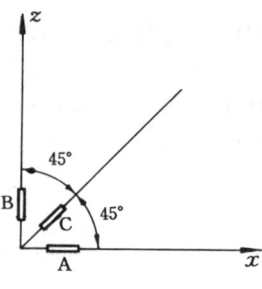

(a) structure of the strainmeter   (b) arrangements of three rosettes on the outer wall   (c) schematic map of a rosette

Figure 1. Schematic diagram of a hollow strainmeter

occur within a range of 400m where the tunnel passes through the faults fractured zone. In this area, the rocks surrounding the tunnel consist mainly of coal, coal stone and soft sandstone. Most rocks look clastic shaped and most coal seams are fragmental and silt-grain shaped.

3 MEASURING PRINCIPLE AND CALCULATION OF STRESS

Shown in Fig. 1 is the structure of a hollow inclusion borehole strainmeter, consisting of a hollow cylinder, a piston, compensating strain gages, a sealed cable joint, etc.. In the middle of the cylinder, three sets of strain gage rosettes are cemented on the outer wall, each containing three strain gages respectively taking the direction of generatrix, circumference and bisector of the formers.

The testing procedure is shown in Fig. 2. Firstly, insert the strainmeter into the small guiding hole in the borehole bottom, then push the piston to squeeze out the epoxy resin previously injected into the hollow cylinder to fill the gap between the cylinder and the guiding hole, as a result, the stain gages are tightly cemented on the guiding hole's wall through a thin layer of the epoxy resin, and finally perform stress relief technique using the overcoring method to measure the strain values during unloading. Based upon the measured strains, the complete strain state of the rockmass can be calculated.

Leeman proposed a borehole wall strain method (Leeman, 1968) to determine the complete strain state of a rockmass using three strain gage rosettes directly cemented on the guiding hole wall in the bottom of a borehole. The measuring principle and formulation for

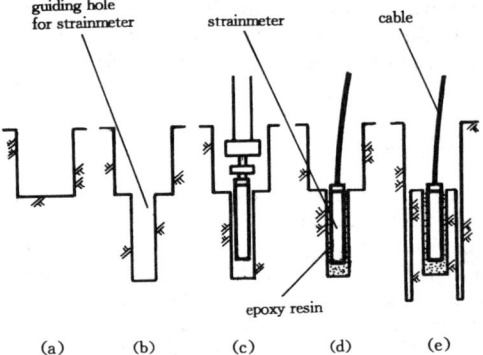

(a) drilling of borehole; (b) drilling of guiding hole; (c) inserting strainmeter; (d) solidification of epoxy resin; (e) stress relief

Figure 2. Testing procedure of stress relief by overcoring method

geostresses of our strainmeter are basically the same as Leeman's.

From the formulation derived based upon the borehole wall strain method, we have the relationship between the measured stress components and those of the initial geostress field at each point ($r = a$) on the guiding hole wall:

$$P_\theta(1) = (\sigma_x + \sigma_y) - 2(\sigma_x - \sigma_y)\cos2\varphi_i - 4\tau_{xy}\sin2\varphi_i \qquad (1)$$

$$P_z(i) = -\mu[(\sigma_x - \sigma_y)\cos2\varphi_i + 2\tau_{xy}\sin2\varphi_i] + \sigma_z \qquad (2)$$

$$\tau_{\theta z}(i) = -2\tau_{zx}\sin\varphi_i + 2\tau_{yz}\cos\varphi_i \qquad (3)$$

$$P_r(i) = \tau_{r\theta}(i) = \varphi_{rz}(i) = 0 \qquad (4)$$

where for three sets of strain gage rosettes, *is*

are respectively 1, 2, 3; φ is the angle between the rosettes.

From the above equations, it can be seen that any point, whatever its location is on the wall, is in a plane stress state. In the case of the rosette shown as in Fig. 1, each strain gage has a strain value of

$$\varepsilon_a = \varepsilon_\theta \cos^2\alpha + \varepsilon_z \sin^2\alpha + \gamma_{\theta_z}\sin\alpha \cdot \cos\alpha \quad (5)$$

where, α is $0, \pi/2, \pi/4$ respectively for $\varepsilon_A, \varepsilon_B$ and ε_C.

Based upon the physical formulation of a plane problem, the relationship between the measured strain and the corresponding stress is

$$\varepsilon_a(i) = \frac{1}{E}\{[P_\theta(i) - \mu P_z(i)]\cos^2\alpha + P_z(i) - \mu P_\theta(i)\sin^2\alpha\} + \frac{2(1+\mu)}{E}\tau_{\theta z}(i)\sin\alpha\cos\alpha \quad (6)$$

In institution of eq. s(1), (2) and (3) into eq. (6), we have the following relation between the measured strain $\varepsilon_a(i)$ and the stress component of the rockmass:

$$\{\varepsilon\} = \{A\}\{\sigma\}/E \quad (7)$$

where:
$\{A\}$ — coefficient matrix calculated from eq. (6)
E — elastic module of core

Then we may use least square method to perform optimization on the monitoring equatin of (7) to obtaion the initial stress of $\{\sigma\}$ and to calculate the principle stresses of $\sigma_1, \sigma_2, \sigma_3$ and their orientations.

4 IN SITE MEASURING AND TESTING RESULTS

In order to assess the effect of both magnitude and acting orientation of initial geostress of the rockmass on the tunnel's large deformations, the measuring points were arranged in the zone where large deformations happened. Bearing two aspects in minds, viz., basic requirements for testing and not interfering with the construction, we arranged the measuring points in the sandstone region surrounding a pilot drift parallel to and 25 meters away from the major tunnel. Altogether three boreholes were horizontally drilled.

Overcoring was very difficult during testing because of well-developed rock joints in the test-

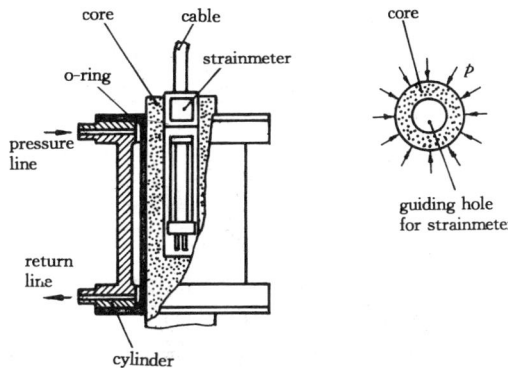

Figure 3. Determination of core elastic module in a specially designed device

ing area. Altogether, 15 stress measurements were conducted and only 3 sets of effect data — quite valueable were obtained.

The cores overcored after stress relief testing, with a hollow strainmeter tightly cemented on its central guiding hole wall, were put into a specially designed elastic-module device to determine the elastic module (E) and Poisson's ratio (μ) of the cores (Fig. 3). In testing, confining pressures were step-wise exerted on a core and the strains in the guiding hole wall were recorded. According to these strains, the core's elastic module, E, and Poisson's ratio, μ, were determined through calculation. This method to determine the physico-mechanical indexes of a core takes into account the comprehensive error effects of comlicated and random factors including the thin epoxy resin layer.

In exerting confining pressures, the stress state is that $\sigma_x = \sigma_t = P$ and the rest is zero. The formulations for E and μ are

$$E = 2P/\varepsilon_A(i) \quad (8)$$

$$\mu = -E\varepsilon_B(i)/2P \quad (9)$$

where: $\varepsilon_A(i)$ and $\varepsilon_B(i)$ are longitudinal and circumferential strains at a measuring point (see Fig. 1(c)).

The calculated elastic module, E, and Poisson's ratio, μ, of the rock in the testing region are:

$$E = 1.45 \times 10^4 \text{MPa} \qquad \mu = 0.28$$

Then majorization treatment was performed on eq. (7) to calculate the magnitude and the orientation of principle stresses, σ_1, σ_2 and σ_3 by

Table 1. Computing results of in site stresses

thickness of overburden above tunnel: 380m			span of testing gallery: 2.5~3.0m	
lithology around measuring points: grey sandstone			depth of borehole: 6.02m	
principle stresses ① (MPa)	azimuths ② D (°)	dip V ③ (°)	stress components ④ (MPa)	
$\sigma_1 = 19.6$	$D_1 = 75.8$	$V_1 = 26.7$	$\sigma_x = 8.3$	$\tau_{xy} = 2.5$
$\sigma_2 = 7.8$	$D_2 = 174.9$	$V_2 = 17.6$	$\sigma_y = 16.1$	$\tau_{yz} = 5.6$
$\sigma_3 = 5.4$	$D_3 = 113.6$	$V_3 = -70.7$	$\sigma_z = 8.6$	$\tau_{zx} = 6.7$
lithology around measuring points: grey sandstone			depth of borehole: 6.5m	
$\sigma_1 = 17.4$	$D_1 = 72.1$	$V_1 = 21.6$	$\sigma_x = 7.81$	$\tau_{xy} = 3.12$
$\sigma_2 = 8.2$	$D_2 = 186.7$	$V_2 = 46.7$	$\sigma_y = 14.96$	$\tau_{yz} = 3.65$
$\sigma_3 = 5.7$	$D_3 = 145.3$	$V_3 = -36.0$	$\sigma_z = 8.71$	$\tau_{zx} = 0.02$

① $\sigma_1, \sigma_2, \sigma_3$ are maximum, medium and minimum principle stresses respectively;
② D_1, D_2, D_3 are the azimuths of maximum, medium and minimum principle stresses respectively;
③ V_1, V_2, V_3 are the dips of max., med. and min. principle stresses respectively, (V is the angle between principle stress and coordinate plane of XOY, positive for elvation angle and negative for depression angle);
④ σ_x, σ_y are horizontal stress components and σ_z is vertical one.

solving a character equation. The calculating results are listed in Table 1.

5 INTERPRETATION OF TESTING RESULTS AND CONCLUSIONS

5.1 The data listed in Table 1 show that the vertical stress components converted from the in site measured one are $\sigma_z = 8.6$MPa at 6.02m — point and $\sigma_z = 8.71$MPa at 6.5m — point, all somewhat greater than the stress caused by the self-weight of the overburden rockmass, which indicates that there exists a structural stress in this region besides the self-weight stress.

5.2 Under the action of the self-weight of the rockmass, the horizontal stress components are equal along any direction in any horizontal plane in the deep part of the rockmass, viz., $\sigma_x = \sigma_y = \mu \cdot \gamma H / (1 - \mu)$. Nevertheless, the in site measuring shows that $\sigma_x \neq \sigma_y$, with an ratio of (σ_y/σ_x) of about 2.0. Probably, the reason is that both distribution and magnitude of stresses in the testing region are strongly affected by the fractured band in major fault F_1.

5.3 The situation revealed by the excavation shows that in the large deformation region, not only does there exist major fault F, but also stratifications and joints are considerably developed. The rockmass in the region is characterized by fragment in structure, poor intactness, low diagenetic degree, low rock strength and structure strength, and low self-supporting capability. In summary, the geological engineering property is quite poor, which is the potential reason causing serious deformation and failure of the rockmass after the excavation of the tunnel. Furthermore, large size excavation creates a spacial condition for the deformation and failure of the rockmass under the action of self-weight and structural stresses.

5.4 The value and azimuth of maximum principle stress *in-situ* measured indicate that the large deformation occuring in the testing region is likely the reflection of the above stated results.

5.5 In view of the above analyses, we have the following conclusion. The interaction between geostress and rock medium is the main reason causing serious deformations and failure after excavation; the mechanism of deformation and failure is that the unloading caused by excavation disturbs the equilibrium state of the rockmass itself and results in redistribution of stresses and inward deformation and displacement of the rockmass surrounding the tunnel; owing to well-developed rock joints and fractured structure, the engineering property of the rockmass is very poor and the structure strength and self supporting capability are very low, as a result, no higher strain energy can be accumulated in the rockmass. So, under the continuing reaction of the rockmass self-weight and the structural stress, the rockmass gradually creeps and deforms towards the tunnel air surface. Large deformations will occur and instability failure will result when the displacement of the rockmass reaches to a certain limitation.

REFERENCES

Bai Shiwei, Fang Zhaoru 1987. Hollow Inclusion Strainmeter, *J. of Rock mechanics*, Vol. 8, No. 4

Leeman E. R. 1968. The Determination of the Complete State of Stress in Rock in Single Borehole-Laboratory and Underground Measurements. *Int. J. Rock Mech. Min. Sci.* Vol. V, pp. 31—56

The Second Design Institution of the Chi. Minstry of Railway, Generalization of Engineering Geology, *Handbook for Railway Design*

Rock Stress, Sugawara & Obara (eds) © 1997 Balkema, Rotterdam, ISBN 90 5410 901 7

Rock stress changes during excavation of a large underground cavern

Keigo Kudoh, Toshihiro Koyama & Yuichi Komatsuzaki
The Tokyo Electric Power Co., Inc., Japan

ABSTRACT: The underground cavern of the Kazunogawa power plant has a cross-sectional area of around 1,500 square meters and an excavated volume of around 250,000 cubic meters. The cavern is located in the Shimanto group where discontinuities such as joints and faults have developed, and at a depth of 500 meters below the surface. Therefore, excavation was carried out while measuring rock stress changes and other items in order to grasp the behavior of the rock near the cavern, and the development of loosened zone during excavation. As a result, rock stress concentration near the cavern with the progress of excavation, and stress redistribution owing to rock failure were confirmed. This paper describes the observed and predicted rock behavior including rock stress changes during excavation of the cavern at the Kazunogawa power plant.

1. INTRODUCTION

The Tokyo Electric Power Co., Inc. has been constructing the Kazunogawa power plant (a pure pumped storage power plant) having the maximum output of 1,600 MW, the maximum discharge of 280 m^3/s and the effective head of 714 m and stretching over Ohtsuki City and Enzan City in Yamanashi Prefecture, since the start of work in January 1993. The plant is scheduled to start service in December 1999 with the capacity of 400 MW.

The underground cavern of the plant was excavated while observing the cavern behavior in real-time using about 1,400 various gauges installed around the cavern, as the cavern is under the high ground pressure of approximately 500 m depth below the ground surface, and the rock around the cavern had highly developed joints due to cleavage in the mudstone belonging to the Shimanto group.

This paper reports the behavior of the underground cavern of the power plant excavated in the rock mass having joints, based on the data obtained during the excavation.

2. OUTLINE OF THE KAZUNOGAWA UNDERGROUND POWER PLANT

The Kazunogawa underground power plant is 54 m high, 34 m wide and 210 m long, and excavated volume is amount to 250 thousand m^3. Four units of water wheel generator having a capacity of 400 MW, and two units of 500 kV transformer will be installed. Excavation was conducted for the period of about 21 months between 1994 and 1996. The generators are now being installed.

3. GEOLOGY AT THE SITE OF POWER PLANT CAVERN AND PROPERTIES OF ROCK MASS

3.1 Geology

The geology at the site of the power plant consists mainly of mixed strata of sandstone and mudstone in the Shimanto group which seems to have been deposited in the Upper Cretaceous through the Paleogene period in the Cenozoic era. The general strike of the rock is nearly east-west, and the rock takes on the homocline structure, steeply dipping northward (Fig. 1).

The number of faults confirmed on the face of the cavern amounts to 42. The maximum fracture width is 80 cm. Most of the faults are considered lateral faults based on the scratches of the fault surface and the slip of the strata. The rock has an east-west strike, and a noticeable steep northward dip.

The joints that are observed on the face of the cavern are classified into three groups according to the strike and the dip (Fig. 2). (1) The joints whose

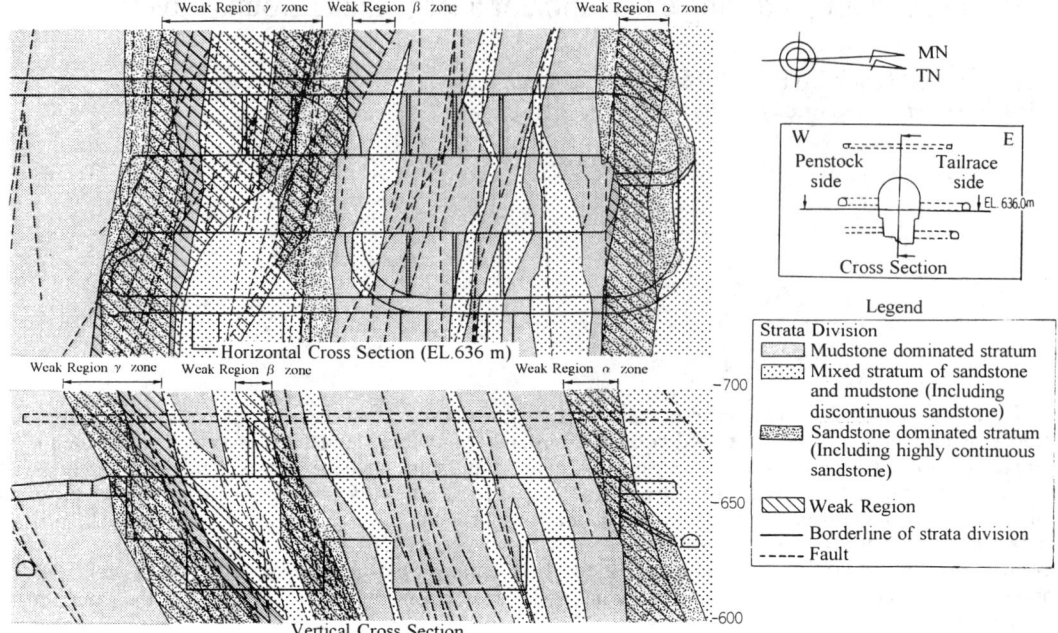

Fig.1 Geological Cross Section of the Site

strike is east-west, perpendicular to the cavern axis of the power plant, and whose dip is steeply northward (J$_{EW}$-h joints) account for 87%. (2) The joints whose strike is north-south, acutely crossing the cavern axis of the power plant, and whose dip is steeply (J$_{NS}$-h joints) account for 9%. (3) The joints whose strike is north-south, almost parallel to the cavern axis of the power plant, and whose dip is gently (J-l joints) account for 4%. Group (1), the most among the three, developed in the mudstone at a few to a dozen cm intervals. This group belongs to what is generally known as the slaty cleavage.

Based on the above findings, zones α, β and γ, where east-west faults and joints have developed, are defined as the weak regions, and management efforts are focused on them in design and construction.

3.2 Rock properties

The results of the rock test, and rock stress measurement conducted in survey adits prior to the construction are as shown in Table 1. Initial stress was measured with the multi-element strain gauge. For measuring the local stress during excavation,

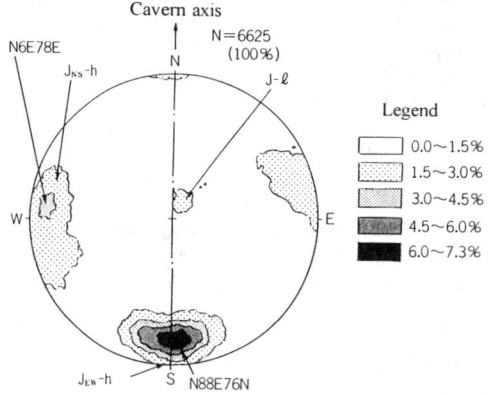

Fig.2 Distribution of Joint Density

Table-1 Rock Properties

	Test Results		
Deformation	[Jack Test]		($\times 10^3$MPa)
	Tangent Elastic Modulus		Modulus of deformation
	Loading	Unloading	
	Average 11.5	7.2	4.0
	(Range) (5.0~22.5)	(2.6~15.0)	(1.0~11.1)
	Ordinary Region E (Unloading) Ave. 12.6 $\times 10^3$MPa		
	Weak Region E (Unloading) Ave. 7.7 $\times 10^3$MPa		
Strength	[Rock Specimen Test]		
	Unconfined Compression Test Ave. 106 MPa		
	(35.3~245 MPa)		
	High Pressure Triaxial Compression Test		
	Peak Strength $\tau = 12.9$MPa $+ \sigma \tan 57°$		
	Residual Strength $\tau = 2.8$MPa $+ \sigma \tan 48°$		
	[Rock Shear Test]		
	Ordinary Region (Peak) $\tau = 1.5$MPa $+ \sigma \tan 58°$		
	Weak Region (Peak) $\tau = 0.8$MPa $+ \sigma \tan 55°$		
	Residual Strength $\tau = 0.5$MPa $+ \sigma \tan 50°$		
Rock Stress	[Initial Rock Stress Measurementt]		
	Overburden : 520 m		
	$\sigma_1 = 14.2$ MPa (N17° E, 68° down)		
	$\sigma_2 = 12.0$ MPa (N191° W, 20° down)		
	$\sigma_3 = 9.4$ MPa (N97° W, 9° down)		

conical-ended borehole technique using the compact overcoring was also used. In addition, a vibrating-wire stress meter was installed in order to measure stress changes around the cavern due to excavation. Redistribution of stress of actual rock was evaluated comparing with the analytical results.

4. PREDICTION OF CAVERN BEHAVIOR AND SUPPORT DESIGN

In order to predict behavior of the cavern, and to design supports, support pattern was calculated in accordance with the deformation and failure mode based on geological conditions. The deformation and failure mode were assumed by geological degradation due to concentration of faults and joints, formation of key blocks attributable to faults and joints, and so on. The specified support pattern is shown in Table. 2.

5. ACTUAL RESULTS OF THE BEHAVIOR OF THE ENTIRE CAVERN

5.1 Measurement management

In managing measurement during excavation, daily management, based on the measurement of displacement (strain) with multistage extensometers installed across the rock around the cavern, was adopted in combination with step management which comprehensively evaluated and analyzed the stability of the cavern in each phase of excavation interrelating the strain, stress and loosening for predetermined typical cross sections (main sections in which measurement is conducted). Allocation of measuring instrument in the main measurement sections is shown in Fig. 3.

Table.2 Support Pattern

			Ordinary Region	Weak Region
Vault	Anchor Pre-stress	MPa	0.21	0.31
	Anchor Length	m	15	20
	Anchor Pitch	m	3.0 × 1.5(4.50m²)	2.5 × 1.2(3.00m²)
	Shotcrete Thickness	cm	32	40
Side Wall	Anchor Pre-stress	MPa	0.18	0.31
	Anchor Length	m	15	20
	Anchor Pitch	m	2.5 × 2.1(5.25m²)	2.5 × 1.2(3.00m²)
	Shotcrete Thickness	cm	24	40
Elastic Modulus of Rock MPa			9,800	4,900

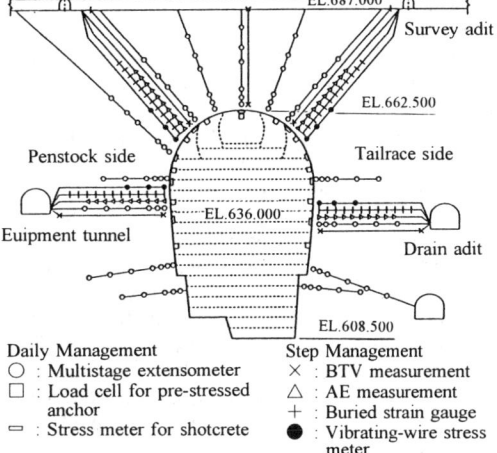

Fig.3 Allocation of Measuring Instruments

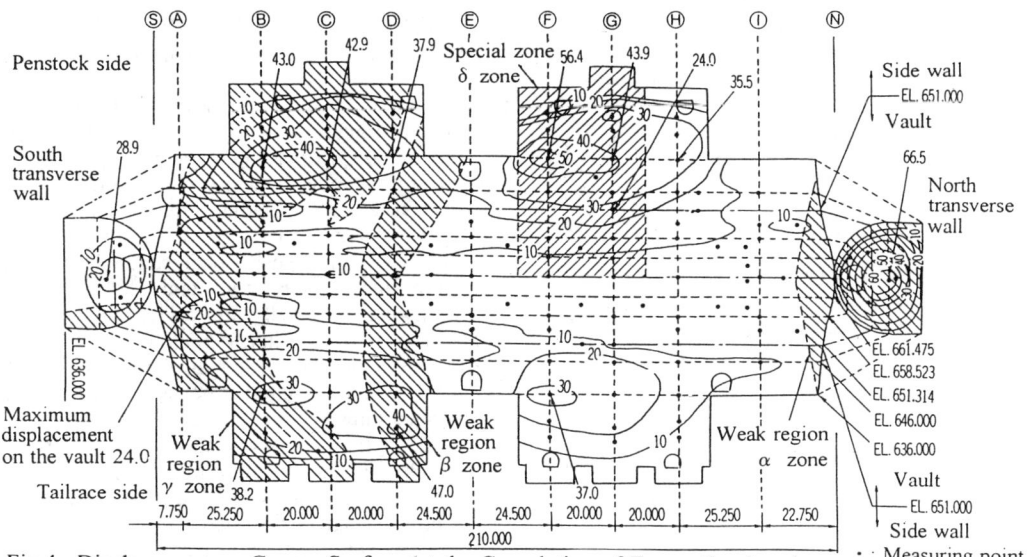

Fig.4 Displacement on Cavern Surface (at the Completion of Excavation)   unit : mm

5.2 Actual behavior of entire cavern

a. Displacement on cavern surface

The behavior of the entire cavern at the completion of excavation is as shown in Fig. 4. If analyzed by zone, displacement was larger in the weak region than in the ordinary region. In the middle level of the cavern (EL.636.0 m), there is a surface displacement of 36 to 43 mm in the weak region as compared with 12 to 37 mm in the ordinary region. In the transverse wall, there occurred a displacement of 67 mm, the largest in the entire cavern. On the side of the penstock in the F and G sections which were initially zoned in the ordinary region, displacement was greater than expected during excavation.

b. Results of measurement of stress and strain in the rock and AE measurement

In the main measurement sections (C and G sections), changes in stress and strain of the rock due to excavation were measured with the extensometers, and vibrating-wire stress meters placed close to one another. Acoustic emissions (AE) were also measured to confirm the evolution of loosened zones with the progress of excavation.

As a typical example, the results of measurement for the middle level of the penstock-side surface of the C section (EL.638.5 m) (Fig. 5) and evaluation are presented below.

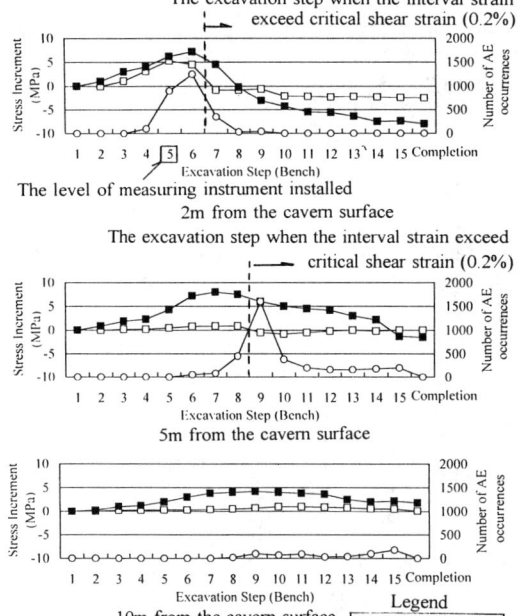

Fig.5 Results of Measurement of Stress and Strain in the Rock and AE Measurement

(i) Changes in tangential stress of the cavern due to excavation were great near the cavern surface, and the value measured at the point 2 m away from the surface duly agreed to the analytical result.

(ii) Tangential stress reached a peak near (2 m from) the cavern surface when excavation was carried out at the level where measurement instrument was installed. The stress peak shifted from the cavern surface to a deeper position with the progress of bench excavation. This was in agreement with the analytical result.

(iii) Tangential stress at the point 2 m or 5 m away from the cavern surface reached a peak almost at the same time as the AE peak and as when the radial interval strain (displacement measured with the multistage extensometers divided by the interval) reached the critical shear strain at this site, equivalent to 0.2% of the axial strain.

Judging from all of the above points, stress was concentrated due to excavation near the cavern surface, and stress was re-distributed as a result of rock failure. The 0.2% excess of radial interval strain and the drastic increase in AE are assumed to indicate the shift of the rock conditions from the sound region to a loosened region. That is, the loosened region is assumed to range from the point at a distance of 2 m or more and less than 5 m from the cavern surface during excavation of the sixth bench to that at a distance of 5 m or more and less than 10 m from the cavern surface at the completion of excavation. Thus the range was slightly smaller than analytical results (5.0 m at the time of excavation of the sixth bench, and 10.0 m at the completion of excavation), but was nearly in agreement with the prediction.

6. BEHAVIOR IN THE PRIORITY ZONE FOR OBSERVATIONAL MANAGEMENT

In zones α (north transverse wall), β (D section) and γ (south transverse wall through C section) in the weak region, displacement greater than in the ordinary region was expected because joints having east-west strike and dipping steeply northward (J$_{EW}$-h joints) were initially so concentrated that the rock was a weak character. Therefore, prestressed anchor was used and shotcrete was applied more substantially for performing support system than in the ordinary region. As a result, each zone experienced greater displacement than in the ordinary region, but the behavior was within the predicted range.

The side of the penstock in the F and G sections was initially zoned in the ordinary region, but specified as the special zone δ during excavation, based on the geological revaluation and the displacement condition, and was managed as a priority zone. The behavior of zone δ (penstock side of the G section) is described below.

6.1 Geological properties and actual behavior

(i) The area near the G section is mudstone dominated, which is constituted with homogeneous and massive rock that have relatively low density of east-west faults and joints. But during the excavation of the vault, a number of long joints (the maximum length on face was 6 m) striking north-south and dipping eastward steeply (J_{NS}-h joints) were confirmed more than other section.
(ii) Wall surface displacement of 17 mm occurred on the shoulder of the penstock side of the cavern in the secondary enlargement of the vault through excavation of the first bench. Thus the deformation behavior was asymmetrical to the side of the tailrace (cavern surface displacement of 3 mm) (Fig. 6)

6.2 Behavior analysis

The displacement which occurred on the shoulder of the cavern in the secondary enlargement of the vault through the excavation of the first bench is analyzed as below.
(i) A back analysis (Sakurai's inverse formulation method) assuming that the surrounding rock was isotropically homogeneous rock revealed that stress of approximately 36.3 MPa was acting horizontally from the side of the penstock at an angle of 69° based on the displacement measured in the vault. The results were much different from the results of back analyses for other sections and the initial stress measured with the multi-element strain gauge in the survey adit (σ_1=12.3 MPa, σ_2=11.0 MPa, an angle of 14°), as for the value and direction of the maximum principal stress (Fig. 7).
(ii) In order to investigate the possibility of local stress concentration, rock stress was measured using the borehole from the survey adit in the upper part of the G section (on the penstock side) with the conical-ended borehole technique using the compact overcoring. As a result, the maximum principal stress σ_1 was 12.1 MPa, and the minimum principal stress σ_2 was 8.6 MPa in the cross-section of the plant. The maximum principal stress acted toward the tailrace at an angle of about 45°

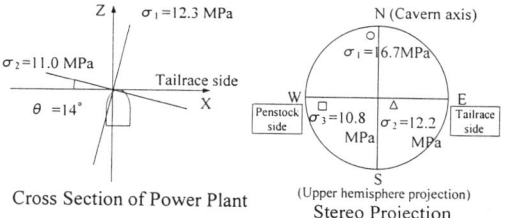

Fig.7 Initial Rock Stress in the Survey Adit with Multi-axial Strain Gauge

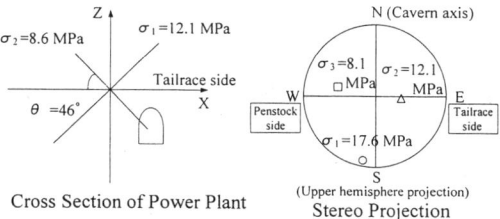

Fig.8 Rock Stress during Excavation with Conincal-ended Borehole Technique

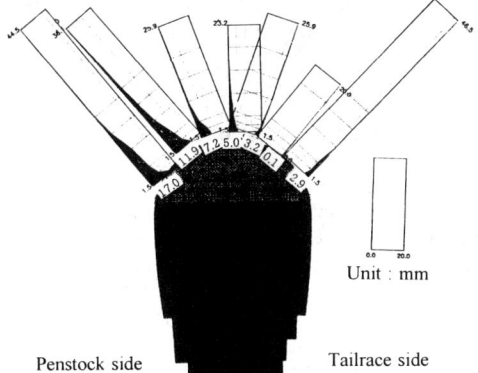

Fig.6 Rock Displacement Distribution in the G-section (at Completion of the first bench)

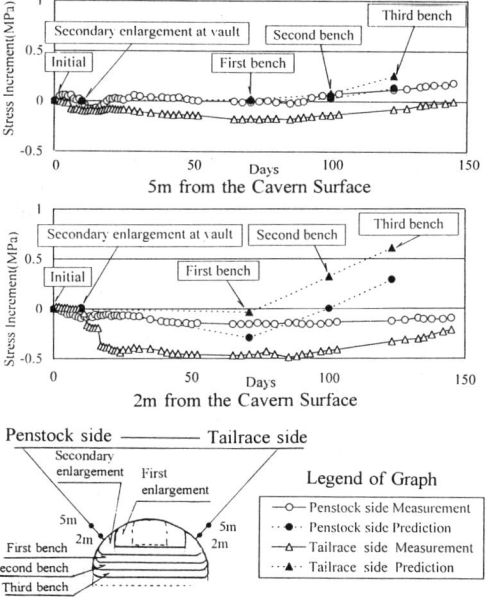

Fig.9 Comparison between Stress Measurement in Rock and Prediction (G-section)

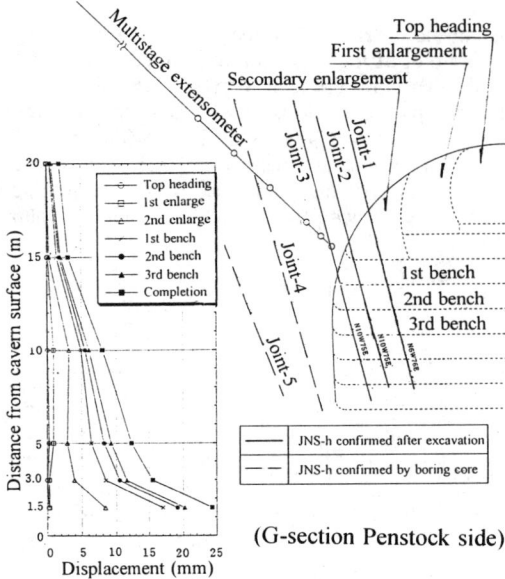

Fig.10 Deformation Behavior

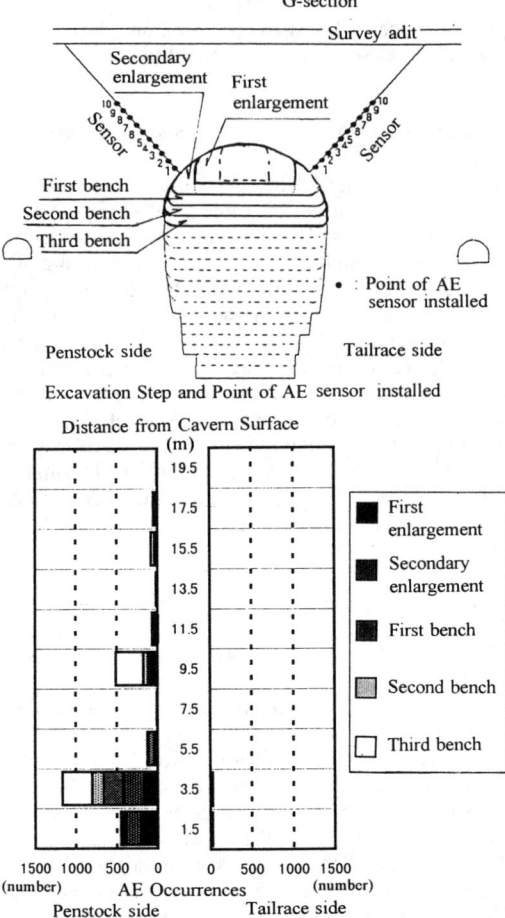

Fig.11 AE Measurement (G-section)

The value and the direction of the maximum principal stress were almost the same as the results of the initial rock stress measurement prior to the excavation (Fig. 8).
(iii) The measurement with a vibrating-wire stress meter installed in the G section from the survey adit through the borehole prior to the excavation of the vault revealed that the tangential stress due to excavation at the depths of 2 m and of 5 m from the cavern surface tended to change more or less the same either for the penstock or tailrace side though there were minor differences (Fig. 9).
(iv) Displacement increased drastically when the place was excavated where J_{NS}-h joints, confirmed at the time of excavation of the first bench, crossed the cavern surface (Fig. 10). AE occurred remarkably on the side of the penstock at the depth of 3.5 m, but no AE observed on the tailrace side (Fig. 11).

Judging from the above, asymmetrical deformation was considered attributable to the J_{NS}-h joints having a steep eastward dip slope toward the penstock side.

7. CONCLUSIONS

Listed below are the conclusions about cavern behavior.
(i) As for the displacement of cavern surface, the deformation behavior was almost as predicted for the weak region with high density of faults and joints (α, β and γ zones) and for the ordinary region.
(ii) Concentration of stress in the rock during excavation, and post-failure stress redistribution were confirmed based on the results of measurement of tangential stress and strain in the rock and AE measurement. These rock stress changes indicated the shift of the rock conditions from the sound region to a loosened region. It was also confirmed from a comparison between the measurement results and predictive analyses that strain softening FEM analyses provided for simulation not only for cavern surface displacement but also for stress in the rock.
(iii) Pre-excavation investigation and classification of joints proved effective in estimating the causes of behavior and studying corrective measures, in relation to slip and delamination behavior of fast joints due to stress release caused by excavation, as shown in zone δ.

Rock Stress, Sugawara & Obara (eds) © 1997 Balkema, Rotterdam, ISBN 90 5410 901 7

Affect of thermal hysteresis on rock mass around openings for storage of heated water

Yoshinori Inada & Naoki Kinoshita
Department of Civil and Environmental Engineering, Ehime University, Japan

Takao Ueda
Office of Energy Engineering, Takenaka Corporation, Japan

Kimio Yamada
Department of Geology, Fuyo Chosa Sekkei Co., Ltd, Japan

ABSTRACT: The authors have proposed temporary storage of heated water in openings excavated in rock mountain. In this case, the rock mass around openings will receive the effects of thermal hysteresis of high temperatures. In this study, strength and deformation characteristics of rocks were examined at high temperatures and after undergoing thermal hysteresis of high temperatures by using a thermal cycle apparatus. From the results, it was found that temperature, number of cycles and porosity etc. were the most important factors which have an influence on strength and deformation characteristics. Using these values, stress distribution around openings was analyzed theoretically, and the affect of thermal hysteresis of high temperatures on rock mass around openings for storage of heated water was discussed.

1 INTRODUCTION

The authors have proposed temporary storage of heated water in openings excavated in rock mountain from the view point of efficient utilization of energy, land and preservation of the environment. Heated water, such as that produced by surplus heat from garbage burning plants, should be used for many purposes such as district heating, heated water supply and green houses etc. The authors have shown in this study by theoretical analysis that thermal stress occurs around openings and compressive stress occurs towards the tangential direction due to the thermal expansion of rock in the case of high temperature materials storage(Inada et al., 1990).

In this case, the quantity of heated water changes on a daily and seasonal cycle according to its use for many purposes. The rock mass around openings will receive the effects of thermal hysteresis of high temperatures. Therefore, obtaining the strength and deformation characteristics of rocks at high temperature and after undergoing thermal hysteresis of high temperatures becomes important for discussing the stability of the openings.

In this study, strength and deformation characteristics of rocks which have low and high porosity were examined at high temperatures and after undergoing thermal hysteresis of high temperatures by using a thermal cycle apparatus.

Using these values, stress distribution around openings was analyzed theoretically, and the affect of thermal hysteresis of high temperatures on rock mass around openings for storage of heated water was discussed.

2 STRENGTH AND DEFORMATION CHARACTERISTICS OF ROCKS AFTER UNDERGOING THERMAL HYSTERESIS

2.1 *Rocks used for experiments*

The rocks used for the experiments were granite obtained in Miyakubo, Ehime, Japan and tuff obtained in Utsunomiya, Japan. In the case of granite, "rift plane", "grain plane" and "hardway plane" were determined by measuring elastic wave propagation velocity of the block of rock. Then a specimen was taken by core drill in the direction of intersecting perpendicularly to the hardway plane. In the case of tuff, the depositional surface was also determined by measuring the elastic wave propagation velocity of the block of rock, and a specimen was taken by core drill in the direction of which is parallel to the depositional surface. Specimens were $\phi 30 \times 60$mm for the uniaxial compression test, and $\phi 30 \times 30$mm for the radial compression test. Specimens were prepared as "Dry" by drying for one week in a desiccator after air drying for a week, and as "Wet" by being kept in a desiccator filled with distilled water for 5 hours using a vacuum pump. The physical properties of these specimens are shown in Table 1.

Table 1 Physical properties of rocks.

Rocks	Porosity (%)	Moisture content ratio (%)	Degree of saturation (%)	Bulk specific gravity	True specific gravity
granite(Dry)	1.99	0.16	20.67	2.625	2.673
granite(Wet)	1.99	0.16	70.86	2.653	2.673
tuff(Dry)	37.09	1.39	5.76	1.560	2.446
tuff(Wet)	37.09	24.01	99.62	1.908	2.446

2.2 Experimental method

The specimens underwent thermal hysteresis of high temperatures by using a thermal cycle apparatus. The schematic diagram of the thermal cycle apparatus is shown in Fig.1. The conditions of thermal hysteresis of high temperatures is as follows. The Wet specimens were set in the thermal cycle box, submerged in distilled water, and the Dry specimens were set in as is. For measuring temperature during the test, the thermometers were set up at one point each in the center of Wet and Dry specimens, at 3 points in the distilled water bath and at 25 points in the thermal cycle box. Then the specimens underwent thermal hysteresis of high temperatures as shown in Fig.2. Heat sources were a heater and a freezer, as the temperature rises and drops linearly. The heating rate was set at 1°C/min for avoiding the effects of thermal impact (Yamaguchi et al., 1970). In this experiment, the maximum temperature was 99°C. However, this temperature was taken as 100°C for the sake of convenience. The specimens were kept at 100°C for 60min after making certain that the temperature at the center of the specimen was 100°C and cooled to 15°C at a rate of 1°C/min and kept at 15°C for 60min. We call the process mentioned above, 1 cycle. Specimens underwent thermal hysteresis of high temperatures for up to 10 cycles.

The uniaxial compression test and the radial compression test were carried out. A schematic diagram of the test is shown in Fig.3. The tests were carried out at room temperature (15°C) and 100°C. When the specimens were heated to 100°C, the heating conditions were the same as those of thermal hysteresis of high temperatures. The tests for Wet specimens were carried out in the water and the tests for Dry were carried out in the air.

2.3 Results and considerations

The compressive strength of rocks after undergoing thermal hysteresis is shown in Fig.4(a),(b). It was found that compressive strength decreases with the increasing number of thermal hysteresis in all cases. It is supposed that microcracks occurred in the rock due to differences of thermal expansion among rock-forming mineral grains when the rocks underwent thermal hysteresis. However, it was found that the ratio of decreasing compressive strength decreases with the increasing number of thermal hysteresis and the values converge to a constant value. The compressive strength of the Wet specimen of both rocks is lower than that of the Dry. In the case of the test for granite, it was found that the compressive strength at 100°C is about the same as that at 15°C, but, in the case of the test for tuff, the value at 100°C is smaller than that at 15°C.

Fig.5(a),(b) show the tensile strength. In all cases, the tensile strength decreases with the

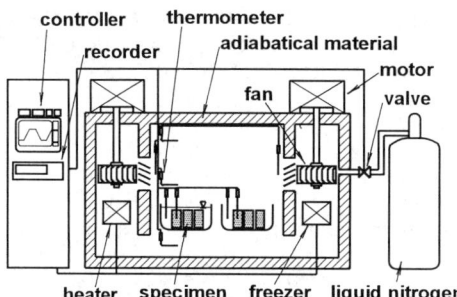

Fig.1 Schematic diagram of thermal cycle apparatus.

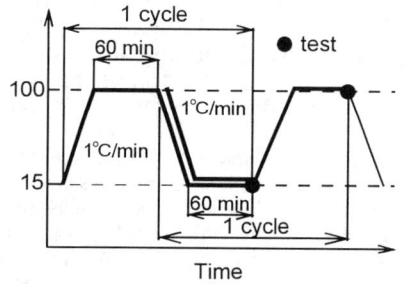

Fig.2 Schematic diagram of thermal hysteresis.

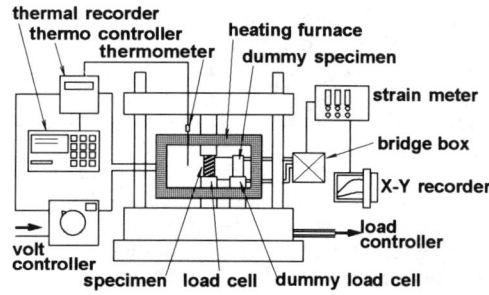

Fig.3 Schematic diagram of the test.

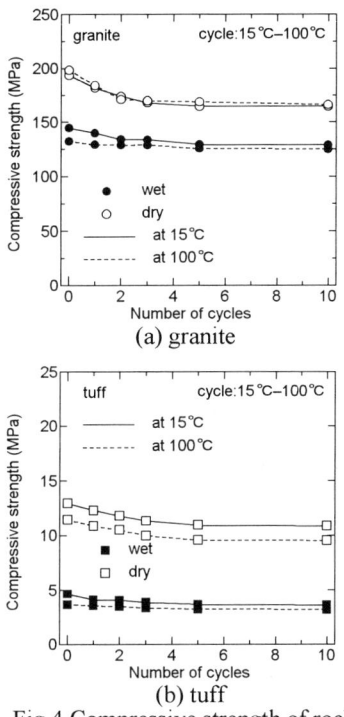

(a) granite

(b) tuff

Fig.4 Compressive strength of rocks.

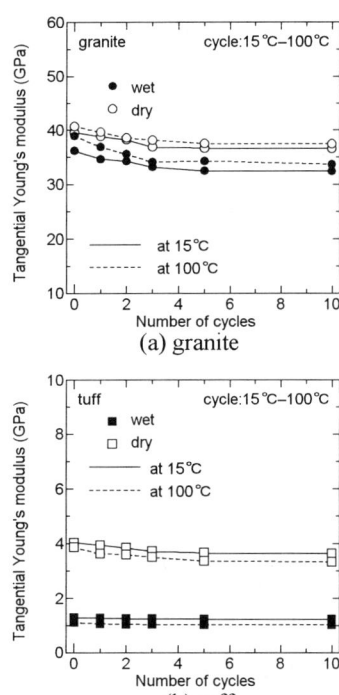

(a) granite

(b) tuff

Fig.6 Tangential Young's modulus of rocks.

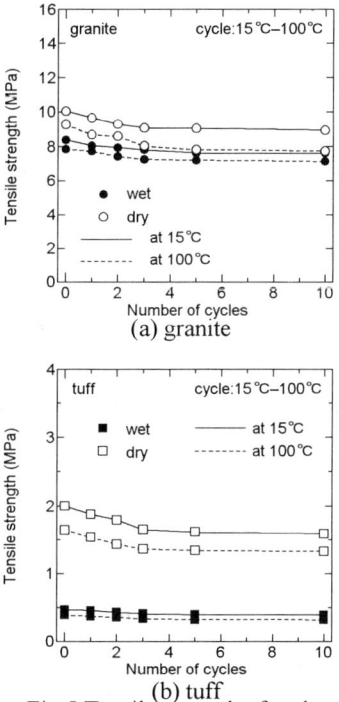

(a) granite

(b) tuff

Fig.5 Tensile strength of rocks.

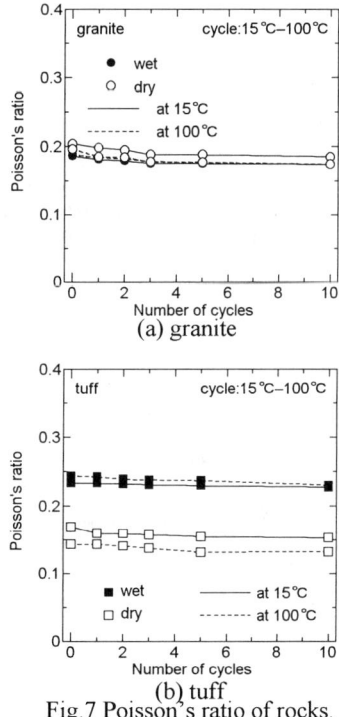

(a) granite

(b) tuff

Fig.7 Poisson's ratio of rocks.

increasing number of thermal hysteresis. It was found that tensile strength at 100°C was slightly smaller than that at 15°C. The strength for Wet rock of both types was lower than that of the strength for Dry.

Fig.6(a),(b) show the tangential Young's modulus at 30% of fracture stress which was obtained from the stress-strain curve of the compression test. In all cases, the tangential Young's modulus decreases with the increasing number of thermal hysteresis. This seems to be due to microcrack expansion in rocks.

Fig.7(a),(b) show the value of Poisson's ratio at 30 % of fracture stress. The value becomes slightly lower with the increasing number of thermal hysteresis, but a large change of the value with temperature is not seen.

2.4 *Strain with thermal hysteresis*

As mentioned above, it is considered that the strength characteristics of rocks were affected by microcracks occurring due to expansion of the rocks which underwent thermal hysteresis. From this, it is considered that thermal strain will also be affected by thermal hysteresis. The thermal expansion of rocks with thermal hysteresis of high temperatures was measured using a comparison method with a quarts glass rod (Inada et al., 1971).

The results of the test of granite are shown in Fig.8 and Fig.9. The residual strains at room temperature can be seen for all specimens after undergoing thermal hysteresis. It can also be seen that residual strain for all specimens tends to converge to a constant value as the thermal hysteresis is repeated. From the results, it is considered that microcracks due to differences of thermal expansion among rock-forming mineral grains did not return to the original state completely at room temperature.

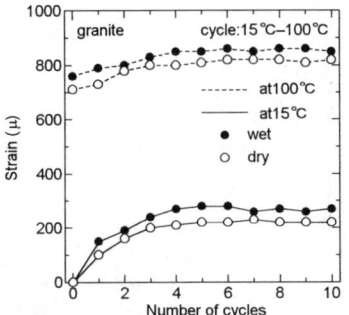

Fig.9 Residual strains of granite.

3 THERMAL BEHAVIOR OF ROCK MASS AROUND OPENINGS EFFECTED BY HEATED WATER

3.1 *Temperature distribution*

In this study, as mentioned previously, it is supposed that the opening is excavated in granite rock mountain at a depth of 100m beneath the ground surface with a diameter of 10m and used to store 100°C heated water. Temperature distribution around opening with time was calculated by FDEM (Inada et al., 1983). The analysis was performed on the following cases.

Case 1: the case in which the temperature of rock mountain is 15°C and 100°C heated water has been stored in the opening until the temperature of the rock mass around the opening reached a semi-steady state.
Case 2: the case in which heated water storage has been stopped during 30 days for maintenance etc. after Case 1. In this case, it is assumed that the temperature of the opening's surface is 15°C.
Case 3: the case in which after Case 2, heated water storage has been begun again until a semi-steady state is reached.

Thermal properties of granite at high temperatures used for analysis obtained by examination were shown in Table 2.

The change of temperature distributions around

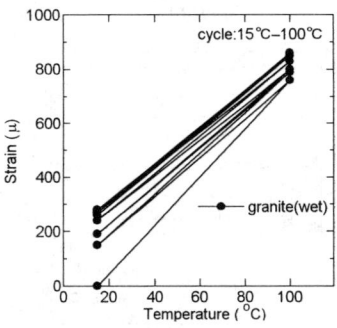

Fig.8 Strain of granite (Wet).

Table 2 Thermal properties of granite.

Heat capacity $(cal/(cm^3 \cdot °C))$	Thermal diffusivity $(\times 10^{-3} cm^2/s)$	Thermal conductivity $(\times 10^{-3} cal/(s \cdot cm \cdot °C))$
0.632	12.3	7.77

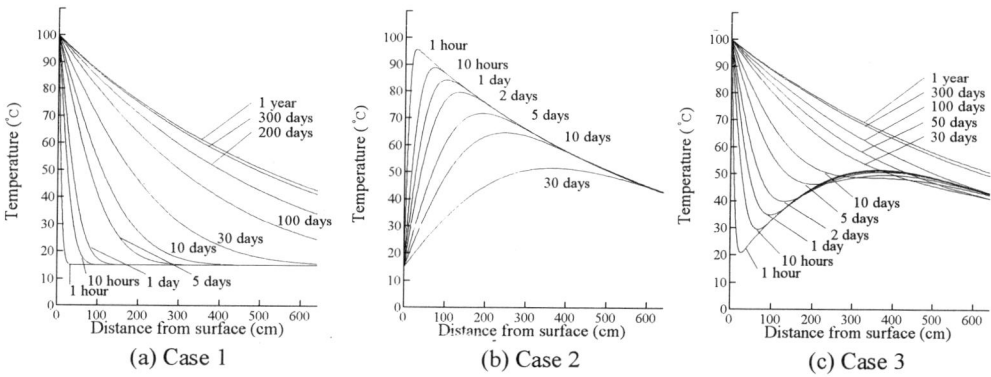

Fig.10 Temperature distribution around the opening.

the opening with time are shown in Fig.10(a)-(c). In Case 1, it is found that the temperature gradient is extremely sharp at the beginning of storage, but become gentler with time. The temperature enters a semi-steady state after 1 year. In Case 2, the temperature of rock mountain drops within the range of the opening's surface to about 6m distance from the surface. In Case 3, the temperature enters a semi-steady state again after about 1 year.

3.2 Stress distribution

Stress changes around openings were analyzed by FEM considered thermal stress using the results of temperature analysis mentioned above. In Case 3, the physical properties of granite used for analysis

Table 3 Physical properties of granite after undergoing thermal hysteresis.

Temperature (°C)	Expansion coefficient (1/°C) × 10^{-5}	Young's modulus (kgf/cm^2) × 10^6	Poisson's ratio	Compressive strength (kgf/cm^2)	Tensile strength (kgf/cm^2)
10~20	0.000	0.323	0.174	−1291.1	76.4
20~30	0.686	0.325	0.174	−1286.1	75.8
30~40	0.686	0.327	0.174	−1281.0	75.2
40~50	0.686	0.328	0.174	−1276.0	74.6
50~60	0.686	0.330	0.174	−1270.0	74.0
60~70	0.686	0.331	0.174	−1265.8	73.4
70~80	0.686	0.333	0.174	−1260.8	72.8
80~90	0.686	0.334	0.174	−1255.7	72.2
90~100	0.686	0.336	0.174	−1250.7	71.6

Table 4 Physical properties of granite

Temperature (°C)	Expansion coefficient (1/°C) × 10^{-5}	Young's modulus (kgf/cm^2) × 10^6	Poisson's ratio	Compressive strength (kgf/cm^2)	Tensile strength (kgf/cm^2)
10~20	0.000	0.360	0.186	−1453.9	84.2
20~30	0.892	0.363	0.186	−1438.5	83.5
30~40	0.892	0.367	0.186	−1423.1	82.8
40~50	0.892	0.370	0.187	−1407.7	82.1
50~60	0.892	0.374	0.187	−1392.4	81.4
60~70	0.892	0.377	0.187	−1377.0	80.8
70~80	0.892	0.380	0.187	−1361.6	80.1
80~90	0.892	0.384	0.188	−1346.3	79.4
90~100	0.892	0.387	0.188	−1330.9	78.7

are those after undergoing thermal hysteresis of 10 cycles from experiments mentioned above. In Case 1 and Case 2, those which had not undergone thermal hysteresis were used. Physical properties of granite used for analysis are shown in Table 3 and Table 4 respectively.

Fig.11(a)-(c) show the change of stress distribution with time for radial and tangential direction along a horizontal line. Fig.12(a)-(c) show the principal stress directions around openings. In Case 1, it is found that stress for tangential direction occurs at the surface of the opening immediately after storage. Stress for radial and tangential direction increase with time. In Case 2, the thermal stress near the surface of the opening decreases and compressive stress for tangential direction at about 3m distance from surface reaches maximum compressive stress at 30 days. In Case 3, at the surface, stress for tangential direction occurs immediately after storage and increases with time as in Case 1. In all cases, the theoretical fracture stress is still not reached and the openings are calculated to remain stable. The reasons for these results are considered to be as follows. The strength of granite decreased after undergoing thermal hysteresis. However, thermal stress occurring in the rock mass decreased because tangential Young's modulus also decreased.

4 CONCLUSION

The main results obtained in this study are as follows :

1. From the results of the experiments, strength and deformation characteristics of rocks decrease with the increasing number of thermal hysteresis. However, it is supposed that the value will converge to a constant value.

2. From the results of measuring the thermal

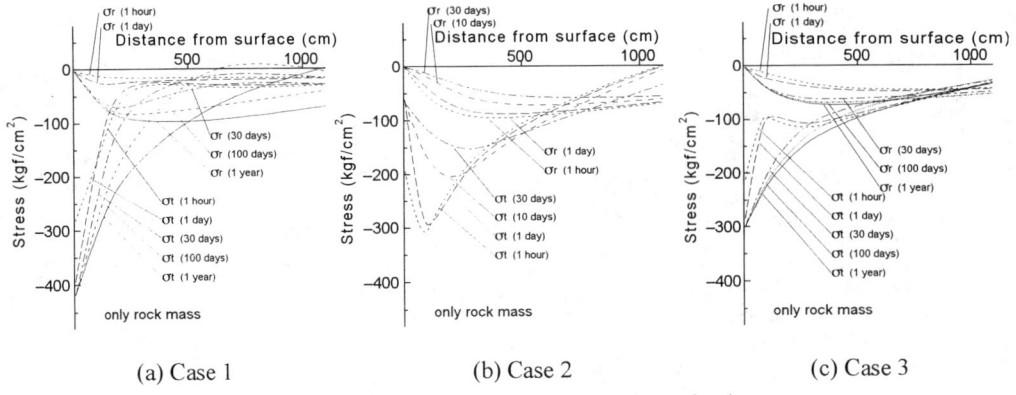

(a) Case 1   (b) Case 2   (c) Case 3

Fig.11 Stress distribution along horizontal axis.

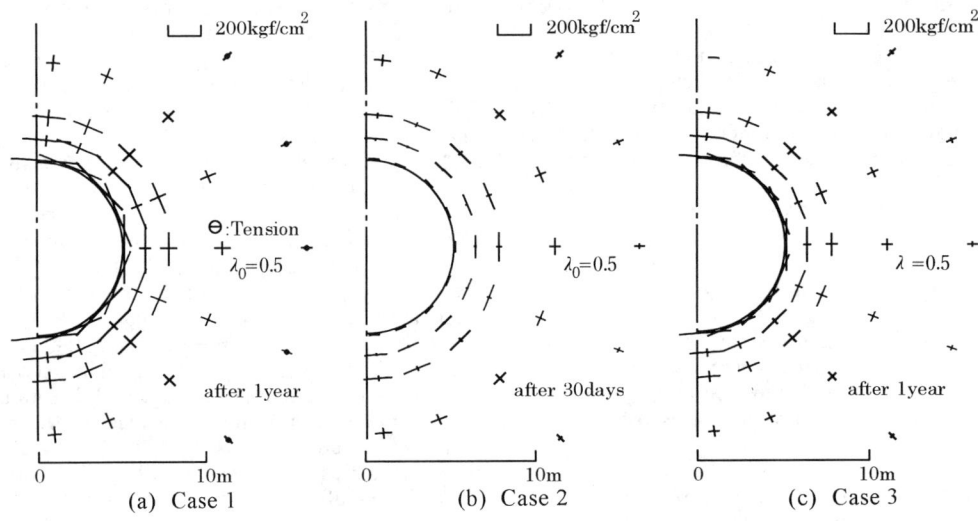

(a) Case 1   (b) Case 2   (c) Case 3

Fig.12 Principal stress direction around opening.

expansion of rocks with thermal hysteresis, the residual strains at room temperature can be seen for all specimens after undergoing thermal hysteresis. It is considered that microcracks due to the difference of thermal expansion among rock-forming mineral grains did not return to the original state completely at room temperature.

3. From the results of stress analysis, theoretical fracture stress is still not reached and the opening is calculated to remain stable after undergoing thermal hysteresis by heated water.

ACKNOWLEDGMENT

The authors would like to express their gratitude to N. Matsushima, graduate student of Ehime University, who extended his kind assistance.

REFERENCES

Inada,Y., Kinoshita,N., Nakazaki,H. & Ueda,T. 1990. A fundamental study on stability and leakage of openings due to storage of heated water. *J. of Japan Soc. of Civil Eng.* 424:227-234.

Yamaguchi, U. & Miyazaki, M. 1970. A study of the strength or failure of rocks heated to high temperature. *J. of Mining and Metallurgical Inst. of Japan.* 86. 986 : 346-351.

Inada, Y., Terada, M. & Ito, I. 1971. On the coefficient of thermal expansion of rocks. *Suiyokwai-shi.* 17.5 : 200-203.

Inada,Y & Shigenobu,J.1983. Temperature distribution around underground openings excavated in rock mass due to storage of liquefied natural gas.*J.ofMin.Meta.Inst.Japan*.99.1141:179-185.

Rock stress behavior of large cavern in underground excavation

K. Ohno
Kajima Corporation, Tokyo, Japan

A. Yada
The Kansai Electric Power Co., Inc., Osaka, Japan

ABSTRACT: Monitoring of various types was performed to grasp ground behavior during the excavation of a large underground powerhouse cavern. This paper reports the results of the two types of rock stress measurement which were especially effective in the control of ground behavior during excavation and in the interpretation of cavern stability. The first is the measurement of three dimensional stress variation by a stress meter imbedded in the center pillar which was formed during the arch excavation. The relationship between excavation progress and stress variation within the pillar is described. Second is the measurement of stress distribution within the rock mass to grasp the cause of an anomaly which developed during the arch excavation. The mechanism of redistribution of stress within the surrounding rock mass accompanying cavern excavation is described.

1 INTRODUCTION

In the construction of a large-scale underground cavern such as that for an underground powerhouse, design is performed with thorough consideration to geological conditions based on detailed investigations and tests. However, due to conditions of nonhomogeneity and discontinuity which are a characteristic of rock, it is extremely difficult in practice to predict with accuracy ground behavior due to excavation through analytical study performed prior to construction. Consequently, in order to secure safety during construction and stability of the underground cavern in the future, observational construction control in which design revision is performed on the basis of quick feedback of construction information obtained through the observation and monitoring of behavior during excavation is indispensable to construction management.

Monitoring of various types was performed to grasp ground behavior during the excavation of a large underground powerhouse cavern. This paper reports the results of two types of rock stress measurement which were especially effective in the control of ground behavior during excavation and in the interpretation of cavern stability.

2 OUTLINE OF UNDERGROUND POWERHOUSE CAVERN

The underground power station where these rock stress measurements were performed is the Ohkawachi Power Plant, a pure pumped storage type power station located in the center of Hyogo Prefecture which was designed to generate a maximum output of 1,280Mw utilizing an effective head of 395m. The powerhouse is a large underground cavern which is 24m wide, 47m high and 135m long.

2.1 Topography and geology

The site of the power plant is at the eastern slope of Mineyama Heights, a plateau at an elevation of 800 to 1000m at the eastern end of the Chugoku Mountain Range. The powerhouse cavern was constructed at a depth of approximately 280m below the surface.

The bedrock at the site belongs to the Ikuno formation of the Cretaceous period and consists of porphyrite, and diorite which exists in the form of an intrusion into this porphyrite. Mottled porphyrite is widely distributed surrounding the powerhouse cavern. This porphyrite is hard and fresh. Although medium hard bedrock is to be found in part, the bedrock is principally hard rock, and having no marked faults or fractured zones, it can be said that the bedrock is in a stable condition. However, because the RQD, an index of crackiness, is rather low at 60 to 70%, it is thought that the ground is relatively cracky.

2.2 Cavern design

In selecting the cross sectional configuration of the

powerhouse cavern, a comparative study was made by performing FEM analyses of cavern stability during excavation for three types of configuration; the often used "mushroom shape" or arch type in which the arch reaction is supported by the rock at the arch abutments, the "egg-shape" or horseshoe type in which stress concentration is small and cavern stability is excellent, and the "bullet head" type which possesses the superior qualities of both. From an overall viewpoint including ease of construction and economy in addition to the results of the comparative study, the "bullet head" configuration was adopted, for the first time in Japan, as being the most rational configuration of the three.

The support structure to secure cavern stability was designed on the basis of the NATM concept of actively utilizing the intrinsic support capability of the rock surrounding the cavern. The principal support members consist of shotcrete, rock bolts and PS anchors. The basic support pattern is shown in Figure 1.

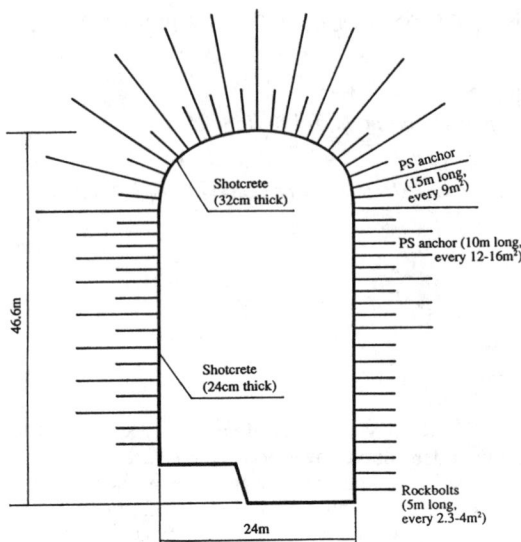

Figure 1. Design support pattern.

2.3 Cavern excavation

In the excavation of the arch, the "large cross section side pilot and arch enlargement excavation method" was employed for the first time. In this method side pilots are first driven on both sides of the arch with support being placed and then the center section is removed by enlargement excavation to complete the arch cross section. In the excavation of the center section, the length of the powerhouse was divided into six blocks of approximately 20m length and each block was carefully excavated with the shotcrete, rock bolts and other support members completed block by block. The sequence of arch excavation is shown in Figure 2.

The excavation of the main body of the powerhouse was performed by bench cut. The standard height of bench was taken as 3m to conform with the vertical pitch of the PS anchors, and the behavior of the arch and side walls was monitored as the excavation progressed downward. In order to minimize damage to the finished walls due to blasting, smooth blasting explosive was used with controlled blasting in the finish excavation at the walls.

3 ROCK STRESS MEASUREMENT

In the excavation of a large cross section underground cavern, stability during the arch excavation is of important significance in securing the stability of the cavern as a whole during the subsequent excavation of the main body of the cavern. On this project, especially careful construction execution and grasping of ground behavior were required during the arch excavation because the "large cross section side pilot and arch enlargement excavation method" which was employed for the excavation of the arch section was a new unexperienced method.

3.1 Behavior of center section ground

Accompanying excavation of the side pilots, a stress concentration develops in the ground left between the two side pilots (center section ground) which is predominant in the vertical direction. It is predicted that if this stress concentration reaches an excess, sudden failure may occur which would have a grave effect on the stability of the cavern. Therefore, an instrument was imbedded in the pillar which would be left until the last, and the variation in three dimensional stress within this pillar was monitored. The method which was employed in monitoring this rock stress was the stress relief method by "hemispherical-ended borehole technique" by which stress can be measured in three dimensions using a single borehole.

As shown in Figure 3, the stress remaining in the center section ground when the side pilot excavation was completed had a predominant stress component in the vertical direction, and in comparison with initial rock stress, a stress concentration has developed which is approximately 20MPa or double in terms of maximum principal stress, and on the order of three times when comparing the vertical component only. On the other hand, looking at the horizontal component of stress in the direction of the short axis of the cavern, the stress was smaller, having been relieved by the excavation of the two side pilots, and in terms of stress condition, a condition had been formed in which failure could easily occur. As shown in Figure

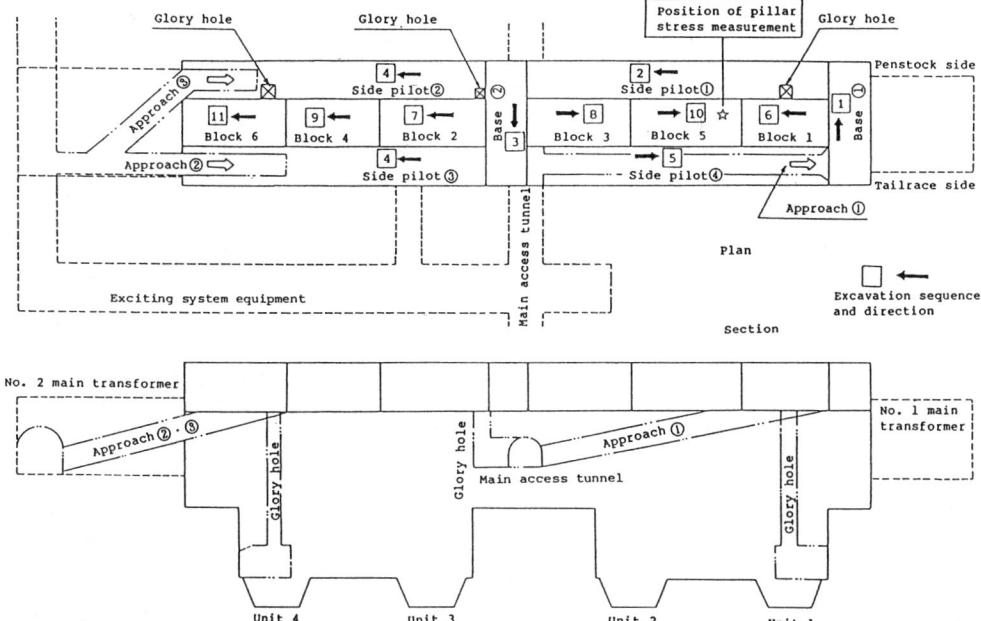

Figure 2. Sequence of arch excavation.

4, variation in rock stress within the center section accompanying the arch enlargement excavation showed a tendency for the vertical component to increase (stress concentration) and the horizontal component to decrease (stress relief) as the excavation face approached.

Stress concentration in the vertical direction showed an increase of approximately 1MPa when the face of the excavation which was advanced from Base No. 1 had approached to about 4.5m from the monitored point. Following this, as the excavation approached from Base No. 2 on the opposite side, the effect began to appear gradually about the time when the face had approached to about 20m from the monitored point, and the stress further increased to a total of 3.5MPa when the face had approached to about 6m from the monitored point. Later when the face advanced to about

	Principal stress (MPa)			Axial stress (MPa)		
	P1 (Maximum)	P2 (Intermediate)	P3 (Minimum)	PX	PY	PZ
Stress within center section	20.7	6.8	4.2	4.4	7.5	19.8
Initial stress	10.0	6.4	3.9	7.9	6.5	5.9

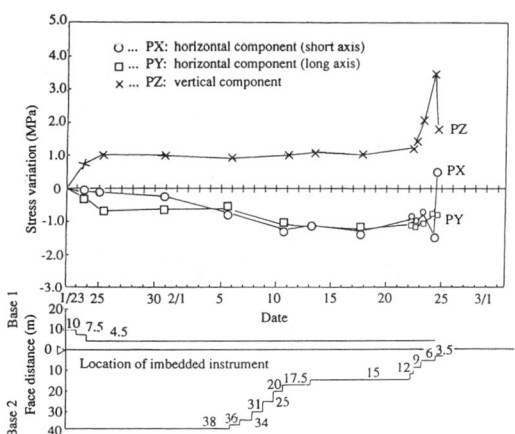

Figure 3. Stress in center section of arch following excavation of side pilots.

Figure 4. Three dimensional stress variation in remaining pillar.

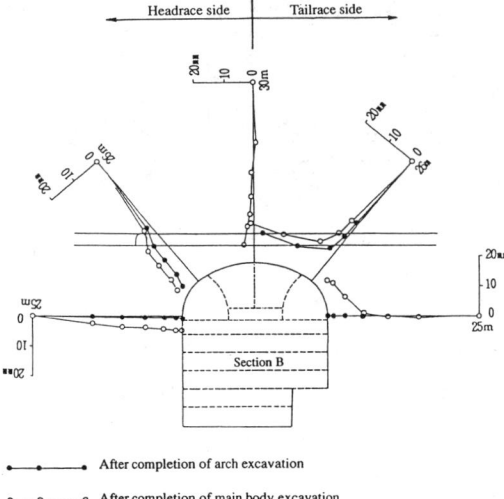

Figure 5. Distribution of displacement in cavern arch.

3.5m from the monitored point, the vertical component of stress decreased through a sudden stress change which is thought to be due to the influence of local joints in the vicinity of the imbedded instrument, but the maximum principal stress showed an increase to 5MPa.

On the other hand, stress relief in the horizontal direction showed a pattern in which that in the direction of the long axis of the powerhouse was predominant at first, but that in the direction of the short axis gradually increased accompanying the approach of the excavation face followed by simultaneous progress of stress relief in both directions. This is thought to be due to the fact that the horizontal shape of the remaining center section which initially is long in the direction of the long axis of the powerhouse approaches the shape of a square as the excavation advances. Also, as mentioned above, when the excavation face approached about 3.5m from the monitored point, the direction of stress relief changed greatly under the influence of the opening of local joints, and tensile stress acted in the direction normal to the predominant joint surfaces.

Accompanying progress of the excavation the direction of maximum principal stress accompanying stress concentration gradually rotated in the clock-wise direction from its direction at the time of completion of the side pilot excavation and came to generally correspond with the direction of the maximum principal stress of initial rock stress immediately prior to being influenced by local joints. From this fact it is thought that although the stress within the center section undergoes a complex three dimensional change due to the excavation, this change is greatly influenced by the initial rock stress naturally existing in the rock mass.

3.2 Behavior during arch excavation

The ground on the penstock side and that on the tailrace side showed contrasting behavior accompanying excavation of the arch. Displacement on the tailrace side was three to four times that on the penstock side (Figure 5.), rock bolts and PS anchors showed increased axial force and local cracking developed in

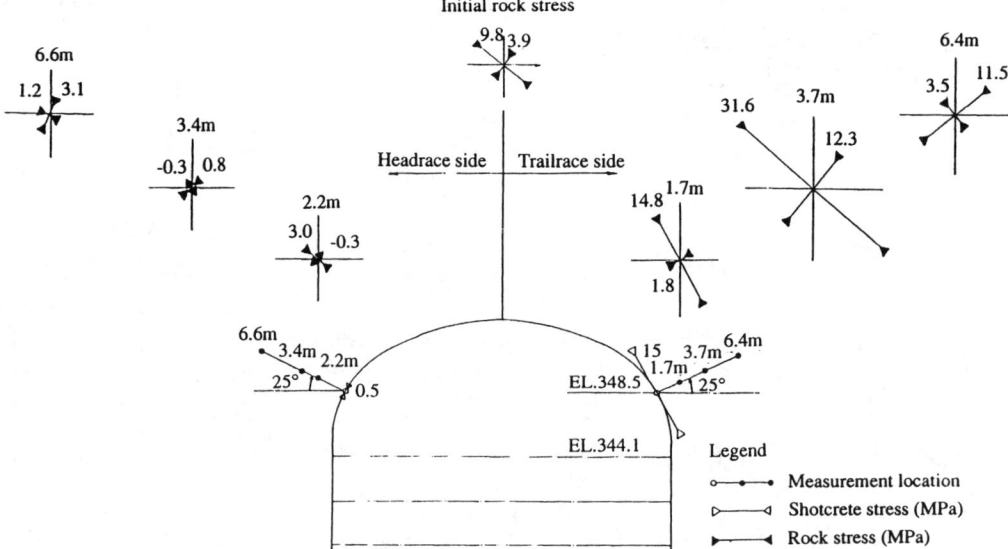

Figure 6. Results of rock stress measurement at arch.

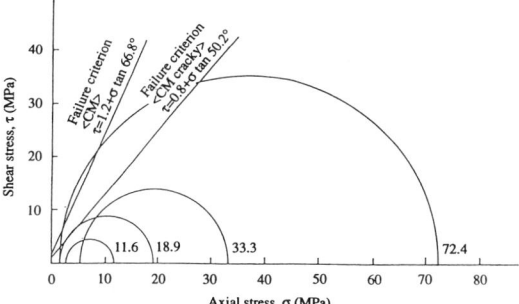

Figure 7. Mohr's stress circle and failure criteria.

the shotcrete. In order to clarify the condition which had caused this behavior, measurements of stress within the rock mass were performed.

As shown in Figure 6, the stresses within the rock are clearly different between the tailrace side and penstock side of the powerhouse cross section; a zone of stress concentration existing on the tailrace side and a zone of stress relief on the penstock side.

Looking at the distribution of stress on the tailrace side which has the zone of stress concentration, a zone of high stress close to the failure criterion of the rock mass shown in Figure 7 is formed in the vicinity of 3 to 4m from the excavated surface, and stress decreases in the vicinity of 6m, approaching the level of initial rock stress. From this stress distribution it is imagined that the zone from the excavated surface to a depth of about 3m is a plastic region (loosened zone), the zone at a depth of 4m and more is an elastic region, and that the elastoplastic boundary exists in the vicinity of 3 to 4m depth, with the ground arch formed there. Further, it is thought that stress on the order of 15MPa exists as residual strength in the zone which is thought to be a plastic region.

Looking at the distribution of stress on the penstock side which has the zone of stress relief, because stress is generally uniform to a depth of about 6m from the excavated surface, it is estimated that the influence of stress relief due to excavation extends to a depth of at least 6m, and with tensile stress acting, although to only a slight extent, in the vicinity of the excavated surface, the stress distribution corresponds well with the results of FEM analysis.

The three dimensional redistribution of stress in the rock mass surrounding the cavern accompanying arch excavation shows a tendency toward concentration in the tangential direction and relief in the radial direction in the powerhouse cross section, and no redistribution in the powerhouse longitudinal direction.

3.3 Mechanism of stress development in shotcrete

From the fact that the tangential stress in the shotcrete measured in the vicinity of the rock stress measurement cross section is 15MPa on the tailrace side where the zone of stress concentration was seen, a value which is generally equal to the tangential stress in the rock near the excavation surface, it is possible to consider that the internal rock stress is transmitted to the shotcrete by action of the shotcrete in union with the rock mass. On the other hand, on the penstock side which has the zone of stress relief, from the fact that only a very small amount of stress has developed, on the order of 0.5MPa, it can be seen that the stress acting in the shotcrete is closely related to the redistribution of stress in the rock mass surrounding the cavern accompanying excavation.

From the above, it is inferred that the cracks which developed in the shotcrete on the tailrace side accompanying the arch excavation are due to an excessive concentration of rock stress in the tailrace side of the arch.

4 RESUME

4.1 Divided excavation and stress redistribution

Accompanying excavation of the side pilots, the vertical component of stress in the remaining center section of the arch becomes predominant, and the stress in the direction of the short axis of the powerhouse is relieved.

Accompanying excavation of the center section, the concentration of stress into the vertical direction proceeds even further. First, the stress in the long axis direction of the powerhouse is relieved, and then as the excavation progresses and the length of the remaining center section becomes shorter, the effect of stress relief in the short axis direction appears.

Variation of rock stress accompanying excavation is also influenced by the behavior of local joints, but viewed on a large scale, this variation is three-dimensionally dominated by the initial rock stress naturally existing in the ground.

Because the amount of stress increase in the vertical direction accompanying excavation of the center section of the arch, on the order of 5MPa at the most, was small in comparison with the 10MPa stress increase due to the excavation of the side pilots, it is judged that stress redistribution due to excavation by the "large cross section side pilot and arch enlargement excavation method" proceeded smoothly and the effect on the stability of the cavern was very small.

4.2 Inferences regarding ground behavior due to arch excavation and support strengthening

As described above, the singular behavior on the tailrace side of the powerhouse is inferred to be the result of stress concentration into the tailrace side of the arch causing failure in the rock mass and the formation of a loosened zone (thought to be due to the opening of latent cracks within the ground and the development of new cracks) which resulted in increased displacement and increased axial force in rock bolts and PS anchors.

Further, it is interpreted that the stress concentration in the rock mass was transmitted to the shotcrete by the process of stress redistribution, causing the development of local cracking.

Among the factors which can be given to explain why contrasting distributions of rock stress were shown on the tailrace and penstock sides of the arch are the fact that the rock on the tailrace side was generally poor and the fact that the side pilot on the tailrace side was excavated before that on the penstock side. Further, another fact which is thought to be a major factor is the fact that the direction of maximum principal stress of initial rock stress was inclined at an angle of 54° from the vertical axis toward the penstock side.

Based on the above inferences regarding rock stress behavior due to arch excavation, additional rock bolts and PS anchors were placed in the tailrace side of the arch and the shotcrete in the zone of cracking was reinforced in order to control the advance of displacement and the zone of loosening in the arch accompanying the excavation of the main body of the cavern which followed.

5 CONCLUSION

In general, monitoring by displacement measurement has been given first importance in observational control of underground cavern construction, including tunnels. However, monitoring of the stress within the rock mass is an extremely effective means of quickly discovering loosening phenomena accompanying unbalanced stress concentration such as that seen so distinctively in the behavior of the rock during the excavation of this powerhouse. Consequently, we believe that it is important that excavation monitoring of a higher degree of precision be performed by also including, from the initial stage of excavation, the measurement of stress in the plan of monitoring in addition to displacement measurement.

Because underground structures will become more and more subject to the effects of rock stress as they come to be constructed in greater size and at greater depth in the future, the further improvement and development of stress measurement technology, including the simplification of measurement techniques and the improvement of techniques of analysis and evaluation, are greatly desired.

REFERENCES

Fukuoka, T. 1992. Rapid construction methods employed at Ohkawachi Underground Power Plant. In L. Vieitez-Utesa & L. Montañez-Cartaxo (eds), *Proc. Int. Cong. Towards New Worlds in Tunnelling, Acapulco, 16-20 May 1992*: Vol 2. Rotterdam: Balkema.

Hoek, E. & E.T. Brown 1980 *Underground excavations in rock*. London: Institution of Mining and Metallurgy.

Katayama, T., A. Yada & Y. Hirakawa 1992. Observational construction control of underground powerhouse excavation at Ohkawachi Power Plant. *Electric Power Civil Engineering* 237.

Mimaki, Y., S. Kuramochi & K. Kudo 1983. Regarding the construction of Imaichi Underground Power Station and the surrounding ground behavior. *Electric Power Civil Engineering* 185.

Ohno, K., et al 1986. Rock cavern stability analysis when considering strain-softening of the surrounding loosened zone. *Annual Report of Kajima Institute of Construction Technology*, Kajima Corp. Vol 34. Tokyo.

Ohno, K. & T. Yamazaki 1989. Mechanism of support action on excavation stability of underground caverns. *Symposium of science and engineering papers of Graduate School of Science and Engineering of Waseda University*: 122. Tokyo.

Sugawara, K. & Y. Obara 1986. Measurement of in-situ rock stress by hemispherical ended borehole technique. *Int. J. Min. Sci. & Tech.* 3: 287-300.

Optimum locations for displacement measurements in underground openings to determine in situ stress by means of back analysis

N. Shimizu, H. Kakihara & K. Nakagawa
Department of Civil Engineering, Yamaguchi University, Ube, Japan

S. Sakurai
Department of Civil Engineering, Kobe University, Japan

ABSTRACT: Indices to evaluate the accuracy of back analysis for determining rock stress are introduced. Numerical simulations are conducted to find the optimum locations for displacement measurements in back analysis using these indices. The appropriate installation angles and lengths of the extensometers and the required accuracy of the measurements are discussed.

1 INTRODUCTION

The *in situ* initial stress of rock masses is fundamental and important knowledge for the design and stress analysis of underground openings. It is needed when evaluating the stability and predicting the mechanical behavior of rock masses. There are various types of methods for determining *in situ* stress; i.e., hydraulic methods, relief methods, jacking methods, etc. (Amadei and Stephansson 1997).

However, the scale effects on *in situ* rock stress are generally found to be due to the heterogeneous properties of rock masses, and their values depend on the rock volume involved in the testing methods (Cuisiat and Haimson 1992). Therefore, the validity of the results determined by such ordinary *in situ* tests is limited to the immediate vicinity of the testing sites.

In the design and stress analysis of excavations, the design/input parameters should be evaluated in relation to the size of the openings. Thus, the average value of initial stress over the whole region around an underground opening is required.

One of the most promising ways to determine the average value of initial stress is a back analysis of the field measurement results obtained during excavations of underground openings. For this purpose, the authors have proposed back-analysis methods (Shimizu and Sakurai 1983; Sakurai and Takeuchi 1983; Sakurai and Shimizu 1986), and those have been improved for monitoring the stability of underground openings (Sakurai et al. 1985; Sakurai 1993; Shimizu et al. 1996; Shimizu et al. 1997). Since the back analysis of field measurements involves a large rock volume, it can provide an average value for the *in situ* initial stress and eliminate the effects of local rock mass properties.

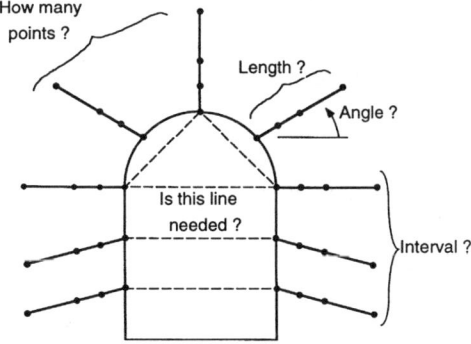

Figure 1: What are the optimum locations for the displacement measurements in underground openings?

On the other hand, the results of back analysis are affected by the locations and the accuracy of the field measurements as are ordinary rock stress measurements. Therefore, problems arise when planning the instrumentation for field measurements; i.e., how are the number of measurement lines, angles, lengths, ... etc. determined? (see Figure 1).

In this paper, a back analysis method for measured displacements is introduced for initial stress determination, and then indices to evaluate the accuracy of the back analysis are proposed. Numerical simulations are conducted to find the optimum locations for the displacement measurements and the appropriate installation angles and lengths of the extensometers, and the required accuracy of the measurements are discussed using the indices.

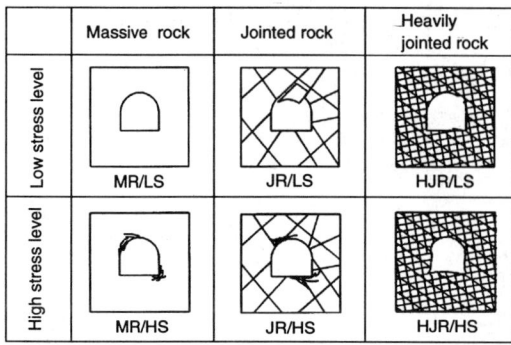

Figure 2: Types of mechanical behavior under different rock mass conditions (Hoek et al. 1995)

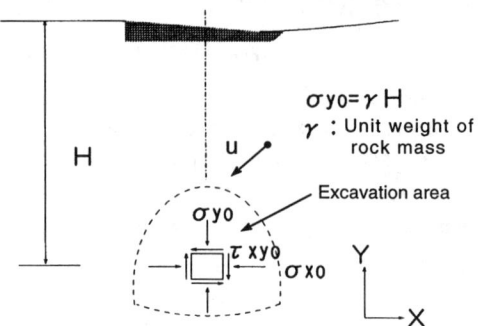

Figure 3: Initial stress and displacement around an underground opening

2 TYPES OF ROCK MASS BEHAVIOR

The back-analysis method used in this research is based on conventional continuum mechanics. Therefore, it is limited in its applicability to the continuum behavior of rock masses. The rock mass behavior treated here is described in this chapter.

Hoek et al.(1995) described the various types of rock mass behavior around underground openings associated with the frequency of discontinuities and the *in situ* stress levels, as shown in Figure 2.

A massive rock subjected to low *in situ* stress levels (type MR/LS) exhibits a linear elastic response. A heavily jointed rock subjected to both low (HJR/LS) and high (HJR/HS) *in situ* stress conditions fails by unraveling into small interlocking blocks and by sliding on discontinuities and being crushed into rock pieces, respectively. Both cases, types HJR/LS and HJR/HS, are modeled by pseudo or equivalent continuum models if the behavior of the rock mass is well controlled by the appropriate support systems.

In the case of a massive rock with relatively few discontinuities, subjected to low *in situ* stress conditions (JR/LS), rock blocks released by intersecting discontinuities fall or slide due to gravity loading.

A massive rock with no or relatively few discontinuities subjected to high *in situ* stress conditions (MR/HS and JR/HS) behaves by spalling, slabbing, crushing, and splitting. In addition, progressive failures may occur in the rock mass.

The back analysis used in this research deals with types MR/LS, HJR/LS, and HJR/HS by using continuum models. Other types are excluded here.

3 BACK ANALYSIS PROCEDURE

The behavior types illustrated as MR/LS, HJR/LS, and HJR/HS in Figure 2 are treated with the continuum mechanics model. A back-analysis method can be formulated based on continuum mechanics.

The mechanical behavior of a rock mass is assumed to be idealized by an isotropic linear elastic model, and the initial state of stress is supposed to be constant all over the region surrounding an underground opening. Then, displacement u is represented by the following equation in two dimensional problems due to the excavation of underground openings:

$$u = f_1(\sigma_x^0/E) + f_2(\sigma_y^0/E) + f_3(\tau_{xy}^0/E) \quad (1)$$

where σ_x^0, σ_y^0 and τ_{xy}^0 are the components of the initial stress, and E is the elastic modulus of the rock mass (see Figure 3). f_1, f_2 and f_3 are functions determined by the locations and the directions of the measured displacements, the geometry of the opening, and Poisson's ratio. The observation equations derived from Equation (1) are applied to the least squares method together with the measured displacements, and the normalized initial stress, $\{\sigma^{0*}\}$, is obtained as follows:

$$\{\sigma^{0*}\} = ([F]^T[F])^{-1}[F]^T\{u_m\} \quad (2)$$

where $[F]$ is composed of f_1, f_2 and f_3, $\{u_m\}$ is the measured displacements, and the normalized initial stress is defined by $\{\sigma_0^*\}^T = \{\sigma_x^0/E \ \sigma_y^0/E \ \tau_{xy}^0/E\}$.

The vertical component of the initial stress is assumed to have the same value as the overburden pressure, namely,

$$\sigma_y^0 = \gamma H \quad (3)$$

where γ and H denote the average unit weight of the rock mass and the overburden height of the opening, respectively. The elastic modulus and the initial stress are obtained from the normalized initial stress as follows:

$$\begin{aligned} E &= \gamma \cdot H/\sigma_y^{0*} \\ \sigma_x^0 &= \sigma_x^{0*} \cdot E \quad (K = \sigma_x^0/\sigma_y^0 = \sigma_x^{0*}/\sigma_y^{0*}) \\ \tau_{xy}^0 &= \tau_{xy}^{0*} \cdot E \end{aligned} \quad (4)$$

where $\sigma_x^{0*} = \sigma_x^0/E, \sigma_y^{0*} = \sigma_y^0/E$ and $\tau_{xy}^{0*} = \tau_{xy}^0/E$.

Equation (1) represents the total displacement due to the excavation. However, the measuring instruments are often installed after the excavation, and the measured displacements are not usually total displacements but displacements measured after the installation of the instruments. Besides, the measured displacements are not absolute displacements either, but relative displacements between two measurement points (e.g. measurements using extensometers, etc.).

In those cases, Equation (1) is modified as follows:

$$\Delta u_{(j-i)} = \{f\}^T_{(j-i)}\{\sigma^{0*}\} \tag{5}$$

where $\Delta u_{(j-i)}$ is a displacement measured at the jth excavation step by instruments installed after the ith excavation step $(j > i)$. $\{f\}_{(j-i)}$ is derived from f_1, f_2 and f_3 for both the i and the jth excavation steps. The initial stress and the elastic modulus of the rock mass are obtained in the same manner as that shown in Equations (2) and (4).

By comparing the back-analyzed initial stress and elastic modulus with the parameters used at the initial design stage, the design parameters can be verified during the construction process. If the design parameters are over- or under-estimated, the original design should be changed to match the actual rock behavior.

In order to assess the stability of underground openings on the basis of the strain control procedure (Sakurai 1981), the strain distribution is calculated by an ordinary analysis method using a back-analyzed initial stress and elastic modulus.

4 INDICES TO DETERMINE OPTIMUM LOCATIONS FOR DISPLACEMENT MEASUREMENTS

There are basically three factors which affect the results of a back analysis; i.e., (1) computational errors, (2) measurement errors, and (3) modeling errors. The first factor involves errors based on numerical calculations, and they can be evaluated by the condition number of the matrix $([F]^T[F])^{-1}$. The second factor is errors based on the accuracy of the instruments. The third factor is errors caused by simplifications of reality; i.e., numerical models adopted for analysis to simplify real behavior of rock masses.

In this paper, focus is placed on the measurement errors to investigate the optimum locations for the measurements. That is, the optimum locations for the back analysis are determined in order to minimize the influence of the measurement errors.

The index representing the accuracy of the displacement measurements is defined by the standard deviation (STD) of the instruments, and it is expressed by $STD(u_m)$ for measured displacements, u_m. The standard deviation of the back-analyzed elastic modulus, E, the coefficient of horizontal initial stress, $K(=\sigma^0_x/\sigma^0_y)$, and the shear component of initial stress, τ^0_{xy}, are obtained by applying the law of error propagation to Equations (2) and (4) as follows:

$$STD(E) = COV(E)\,\overline{E} \tag{6}$$
$$STD(K) = COV(K)\,\overline{E} \tag{7}$$
$$STD(\tau^0_{xy}) = COV(\tau^0_{xy})\,\overline{\tau^0_{xy}}, \tag{8}$$

where

$$COV(E) = \{COV^2(\sigma^0_y)+(1/\overline{\sigma^{0*}_y})^2(F^TF)^{-1}_{22}(STD(u_m))^2\}^{1/2} \tag{9}$$

$$COV(K) = (STD(u_m))\{(1/\overline{K}/\overline{\sigma^{0*}_y})^2(F^TF)^{-1}_{11}$$
$$+ (1/\overline{\sigma^{0*}_y})^2(F^TF)^{-1}_{22} + 2(1/\overline{K}/\overline{\sigma^{0*}_y}^2)(F^TF)^{-1}_{12}\}^{1/2} \tag{10}$$

$$COV(\tau^0_{xy}) = \{(1/\overline{\tau^{*0}_{xy}})^2(F^TF)^{-1}_{33}(STD(u_m))^2+COV^2(E)\}^{1/2} \tag{11}$$

$COV(\cdot)$ is the coefficient of variance and $\overline{\cdot}$ is the average value. The average value $\overline{\cdot}$ is assumed to be known. $(F^TF)^{-1}_{ij}$ is a component of the matrix $([F]^T[F])^{-1}$ in Equation (2), and it is determined by giving the locations and directions of the displacement measurements, the geometry of the opening, and Poisson's ratio of the rock mass. It should be noted that $COV(E), COV(K)$ and $COV(\tau^0_{xy})$ are also functions of the standard deviation of measured displacements, $STD(u_m)$.

Equations (6) ~ (8) represent the accuracy of the back-analyzed parameters, E, K and τ^0_{xy}, and those are functions of the measurement locations. Therefore, the optimum locations for the measurements can be determined to minimize those standard deviations.

On the other hand, the accuracy of the displacements and the maximum shear strain estimated by the results of the back analysis is evaluated by the following equations:

$$STD(u) = (STD(u_m))\{f_1^2(F^TF)^{-1}_{11} + f_2^2(F^TF)^{-1}_{22}$$
$$+ f_3^2(F^TF)^{-1}_{33} + 2f_1f_2(F^TF)^{-1}_{12}$$
$$+ 2f_2f_3(F^TF)^{-1}_{23} + 2f_3f_1(F^TF)^{-1}_{13}\}^{1/2} \tag{12}$$

$$STD(\gamma_{max}) = (STD(u_m))\{g_1^2(F^TF)^{-1}_{11} + g_2^2(F^TF)^{-1}_{22}$$
$$+ g_3^2(F^TF)^{-1}_{33} + 2g_1g_2(F^TF)^{-1}_{12}$$
$$+ 2g_2g_3(F^TF)^{-1}_{23} + 2g_3g_1(F^TF)^{-1}_{13}\}^{1/2} \tag{13}$$

where $STD(u)$ and $STD(\gamma_{max})$ are standard deviations of the predicted displacement and maximum shear strain, respectively. They are obtained by applying the law of error propagation to Equation (1) and maximum shear strain equation $\gamma_{max} = \sqrt{(\varepsilon_x - \varepsilon_y)^2 + \gamma^2_{xy}}$. g_1, g_2 and g_3 in Equation (13) are the differential coefficients of γ_{max} with respect to the normalized initial stress, $\partial\gamma_{max}/\partial\{\sigma^{0*}\}$.

The optimum measurement locations for the predicted displacements and maximum shear strain can be determined to minimize the indices defined by Equations (12) and (13), respectively.

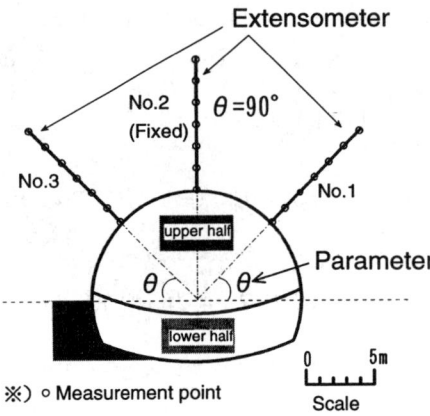

Figure 4: Installation of the extensometers

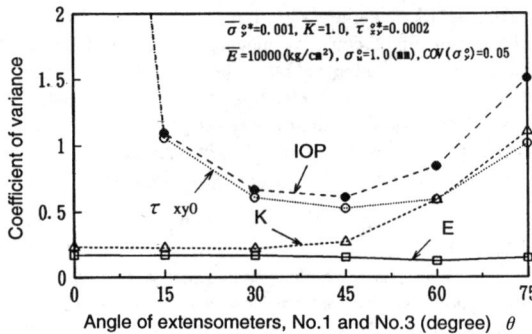

Figure 5: Optimum installation angles of the extensometers

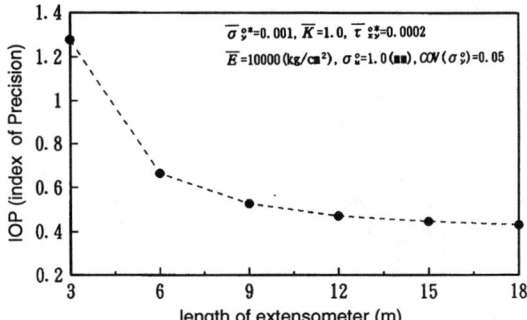

Figure 6: Optimum length of the extensometers

5 NUMERICAL SIMULATIONS

Numerical simulations are conducted to discuss the optimum locations for the measurements in the back analysis using the indices defined in the last section. The boundary element method is used for the numerical implementation (Shimizu and Sakurai 1983).

5.1 Installation angle

The installation direction of the multi-rod borehole extensometers is discussed in a tunnel example (see Figure 4). Angle θ is taken as a parameter for the installation of three extensometers. The vertical extensometer (No. 2 in Figure 4) is supposed to be fixed at the angle. The other extensometers are assumed to be installed symmetrically. Therefore, θ is a parameter for determining the locations of the measurement points in this case.

Figure 5 shows the results of $STD(E), STD(K)$ and $STD(\tau_{xy}^0)$ v.s. installation angle θ. The accuracy of the displacement measurements is given as $STD(u_m) = 1\ mm$ in this case. $\overline{\sigma_y^{0*}} = 0.001, \overline{\tau_{xy}^{0*}} = 0.0002$, and $COV(\sigma_y^0) = 0.005$ are assumed here.

$\theta < 30° \sim 45°$ is a suitable range for the coefficient of horizontal initial stress, K, and $30° < \theta < 60°$ for the initial shear stress, τ_{xy}^0. The elastic modulus is back-analyzed with the same accuracy as any installation angle. It is caused by the assumption of the isotropic rock mass.

In order to evaluate the optimal angle, the following index is defined:

$$IOP = \{COV^2(E) + COV^2(K) + COV^2(\tau_{xy}^0)\}^{1/2} \quad (14)$$

As the IOP (Index of Precision) takes its minimum value around $\theta = 30° \sim 45°$, this is the most suitable range for the installation angles of the extensometers.

5.2 Installation length

Figure 6 shows the variation in IOP to the length of the extensometers. In this case, the installation angle is fixed at $\theta = 30°$. The value of the IOP decreases as the length increases, but it becomes almost stable at more than 9 m in length. It may be concluded that $6 \sim 9$ m is a sufficient length to obtain a precise back-analyzed initial stress and elastic modulus.

Displacements can be predicted using the back-analyzed initial stress and elastic modulus. Figure 7 exhibits the distribution of the standard deviation of the predicted displacements around a tunnel for $\theta = 30°$ and $L = 6$ m. The accuracy of the displacement measurements is given as $STD(u_m) = 1$ mm. It is found that displacements can be predicted with an accuracy of $0.4 \sim 0.6$ mm around the upper half of the section (the depth being $1 \sim 2$ m) and the bottom area (the depth being $2 \sim 3$ m), and with an accuracy of less than 0.4 mm for areas far from the tunnel.

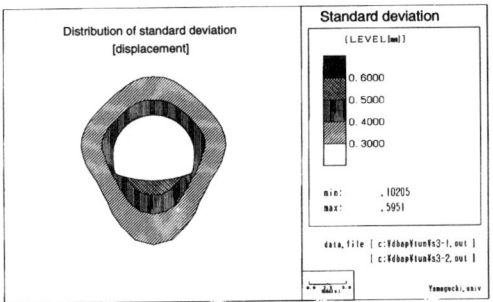

Figure 7: Distribution of the standard deviation of estimated displacements ($L = 6\ m, \theta = 30°$)

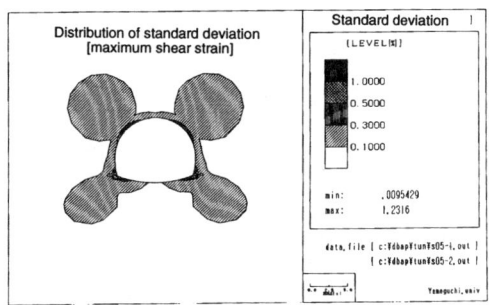

Figure 9: Distribution of the standard deviation of estimated maximum shear strain ($L = 6\ m, \theta = 30°$)

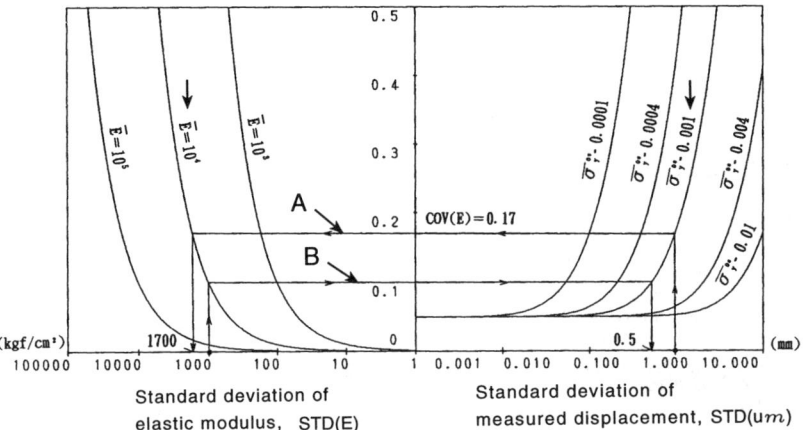

Figure 8: Coefficient of variance of back-analyzed elastic modulus ($L = 6\ m, \theta = 30°$)

5.3 Required accuracy in measurements

Figure 8 shows the coefficient of variance for the elastic modulus v.s. the accuracy of the displacement measurements when three extensometers with six measurement points are installed at $\theta = 30°$ and $L = 6$ m. If the accuracy of the displacement measurements is given as $STD(u_m) = 1$ mm, the elastic modulus can be back-calculated with an accuracy of $COV(E) = 0.17$ on the line of $\overline{\sigma_y^{0*}} = 0.001$ in Figure 8. Therefore, the elastic modulus is obtained approximately with 1700 kg/cm^2 of the standard deviation in the case of $\overline{E} = 10000\ kg/cm^2$ (see procedure line A in Figure 7).

On the other hand, if it is necessary for the elastic modulus to be back-analyzed with $STD(E) = 1000$ kg/cm^2, the displacements have to be measured within $STD(u_m) = 0.5$ mm (see procedure line B in Figure 8).

In a similar manner to that described above, the minimum requirement for the accuracy of the measurements can be determined.

5.4 Maximum shear strain

In order to assess the stability of underground openings based on the strain control method (Sakurai 1981), the maximum shear strain distribution is calculated with the back analysis results. Extensometers should be installed to evaluate the maximum shear strain with an appropriate amount of accuracy.

Figure 9 shows the distribution of the standard deviation of the estimated maximum shear strain around a tunnel. The $STD(\gamma_{max})$ is less than 0.3% in almost the entire area except for the vicinity of the tunnel surface. If the critical shear strain, which is a critical value for assessing the stability of the rock in the strain control method, is 1.0%, this measurement location provides enough accuracy of γ_{max} to evaluate the tunnel stability.

6 CONCLUTIONS

In this paper, a back analysis was described to determine the *in situ* initial stress from displacement measurements, and the optimum locations for the measurements was discussed. The conclusions can be summarized as follows:

1. Indices for evaluating the accuracy of back-analysis results (i.e., initial stress and elastic modulus of rock masses) were proposed. The optimum locations for measurements can be discussed quantitatively using the indices.

2. The optimum locations can be determined by minimizing the above-mentioned indices.

3. Numerical simulations proved the effectiveness of the indices for discussing optimum measurement locations.

ACKNOWLEDGEMENTS

The authors wish to thank Ms. H. Griswold for proofreading this paper.

REFERENCES

Amadei, B. and O. Stephansson, 1997. *Rock Stress and Its Measurement*. Chapman & Hall.

Cuisiat, F. D. and B. C. Haimson, 1992. Scale effects in rock mass stress measurements. *Int. J. Rock Mechanics and Mining Science & Geomechanics Abstract*, **29**(2):99–117.

Hoek, E., P. K. Kaiser and W. F. Bawden, 1995. *Support of underground excavations in hard rock*. Balkema.

Sakurai, S., 1981. Direct strain evaluation technique in construction of underground openings. In *Proc. 22nd U.S. Sympo. Rock Mech.*, pp. 278–282.

Sakurai, S., 1993. Back analysis in rock engineering. *Comprehensive Rock Engineering*, **4**:543–569. Pergamon Press.

Sakurai, S. and N. Shimizu, 1986. Initial stress back analyzed from displacements due to underground excavations. In *Proc. Int. Sympo. Rock Stress and Rock Stress Measurements*, pp. 679–686, Stockholm.

Sakurai, S., N. Shimizu and K. Matsumuro, 1985. Evaluation of plastic zone around underground openings by means of displacement measurements. In *Proc. 5th Int. Conf. Numerical Methods in Geomechanics*, vol. 1, pp. 111–118, Nagoya.

Sakurai, S. and K. Takeuchi, 1983. Back analysis in measured displacements of tunnels. *Rock Mechanics and Rock Engineering*, **16**:173–180.

Shimizu, N., H. Kakihara and K. Nakagawa, 1996. A back analysis method for predicting deformational behavior of discontinuous rock mass. In *The 2nd North American Rock Mechanics Symposium: NARMS'96*, pp. 2001–2008, Montréal.

Shimizu, N., K. Nakagawa and S. Sakurai, 1997. An integrated back-analysis system for monitoring underground openings. In *The 1st Asian Rock Mechanics Symposium: ARMS'97*, Seoul. (in print).

Shimizu, N. and S. Sakurai, 1983. Application of boundary element method for back analysis associated with tunnelling problems. In *Proc. 5th Int. Conf. Boundary Elements*, pp. 645–654, Hiroshima.

Application of in situ stresses measured by hydraulic fracturing to a tunnel design in Korea

Sung-Oong Choi & Hee-Soon Shin
Korea Institute of Geology, Mining and Materials, Taejon, Korea

ABSTRACT: A rock mass is usually classified by the results of geological survey and laboratory tests on rock specimens in order to obtain the adequate properties for the numerical analysis. For those purposes a rock mass strength is estimated based on the empirical criterion proposed by Hoek and Brown, and a modulus of deformation is taken with the empirical relations developed by Bieniawski, Serafim and Pereira. In addition, the K_0 value which is the ratio of the horizontal stress to the vertical stress is one of the most important input data in the numerical analysis. Its role on a tunnel stability analysis could be verified with the numerical results taken by a finite difference code or a distinct element code.

However, a deduced value used to be applied for the K_0 value in most of tunnel designs, even though the patterns of stress tensor are variable with regions and depths. Thus in-situ stresses were measured by a hydraulic fracturing technique on several tunnel sites in Korea, and applied directly to the tunnel design for the enhancement of its precision. With those informations on in-situ stresses, the safe design could be obtained economically on the road or subway tunnels.

1 INTRODUCTION

Up to recently, a deduced value for the K_0 used to be applied for the tunnel design. But these made the underground openings unstable owing to the unconsideration of the stress changes in a tunnel face during the excavation.

However it is reported that the horizontal stresses are relatively larger than the vertical stresses at the shallow depth in the world(Brown and Hoek, 1978), and in-situ stresses are variable in the vicinity when these were effected by the topographical or geological conditions(Goodman, 1989).

Therefore the K_0 value which is the essential input datum in the numerical analysis for the design of tunnel or underground facilities should be measured directly. In addition to the magnitude of in-situ stresses, its direction has a large influence on the tunnel stability, even though the directions of tunnel are decided not by the engineering condition but by the public condition in most cases. So the patterns of excavation and support should be decided for the assurance of the tunnel stabilities, regarding for the directions of the tunnel and the horizontal stresses.

In this paper, consequently, we would like to emphasize the importance of the K_0 value in the tunnel design with the results of the analysis of the field data measured by hydraulic fracturing method in 1996 in Korea.

2 IN-SITU STRESS MEASUREMENT

In-situ stresses which are very important not only in the analysis of the ground movement but also in the analysis of the underground facility are very complicated in evaluating its quantity because there are many factors influencing to the horizontal stress field such as the tectonic stress, erosion or rising of the ground surface, the thermodynamic anomalies, and so forth. So these stresses should be measured directly in the field(Haimson, 1988).

Methods for measuring the in-situ stresses can be generally divided into 4 methods, based on ISRM in 1987.

2.1 *Flat jack method*

With the flat jack method, the stress field parallel to

the wall of tunnel can be measured in the vicinity of the tunnel face. But six tests should be performed in the different directions in order to determine the stress tensor. This method is known that it is not easy to accept for the determination of undisturbed in-situ state of stress, but generally it can be applied for the determination of the stress generated in the tunnel lining after the construction.

2.2 Borehole deformation gage method

This method was developed in USBM, and its principle is measuring the changes of borehole diameter during the overcoring. Measured data is used for determination of the two dimensional state of stress in the plane normal to the borehole axis with the elastic modulus of rock mass. For determining the total stress tensor, three tests should be at least conducted on the different directional boreholes.

2.3 Soft inclusion strain cell method

This is very similar to the borehole deformation gage method in the principles, but it can measure the total stress tensor with just one test because the stain cell has 9 or 12 strain gages. The key point in this method is the stickiness of the strain cell onto the rock mass.

2.4 Hydraulic fracturing method

The elastic modulus of rock mass is not needed for the determination of the stress tensor in hydraulic fracturing method. And with the characteristics of using the borehole in testing, the stress field can be measured prior to the excavation. But it has a weak point that the direction of the borehole is assumed to be one of the directions of the principal stresses. Before the hydraulic fracturing test, the borehole wall is examined in order to select the test intervals with the borehole TV camera or the borehole televiewer. After testing, the hydraulic fractures are looked into by the borehole televiewer or the impression packer together with the orientation tool.

3 HYDRAULIC FRACTURING TESTS

There were many tests for the determination of in situ stresses by hydraulic fracturing in 1996. Most of them was for a design of a road tunnel, but we have experienced on the subway tunnel or underground storage cavern.

To evaluate in situ stresses from the field data obtained by hydraulic fracturing, we should convince ourselves of the parameters such as the shut-in pressure, the reopening pressure and the fracture orientation.

In general, the graphical methods used to be applied for determining these parameters, but there are many possibilities of ambiguities in determining them owing to the subjectivity of the interpreter. Consequently we analyzed the field data with the new developed program HYDFRAC which is an integrated hydrofracturing data processing code.

By using this program, in situ stresses could be determined successfully in several areas. Table 1 shows the summarized results.

4 NUMERICAL ANALYSIS

To evaluate the stability of underground facilities, the state of stress in the rock mass used to be estimated by theoretical solutions. Then the behavior of the rock mass was investigated empirically during the excavation, and compared with the analytical solutions. Recently, however, it became popular to analyze the stability of the underground structures by a numerical analysis with the aid of the computer.

There are so many geotechnical programs for the prediction of the rock mass behaviors, but the numerical results are dependent on the accuracy of the input data than the program itself.

Main input data which can affect the results of the numerical analysis are the characteristics of the strength / deformation of rock mass, the state of in situ stress, the tunnel shape, the support pattern, and so forth. Among them, in order to emphasize the importance of in situ stresses as an input data, the finite difference code and the distinct element code were applied to the numerical analysis with a various K_0 value.

4.1 Finite difference analysis

Regarding for the excavation steps of tunnel, the numerical analysis was performed with 3 steps such as the initial equilibrium state, the excavation of right tunnel, and the excavation of left tunnel.
The rock mass was modeled with the residual soil, the weathered rock, and the moderate rock from the surface. The properties of them are assumed as

Table 1. Results for the hydraulic fracturing stress measurements in several areas.

Site	Depth (m)	S_v (MPa)	S_h (MPa)	S_H (MPa)	T* (MPa)	K_0	Orientation**
Kyung-Nam	10.0	0.27	0.24	0.33	0.35	0.89~1.22	60°±10°
	18.0	0.48	0.54	0.73	0.50	1.12~1.52	
Kyung-Buk	11.0	0.30	0.61	0.63	1.08	2.03~2.10	76°±6°
	15.0	0.40	0.84	0.99	0.87	2.10~2.48	
	16.0	0.43	1.85	2.78	0.76	2.85~3.52	
Jeon-Nam	39.5	1.06	2.38	3.26	4.78	2.25~3.08	85°±5°
	69.5	1.86	3.97	6.65	3.73	2.13~3.58	
	81.5	2.18	4.50	6.16	1.01	1.78~2.83	
	87.5	2.35	4.19	4.59	4.61	1.78~1.95	
	93.5	2.51	3.17	3.46	1.20	1.26~1.38	
Jeon-Buk	11.0	0.30	0.54	-	0.93	1.80~?	63°±3°
	14.5	0.39	0.74	0.96	1.12	1.89~2.46	
Choong-Nam	25.5	0.68	1.92	2.29	3.18	2.82~3.37	85°±5°
	27.0	0.72	1.25	2.12	1.18	1.74~2.94	
	28.5	0.76	1.55	2.32	1.50	2.04~3.05	
	45.0	1.21	2.28	2.56	3.49	1.88~2.12	
	48.0	1.29	2.01	2.65	4.52	1.56~2.05	
Choong-Buk	22.5	0.60	0.88	1.14	1.22	1.46~1.90	95°±5°
	28.0	0.75	1.39	1.53	1.03	1.86~2.02	
	33.5	0.90	1.42	1.57	1.19	1.57~1.75	
Kyung-Ki(I)	19.2	0.52	0.68	1.07	0.53	1.31~2.06	45°±5°
	25.5	0.68	1.12	2.05	0.71	1.64~3.01	
	27.1	0.73	1.34	1.86	0.90	1.84~2.55	
Kyung-Ki(II)	34.5	0.93	2.48	2.64	4.31	2.67~2.84	100°±10°
	36.0	0.97	3.03	4.77	5.86	3.12~4.85	
	40.5	1.09	3.10	5.25	3.75	2.84~4.82	
	48.0	1.30	3.27	4.47	6.83	2.52~3.44	
Kyung-Ki(III)	121.0	3.27	4.16	4.35	3.33	1.27~1.33	95°±5°
	130.0	3.51	3.37	4.14	3.95	0.96~1.18	
	136.0	3.67	3.64	3.88	3.90	0.99~1.05	
Kang-Won	120.5	3.23	1.71	3.01	3.64	0.53~0.93	65°±10°
	126.5	3.39	2.11	2.77	2.68	0.62~0.82	
	132.5	3.55	2.68	4.89	2.78	0.76~1.36	
	138.5	3.71	2.33	2.99	4.08	0.62~0.82	

* In situ tensile strength calculated by the initial breakdown pressure and the reopening pressure.
** Clockwise from the true north

shown in Table 2. It is general to follow the series of procedures suggested by Hoek & Brown in order to evaluate the in situ strength from the results of the laboratory tests. But in the laboratory tests, there are tendencies to overestimate the internal friction angle in the low confining pressure. Regarding the inhomogeneities or uncertainties of the rock mass and the declines of strength due to the creep, therefore, the strength parameters should be determined by Mohr-Coulomb criterion which has a tension cut-off.

Numerical model consists of 3,500 elements. Each tunnel width is 10m at intervals of 20m, and overburden height of the tunnel is 75m. For the efficiency of the analysis, the element size adjacent to the tunnel is 1m×1m and becomes larger to the boundary in which the maximum element size is 2.5m×3.5m. The left and right boundaries of the numerical model are fixed to the horizontal direction, and the bottom boundary is fixed to horizontal and vertical direction. The vertical stress is assumed equal to the overburden stress, but the horizontal stresses are assumed

Table 2. Input data for in situ properties used in the numerical analysis by finite difference code.

	Residual soil	Weathered rock	Moderate rock
Density(kg/cm³)	2,000	2,200	2,400
Bulk modulus(Pa)	4.90e9	12.25e9	65.33d9
Shear modulus(Pa)	1.05e9	5.65e9	39.20e9
Friction angle(°)	25	30	35
Cohesion(Pa)	0.10e6	0.50e6	0.80e6
Tensile strength(Pa)	0.05e6	0.20e6	0.30e6

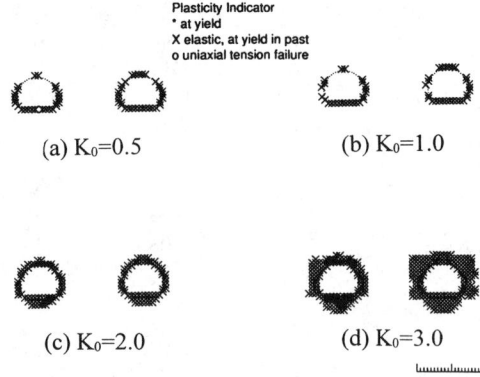

(a) $K_0=0.5$ (b) $K_0=1.0$

(c) $K_0=2.0$ (d) $K_0=3.0$

Figure 1. Variance of plasticity indicator with the various K_0 values.

with various K_0 values to investigate the influences of its value. Figure 1 shows its influence by the plasticity indicator.

When the K_0 value was assumed to be 0.5, the shear failure happened in the tunnel boundaries such as the side-wall or the bottom. Asymmetry of its pattern can be concluded by the step difference between the excavations of left and right tunnels. In most cases of tunnel, this kind of plastic zone can be ignored because of the permanent lining for the drainage and roof support. With increasing the K_0 values from 1.0 to 3.0, it is shown that the plastic zones are developed nearby the tunnel. Regarding the only elasticity, the ratio between the width and height of the tunnel should be equivalent to the K_0 value. But it may be impossible when the tunnel shape is designed according to not only the stability but also the economy and the efficiency.

4.2 *Distinct element analysis*

Distinct element code is a numerical technique for the prediction of the behaviors of the block with the results of the stress and the deformation generated between the blocks which represents the joints or the fractures in the rock mass. In this numerical analysis, the block was assumed to be deformable in order to reveal the major geological condition such as the joint or fracture.

The model has a single tunnel of 15m width which lies under 60m depth from the surface. The physical properties were adopted as shown in Table 3, assuming that the RMR is 50.

There are two sets of joint in the numerical analysis, one is 60° counterclockwise from the horizon and the other is 140°. The joint space was 6m and 5m, respectively, with the standard deviation of 1.5m. The in situ stress condition was same to the finite difference analysis.

As shown in figure 2, the compressive stress was

Table 3. Input data for in situ properties used in the numerical analysis by distinct element code.

	Weathered rock	Moderate rock
ensity (kg/cm³)	2,200	2,700
ulk modulus (Pa)	5.55e9	5.55e9
hear modulus (Pa)	4.14e9	4.14e9
riction angle (°)	30	35
ohesion (Pa)	7.17e5	7.17e6
ensile strength (Pa)	5.26e3	5.26e4
oint normal stiffness(GPa/m)		2.0
oint shear stiffness(GPa/m)		2.0
oint friction angle(°)		30
oint cohesion (GPa)		10.0
oint tensile strength(GPa)		10.0

concentrated in the roof and bottom of the tunnel in case of $K_0=0.5$. Being increased the K_0 values from 1.0 to 3.0, the tension zones are found in the side-wall or the center of the bottom, and the magnitude and influencing zone of the tension failure seemed to be increased. The larger tensile strength in the left side of the tunnel might be due to the larger over-burden than the right side of the tunnel.

CONCLUSIONS

A geological survey and a laboratory test on rock specimens are conducted for the evaluation of the in situ rock mass properties which will be used as an input data for a numerical analysis. Among these input data, the K_0 value is very important for the analysis of tunnel stability.

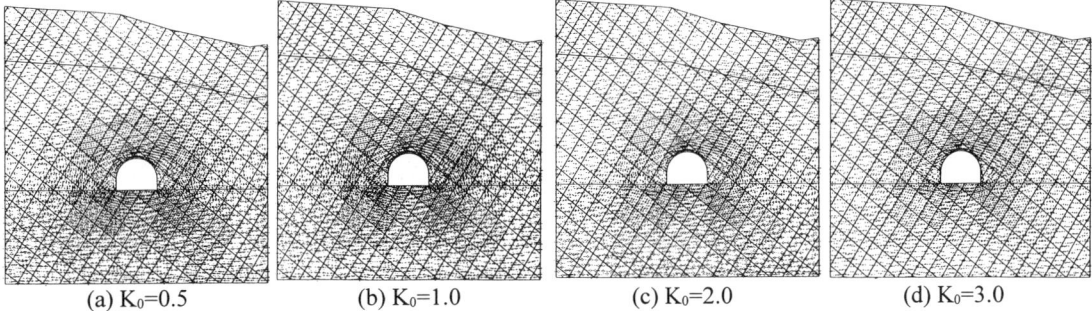

(a) $K_0=0.5$ (b) $K_0=1.0$ (c) $K_0=2.0$ (d) $K_0=3.0$

Figure 2. Different patterns of principal stresses according to the different K_0 values as an input data.

However, an estimated value used to be adopted for the designs of most tunnels up to recently in Korea. But it has been reported that the in situ stress field is various in its magnitude and orientation with respect to a region or a depth. In situ stress field, therefore, should be measured before excavations at the rock mass in which the underground spaces will be sited, and applied to the stability analysis. Especially regarding that the three dimensional analysis code becomes popular in the design of the underground facilities, the magnitude and direction of in situ stress field as a boundary condition should be dealt with a more importance in generating the mesh or in the whole procedure of analysis.

REFERENCES

Amadei, B. And O. Stephansson 1997. Rock stress and its measurement. *Chapman & Hall.*

Bieniawski, Z. T. 1978. Determining rock mass deformability: Experience from case histories. *Int. J. Rock Mech. Min. Sci. & Geomech. Abstr.* 15:237-247.

Choi, S. O. 1994. Fracture propagation analysis on artificial slot model and in situ stress measurement by hydraulic fracturing. *Ph.D. thesis. Seoul Nat'l University.*

Cornet, F. H. 1986. Stress determination from hydraulic tests on preexisting fractures - the H.T.P.F. Method. *Proc. Int. Symp. Rock Stress and Rock Stress Mea.*:301-311.

Goodman, R. E. 1989. Introduction to rock mechanics. 2nd ed. *John Wiley & Sons.*

Haimson, B. C. 1988. Current hydraulic fracturing interpretation, How correctly does it estimate the maximum horizontal crustal stress? *Trans. Am. Geophys.* 69:1454.

Hoek, E. and E. T. Brown 1988. The Hoek-Brown failure criterion - A 1988 update, Rock engineering for underground excavation. *Proc. 15th Candian Rock Mechanics Symp.* pp.31-38.

Hubbert, M. K and D. G. Willis 1957. Mechanics of hydraulic fracturing. *Trans. AIME.* 210:153-166.

ISRM 1987. Suggested methods for rock stress determination. *Int. J. Rock Mech. Min. Sci. & Geomech. Abstr.* 24:53-73.

Ryu, D. W., H. K. Lee and S. O. Choi 1996. Development of integrated hydrofracturing data processing program by statistical approach. *Proc. the Korea-Japan Joint Symp. on Rock Engineering.* 225-230.

Serafim, J. L. And J. P. Pereira 1983. Considerations of the geomechanical classification of Bieniawski, *Proc. Int. Symp. on Eng. Geology and Underground Constr.* 1: II.33-42.

Rock behavior estimated by field measurements during large underground cavern excavation

Y.Uchita & Y.Hirakawa
NEWJEC Inc., Osaka, Japan

T.Ishida
Yamaguchi University, Ube, Japan

ABSTRACT: The behavior of the rock mass was monitored during the excavation of a large underground cavern for a power station in a mountain area in Hyogo Prefecture, Japan. The results by three monitoring techniques, which are the observation of discontinuities in the borehole, the measurements of the horizontal displacement and the vertical stress increment, are presented here. It was found that the rock deformation was dominated by the extending apertures caused with the local sliding in the discontinuity planes. The stress redistribution caused by the excavation did not indicate regular distribution as expected by an elastic theory and made alternately the increased zones and the decreased zones in the vertical stress toward deeper portion from the cavern wall. The loosening region was extended to be more than three fifths of the cavern width at the last stage of the excavation. However, the region was prevented from failing down by the support system.

1 INTRODUCTION

Since the many rock masses in Japan are highly jointed, it is very important in the design and construction of the underground caverns that loosened regions caused by excavation are assessed and worked out countermeasures for their stabilization beforehand. It has generally been understood that the loosening region in a rock mass is caused by direct damage from blasting and developments with openings of hidden cracks and/or increasing of apertures of existing discontinuities with the progress of the excavation. Although various monitoring techniques have been applied to detect developing of the loosened regions, the mechanism has not been clarified. Thus, the lack of the knowledge makes it difficult to confirm a design of the countermeasures to prevent the failure of the cavern stability under the excavation.

For the purpose of clarifying the mechanism, at the site of a large underground cavern excavation for a power station, the following six monitoring techniques were adopted, ① the observation of discontinuities in the borehole, ② the measurements of the horizontal displacement, ③ the increments of vertical stress, ④ acoustic emissions (AE), ⑤ the seismic wave velocities between boreholes and ⑥ the air and water permeability around the boreholes (Uchita 1993,1995,1997),(Ishida 1995).

In this paper, outline of the system measuring the changing process of the discontinuity state, the horizontal displacement and the vertical stress and these measurement results obtained will be shown in the following sections.

2 SITE DESCRIPTION

The Ohkawachi pumped storage power station with a maximum output of 1.28MW (0.32MW×4 units) was constructed since 1988 to 1995. The measurement was conducted in the construction site of a large underground cavern of the power house locating in the middle of Hyogo Prefecture, Japan. The underground powerhouse cavern is located at about 280m below the surface of the slope. The geological cross section and the initial stress state is indicated in Fig.1.

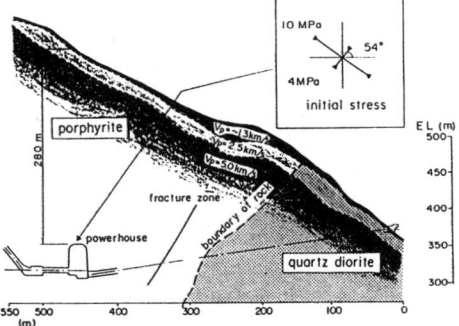

Fig.1. Geological cross section.

Table 1. Mechanical properties of porphyrite.

Mechanical properties	Mean value	numbers of data
Intact:		
Specific gravity	2.75	69
Water absorption	0.34 %	69
Unconfined compressive strength	236.7 MPa	76
Tensile strength	11.8 MPa	49
Young's modulus	76 MPa	71
Poisson's ratio	0.25	31
P wave velocity	5.71 km/s	36
S wave velocity	3.69 km/s	36
Critical strain	0.3 %	69
Rock mass:		
Young's modulus	24 GPa	18
P wave velocity	5 to 6 km/s	—
Shear strength	4.53 MPa	—
Internal friction angle	60.9 deg.	—

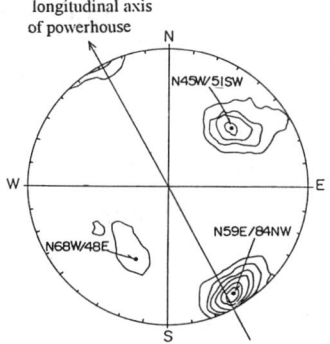

Fig.2. Stereo plots of main joint system. (lower hemisphere).

The rock mass surrounding the cavern is porphyrite of the Mesozoic era, which is fresh and hard. The Q values were about 4 to 20. The mechanical properties obtained from the laboratory and in-situ tests are shown in Table 1. There is no weak layer such as a fractured zone or fault. However, three joint sets exist. Two of them have strikes which are approximately parallel to the longitudinal axis of the cavern. The other set has a strike which is perpendicular to the axis of the cavern (See Fig.2).

The cavern has a width of 24m, a height of 46.6m and a length of 134.5m, its cross section has a bullet-like shape as shown in Fig.3. The excavation was started at the top oval portion and the rock mass was removed in the order of ① through ④ indicated in Fig.3. Thereafter, the floor was excavated downward by 10 lifts of about 3m height using the bench cutting method.

The support system of the cavern, based upon the fundamental concepts of NATM, was installed on the excavated wall was covered with the shotcrete of 24cm thick, and the fully grouted rock bolts of 5m long and the PS anchors of 10m long with a fixation length of 4m were installed in it (Yada 1994).

3 OUTLINE OF MEASUREMENT SYSTEM

The purpose of the measurements is to monitor the behavior of the side wall rock during the excavation process. Therefore six horizontal boreholes with a length of 20m were bored perpendicular to the axis of the cavern from an access tunnel in the tailrace side rock, to install many kind pieces of apparatus in it, as shown in Fig.3. The tunnel was previously excavated at 20m away from the cavern wall. The elevation of the boreholes was approximately at the same elevation of lift No.3. The initial values were taken at the time when the excavation of side pilot tunnels ①, shown in Fig.3, was completed.

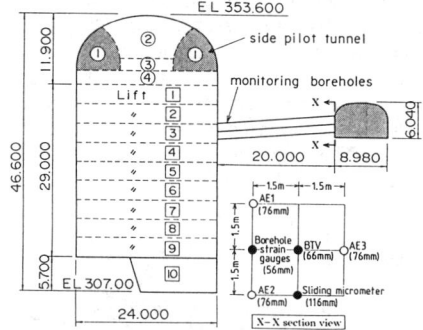

Fig.3. Cavern cross section, its excavation steps and location of monitoring boreholes.

After that, the measurements were carried out at each stage with progressive cavern excavation. The method of these measurements are as follows.

The observation of discontinuities was performed by means of Borehole Television (BTV)(Kamewada 1990), in order to directly detect the location, the direction and opening width of the discontinuities in the borehole, which was arranged in the center of six holes. The relative horizontal displacement was measured with Sliding Micrometer (SMM)(Kovari 1979), providing the relative displacement every 1m section with a precision of 0.003mm.

The measurement of the vertical stress increment was carried out to assess the process forming the loosening region of surrounding rock mass. The stress increment was measured by using the eleven strain gauges (Ishida 1992) buried with cement grouting in a borehole. These gauges were set at the locations where discontinuities were not found with BTV. The stress increments were calculated with the measured strains multiplying by the average coefficient (0.013×10^6 MPa) which was represented an apparent Young's modulus. The coefficient was obtained in the calibration test of the overcored rock with four strain gauges oriented in the radial

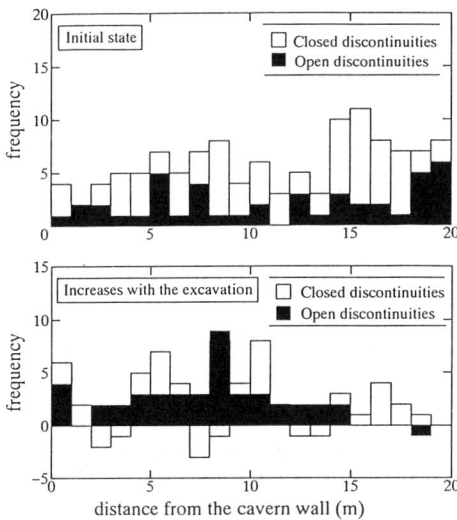

Fig.4. The frequency distribution of discontinuities.

direction of the hole for the measurement of in-situ initial rock stress.

4 ROCK MASS BEHAVIOR DURING UNDERGROUND CAVERN EXCAVATION

4.1 *Behavior of discontinuities*

The state of discontinuities in relation to the excavation was directly observed by the BTV. The existing discontinuities were defined as open or closed ones by whether an aperture width could be recognized or not. Fig.4 shows the frequency distribution of closed and open discontinuities under initial state (before the cavern excavation, that is just after the excavation of side pilot tunnels ①, shown in Fig.3, was completed) and the increased ones caused by the excavation. From the lower figure, it is recognized that a number of open discontinuities in the region from cavern wall surface to 15m increased about two times with the excavation. Also, it is estimated that apparent Young's modulus of the rock mass surround the cavern decreased with the excavation because a number of open discontinuities increased.

Fig.5 shows the accumulative amount of horizontal displacement measured by SMM and of increase apertures with the excavation from arch portion through lift No.3. After the excavation of lift No.2 completed, the accumulative amount of horizontal displacement was 13.8mm, which was calculated as 0.09% in average strain, in the measured section of 16m. As compared with this, the accumulative amount of aperture increments was quite small, therefore it is considered that the rock mass behavior in the section was dominated by elastic deformation.

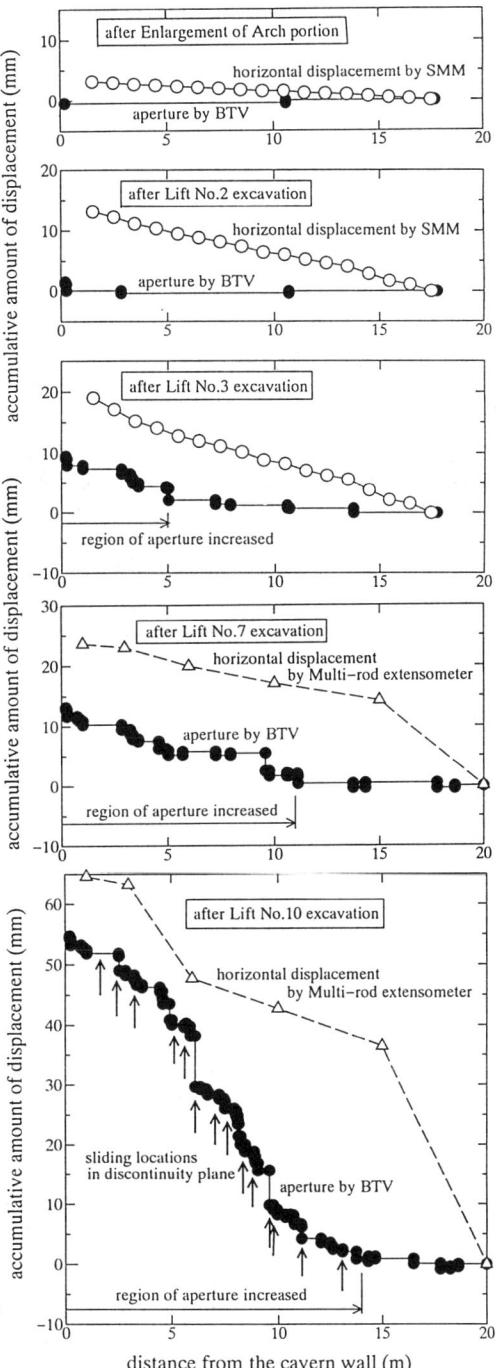

Fig.5. Comparison of accumulative amount between horizontal displacement and aperture increment.

After the excavation of lift No.3 completed, the accumulative amount of the displacement and the average strain were 19.1mm and 0.12% respectively. As compared with this, the accumulative amount of aperture increments was 7.9mm. It should be noted that aperture increment in the region near the cavern wall surface from 1.5m to 5m was 5.5mm, occuping about 80% of 7.0mm in the displacement and 70% of whole aperture increment. Such region where the aperture increment dominated the displacement of the rock mass was definited as loosening region, here. The loosening region was identical to a region bounded by a discontinuity in which a rock mass slided, with around 18mm offset displacement across the borehole and with making it difficult to install the measuring probe for SMM into the borehole after the excavation of lift No.4. Due to the lack of SMM data, in the excavation of lift Nos.7 and 10, the data measured by multi-rod extensometer (ETM) for construction monitoring was used as the accumulative amount of horizontal displacement. The measuring position of the ETM was 22m away from the position of SMM. After the excavation of lift No.7, since the aperture increment indicated a little increase, the loosening region, where aperture increment dominated the displacement, was recognized to extend to the location of 11m. After the excavation of lift No.10, the accumulative amount of aperture increments exceeded 50mm and the loosening region was recognized to extend to the location of 14m. Also, many local slidings in the discontinuity planes were found at the points of the borehole as shown with short arrows in the figure. From the above figure, it is estimated that the deformation in highly jointed rock mass with the excavation was dominated by the slidings in the discontinuity plane.

4.2 Distribution of vertical stress increments

Fig.6 shows a distribution of the vertical stress increments along the hole as an accumulative amount at the some excavation steps from the arch portion through lift No.7. The stress increments made an irregular distribution and indicated the peaks in the compressive stress at the two locations. This phenomena were estimated that the stress concentration acted on a piece of rock in which the gauge was buried. The characteristic shape of the stress distribution had been kept after the excavation of lift No.2. However, by the excavation of lift Nos.3 through 7, the stress increment at the location of 4.5m turned to peak a tension side and the location indicating the compressive stress moved from 4.5m to 5.5m. This behavior seems to indicate that the region to the depth of about 5m from the cavern wall lost the load support ability, i.e. became the loosened region. The two peaks of compressive stress suggest that the stress redistribution caused by the excavation did not indicate regular distribution as expected by an elastic theory.

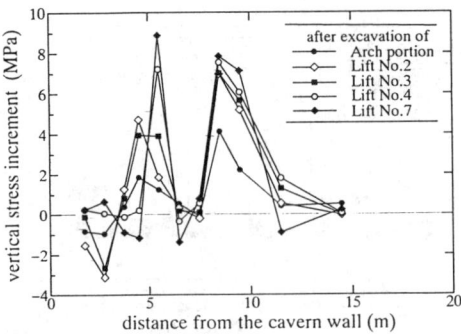

Fig.6. Distribution of the vertical stress increments along the borehole.

Fig.7 shows the vertical stress increment compared with the discontinuities changing their state at the excavation steps. Fig.7(1) shows the changes with the enlargement of the arch portion. The stress increments already made an irregular distribution when this excavation step was completed(Arch ② in the Fig.3). In this figure, the region from the cavern wall to the location of 2.7m indicated the stress reduction, and the two locations at the depths of 4.5m and 8.5m indicated the peaks in the compressive stress. At this step, the number of the discontinuities changing their state was a few, but it is estimated that the stress concentrated nearby the location of 17m because a newly crack was found and an aperture of an existing discontinuity was extended. Fig.7(2) shows the changes with the excavation of core portion ③ through lift No.2. At this step, the compressive stress increased still more at the two locations where it had concentrated and a few discontinuities increased their apertures. Fig.7(3) shows the changes with the excavation of lift No.3 where is just beside the location of the measurement system. At this step, the stresses increased a little over the whole measuring region. Against this, a lots of cracks newly occurred. Because of the phenomena, it is estimated that the release of horizontal confined stress and the vertical stress concentration at a particular location occurred with the excavation. Fig.7(4) shows the changes with the excavation of lift Nos.4 through 7. At this step, the remarkable stress changes and the extension of aperture in many discontinuities occurred over the whole measuring region with the excavation. The increased zones and the decreased zones in the vertical stress took place alternately along the borehole. Particularly, the locations of 4.5m and 11.5m where the remarkable stress reduction occurred correspond to the locations where many new cracks and extension of aperture in many discontinuities induced by the excavation of lift No.3. The characteristic behavior may be, resulted from local shear failure in the existing and/or hidden

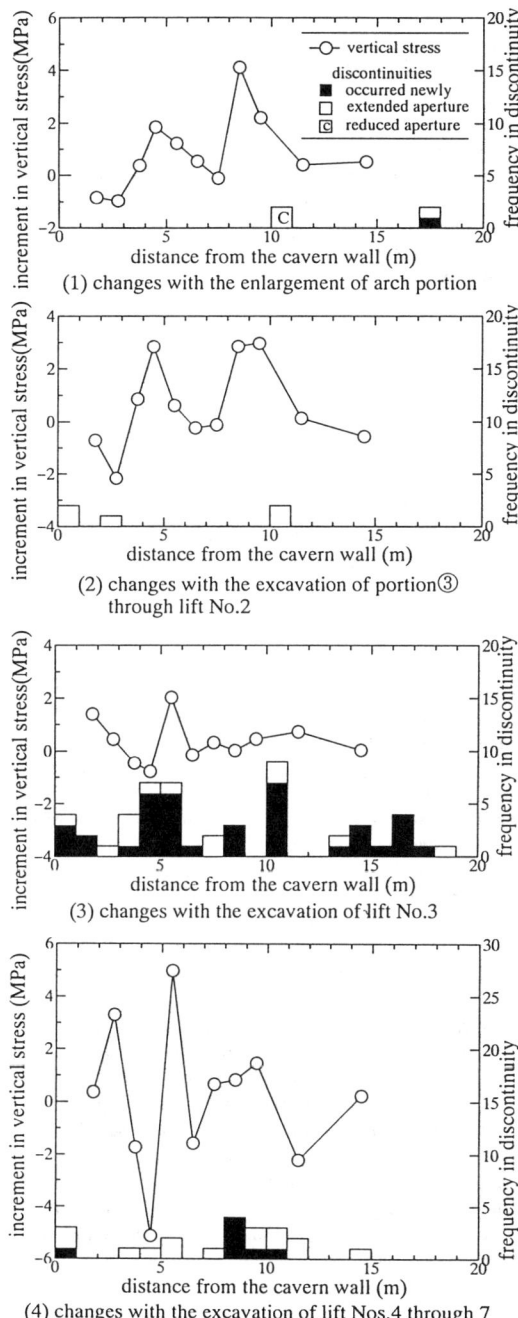

Fig.7. Coresspondence between the vertical stress increments and the discontinuities changing their state at the excavation steps

discontinuity planes. The stress reduction zone could not support an increased load, the load should be supported at the either side of the zones.

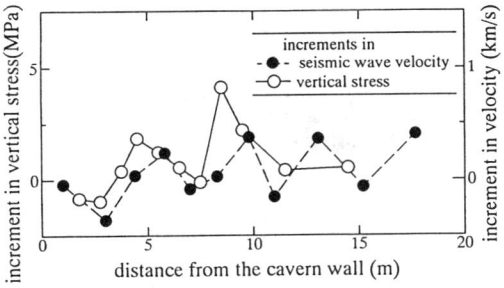

Fig.8. Distribution of the vertical stress increment with the enlargement of the arch portion compared with increments in the sesmic wave (P wave) velocity.

5 DISCUSSION

Fig.8 shows the distribution of the vertical stress increment with the enlargement of the arch portion compared with the velocity increments in the seismic wave(P wave) measured nearby the borehole at the same time (Uchita 1997). They shows similar distributions. The velocity increments shows four peaks at intervals of 3 to 5m except the portion nearby 3m from the cavern wall. The velocity increments suggest existing apertures and micro cracks to close due to the stress redistribution with the excavation, if the velocity represents the aperture states in the rock mass. Still more, the initial velocities measured after the excavation of the side pilot tunnels has already indicated an irregular distribution with two peaks. From these results, it is considered that the stress concentration had already occurred when the initial velocities were measured.

Fig.9 shows a model of the rock behavior near the monitoring boreholes with the process of the cavern excavation. It estimated to take the above results into account in addition to the behavior of the discontinuities and the distribution of the stress increments.

When the upper portion was excavated, the stress distribution nearby the monitoring boreholes should be strongly influenced by the both orientations of the principal stress and the dominant discontinuities as shown Fig.9(1),(2). In these stages, the behavior of the discontinuities were not active.

In contrast to these stages, in the excavation stages below the monitoring boreholes, the rock mass behavior should be dominated by the local sliding in the discontinuity planes as shown Fig.9 (3),(4). These phenomena suggest that locations of the portions supporting the redistributed stress increment are controlled by the geological structure including discontinuities, even for small stress increments.

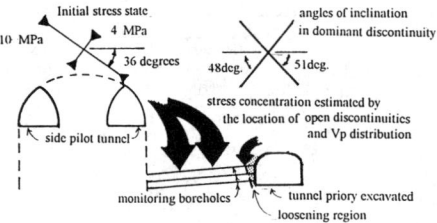

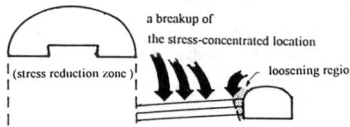

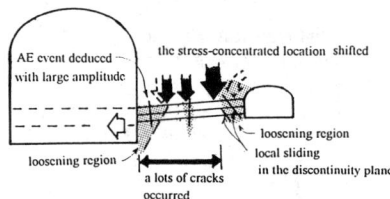

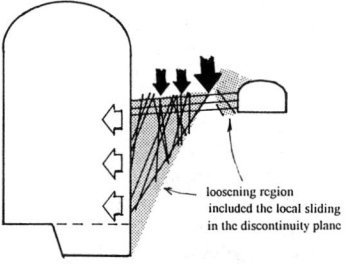

Fig.9. Model of the rock behavior near the monitoring boreholes with the process of the cavern excavation.

6 CONCLUSION

Through the measurements and discussion, the following conclusions were obtained.
1) The rock deformation in the horizontal direction indicated an elastic behavior in the region where the average strain was less than 0.1%, but it was dominated by increase of aperture width of discontinuities in the region where the average strain was more than 0.1%. Such region where the aperture increment dominated the displacement of the rock mass was definited as loosening region, here.
2) The horizontal depth of the loosening region at the monitoring portion was extended to more than three fifth of the cavern width when the excavation completed. However, the region was prevented from failing down by the support system.
3) The vertical stress increments with the progressive excavation showed an irregular distribution along the borehole. In the case of stress redistribution with the excavation, the stress concentration zones and the reduction zones appeared alternately in the monitoring portion. This suggests that the stress redistribution in a real rock mass around a cavern is much different from an one expected from an elastic theory.
4) The characteristic behavior may be resulted from local shear failure in the discontinuity planes.

ACKNOWLEDGMENT

During this study, we were grateful to obtain advice and support from Mr.T.Kanagawa of CRIEPI, and comments on the data and kind help in our field work from Mr.A.Yada of the Kansai Electric Power Co.,Inc. and Mr.T.Nakamura of Toda Construction Co.,Ltd. We would like to express our warmest thanks to all of them for their contributions.

REFERENCES

Ishida,T. et al. 1992. Proposing of a new method to detect loosened regions around a rock chamber, taking note of stress redistribution due to excavation. *Journal of Geotechnical Engineering, JSCE:No.457/III-21, pp.41-50.* (in Japanese)

Ishida,T. et al. 1995. Acoustic emission mechanism and rock mass behavior as deduced from in situ measurements during progressive excavation of an underground powerhouse. *8th Congress in International Society for Rock Mechanics*: 593-596. Tokyo.

Kovari,K. & Ch.Amstad. 1979. Decision making and field measurements in tunneling. *25th OYO Anniversary Lecture Meeting*. Tokyo.

Kamewada,S. et al. 1990. Application of borehole image processing system to survey of tunnel. *International Symposium on Rock Joints* :51-58. Loen.

Uchita,Y. et al. 1993. Behavior of discontinuous rock during large underground cavern excavation. *International Symposium on Assessment and Prevention of Failure Phenomena in Rock Engineering*: 807-816: Istanbul.

Uchita,Y. et al. 1995. Rock behavior measured by borehole strain gauges during large underground cavern excavation. *4th International Symposium on Field Measurements in Geomechanics*: 89-96. Bergamo.

Uchita,Y. et al. 1997. Loosening rock region estimated by field measurements during large underground cavern excavation. *1st Asian Rock Mechanics Symposium*: Seoul.(in print)

Yada,A. et al. 1994. Excavation control of underground powerhouse cavern. *IV CSMR, Integral Approach to Rock Mechanics* :523-534. Santiago.

Author index

Abdrakhimov, M.Z. 409
Alheib, M. 211
Andersson, J. 223
Ardito, J.A. 423
Aydan, Ö. 369, 385

Bai, S. 511
Batchelor, A.S. 265, 299
Bawden, W.F. 229
Bigarre, P. 211
Bouhlel, M.S. 305

Cai, M. 89
Campos Fernandes, A.C. 451
Cartwright, P.B. 469
Chan, C.F. 391
Chen, G. 259
Cheng, H. 133, 137
Cheung, L.S. 391
Chkouratnik, V.L. 193
Choi, S.-O. 539
Chou, W. 133, 137
Choy, H.H. 391
Cornet, F.H. 43
Corthésy, R. 59, 65, 71

Davies, N. 265
Davies, P.J. 181
De-La-Sota, G. 423
Demboya, N. 83
Dimova, V.Iv. 417
Du, S. 321
Dusseault, M.B. 111
Dyskin, A.V. 235

Enever, J. 181
Esaki, T. 321

Fang, Z. 511
Fehler, M. 247
Feng, X.-T. 279
Fouial, K. 211
Fujimura, F. 451
Fujimura, H. 499
Fujiwara, Y. 171
Fukuhara, A. 83
Fukui, K. 327

Galybin, A.N. 235
Gill, D.E. 65, 71
Giraud, A. 101

Haimson, B.C. 35
Haque, A. 315
Hatakeyama, N. 333
Hayashi, K. 107, 167
Hirakawa, Y. 171, 545
Hirata, A. 505
Homand, F. 101, 205
Hongo, K. 343
Horie, M. 171

Ichikawa, Y. 309
Ichinose, M. 475
Ikezoe, Y. 499
Inaba, T. 505
Inada, Y. 521
Indraratna, B. 315
Ishida, T. 545
Ishiguro, Y. 491
Ishihara, H. 117
Ishii, H. 253, 259
Ito, H. 351, 355, 359
Ito, T. 107, 167
Ito, Y. 171

Jeong, G.-C. 309
Jewell, R.J. 235
Jha, P.C. 457
Jia, J. 217
Jiang, Y. 321
Joseph, D. 397

Kakihara, H. 533
Kaneko, K. 429
Kar, A. 397
Karakin, A.V. 363, 381
Kato, M. 429
Katsuyama, K. 187, 279
Kawamoto, T. 369, 385
Kinoshita, N. 521
Kiyama, H. 499
Kobayashi, H. 479
Kobayashi, S. 161
Komatsuzaki, Y. 515

Koyama, T. 515
Kudo, R. 359
Kudoh, K. 515
Kuriyagawa, M. 117
Kusumoto, F. 253
Kuwahara, Y. 351, 359
Kuznetsov, Yu.I. 363, 381
Kwakwa, K.A. 265, 299

Lavrov, A.V. 193, 197
Leite, M.H. 59, 65, 71
Li, C. 89, 289
Li, F. 121, 485
Liepin, Y.I. 403
Liu, T. 447
Ljunggren, C. 223

Matsui, H. 95
Matsui, K. 475
Matsuki, K. 343
Matsunaga, I. 177
Mills, K.W. 149
Miyazaki, S. 177
Mizuta, Y. 51, 241
Moriya, H. 247
Murakami, T. 241
Muzo, M.C. 283

Nag, D.K. 463
Nagaraj, C. 397
Nakagawa, K. 533
Nakamura, N. 95, 429
Nakanishi, A. 143
Narita, T. 479
Nawrocki, P.A. 111
Nechnech, A. 101
Nguyen, D. 71
Nieble, C.M. 451
Niitsuma, H. 247
Nishimura, H. 491
Nishimura, T. 499
Nishino, K. 491
Nishizawa, O. 351, 355, 359
Noguchi, Y. 429
Nunomura, S. 333

Obara, Y. 77, 83, 505

Ohnishi, Y. 259
Ohno, K. 527
Ohtsu, M. 283
Oikawa, Y. 177, 479
Okubo, S. 121, 327
Özbay, M. 279

Proughten, A.J. 265
Pun, W.K. 391

Qiao, L. 89

Raju, N.M. 457
Read, R.S. 65
Rossmanith, H.P. 27, 283
Rouis, M.J. 305
Rowley, J.C. 339
Rutledge, J.T. 247
Rutqvist, J. 127

Sakaguchi, K. 343
Sakurai, S. 533
Sano, O. 241, 355
Sato, A. 107
Sato, T. 95
Seiki, T. 309, 385
Sengupta, S. 397
Seto, M. 187, 279, 463
Shao, J.F. 101
Sharma, P. 441
Shen, B. 289

Shimada, H. 475
Shimizu, N. 533
Shimizu, Y. 333
Shin, H.-S. 539
Shin, K. 121
Souley, M. 205
Srinivasan, C. 457
Stephansson, O. 3, 127, 289
Sugawara, K. 15, 77, 83, 171, 491
Sugihara, K. 95
Sukirman, Y.B. 435
Sun, J. 133, 137, 321
Suzuoki, S. 333

Takahashi, H. 333
Takehara, T. 117
Tan, X. 289
Tanaka, Y. 241
Tani, K. 155
Thompson, P.M. 59
Tod, J.D. 229
Traskin, V.Yu. 409
Tubagus, N.H. 327

Uchita, Y. 545
Ueda, T. 521
Uenishi, K. 27
Utagawa, M. 187

Vutukuri, V.S. 463

Wang, D.F. 181
Wang, S. 89
Watanabe, K. 167
Webber, S. 279

Xue, Z. 171, 355

Yabe, Y. 375
Yada, A. 527
Yamada, K. 521
Yamaguchi, T. 117, 161, 479
Yamamoto, H. 375
Yamamoto, K. 359, 375
Yamamoto, M. 505
Yamashita, M. 117
Yamauchi, T. 253
Yang, M. 217
Yassir, N. 181
Yokoyama, T. 143, 359
Yoshida, Y. 155
Yoshikawa, T. 161
Yu, B. 89

Zairi, M. 305
Zhang, B. 121
Zhang, J. 217
Zhang, S. 217
Zhang, X.M. 479
Zhou, C. 447
Zoubkov, A.V. 403